Advanced Emergency Medical Technician

Transition Manual

Bridging the Gap to the National EMS Education Standards

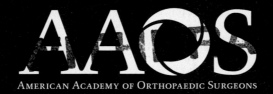

American Academy of Orthopaedic Surgeons

Series Editor:
Andrew N. Pollak, MD, FAAOS

Author:
Rhonda J. Beck, NREMT-P

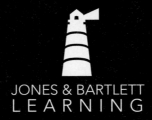

JONES & BARTLETT
LEARNING

1842672

OCT 3 2013

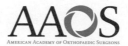

AMERICAN ACADEMY OF ORTHOPAEDIC SURGEONS

World Headquarters
Jones & Bartlett Learning
5 Wall Street
Burlington, MA 01803
978-443-5000
info@jblearning.com
www.jblearning.com

Jones & Bartlett Learning books and products are available through most bookstores and online booksellers. To contact Jones & Bartlett Learning directly, call 800-832-0034, fax 978-443-8000, or visit our website, www.jblearning.com.

Substantial discounts on bulk quantities of Jones & Bartlett Learning publications are available to corporations, professional associations, and other qualified organizations. For details and specific discount information, contact the special sales department at Jones & Bartlett Learning via the above contact information or send an email to specialsales@jblearning.com.

Production Credits
Chief Executive Officer: Ty Field
President: James Homer
SVP, Editor-in-Chief: Michael Johnson
Executive Publisher: Kimberly Brophy
Executive Acquisitions Editor—EMS: Christine Emerton
Editor: Alison Lozeau
Production Editor: Jessica deMartin
Associate Production Editor: Nora Menzi
Vice President of Sales, Public Safety Group: Matthew Maniscalco
Director of Sales, Public Safety Group: Patricia Einstein
VP, Marketing: Alisha Weisman
VP, Manufacturing and Inventory Control: Therese Connell
Composition: Publishers' Design and Production Services, Inc.
Cover Design: Michael O'Donnell
Director of Photo Research and Permissions: Amy Wrynn
Cover Image: Courtesy of Rhonda Beck
Printing and Binding: Courier Companies
Cover Printing: Courier Companies

Library of Congress Cataloging-in-Publication Data
American Academy of Orthopaedic Surgeons.
    Advanced emergency medical technician transition manual : bridging the gap to the national EMS education standards / American Academy of Orthopaedic Surgeons, Rhonda Beck. — 1st ed.
        p. ; cm.
    Includes bibliographical references and index.
    ISBN 978-1-4496-5019-3
    I. Beck, Rhonda J. II. Title.
    [DNLM: 1. Emergency Medical Services—standards—United States. 2. Emergency Medical Services—legislation & jurisprudence—United States. 3. Emergency Medical Technicians—education—United States. 4. Emergency Medical Technicians—standards—United States.
WX 215]
    616.02'52—dc23
                                                2012051514

6048
Printed in the United States of America
17   16   15   14   13   10 9 8 7 6 5 4 3 2 1

Brief Contents

Contents

CHAPTER 1

Preparatory

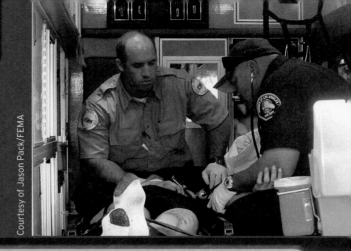

Courtesy of Jason Pack/FEMA

National EMS Education Standard

Preparatory

Applies fundamental knowledge of the EMS system, safety/well-being of the AEMT, and medical/legal and ethical issues to the provision of emergency care.

Public Health

Uses simple knowledge of the principles of illness and injury prevention in emergency care.

Review

Emergency care is just one component of the emergency medical services (EMS) system. Other components include transportation, facilities (such as trauma and burn centers), communications, public information and education, medical direction, regulation and policy, human resources management, and evaluation of the EMS system. Advanced emergency medical technicians (AEMTs) function within the system to provide basic and some advanced life support. To be effective, an AEMT must exhibit certain personal and professional characteristics, including integrity, empathy, self-motivation, self-confidence, and effective communication and time management skills.

What's New

Formerly, there were two EMT-I curricula: 1985 and 1999. The AEMT role resembles the EMT-I 1985 curriculum. While EMT-Is at the 1999 level were trained to perform certain skills such as intubation and manual defibrillation, these skills are not performed in the AEMT role. Also, AEMTs can assist with administering certain medications but not others. Although specific training and licensure requirements for AEMTs vary from one state to another, almost every state's requirements follow or exceed the guidelines recommended in the current National Highway Traffic Safety Administration (NHTSA) 2009 *National EMS Education Standards*. Public health and research in EMS are new concepts that will be discussed in this chapter. The AEMT's role in illness and injury prevention is now expanded. Finally, well-being of the AEMT, including the effects of stress on a person's body and steps to help alleviate stress, are discussed in greater detail.

▌Introduction

EMS has finally moved out of its infancy. Over the past 40 years, it has developed into an integrated system of care, beginning with the general public and ending with specialized emergency medicine in trauma centers. Helicopters staffed with flight medics, training emphasizing the speed of care at the scene of a traumatic injury, and an increase in the number of trauma centers in the United States have all decreased the length of time from onset of illness or injury to delivery of definitive care. Paramedics now equipped with life-saving medication such as tissue plasminogen activator (tPA), a thrombolytic agent (clot-busting drug) that can dissolve a blood clot in the coronary or cerebral arteries, have had a significant impact on the morbidity and mortality rates of persons experiencing strokes or heart attacks.

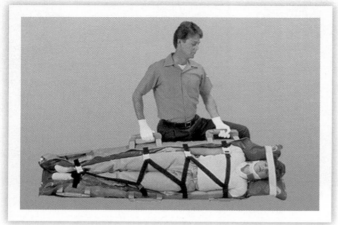

Courtesy of Hartwell Medical

FIGURE 1-1 The EVAC-U-SPLINT mattress can provide full-body immobilization using a vacuum to conform to the exact contour of the patient's body.

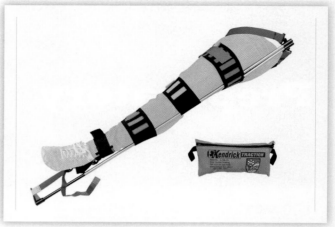

Courtesy of Life Medical Supplier

FIGURE 1-3 The Kendrick Traction Device (KTD) is a compact, light-weight, easy-to-apply traction device small enough to fit into a trauma pack or first aid kit.

Through research and a system-wide approach, EMS continues to make new advances on a daily basis. A visit to any EMS convention will reveal numerous new equipment and technology options. EMS personnel are now able to communicate virtually with emergency department (ED) physicians, document calls via a personal digital assistant (PDA) with run reports automatically transmitted to ED personnel, and track supply use and be automatically notified when items need to be reordered.

Equipment has advanced from the day of the rickety old stretcher that required significant lifting ability, to stretchers that virtually load themselves and vacuum splints that can fully immobilize a patient effortlessly **FIGURE 1-1**. Suction units no longer need batteries and have become so portable that they can be included in every medical and trauma bag, eliminating the excuse that this technology was not available when needed **FIGURE 1-2**. Traction devices are now portable enough to fit into a trauma bag **FIGURE 1-3**. Long backboards now include integrated cervical immobilization devices (CIDs), ruling out the need to carry bulky blocks along with the rest of the equipment needed at the scene of an accident or mass-casualty incident **FIGURE 1-4**. Cryogenics has entered the world of EMS, with devices available to aid in the therapeutic cooling of patients and to provide comfort during transport **FIGURE 1-5**. In summary, the advances made in recent years are astounding.

Throughout this text, we will highlight some of the newer equipment now available to AEMTs—equipment that might not have been available when you took your initial EMT-I course. One of the responsibilities of any AEMT is continuing education, and an important part of that continuing education is knowledge of new equipment that can not only help the patient, but also make the AEMT's life easier.

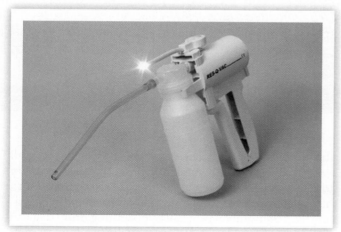

Courtesy of RMS Medical Products

FIGURE 1-2 The RES-Q-VAC is a lightweight, hand-powered suction device that provides as much suction as battery-operated units but is compact enough to fit in a trauma bag.

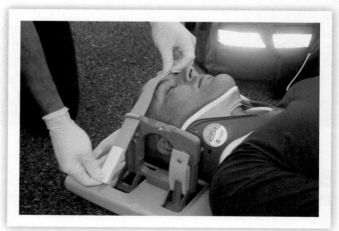

Courtesy of Tomcat EMS

FIGURE 1-4 The Tomcat Integral Cervical Immobilization Device (ICID) utilizes an integrated disposable cervical immobilization device system to provide a quick and efficient method of immobilization without the need to carry or store multiple pieces of equipment.

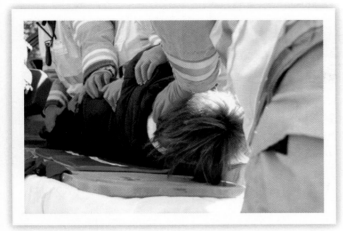

Courtesy of The Turley Backboard Pad Co.

FIGURE 1-5 The Turley Backboard Pad is a reusable multi-purpose gel pad that can be heated and cooled according to patient needs.

New Levels of EMS Training

The *National EMS Scope of Practice Model* document was created by experts throughout the United States and is designed to provide guidelines regarding the skills each level of EMS provider should be able to accomplish. This document categorizes responders into four training and licensure levels: *emergency medical responder (EMR)*, formerly called first responder; *emergency medical technician (EMT)*, formerly called EMT-Basic; *advanced EMT (AEMT)*, formerly called EMT-Intermediate; and *paramedic*, formerly called EMT-P. EMRs include law enforcement officers, fire fighters, park rangers, ski patrollers, or other organized rescuers who often arrive at the scene before the ambulance and other EMS providers. EMR training focuses on providing basic life support (BLS) and urgent care with limited equipment. EMTs are trained in BLS, including automated external defibrillators (AED), the use of airway adjuncts, and assisting patients with certain medications. AEMTs are trained in specific aspects of advanced life support (ALS), such as intravenous (IV) therapy and administration of certain emergency medications. Paramedics have extensive training in ALS, including endotracheal intubation, emergency pharmacology, cardiac monitoring, and other advanced assessment and treatment skills.

> *National EMS Scope of Practice Model* A document created by the National Highway Traffic Safety Administration (NHTSA) that outlines the skills performed by various EMS providers.
> *Emergency medical responder (EMR)* The first trained individual, such as a police officer, firefighter, lifeguard, or other rescuer, to arrive at the scene of an emergency to provide initial medical assistance.
> *Emergency medical technician (EMT)* An individual who has training in basic life support, including automated external defibrillation, use of a definitive airway adjunct, and assisting patients with certain medications.

> *Advanced EMT (AEMT)* An individual who has training in specific aspects of advanced life support, such as intravenous therapy, and the administration of certain emergency medications.
> *Paramedic* An individual who has extensive training in advanced life support, including endotracheal intubation, emergency pharmacology, cardiac monitoring, and other advanced assessment and treatment skills.

Changes in AEMT Skill Requirements

According to the 2009 *National EMS Education Standards*, AEMTs are no longer taught the following skills:

- Insertion of esophageal airways
- Performance of needle chest compression
- Performance of needle cricothyrotomy
- Insertion of nasogastric and orogastric tubes
- Insertion of an orotracheal tube
- Performance of direct laryngoscopy
- Tracheobronchial suctioning (AEMTs are permitted to perform suction only in patients who are already intubated)
- Interpretation of single-lead electrocardiograms (ECGs)
- Performance of manual defibrillation attempts
- Application of ECGs to monitor cardiac pacing
- Performance of transcutaneous cardiac pacing
- Rectal medication administration

TABLE 1-1 shows the skill guidelines for each level of training, as defined in the National EMS Scope of Practice Model.

Certification and *licensure* of AEMTs remains a state function, subject to the laws and regulations of the state in which the AEMT practices. Each state retains the ability to control the functions of its licensed individuals. For this reason, there remains some variation from state to state on the scope of AEMT practice as well as training and recertification requirements. Keep in mind that you must follow the guidelines specific for your area.

> *Certification* A process in which a person, an institution, or a program is evaluated and recognized as meeting certain predetermined standards to provide safe and ethical care.
> *Licensure* The process by which a competent authority, usually the state, grants permission to practice a job, trade, or profession.

The 2009 *National EMS Education Standards* are national guidelines intended to create more consistent delivery of EMS across the country. The only way a medical director can allow an AEMT to perform a skill is if the state has already approved performance of that skill. The medical director can limit the scope of practice but cannot expand it beyond state law. Expanding the scope of practice requires state approval.

Table 1-1
National EMS Scope of Practice Model Guidelines for Levels of Training*

EMR	EMT	AEMT	Paramedic
Airway and Breathing Minimum Psychomotor Skill Set			
Oral airway	Humidifiers	Esophageal-tracheal intubation	BiPAP/CPAP
Bag-mask device	Partial rebreathing mask	Multi-lumen airways	Needle chest decompression
Head tilt–chin lift maneuver	Venturi mask		Chest tube monitoring
Jaw-thrust	Manually triggered ventilators		Percutaneous cricothyrotomy
Modified chin-lift	Automatic transport ventilators		$ETCO_2$/capnography
Obstruction, manual	Oral and nasal airways		NG/OG tube
Oxygen therapy			Nasal and oral endotracheal intubation
Nasal cannula			Airway obstruction removal by direct laryngoscopy
Nonrebreathing mask			Positive end-expiratory pressure
Upper airway suctioning			
Assessment Minimum Psychomotor Skill Set			
Manual BP	Pulse oximetry	Blood glucose monitoring	ECG interpretation
	Manual and auto BP		Interpretive 12-lead
			Blood chemistry analysis
Pharmacologic Intervention Minimum Psychomotor Skill Set			
Medication Administration Routes ■ Unit dose auto-injector for self or peer care (such as the MARK 1)	*Assisted Medications* ■ Assisting a patient in administering his or her own prescribed medications, including auto-injector	■ Peripheral IV insertion ■ IV fluid infusion ■ Pediatric IO insertion	■ Central line monitoring ■ IO insertion ■ Venous blood sampling
	Medication Administration Routes ■ Buccal ■ Oral	*Medication Administration Routes* ■ Aerosolized ■ SQ ■ IM ■ Nebulized ■ SL ■ Intranasal ■ IV push or D_{50} and narcotic antagonist only	*Medication Administration Routes* ■ Endotracheal ■ IV (push and infusion) ■ NG ■ Rectal ■ IO ■ Topical ■ Accessing implanted central IV port
	Medications to be Administered ■ Physician-approved over-the-counter medications (oral glucose, aspirin for chest pain of suspected ischemic origin)	*Medications to be Administered* ■ SL nitroglycerin for chest pain of suspected ischemic origin ■ SQ and IM epinephrine for anaphylaxis	*Medications to be Administered* ■ Physician-approved medications ■ Maintenance of blood administration

Table 1-1
National EMS Scope of Practice Model Guidelines for Levels of Training* (continued)

EMR	EMT	AEMT	Paramedic
Emergency Trauma Care Minimum Psychomotor Skill Set			
Manual cervical stabilization	Spinal immobilization		Morgan lens
Manual extremity stabilization	Seated spinal immobilization		
Eye irrigation	Long board		
Direct pressure	Extremity splinting		
Hemorrhage control	Traction splinting		
Emergency moves for endangered patients	Mechanical patient restraint		
	Tourniquet		
	MAST/PASG		
	Cervical collar		
	Rapid extrication		
Medical/Cardiac Care Minimum Psychomotor Skill Set			
CPR	Mechanical CPR		Cardioversion
AED	Assisted complicated delivery of an infant		Carotid massage
Assisted normal delivery of an infant			Manual defibrillation
			TC pacing

Abbreviations: AED, automated external defibrillator; BiPAP/CPAP, bilevel positive airway pressure/continuous positive airway pressure; BP, blood pressure; CPR, cardiopulmonary resuscitation; D50, 50% dextrose in water; ECG, electrocardiogram; IM, intramuscular; IO, intraosseous; IV, intravenous; MAST/PASG, military antishock trousers/pneumatic antishock garments; NG, nasogastric; OG, orogastric; SL, sublingual; SQ, subcutaneous; TC, transcutaneous.

Note: The 2005 National EMS Scope of Practice Model serves as a foundation for states to build their own model. It is intended to illustrate the operation of each level of EMS provider and the progression from one level to another. It is not inclusive of every skill a state may allow.

*Substantial variation exists state to state, and you must be sure to understand which skills are within the scope of any given certification level in your own state.

The National Registry of Emergency Medical Technicians (NREMT) is a nongovernmental agency that provides a national standard for AEMT testing and certification throughout the United States. Many states use the NREMT testing process for licensing their AEMTs and grant licensing reciprocity to NREMT-certified AEMTs. It is important to remember, however, that EMS is regulated entirely by the state in which you are licensed.

Transition Tip

The EMR, EMT, AEMT, and paramedic curricula can be downloaded from NHTSA's website at www.ems.gov.

Transition Tip

Some states provide certification, licensure, or credentialing of individuals who perform emergency medical care. Sometimes this terminology is confusing. Certification is the process by which an individual, institution, or program is evaluated and recognized as meeting certain predetermined standards to ensure safe and ethical patient care. Once certified, you are obliged to conform to the standards that are generally recognized nationally by various registry groups and provide an important link in nationwide EMS. Licensure is the process by which a competent authority, usually the state, grants permission to practice a job, trade, or profession.

Components of the EMS System

The *EMS Agenda for the Future* is a multidisciplinary, national review of all aspects of EMS delivery, undertaken with the goal of developing a more cohesive and consistent system across the United States. This document outlines 14 components of an EMS system **TABLE 1-2**.

Medical Direction and Quality Control

Information and skills in emergency medical care change constantly. Your medical director is responsible for ensuring that all providers who care for patients meet the appropriate standards on each call. This is done with regular evaluations of all aspects of an EMS call **FIGURE 1-6**. Improved technology allows EMS providers to electronically document the care that has been provided. The data can then be analyzed to improve care. For example, you will have data on the average on-scene time for major trauma patients or how many AED runs the department has made. On the basis of the information gathered, your medical director might establish a continuous quality improvement process to target ways to improve patient care and ensure that your skills and knowledge are current.

Table 1-2 *EMS Agenda for the Future* Components of an EMS System	
EMS System	
1. Public Access	8. Communication Systems
2. Clinical Care	9. Human Resources
3. Medical Direction	10. Legislation and Regulation
4. Integration of Health Services	11. Evaluation
5. Information Systems	12. System Finance
6. Prevention	13. Public Education
7. EMS Research	14. Education Systems

> **Transition Tip**
>
> Handing patients off is a high-risk activity. You must deal with issues of the physical transfer of the patient from your stretcher as well as communication issues with the next caregiver in line. Providing a written copy of your assessment and treatment along with a verbal report helps to ensure coordinated care. It is imperative that you give a report of your care of the patient and any changes that may have occurred since you took over care. Other safety issues revolve around safe transport (such as avoiding ambulance crashes) and providing proper immobilization of patients who may have potential traumatic injuries.

Another function of the evaluation process is to determine ways to eliminate human error. It is important that the AEMT strive to eliminate errors as much as possible. Understanding the circumstances behind these errors helps to minimize them. There are three main sources of errors. They can occur as a result of a rules-based failure, a knowledge-based failure, or a skills-based failure (or any combination of these). For example, does an AEMT have the legal right to administer the particular medication needed by the patient? If not, a rules-based failure occurs if an AEMT assists with the administration. Does an AEMT know all of the pertinent information about the medication being delivered? If not, a breakdown at this point, such as the administration of the wrong medication, would be a knowledge-based failure. Finally, is the equipment operating and being used properly? If not, a skills-based error has occurred. Any error can come from multiple sources.

The environment can also contribute to errors. Are there ways to limit distractions? Can AEMTs find what they need in a timely manner? Sometimes the solution is as easy as ensuring flashlights are available on all ambulances and making sure all medications and equipment are properly labeled and organized.

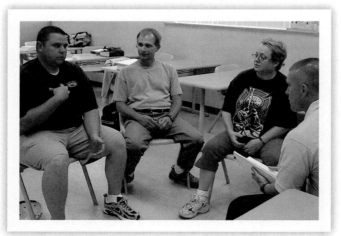

FIGURE 1-6 Regular discussions to review patient care, run reports, and discuss any areas of care that seem to need change or improvement help reduce the chances for error.

> **Transition Tip**
>
> To cut down on the potential for errors, ensure adequate lighting when handling medications and keep interruptions to a minimum. Keeping medications in a specific location and in their original packaging can also reduce the potential for errors.

When you are about to perform a skill, ask yourself, "Why am I doing this?" Considering the reason for your actions allows you time to reflect and make a more informed decision. If you have considered what to do and cannot come up with a solution, ask for help. Talk with your partner, contact medical control, or call your EMS supervisor.

Another way to help limit medical errors is to use cheat sheets. Have a copy of your protocol book with you. Emergency physicians have many reference materials available to them. Physicians recognize they cannot memorize everything, so referencing a book or a reliable Internet resource helps ensure the use of accurate information.

Preventing errors requires AEMTs to be conscientious of protocols, not allowing interruptions while providing patient care. Use down time to refresh skills that are used less often. Use decision-making aids such as algorithms and reflect on what has been done as an informal critique for future improvement of performance. Finally, after a troublesome call, talk with your partner and/or your supervisor. Discussing events that just happened provides an excellent avenue for learning. Your discussions can help lead to changes in protocol, how equipment is stocked, or even the purchase of new equipment.

> **Transition Tip**
>
> Agencies need to have clear protocols, or detailed plans, that describe how certain patient issues such as chest pain or shortness of breath are to be managed. As an AEMT, it is your responsibility to learn and understand these protocols.

Disease Prevention and Public Education

Disease prevention and public education are often closely associated. They are aspects of EMS where the focus is on public health. *Public health* examines the health needs of entire populations with the goal of preventing health problems.

> *Public health* A branch of health care focused on examining the health needs of entire populations with the goal of preventing health problems.

Public health works to prevent illness and injury by being proactive. A good example of public health at work is the common product, salt. The next time you buy salt, check the contents. In the United States, salt is sold with the additive iodine. It was discovered years ago that certain thyroid diseases such as goiter are caused by a decrease in iodine levels within people's diets. The solution was to add this important element into a commonly used food source. Today, goiters are rare within the United States.

EMS is able to work with public health agencies on both primary and secondary prevention strategies. *Primary prevention* focuses on strategies that will prevent the event from ever happening. For example, polio was a devastating disease causing death and disability for thousands of Americans. A vaccine was discovered that could prevent the disease. In the span of one generation, the disease was virtually eliminated. Vaccinations are a good example of primary prevention within public health.

> *Primary prevention* Efforts to prevent an injury or illness from ever occurring.

In 2009, the World Health Organization declared the swine flu (H1N1) virus to be at pandemic levels, which meant that the virus had spread throughout the world. At the writing of this text, the Centers for Disease Control and Prevention has determined that the outbreak of this virus within the United States is limited. If a major outbreak of this virus were to occur in the United States, EMS providers may be called on to assist in the administration of vaccinations. Other examples of primary prevention include ensuring that people know the dangers of drinking and driving and understanding the harmful effects of using tobacco and other drugs.

> **Transition Tip**
>
> Be an active member of your community! However handy a GPS's turn-by-turn directions are, being active in your community is the best way to keep on top of the best local resources. When you are developing a potential care plan, you will ask yourself, "Does the receiving facility have the resources needed for this patient?" When you are active in your community, you will know the answer. If the answer is no, the answer to the next question, "Is there an appropriate facility within a reasonable distance?" will also be a part of your community knowledge.

In a *secondary prevention* strategy, the event has already happened. The question is, how can we decrease the effects of the event? Helmets and seatbelts do not prevent the accident from happening, yet they may prevent serious injuries from occurring. The next time you drive down a major road, note the construction of the guardrails. There have been significant changes in their construction over the years as more information has become available on what happens during a vehicle collision.

> *Secondary prevention* Efforts to limit the effects of an injury or illness that cannot be completely prevented.

AEMTs may also be involved in the surveillance of illnesses and injuries. The patient care reports generated by

EMS personnel can be used to determine if a serious, widespread condition exists. For example, EMS is in a perfect position to provide statistical information to the local government about collisions. Injury surveillance data can be used to determine ways to improve a dangerous intersection, to prevent accidents from ever happening, or to limit the severity of injuries to drivers.

AEMTs can help educate the public. People may not understand why an accident has happened. A parent allows her 15-month-old child to play outside with other children unsupervised. The child falls and cuts her hand. EMS arrives and the cause of the injury is obvious. AEMTs can work with the parents professionally, respectfully, and kindly to help educate them on how to prevent this injury from occurring in the future.

The public may not understand the education that EMS providers have and what services they can provide. AEMTs can go to local schools and teach children to call 9-1-1 when there is a medical emergency. EMS personnel can work with local health care institutions to teach local residents when to call for an ambulance and when other transportation methods are more appropriate.

Teaching people how to perform cardiopulmonary resuscitation (CPR), how to help a choking victim, or even how to assist in the delivery of a baby are all aspects of public education **FIGURE 1-7**. One of the important effects of public education is an increase in respect for EMS. When people understand what it means to work on an ambulance and provide care to the sick and injured, they are more likely to consider EMS a vital part of the public health care system. This change in attitude can be powerful and lead to increased EMS funding and greater respect for EMS as a profession.

EMS Research

Traditional medical practice is based on medical knowledge, intuition, and judgment. In the early years of EMS, many standards relating to professionalism, protocols, training,

and equipment were developed from the direct experience of EMS providers. Now, ongoing EMS research provides a scientific basis for standards, the same as research in any other health care profession. For example, prehospital EMS research has shown that it is more important to rapidly transport major trauma patients to an operating room than for them to receive certain prehospital procedures, such as insertion of an IV line. Now EMS providers provide rapid transport of major trauma patients to trauma centers where the patients can receive the surgical care they need. This is the power of EMS research.

Evidence-based decision making is becoming an integral part of functioning as an EMS provider. Patient care should be focused on the procedures that have proven useful in improving patient outcomes. There is a limited amount of prehospital EMS research relative to other areas of medical research; however, as EMS research continues, evidence-based decision making will have a correspondingly greater role in EMS practice.

EMS research may be performed by EMS providers or other individuals studying a particular branch of medicine. AEMTs typically will be involved in research through gathering data. You may be part of a study to determine how much oxygen should be given to patients with shortness of breath. You may be involved in a study to track the time it takes to transport serious trauma patients to the ED. Your job will be to ensure that you carefully record all of the information about the patients. The information gathered will then be analyzed by others to answer the question(s). The results may then be shared with the rest of the EMS community to improve patient care practices. Traditional medical practice is based on such research.

Research can also be done at each EMS facility. EMS personnel can examine patient care records to determine where the department can improve. This information is then used to generate educational sessions for AEMTs or may be used to plan public education and prevention strategies. High-quality patient care should focus on procedures useful in improving patient outcomes through sound research.

It is important for EMS providers to stay up-to-date on the latest advances in health care. Every 3 to 5 years, the American Heart Association (AHA) unveils a revised set of guidelines based on large amounts of evidence. AHA is an excellent example of evidence-based medical decision making in progress. These changes occur because more information is known. One word of caution: when reading new research results, make sure you understand what the results mean. Ask questions and conduct some of your own research. Conclusions that seem too good to be true usually are.

Illness and Injury Prevention

Grouping injuries into common health problems makes it possible to consider the breadth and depth of the problem and has enabled public health officials and other care

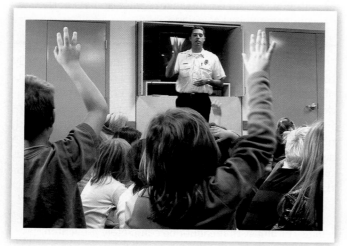

Courtesy of Captain David Jackson, Saginaw Township Fire Department

FIGURE 1-7 Part of your role as a public servant is to interact with and educate the public.

providers to call attention to important problems and target more effective interventions. Intentional injuries such as assaults or suicide are one such group of injuries. EMS can play a role in preventing intentional injuries but can usually have a greater impact in preventing unintentional injuries.

How big is the problem of injuries in the United States? To many health experts, injuries are the largest public health problem facing the country today. From ages 1 to 44 years, unintentional injuries are the leading killer. For all ages combined, unintentional injuries are the fifth leading killer behind heart disease; cancer; cerebrovascular events (stroke); and the effects of bronchitis, emphysema, and asthma.

In most areas, EMS providers are considered high-profile role models. They generally reflect the composition of the community and, in a rural setting, may be the most medically educated people. EMS providers are often considered advocates of the injured or ill and, as such, are welcomed into schools and other environments. They are considered authorities on injury and prevention. An AEMT can be involved in many prevention strategies. Patient education can help prevent the occurrence of injuries. EMS providers are in a good position to recognize signs and symptoms of suspected abuse and abusive situations. When an EMS provider recognizes such signs, he or she can report these suspicions to local law enforcement or other appropriate authorities. EMS providers can also refer patients to care and rehabilitation services to help prevent further problems as a result of an event that has already occurred. Such services may include child protective services; shelters for sexual, spousal, or elder abuse; food; clothing; counseling; alternative sources of health care such as free clinics; grief support; and numerous others. Keeping a list of resources or a few pamphlets from a local shelter in your ambulance can be very beneficial in a time of crisis.

Other situations include recognizing signs and symptoms of exposure to hazardous materials, temperature extremes, vectors, communicable diseases, assault and battery, and structural risks. Remember, personal safety first! Each of these situations may be detrimental to the AEMT and must be considered as such. Always ensure safety before entering the scene and take necessary standard precautions.

Scene Safety and Personal Protection

The personal safety of all people involved in an emergency situation is very important—so important, in fact, that the steps you take to preserve personal safety must become automatic. Anticipate danger based on the type of scene you are about to enter. Drivers who gawk at the scene of a crash may run into you or another vehicle. A second accident at the scene or an injury to you or your partner creates more problems, delays emergency medical care for patients, increases the burden on the other AEMTs, and may result in unnecessary injury or death.

You should begin protecting yourself as soon as you are dispatched. Before you leave for the scene, begin preparing yourself both mentally and physically. Make sure you wear seat belts and shoulder harnesses en route **FIGURE 1-8**. Be sure to wear seat belts and shoulder harnesses at all times during transport unless patient care makes it impossible. It is important to ensure that all equipment is restrained so it does not become a hazard to you or the patient during transport. Finally, remember to don the appropriate personal protective equipment (PPE) when you arrive on scene.

Protecting yourself at the scene is also very important. A second accident may damage the ambulance and may result in injury to you or your partner or additional injury to the patient. Crash scenes must be well marked. If law enforcement has not already done so, you should make sure that proper warning devices are placed at a sufficient distance from the scene to alert motorists coming from both directions that a crash has occurred. You should park the ambulance at a safe but convenient distance from the scene. Before attempting to access patients trapped in a vehicle, check the vehicle's stability. Then take the necessary measures to secure it if possible. Do not rock or push on a vehicle to find out whether it will move. This can overturn the vehicle or send it crashing into a ditch. If you are uncertain about the safety of a crash scene, wait for appropriately trained individuals to arrive before approaching.

When working at night, you must have plenty of light. Poor lighting increases the risk of further injury to you and the patient and results in poor emergency medical care.

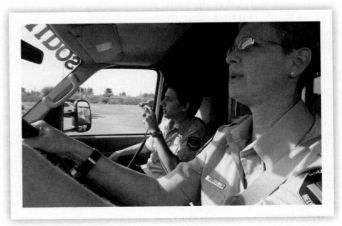

FIGURE 1-8 Wear seat belts and shoulder harnesses en route to the scene.

Reflective emblems or clothing helps to make you more visible at night and decreases your risk of injury.

> ### Transition Tip
>
> Your continued health, safety, and well-being are vital if you are to fully contribute to your EMS operation. Your training will continue to aid you in recognizing and protecting yourself from hazards ranging from personal neglect to environmental and man-made threats to your health and safety.

Wellness of the AEMT

It is essential that you take care of yourself, both physically and mentally. Anyone can respond to a sudden physical stress for a short time. If stress is prolonged, especially if physical action is not a permitted response, your body can quickly be drained of its reserves. This can leave it depleted of key nutrients, weakened, and more susceptible to illness.

Stress

EMS is a high-stress job. Understanding the causes of stress and knowing how to deal with them are critical to your job performance, health, and interpersonal relationships. Stressors include emotional, physical, and environmental situations or conditions that may cause of variety of physiologic, physical, and psychological responses. The body's response to stress begins with an alarm response, followed by a stage of reaction and resistance, and then recovery or, if the stress is prolonged, exhaustion.

There are many methods of handling stress. Some are positive and healthy; others are harmful or destructive. The term, stress management, refers to tactics that have been shown to alleviate or eliminate stress reactions. These may involve changing a few habits, changing your attitude, and perseverance **TABLE 1-3**.

It is important to note that it is not the event itself but the person's reaction to it that determines how much it will tax the body's resources. Remember that stress results from anything you perceive as a threat to your equilibrium. Stress is an undeniable and unavoidable part of everyday life. Understanding how it affects you can help you manage it more successfully.

Nutrition

To perform efficiently, you must eat nutritious food. Food is the fuel that makes the body run. The physical exertion and stress that are part of your job require a high-energy output. If you do not have a readily available source of fuel, your performance may be less than optimal. This can be dangerous for you, your partner, and your patient.

Candy and soft drinks contain sugar. These foods are quickly absorbed and converted to fuel by the body.

Table 1-3 Strategies to Manage Stress
Minimize or eliminate stressors.
Change partners to avoid a negative or hostile personality.
Change work hours.
Cut back on overtime.
Change your attitude about the stressor.
Talk about your feelings with people you trust.
Seek professional counseling if needed.
Do not obsess over frustrating situations such as relapsing alcoholics and nursing home transfers; focus on delivering high-quality care.
Try to adopt a more relaxed, philosophical outlook.
Expand your social support system apart from your coworkers.
Sustain friends and interests outside emergency services.
Minimize the physical response to stress by using various techniques, including: <ul><li>A deep breath to settle an anger response</li><li>Periodic stretching</li><li>Slow, deep breathing</li><li>Regular physical exercise</li><li>Progressive muscle relaxation and/or meditation</li><li>Limit intake of caffeine, alcohol, and tobacco</li></ul>

However, simple sugars also stimulate the body's production of insulin, which reduces blood glucose levels. For some people, eating a lot of sugar can actually result in lower energy levels.

Complex carbohydrates rank next to simple sugars in their ability to produce energy. Complex carbohydrates such as pasta, rice, and vegetables are among the safest and most reliable sources of long-term energy production. However, some carbohydrates take hours to be converted into usable body fuel.

Fats are also easily converted to energy, but eating too much fat can lead to obesity, cardiac disease, and other long-term health problems. The proteins in meat, fish, chicken, beans, and cheese take several hours to convert to energy.

Carry high-energy bars to help you maintain your energy levels. Try eating several small meals throughout the day to keep your energy resources at constantly high levels. Remember, however, that overeating may reduce your physical and mental performance. After a large meal, blood that is needed for the digestive process is not available for other activities.

Adequate hydration is also important for proper functioning. Fluids can be easily replenished by drinking any nonalcoholic, noncaffeinated beverage. Water is generally the best choice because the body absorbs it faster than any other fluid. Avoid fluids that contain high levels of sugar because they can actually slow the rate of fluid absorption by the body and cause abdominal discomfort. One indication of adequate hydration is frequent urination. Infrequent urination or urine that is dark yellow indicates dehydration.

Exercise and Relaxation

A regular program of exercise will enhance the benefits of good nutrition and adequate hydration and allow you to handle job stress better. To be healthy, you should engage in at least 30 minutes of physical activity at least 5 days a week.

Exercise routines should address aspects of cardiovascular endurance, muscular strength building, and muscle flexibility. Building up your endurance will ensure that your cardiovascular system is able to provide your muscles and brain with needed oxygen when you face a stressful situation. Having strength and flexibility ensures that your body will be able to handle lifting patients, performing CPR, and moving heavy equipment.

Relaxation techniques, meditation, and visual imagery are all means that can help reduce stress. In general, relaxation techniques involve refocusing your attention to something calming and increasing awareness of your body. Repeat words or suggestions in your mind to help relax and reduce muscle tension. Take slow, deep breaths to reduce tension and anxiety. Other relaxation techniques include yoga, tai chi, hypnosis, biofeedback, exercise, massage, and listening to music. Many of these forms of relaxation take practice to obtain the desired effect.

Safe Lifting Practices

Lifting is a task that AEMTs perform every day. As such, safe lifting techniques are critical to your health and well-being. Back injuries are a common cause of on-the-job injuries within EMS. For your health and well-being, remember these tips:

- Preplan the move.
- Bend your legs, not your waist.
- Keep the weight close to your body.
- Lift straight up using your legs, not your back.

Sleep

Good productive sleep is as important as eating well and exercising to maintain good health. Sleep should be regular and uninterrupted. The number of hours is not nearly as important as the quality of sleep. Unfortunately, you may not have the luxury of sleeping throughout the night.

The signs that your sleep pattern is ineffective include:

- You fall asleep within seconds of lying down.
- Within an hour or so after an EMS call, you find yourself routinely fatigued. The excitement is over and now your adrenaline rush crashes.
- You are unable to make it through an entire day without severe fatigue.
- You are unable to concentrate on repetitive tasks such as driving or completing paperwork.

Limiting your caffeine intake and tobacco use can help improve your sleep habits. Both agents have stimulating effects that can interrupt sleep. Limit your alcohol use. Alcohol is a depressant and encourages sleep. However, routine or excessive use of alcohol can change your sleep pattern, preventing deep sleep. Try to create as consistent a sleep cycle as possible. This may require naps. Many EMS providers are able to change their sleep pattern into several sleep episodes throughout the day.

Do not worry if you are unable to get eight straight hours of sleep. Three sleep episodes of 2 to 3 hours each will provide similar effects. Each sleep episode needs to be more than 1 hour in length to encourage deep sleep. Finally, do not forget the effects of exercise and sleep. Routine exercise will promote the needed fatigue to slip into a restful sleep.

Disease Prevention

Besides sleep, diet, exercise, hydration, and all the other things that make up a healthy lifestyle, you need to be aware of hereditary factors that may predispose you to certain diseases. Consider what you might know about your immediate family's and your ancestors' health. Alzheimer disease, chemical addiction, cancer, cardiac illness, hypertension, migraine, mental illness, and stroke all feature prominent hereditary factors. The most common of all hereditary health factors are heart disease and cancer.

Share this information with your personal physician. Your physician is bound by the same oath of confidentiality that you are. Work with him or her to set up a schedule for health assessments, building them into your routine physical checkups. Your physician should be your ally in screening for these diseases and in assessing your lifestyle as well as any hereditary factors.

Knowing your hereditary factors may help you adjust your lifestyle to help prevent disease. For example, if diabetes runs in your family, exercise and diet are critical to your well-being. Maintaining a healthy weight and sustaining a consistent exercise routine will help minimize your risk of developing this disease.

If you don't already smoke, don't start! If you do, please stop! Not only does this habit fly in the face of everything that EMS stands for, it also produces many of the worst cardiovascular and lung disasters that you will confront during your career. In addition, it sets an awful example for the public—especially to people who have breathing disorders such as asthma. And it makes you look and smell like anything but a professional caregiver.

Are you a smoker who is trying to quit? Several strategies can help. First, try to cultivate a relationship with a mentor who was once truly addicted to smoking but who has successfully quit. Use that person as a support and draw on his or her advice and encouragement. There are also programs that attack a smoker's psychological dependency. These programs may include instructions and audio that provide ongoing support. Other options include therapy, hypnotism, and acupuncture.

Talk to your primary care physician. Your physician should be familiar with more techniques. All of these solutions are cheaper than cigarettes and their associated health risks.

Death and Dying

Working With Family Members

Although you must treat all patients with respect and dignity, you should use special care with dying patients and their families **FIGURE 1-9**. Be concerned about their privacy and their wishes, and let them know that you take their concerns seriously. However, it is best to be honest with patients and their families; do not give them false hope.

When working with the family of a patient who has died, ask whether there is anything you can do that will be of help, such as calling a relative or religious advisor. Provide gentle and caring support. Reinforcing the reality of the situation is important. This can be accomplished by merely saying to a grieving person, "I am so sorry for your loss." It is not important that you have a well-rehearsed script, for it is not likely that your exact words or consolations will be remembered. It is important to be honest and sincere.

Some statements of consolation may sound trite, and some suggest a kind of silver lining behind the clouds. Although they may be intended to make the person feel better about a situation, they also can be viewed as an attempt to diminish the person's grief. The grieving person needs to grieve. Statements like these can also indicate our inability to comprehend the profound sadness of grief because we have not experienced that kind of loss.

Each person will experience grief and respond to it in his or her own way. Attempts to take grief away too quickly may not be helpful. If you do not know how the person really feels, you should not say that you do. People may be offended by responses that give advice or explanations about the death. Statements such as "Oh, you shouldn't feel that way," are judgmental. If you judge what the grieving person is feeling, it is likely that he or she will stop talking with you. There is no right or wrong way to grieve. Remember that anger is a stage of grieving. Patients or family members may express rage, anger, and despair. The anger may be directed at you. The anger seems irrational to everyone but the person grieving. A professional attitude is a necessity, and you must not take this anger as a personal attack. Their concerns will usually be relieved by your calm, efficient manner.

Statements and comments that suggest action on your part are generally helpful. These statements imply a sense of understanding; they focus on the grieving person's feelings. It is not necessary to go into an extensive discussion. You might say, "I am so sorry. I just want you to know that I am thinking about you." What people really appreciate is somebody who will listen to them. Simply ask, "Would you like to talk about how or what you are feeling?" Then accept the response.

Working With the Patient

Even though the event (death) has not yet occurred, the patient knows that it will happen. The patient has no control over this process. The patient will die whether or not he or she is ready. Furthermore, being ready to die does not mean that the patient will be happy about dying. You may encounter situations in which the patient is close to death, and you may need to provide reassurance and emotional care.

Individuals who are in the process of dying as a result of trauma, an acute medical condition, or a terminal disease will feel threatened. That threat may be related to their concern about survival. These concerns may involve feelings of helplessness, disability, pain, and separation.

Many factors influence how a patient reacts to the stress of an emergency incident. Among these factors are:

- Personality
- Socioeconomic background
- Fear of health care personnel
- Alcohol or substance abuse
- History of chronic disease
- Mental disorders
- Reaction to medication
- Age
- Nutritional status
- Feelings of guilt
- Past experience with illness or injury

Do not make light of a patient's pain and fear. Instead, you may say, "I'm sure you are really scared right now, but you should know that I am doing everything I can to help you." Making a connection with your patient through eye contact and the squeeze of a hand can often do more to allay fear than the most eloquent words.

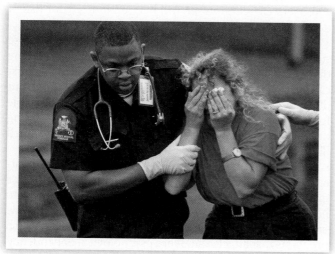

© Craig Jackson/In the Dark Photography

FIGURE 1-9 While you must treat all patients with respect and dignity, use special care with dying patients and their families.

Caring for Critically Ill and Injured Patients

When you are caring for a critically ill or injured patient, the patient needs to know who you are, what you are doing, and that you are attending to his or her immediate needs. Confusion, anxiety, and other feelings of helplessness will be decreased if you keep the patient consistently informed.

Many situations such as mass-casualty scenes, serious automobile crashes; excavation cave-ins; house fires; infant and child trauma; amputations; abuse of an infant, child, spouse, or older person; and death of a coworker or other public safety personnel will be stressful for everyone involved. During these situations, exercise extreme care in both your words and your actions. Always present a professional demeanor in terms of what you say and what you do.

Some patients, especially children and elderly people, may be terrified or feel rejected when separated from family members by the uniformed EMS provider team. Other patients may not want family members to share their stress, see their injury, or witness their pain. It is usually best if parents are transported with their children and if relatives accompany elderly patients. Because medical attention for a child often requires adult consent, treatment may be delayed if a caregiver is not transported with a child.

The religious customs or needs of the patient must also be respected. Some people will cling to religious medals or charms. Others will express a strong desire for religious counsel, baptism, or last rites if death is near. Try to accommodate these requests. Some people have religious convictions that strongly oppose the use of medications, blood, and blood products. If you obtain such information about your patient, it is imperative that you report it to the next level of care.

Ready for Review

- The standards for prehospital emergency care and the individuals who provide it are governed by the laws in each state and are typically regulated by a state office of EMS.
- EMRs, such as law enforcement officers, firefighters, park rangers, ski patrollers, or other organized rescuers, often arrive at the scene before the ambulance and other EMS personnel.
- An EMT has training in BLS.
- An AEMT has training in specific aspects of ALS such as IV therapy and the administration of certain emergency medications.
- A paramedic has extensive training in ALS.
- The *EMS Agenda for the Future* is a multidisciplinary national review of all aspects of EMS delivery that encourages the creation of systems to help protect the well-being of EMS providers. It includes 14 components that make up an EMS system.
- Public health involves activities targeted toward the prevention of illness and injuries.
- It is through research that we learn methods for improving both EMS as a system and specific aspects such as patient outcomes.
- Understanding the causes of stress and knowing how to deal with them are critical to an AEMT's job performance, health, and interpersonal relationships.
- It is essential that EMS personnel get adequate nutrition, exercise, relaxation, and sleep to stay healthy.
- AEMTs must be familiar with the available resources to deal with the emotional issues surrounding death and dying.
- When an AEMT is caring for critically ill or injured patients, he or she needs to consistently inform the patient about what is going on to decrease the patient's confusion, anxiety, and feelings of helplessness.

Case Study

You are dispatched to an intersection known for traffic accidents. As you listen to the additional information from the dispatcher, you remember that a traffic light was just installed there last week because of the high number of crashes. You arrive on the scene and find two vehicles with significant damage. There is a person lying in the street, and you notice a driver in each of the vehicles. A bystander tells you that a pedestrian attempted to cross the street while the traffic had a green light and was hit. The driver of one of the vehicles has blood all over her face and is screaming hysterically.

1. Placing a traffic light at an intersection known for frequent collisions is an example of a primary prevention strategy. Explain the difference between primary and secondary prevention strategies.

2. As your ambulance approaches the scene, what are some important items that you need to consider?

3. Upon delivering your patient(s) to the hospital, you must provide oral as well as written documentation to the receiving personnel. Why is this important?

4. EMS research is an important part of prehospital care. As an AEMT, how might you help in this area?

5. List some of the factors that may influence how a patient reacts to the stress of an emergency incident.

CHAPTER 2

Medical, Legal, and Ethical Issues

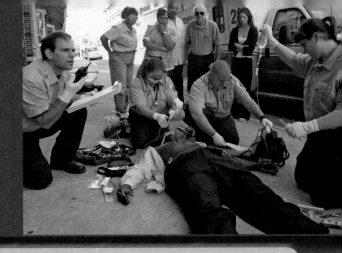

National EMS Education Standard

Preparatory

Applies fundamental knowledge of the EMS system, safety/well-being of the AEMT, and medical/legal and ethical issues to the provision of emergency care.

Review

AEMTs have a duty to act in a professional manner at all times. The *scope of practice* is most commonly defined by state law and outlines the tasks that the AEMT is legally authorized to perform. The *standard of care* comprises how a reasonably prudent person with similar training and experience would act under similar circumstances, with similar equipment, and in the same or similar environment. AEMTs are mandated reporters for certain types of calls, such as suspected child and elder abuse, dog bites, injuries involving criminal activity such as gunshot wounds or sexual assault, and certain infectious or communicable diseases.

What's New

New legal terminology is included in the 2009 *National EMS Education Standards* that will be presented in this chapter, including kidnapping and false imprisonment. The concept of negligence is reviewed in conjunction with certain new concepts that could make EMS personnel more susceptible to a lawsuit. Enhanced content about advance directives, assault and battery, ethical principles and moral obligations, and the Health Insurance Portability and Accountability Act (HIPAA) is included.

Introduction

A basic principle of emergency care is to do no further harm. As the scope and nature of EMS become more complex and widely available, litigation involving participants continues to increase. Providing competent emergency medical care that conforms to the standard of care taught continues to be the best defense to avoid both civil and criminal actions. Consider the following situations:

- You are transporting a patient, and while the stretcher is being loaded into the ambulance, your partner slips, the stretcher crashes to the ground, and the patient is injured.
- You are about to begin treating a child and the father commands you to stop.

What should you do?

An understanding of not only the various legal aspects of emergency care but also the ethical issues is essential for an AEMT. Should you stop and treat patients who were involved in an automobile crash while you are en route to another emergency call? Should you begin CPR on a patient who, according to the family, has terminal cancer? Should patient information be released to a patient's attorney on the telephone? Delivery of patient care involves more than just lifesaving skills; it also requires that you understand the laws and serve as a patient advocate.

> *Scope of practice* A document that outlines the tasks the AEMT is legally authorized to perform.
> *Standard of care* How a reasonably prudent person with similar training and experience would act under similar circumstances, with similar equipment, and in the same or similar environment.

Consent

Under most circumstances, consent is required from every conscious, mentally competent adult before care can be started. A person receiving care must give permission, or *consent*, for treatment. If a person is alert, rational, and capable of making informed decisions, he or she has a legal right to refuse care, even if ill or injured. A patient may also consent to some aspects of care and deny consent to others. If a patient refuses care, you may not care for the patient. In fact, doing so may be grounds for criminal and civil action. Consent can be expressed or implied and can also apply to the care of a minor or a mentally incompetent patient.

Four types of consent exist: *expressed consent*, *implied consent* (emergency doctrine), consent of a minor, and involuntary consent. Consent of a minor is discussed in further detail.

> *Consent* Permission to render care.
> *Expressed consent* A type of consent in which a patient gives specific and direct authorization for provision of care or transport.
> *Implied consent* A type of consent in which a patient who is unable to give consent is given treatment under the legal assumption that he or she would want treatment.

Minors and Consent

Because a minor might not have the wisdom, maturity, or judgment to give valid consent, the law requires that a parent or legal guardian give consent for treatment or transport of a minor **FIGURE 2-1**. However, in some states, a minor can give valid consent to receive medical care, depending on the minor's age and maturity. Many states also allow emancipated, married, or pregnant minors to be treated as adults for the purposes of consenting to medical treatment. An *emancipated minor* is a person who, despite being under the legal age in a given state (in most cases the age is 18 years), can be legally treated as an adult based on certain circumstances. For example, many states consider minors to be emancipated if they are married, if they are members of the armed services, or if they are parents. A minor may also be considered emancipated if he or she is living away from home and no longer relying on his or her parents for support. A minor who is a parent may also give consent for his or her own child.

You should obtain consent from a parent or legal guardian whenever possible; however, if a true emergency exists and the parent or legal guardian is not available, the consent to treat the minor is implied, just as with an adult. You must never withhold lifesaving care.

> *Emancipated minor* A person who is under the legal age in a given state but, because of other circumstances, is legally considered an adult.

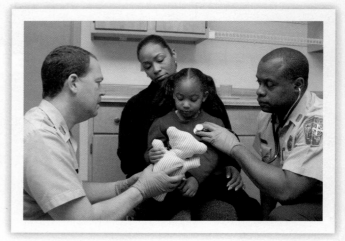

FIGURE 2-1 The law requires that a parent or legal guardian give consent for treatment or transport of a minor. However, you must never withhold lifesaving care.

> ### Transition Tip
>
> You should know your state's laws concerning the issues surrounding involuntary consent and emancipation.

Forcible Restraint

Forcible restraint of a patient who is mentally incompetent or physically violent is the act of physically subduing the patient to prevent any physical action on his or her part. This may help to prevent the patient from harming himself, herself, or the AEMT if the patient is suicidal or homicidal. Forcible restraint of a mentally disturbed person may be required before emergency care can be given. If you believe that a patient will injure himself, herself, or others, you can legally restrain the patient. However, you must consult medical control, online or off-line, depending on local protocol, for authorization to restrain, or contact law enforcement personnel who have authority to restrain people. In some states, only a law enforcement officer may forcibly restrain a person **FIGURE 2-2**. You should clearly understand local laws. Restraint without authority exposes you to civil and criminal penalties. Restraint may be used only in circumstances of risk to the patient, yourself, or others, and must be nonpunitive.

> *Forcible restraint* The act of physically preventing a person from taking physical action.

Your service should have clearly defined protocols pertaining to situations involving restraint. After restraints are applied, they must not be removed en route even if the patient promises to act calmly. It is also important to monitor

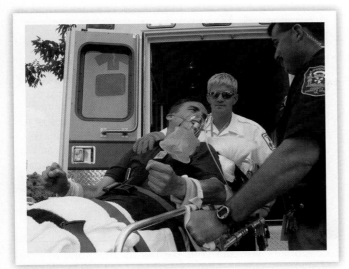

FIGURE 2-2 Be sure that you know the local laws about forcible restraint of a patient. In some states, only a law enforcement officer has the authority to restrain a patient.

the restrained patient closely for any signs of breathing difficulty. It is possible to suffocate the patient if he or she is face down, creating positional asphyxia, or if a mask placed over the patient's face occludes airflow.

Remember that if the patient is responsive and the situation is not urgent, consent is required. Adults who appear to be in control of their senses cannot be forced to submit to care or transportation.

The Right to Refuse Treatment

Adults who are conscious, alert, and appear to have decision-making capacity have the right to refuse treatment or withdraw from treatment at any time, even if doing so may result in death or serious injury. Such patients present you with a dilemma. Should you provide care against their will? Should you leave them alone? Calls involving refusal of treatment are commonly litigated in EMS and require you to proceed cautiously. If you leave patients alone, you risk being accused of negligence or abandonment if their condition becomes worse. You may also face charges of false imprisonment if you transport a patient against his or her wishes.

Refusal of Care for a Minor

You may be faced with a situation in which a parent refuses to permit treatment of an ill or injured child. In this situation, you must consider the emotional impact of the emergency on the parent's judgment. In this and virtually all cases of refusal, you can usually resolve the situation with patience and calm persuasion. You may also need the help of others, such as your supervisor or law enforcement officials. In most states, consent to treat a minor is required from only one parent.

Documentation of Refusal of Care

When you are not able to persuade the patient, guardian, conservator, or parent of a minor or mentally incompetent patient to proceed with treatment, you must obtain the signature of the person who is refusing treatment on an official release form that acknowledges refusal. Be sure to document any assessment findings and any emergency care that you provided. You must also obtain a signature from a witness to the refusal. You should then keep the release form with the patient care report. In addition to the release form itself, you should write a note about the refusal on the patient care report. If the patient refuses to sign the release form, the best you can do is inform your medical director and thoroughly document the situation and the refusal. Report to medical control and follow your local protocols with regard to this situation.

> ### Transition Tip
>
> Be sure to retain documents of refusal with your records, as they will be important if a legal claim is filed later. In some cases, parents who have refused to provide medical care for a child have been charged with child neglect. Such a situation is especially likely to occur during custody battles where one parent refuses treatment without the other parent's knowledge. Given that you might be called as a witness in such cases, you must be sure that all documentation is thorough and accurate.

Confidentiality

Communication between you and the patient is considered confidential and generally cannot be disclosed without permission from the patient or a court order. Confidential information includes the patient history, assessment findings, and treatment provided. You cannot disclose information regarding a patient's diagnosis, treatment, or mental and physical condition without consent; if you do, you may find yourself liable for breach of confidentiality.

To protect yourself, be sure to document only objective findings and omit personal opinions. Do not give information to anyone other than health care professionals directly involved in the patient's continuing care. Briefly but politely explain to others such as family members and concerned friends that you cannot give out information regarding the patient's condition. Instead, suggest that they follow up with immediate family members once the patient has been seen in the emergency department.

HIPAA

HIPAA is the acronym for the Health Insurance Portability and Accountability Act of 1996. This act provides for criminal sanctions as well as civil penalties for releasing a patient's private medical information in an unauthorized manner. Although this act had many aims, including improving the portability and continuity of health insurance coverage and combating waste and fraud in health insurance and the provision of health care, the section of the act that most affects EMS relates to patient privacy. The aim of this section was to strengthen laws for the protection of the privacy of health care information and to safeguard patient confidentiality. As such, it provides guidance on what types of information are protected, the responsibility of health care providers regarding that protection, and penalties for breaching that protection. Medical information can be disclosed only if it is necessary for a patient's treatment or for payment or medical/billing operations.

Transition Tip

HIPAA considers all patient information that you obtain in the course of providing medical treatment to a patient to be protected health information. As an AEMT, you have an obligation to guard all protected health information from unlawful disclosure, either written or verbal.

Protected health information may be disclosed for the purposes of treatment, payment, or operations (including quality assurance activities). Specifically, you are permitted to report your assessment findings and treatment to other health care providers directly involved in the care of the patient. You may also release protected health information for third-party billing. Although patient information may be used for internal quality improvement and training programs, all identifying information must first be removed before sharing it for training purposes with those not involved in the patient's care. In certain situations you may be legally mandated to report your findings, such as in the case of child abuse or when you receive a subpoena. Failure to abide by the provisions of the HIPAA laws can result in civil and/or criminal action against your response agency and against you personally.

If you are unsure, do not give any information to anyone other than those directly involved in the care of the patient. For specific policies, each EMS service is required to have a manual and a compliance officer who can answer questions. You should have received specific training on how the HIPAA legislation affects your specific organization. If not, take the time to ask questions and get training specific to the policies and procedures you are to follow.

> *Protected health information* Any information about health status, provision of health care, or payment for health care that can be linked to an individual. This is interpreted rather broadly and includes any part of a patient's medical record or payment history.

Transition Tip

Duty to act is a person's responsibility to provide patient care. Once your ambulance responds to a call or treatment is initiated, you have a legal duty to act. If you are off duty and come upon a crash, you are not legally obligated to stop and assist patients in most cases. There may be some circumstances where this is not true and you should be familiar with the laws and policies that apply in your service area.

Advance Directives

Occasionally, you and your partner may respond to a call in which a patient is dying of an illness. When you arrive at the scene, you may find that family members do not want you to try to resuscitate the patient. Without valid written documentation such as an advance directive, living will, or do not resuscitate (DNR) order (also known as a Do Not Attempt Resuscitation order), this type of request places you in a difficult position. An *advance directive*, or living will, is a written document that specifies medical treatment for a competent patient, should he or she become unable to make decisions. In this situation, a competent patient is able to make rational decisions about his or her well-being. DNR orders give you permission to not attempt resuscitation. Although laws might differ from state to state, generally speaking, to be valid, DNR orders must meet the following requirements:

- Clearly state the patient's medical problem(s)
- Signature of the patient or legal guardian
- Signature of one or more physicians

> *Advance directive* Written documentation that specifies medical treatment for a competent patient should the patient become unable to make decisions; also called a living will.

In some states, DNR orders contain expiration dates, whereas in others, no expiration date is included. DNR orders with expiration dates must be dated in the preceding 12 months to be valid.

However, even in the presence of a DNR order, you are still obligated to provide supportive measures (oxygen, pain relief, and comfort) whenever possible to a patient who is not in cardiac arrest. Each ambulance service, in consultation with its medical director and legal counsel, must develop a protocol to follow in these circumstances.

In the absence of an advance directive or DNR, the patient may have a durable power of attorney or a health care proxy. There are many different types of powers of attorney and not all authorize the exercise of medical decision making. Some powers of attorney simply authorize someone to handle the financial affairs of the person executing the power and others will apply only if the person executing the power is still competent. Also, remember that a patient who remains conscious and competent has the right to make medical decisions; the person named as the power of attorney or health care proxy is authorized to make decisions only when the patient is no longer capable of doing so. When presented with a power of attorney at the scene of a medical emergency, you must read it carefully to ascertain its meaning. If there is any question, you should contact online medical control for assistance. Do not delay emergency care while efforts to interpret the power of attorney are made.

Because of terminal nursing home placement, hospice, and home health programs, you may often be faced with this situation. Specific guidelines vary from state to state, but the following four statements may be considered general guidelines:

1. Patients have the right to refuse treatment, including resuscitative efforts, provided that they are able to communicate their wishes in a competent manner. Patients also have the right to withdraw a DNR for themselves and request emergency care.
2. A written order from a physician is required for DNR orders to be valid in a health care facility.
3. You should periodically review state and local protocols and legislation regarding advance directives.
4. When you are in doubt or the written orders are not present, begin basic life support and contact medical control for guidance.

When resuscitative efforts will be useless and the patient has less than a 1% chance of survival, resuscitation is considered to be medically futile. This includes situations where death is imminent, such as resuscitative efforts for those patients who are terminally ill, life-sustaining interventions for patients in a persistent vegetative state, or use of chemotherapy in patients with cancer in advanced stages. This is a controversial area because it often puts the physician on the opposite side of the table from the patient's family. Generally the physician feels it is unethical to provide futile treatment and give false hope, yet the family may not be ready to let go.

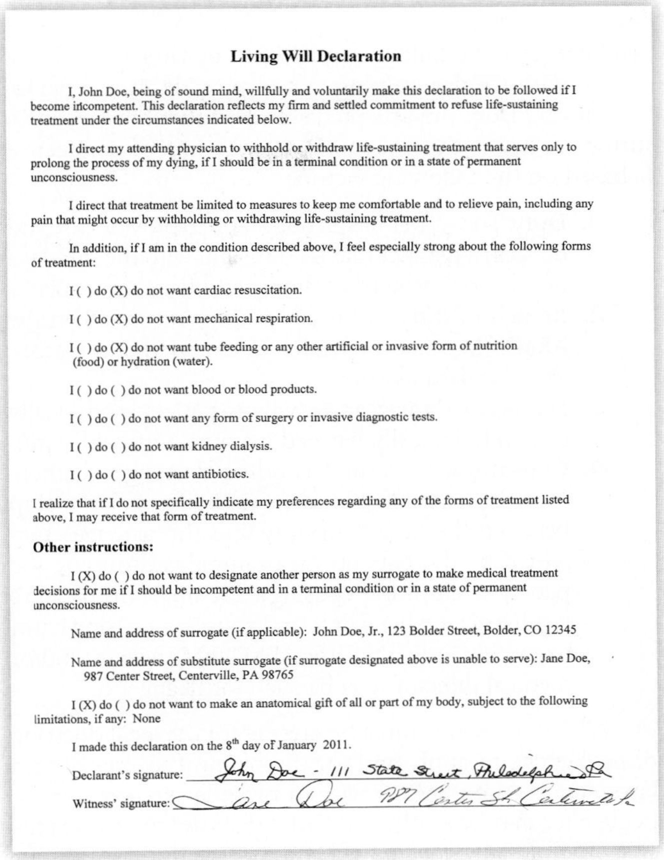

Living Will Declaration

I, John Doe, being of sound mind, willfully and voluntarily make this declaration to be followed if I become incompetent. This declaration reflects my firm and settled commitment to refuse life-sustaining treatment under the circumstances indicated below.

I direct my attending physician to withhold or withdraw life-sustaining treatment that serves only to prolong the process of my dying, if I should be in a terminal condition or in a state of permanent unconsciousness.

I direct that treatment be limited to measures to keep me comfortable and to relieve pain, including any pain that might occur by withholding or withdrawing life-sustaining treatment.

In addition, if I am in the condition described above, I feel especially strong about the following forms of treatment:

I ( ) do (X) do not want cardiac resuscitation.

I ( ) do (X) do not want mechanical respiration.

I ( ) do (X) do not want tube feeding or any other artificial or invasive form of nutrition (food) or hydration (water).

I ( ) do ( ) do not want blood or blood products.

I ( ) do ( ) do not want any form of surgery or invasive diagnostic tests.

I ( ) do ( ) do not want kidney dialysis.

I ( ) do ( ) do not want antibiotics.

I realize that if I do not specifically indicate my preferences regarding any of the forms of treatment listed above, I may receive that form of treatment.

Other instructions:

I (X) do ( ) do not want to designate another person as my surrogate to make medical treatment decisions for me if I should be incompetent and in a terminal condition or in a state of permanent unconsciousness.

Name and address of surrogate (if applicable): John Doe, Jr., 123 Bolder Street, Bolder, CO 12345

Name and address of substitute surrogate (if surrogate designated above is unable to serve): Jane Doe, 987 Center Street, Centerville, PA 98765

I (X) do ( ) do not want to make an anatomical gift of all or part of my body, subject to the following limitations, if any: None

I made this declaration on the 8th day of January 2011.

Declarant's signature: _John Doe - 111 State Street, Philadelphia, PA_

Witness' signature: _Jane Doe, 987 Center St, Centerville_

Courtesy of Catherine Parvensky Barwell

FIGURE 2-3 A sample advance directive (living will).

▋Civil Torts

Civil torts are simply defined as civil wrongs, meaning that they are not within the jurisdiction of US criminal courts. Examples of tort actions include suits for abandonment, negligence, and defamation of character. The goal of tort law is to provide compensation to victims for wrongdoings against them.

> *Civil tort* A wrongful act that gives rise to a civil suit.

Abandonment

Abandonment is the unilateral termination of care by the AEMT without the patient's consent and without making any provisions for continuing care by a medical professional with the skills at the same or a higher level. Once you have started care, you have assumed a duty that must not stop until an equally competent person with an equal or higher level of training assumes responsibility. Not fulfilling that duty exposes the patient to harm and is a basis for a negligence suit. Abandonment is a legally and ethically serious matter that can result in civil and criminal actions against an AEMT.

Transition Tip

An advance directive **FIGURE 2-3** specifically states what type of care the patient wishes to receive in a given situation. This may include the desire to have basic life support performed, but no advanced procedures or life-support equipment.

DNR orders typically state that if the patient is apneic and pulseless, no resuscitative measures are to be taken.

Negligence

Negligence is the failure to provide the same care that a person with similar training would provide. It is a deviation of care from the accepted standard that may result in further injury to the patient. Determination of negligence is based on the following factors:

1. **Duty.** The AEMT has an obligation to provide care and do so in a manner that is consistent with the standard of care established by training and local protocols.
2. **Breach of duty.** A breach of duty occurs when the AEMT does not act within an expected and reasonable standard of care.
3. **Damages.** Damages arise when a patient is physically or psychologically harmed in some noticeable way.
4. **Causation.** To warrant a finding of negligence, there must be a reasonable cause-and-effect relationship between the breach of duty and the damages sustained by the patient. An example is dropping the patient while lifting, causing a fracture of the patient's leg. If a person has a duty and abuses it, causing harm to another individual, the AEMT, EMS agency, and/or medical director may be sued for negligence.

All four elements must be present for the legal doctrine of negligence to apply and for the plaintiff to prevail in a lawsuit against an EMS service or provider. In some cases, negligence may be so obvious that it does not require extensive proof. *Res ipsa loquitur* is Latin for "the thing speaks for itself." The injury could only have been caused by negligence, such as in the case of dropping a patient on a stretcher.

In rare cases the plaintiff may be able to establish liability by using the theory of negligence per se, which means that the conduct of the person being sued is alleged to have occurred in clear violation of a statute. For example, if an AEMT performs a paramedic skill, there is no need to show that the procedure was inappropriate for the patient or that the AEMT administered it incorrectly. An AEMT who carries out procedures for which he or she is not authorized under the enabling legislation is practicing outside his or her scope of practice, which may be considered negligence.

Transition Tip

All forms of negligence come under the general category of law known as tort. Torts are simply defined as civil wrongs. They are not within the jurisdiction of our criminal courts. Examples of tort actions other than negligence are suits for defamation of character and invasion of privacy.

Intentional Torts or Criminality

Criminality, or intentional torts, involves actual crimes. In a criminal case, the focus is on whether the individual committed a crime against society for which he or she should be punished. As a general rule, in a criminal case the issue is not financial compensation for the criminal act. Instead, it is assumed that a civil tort exists to compensate the victim for any financial harm. Assault, battery, kidnapping, false imprisonment, and driving under the influence would all fall under the classification of crimes.

Assault and Battery

Assault is defined as threatening a person or causing a person fear of immediate bodily harm without the person's consent. Battery is unlawfully touching a person; this includes providing emergency care without consent. Assault and battery can be either civil or criminal in nature. Civil lawsuits for battery are common in health care. To sustain a criminal case of assault or battery, it is generally necessary to prove intent to cause harm. The element of intent is rarely present in the case of an EMS provider; therefore, criminal cases of assault and/or battery are rare. *Kidnapping* is the seizing, confining, abducting, or carrying away of a person by force. In theory, this might include a situation where a patient is transported against his or her will. In reality, criminal charges of kidnapping are almost unheard of in EMS because the EMS provider is almost always acting in a good faith effort to provide care to the patient. It is far more likely that an EMS provider could be the target of a civil suit for *false imprisonment*. This is defined as the unauthorized confinement of a person that lasts for an appreciable period of time.

> *Kidnapping* The seizing, confining, abducting, or carrying away of a person by force.
>
> *False imprisonment* The unauthorized confinement of a person that lasts for an appreciable period of time.

Serious legal problems may arise in situations in which a patient has not given consent for treatment. Battery could be charged if you apply a splint to a suspected fracture of the lower leg or use a prefilled epinephrine syringe (for example, an EpiPen) on a patient without the patient's consent. The patient may have grounds to sue you for assault, battery, false imprisonment, or all three. To protect yourself from these charges, make sure that you obtain expressed consent or that the situation allows for implied consent. Consult your medical director if you have questions or doubts about a specific situation.

Transition Tip

Good Samaritan laws are based on the common law principle that when you reasonably help another person, you should not be liable for errors and omissions made in giving good-faith emergency care. Good Samaritan laws vary from state to state. Be familiar with the laws in your state.

Ethical Principles and Moral Obligations

In addition to legal duties, EMS providers have certain ethical responsibilities as health care providers. These responsibilities are to themselves, their coworkers, the public, and the patient. Ethics are related to action, conduct, motive, and character and how they relate to the EMS provider's responsibilities. *Ethics* is the philosophy of right and wrong, of moral duties, and of ideal professional behavior. It is often referred to as the study of morality. *Morality* is a code of conduct that can be defined by society, religion, or a person, affecting character, conduct, and conscience. From an EMS standpoint, ethics are associated with what the EMS profession deems right or fitting conduct. Treating a patient ethically means doing so in a manner that conforms to professional standards of conduct and keeping the patient's best interests at the forefront of decision making. The manner in which principles of ethics are incorporated into professional conduct is known as *applied ethics*.

> *Ethics* The philosophy of right and wrong, of moral duties, and of ideal professional behavior.
> *Morality* A code of conduct that can be defined by society, religion, or a person, affecting character, conduct, and conscience.
> *Applied ethics* The manner in which principles of ethics are incorporated into professional conduct.

How can you make sure that you are acting ethically, especially with all the decisions you have to make in the field? **TABLE 2-1** offers a set of guidelines.

You must meet your legal and ethical responsibilities while caring for your patients' physical and emotional needs. Patient needs vary depending on the situation. Your responsibility also includes supervising care given by EMRs and others on the scene to ensure that the patient is receiving proper attention.

One unquestionable responsibility you have is honest reporting. Absolute honesty in reporting is essential. You must provide a complete account of the events and the details of all patient care and professional duties. Accurate records are also important for quality improvement activities.

To provide the best level of care, it is necessary to maintain mastery of skills. Participating in continuing education and refresher training not only provides updates on changes and new procedures in EMS, but also keeps you current in the areas you deal with infrequently such as obstetrics and pediatrics. As an AEMT, you have a moral obligation to make sure that you are knowledgeable in all areas of emergency care to ensure that you can care for patients to the best of your ability. Critically reviewing your performance and seeking improvement are ethical concerns. **TABLE 2-1** provides guidelines to help you make appropriate ethical decisions.

Table 2-1 Ethical Decision Making
1. Consider all options available to you and the consequence of each option.
2. Which decisions have been made in the past regarding a similar situation? Is this a type of problem that reflects a rule, a law, or a policy? Can an existing policy or rule be applied? This guideline is based on the concept of *precedence*, defined as basing current action on lessons, rules, or guidelines derived from previous similar experiences.
3. How would this action affect you if you were in your patient's place? This is a form of the Golden Rule. Was your decision one that was made in the best interest of the patient?
4. Would you feel comfortable if all prehospital care providers applied this action in all similar situations?
5. Can you supply a good justification for your action to: ■ Your peers? ■ The public? ■ Your supervisor?
6. How will the consequences of your decision provide the greatest benefit in view of all the alternatives?
7. Involve online medical control in your decision making.

> *Precedence* The practice of basing current action on lessons, rules, or guidelines derived from previous similar experiences.

Ethical conflicts may arise during your work as an AEMT, causing distress. Futility of care becomes an issue when faced with a situation in which attempts to provide life support may be useless because of location. An example would be the case of a cardiac arrest in the wilderness, in which time to definitive care makes the attempt at resuscitation futile. Allocation of resources becomes an ethical decision-making process in the event of a triage situation in which the demand for care exceeds your resources. Triage is the practice of doing the most good for the greatest number of patients. This means making the decision to leave patients who under other circumstances might have been viable. Professional misconduct presents yet another conflict when there is evidence of patient abuse by EMS professionals. And finally, there is the practice of economic triage or patient dumping, where patients are left because they may not generate as much income as another or a patient is denied medical treatment because of the inability to pay.

Failing to live up to legal or ethical standards may result in the AEMT being charged civilly, criminally, or both. The best legal protection is to perform an appropriate assessment and provide care that is safe, effective, and competent, coupled with accurate and complete documentation. Laws differ from state to state and area to area, so be sure to seek legal advice if needed. By staying up-to-date on skills and information and treating patients with the same consideration and respect that you would give one of your close family members, you can limit possible complications that might have legal ramifications.

Ready for Review

- Under most circumstances, consent is required from every conscious adult before EMS care can be started. The foundation of consent is decision-making capacity.
- A minor might not have the wisdom, maturity, or judgment to give valid consent. Therefore, the law requires that a parent or legal guardian give consent for treatment or transport of a child.
- Adults who are conscious and alert and who appear to have decision-making capacity have the right to refuse treatment or withdraw from treatment at any time, even if doing so may result in death or serious injury.
- Communication between you and the patient is considered confidential and generally cannot be disclosed without permission from the patient or a court order.
- Advance directives, living wills, and health care directives are most commonly used when a patient becomes comatose.

- Civil torts are defined as civil wrongs; they are not within the jurisdiction of the US criminal courts.
- Abandonment is the termination of care without the patient's consent and without making provisions for the transfer of care to a medical professional with skills at the same level or at a higher level than your own skills.
- Determination of negligence is based on four factors: duty, breach of duty, damages, and causation. All four elements must be present for the legal doctrine of negligence to apply and for a plaintiff to prevail in a lawsuit against an EMS system provider.
- Intentional torts, or criminality, are actual crimes. Assault, battery, kidnapping, false imprisonment, and driving under the influence would all fall under the classification of crimes.
- EMS providers have ethical responsibilities as health care providers. Treating a patient ethically means doing so in a manner that conforms to professional standards of conduct and keeps the patient's best interests at the forefront of decision making.

Case Study

You arrive at the home of a woman who is unresponsive. A paramedic unit was dispatched and is on its way to the scene. You direct your partner to grab the AED as you carry the oxygen and medical bag into the house. A woman greets you at the door. She is crying and says, "I didn't know what else to do, so I called 9-1-1." She tells you that she came to visit her elderly mother that afternoon and found her unresponsive on the floor. As you listen to the woman and offer support, your partner performs a patient assessment. There is no pulse and no obvious breathing noted. The woman tells you the patient has cancer and that her wishes are to not be resuscitated. You inquire about a legal DNR, but the woman says she does not believe the patient has one. On closer examination, you notice ecchymosis along the patient's back that appears to be consistent with dependent lividity.

1. On the basis of the information presented, should resuscitation efforts be initiated on this patient? Explain your reasoning.

2. A neighbor comes over to the scene and asked what happened to the patient. Can you disclose information to the neighbor? Explain your answer.

3. In the event that this patient was viable and treatment was initiated, what is the proper procedure for transferring her for further care to avoid civil and/or criminal charges of abandonment?

4. What is the difference between assault and battery?

5. Failing to respond or provide proper treatment may result in a charge of negligence. What are the four requirements to prove negligence?

CHAPTER 3

Therapeutic Communication

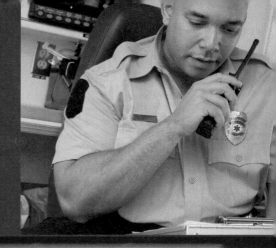

Introduction

Effective communication is an essential component of prehospital care. Verbal communication skills are vital for AEMTs. Your verbal skills will enable you to gather information from the patient and bystanders at an emergency scene. Excellent verbal communication is also an integral part of organizing, summarizing, and transferring information about the patient's care to ensure continued high-quality care after you hand off the patient to other health care workers.

The answer to the simple question of how we communicate can be surprisingly complex **FIGURE 3-1**. People communicate in a variety of ways, such as through eye contact, body position, and facial expressions. Factors such as culture and age need to be taken into consideration during communication. Patients with special needs such as those who are deaf may require you to use alternative forms of communication. Effective communication also requires you to have good listening skills that allow you to fully understand the nature of the scene and the patient's problem.

Therapeutic communication uses various communication techniques and strategies, both verbal and nonverbal, to encourage patients to express how they are feeling and to achieve a positive relationship with the patient. This chapter will discuss the factors and strategies necessary for therapeutic communication.

> *Therapeutic communication* Verbal and nonverbal communication techniques that encourage patients to express their feelings and to achieve a positive relationship with the patient.

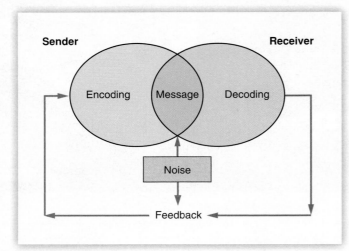

FIGURE 3-1 The Shannon-Weaver communication model is a valuable tool in understanding the variables involved in human communications. The sender must take a thought, encode it into a message, and send the message to the receiver. The receiver then decodes the message and sends feedback to the sender.

The Effects of Age, Culture, and Personal Experience on Communication

The thoughts of people are greatly influenced by their personal experiences. For example, an elderly person who often experiences great pain may view pain as more of an inconvenience than a problem. A child with limited experience of pain would likely react much differently. People are taught to handle pain differently. How do people in certain cultures view illness and injury? Some cultures encourage people to express their emotions; others see it as a sign of weakness. These social and personal pressures will shape a person's thoughts.

People may talk, make gestures, or write a note to express how they are feeling. The tone, pace, and volume of the language tell us about the mood of the person with whom we are communicating. They also provide some insight into the perceived importance of the message. For example, a patient who is yelling at you may be angry, scared, or both. Take note not only of the words being spoken but also how they are said.

People tend to translate the messages they receive using their own world view. *Ethnocentrism* occurs when you consider your own cultural values as more important when you are interacting with people of a different culture. If you are American, for example, you expect that a patient is hiding something, afraid, or untrustworthy if the patient looks away from you while you are talking. These conclusions may be true if the two people communicating are from the same culture. All aspects of communication—eye contact, social distances, body language, and even touching—have a cultural foundation. In Thailand, for example, the touching

of the head is reserved for those who are very intimate. This cultural belief can present a problem for an AEMT if the patient's head is bleeding.

Cultural imposition takes this idea to an extreme. Some health care providers may consciously or subconsciously force their cultural values onto their patient because they believe their values are better. For example, consider a child who is brought to the emergency department with red marks on his back from a traditional Asian practice called coining—rubbing hot coins on the child's back as a treatment for medical illness. The parents explain to the physician that the coining helped for a short time, but now the child seems to be ill again. The physician responds angrily to the parents, accusing them of poor parenting and insisting that their practices are harmful (although they are not). This accusation reflects cultural imposition.

> *Ethnocentrism* A situation in which a person considers his or her own cultural values to be more important when interacting with people of a different culture.
>
> *Cultural imposition* A situation in which one person imposes his or her beliefs, values, and practices on another person because the first person believes his or her ideals are superior.

Forms of Communication

Effective communication—verbal or nonverbal—is essential when gathering information from the patient. Communication skills are put to the test during every patient encounter, not only with the patient, but also with family members and bystanders as well. Remember that someone who is sick or injured is scared and might not understand what you are doing or saying. As such, your gestures, body movements, and attitude toward the patient are critically important in gaining the trust of both the patient and the family.

Verbal Communication

You have most likely mastered many communication skills, including those associated with radio operations and written communication. Skilled verbal communication with the patient and family, bystanders, and the rest of the health care team are an essential part of high-quality patient care.

You may recall that when questioning a patient, there are two types of questions: (1) *open-ended questions*, for which a patient needs to provide some level of detail to give an answer, and (2) *closed-ended questions*, which can be answered in very short or single-word responses. When first approaching your patient, use open-ended questions: "Good day. My name is Chuck and I am an AEMT. What made you call for the ambulance today?" Open-ended questions allow a free flow of conversation and let the patient direct you to what is bothering him or her.

Closed-ended questions are used when a patient is unable to provide long or complete answers to questions, such as an adult patient with severe breathing problems or a child who is scared and does not know what to say. In these situations, closed-ended questions—such as "Are you having trouble breathing?" and "Do you take medications for your heart?"—would be appropriate.

> *Open-ended questions* Questions for which the patient must provide detail to give an answer.
> *Closed-ended questions* Questions that can be answered in short or single-word responses.

You have many powerful communication tools at your disposal when trying to obtain information from patients. Sometimes patients will hide information, either consciously or subconsciously. In such cases, patients may be afraid or confused. The techniques in **TABLE 3-1** can assist you in gathering patient information. They can be helpful to use not only in patients who are willing to share but also in those who are resistant to sharing information.

When interviewing a patient, consider using touch as a means to communicate care and compassion. Although touch is a powerful tool, it should be used consciously and sparingly **FIGURE 3-2**. Many people will be uncomfortable with a stranger touching them suddenly. If you are going to touch the patient, approach slowly and touch the patient's shoulder or arm. You may hold the patient's hand. This allows you to touch the patient, showing you care about what they are telling you, and also allows you to remain at a slight distance.

Avoid touching the patient's torso, chest, or face simply as a means of communication, because these areas are often viewed as intimate. Touching these areas also requires getting closer to the patient, potentially invading intimate space. **TABLE 3-2** provides other tips on what to avoid when communicating with patients.

The presence of family, friends, and bystanders during an interview can be valuable. Sometimes, however, well-meaning family members will speak for the patient; at times

Table 3-1
Communication Tools

Communication Tools	Definition	Example
Facilitation	Encouraging the patient to talk more or provide more information	EMT: "Can you tell me more? I am listening to you."
Silence	Not speaking	Giving your patient space and time to think and respond.
Reflection	Restating a patient's statement made to you to confirm your understanding	Patient: "I am so depressed that I could die." EMT: "I understand that you are feeling sad."
Empathy	Being sensitive to the patient's feelings and thoughts	Using eye contact and touching to reinforce your communication; adjusting tone and pace to allow for open communication.
Clarification	Asking the patient to explain what he or she meant by an answer	Patient: "I just feel sick." EMT: "Can you please tell me what is feeling sick? Can you help me to understand what is going on?"
Confrontation	Making the patient who is in denial or in a mental state of shock focus on urgent and life-critical issues	Patient: "I am having pain in my chest, my back has been hurting me, I feel nauseated, and I ran out of my blood pressure medication." EMT: "Please tell me about your chest pain. We will talk about your other concerns in a moment."
Interpretation	Summing up your patient's complaint	EMT: "If I understand correctly, you have been feeling pain for the past 3 days, and it has gotten worse today." Patient: "That's right."
Explanation	Providing factual information to support a conversation	Patient: "I do not understand what is happening." EMT: "We have checked your blood sugar and blood pressure and both appear to be normal."
Summary	Providing the patient with an overview of the conversation and the steps you will be taking	EMT: "We will be taking you to the emergency department to care for your chest pain. I will be giving you some medication that should make you feel better."

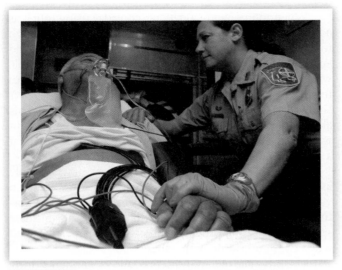

FIGURE 3-2 Using touch can portray care and compassion.

you may need to ask the family member to allow the patient to answer. Ultimately, you will need to assess the situation to determine whether the additional people are helping you care for the patient or hindering your efforts. Do not be afraid to ask others to step outside or step aside for a moment while you talk with the patient. However, take into account how the patient will feel without his or her loved ones nearby—removing them may make the patient more anxious.

> **Transition Tip**
>
> AEMTs need to be dressed professionally. When you have a well-groomed, professional appearance, you send the message that you care without speaking a word. For example, your uniform should be pressed and your shirt tucked in.

Nonverbal Communication

Eye contact and body language are powerful means of communication. Consider how dogs interact. When two dogs meet for the first time, they look at each other. The position of the head, shoulder, tail, and back all help to communicate

Table 3-2
Interview Techniques to Avoid

Improper Technique	Example	Comment
Providing false assurance or reassurance	EMT: "It will be okay." "This is nothing to worry about."	You really do not know that everything will be okay.
Giving unsolicited advice	EMT: "Well, if I were you, I wouldn't have called the ambulance at all."	This statement demeans the patient.
Asking leading or biased questions	EMT: "Are you telling me that this cut is the only reason you called the ambulance?"	Your patient deserves respectful communication. It is inappropriate for you to communicate in a way that suggests to the patient that an ambulance was not needed, even if that is what you believe.
Talking too much	The EMT talks to the patient without really listening to the patient, simply going through the motions.	You should guide the patient through the conversation. When the patient provides information, you need to consider that information and move the conversation toward a goal.
Interrupting	Patient: "Well, I was having trouble breathing last month and ..." EMT: "Can we move on to how you are feeling now?"	You may seem bored or annoyed that the patient is taking up your time.
Using "why" questions	EMT: "Why did you call the ambulance today?"	You may seem annoyed that the patient called you.
Using authoritative language	EMT: "Tell me what is wrong with you." "Just give me the details."	This language does not encourage open communication.
Speaking in professional jargon	EMT: "I think we will need to take you to the ED stat. We will give you ASA and NTG en route. Any questions?"	This type of communication confuses the patient. Most patients do not understand medical jargon.

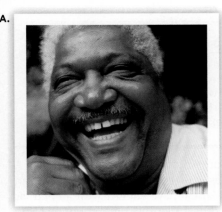

©PhotoDisc/Getty Images

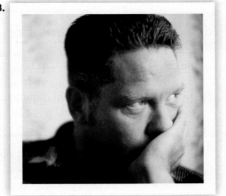

©LiquidLibrary

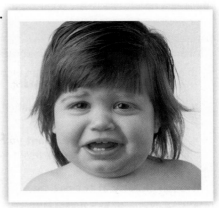

©PhotoDisc/Getty Images

FIGURE 3-3 The effectiveness of body language. **A.** Happy. **B.** Angry. **C.** Sad.

to the other dog. Before they get any closer, the dogs need to understand their new relationship. Who is dominating? Will you hurt me? These questions must be answered quickly.

People communicate using a similar technique. The body language we consciously or subconsciously choose provides more information than words alone. Consider the images in **FIGURE 3-3**. Even without any words, it should be clear what the mood is of each of these people.

For the AEMT, it is important to be attentive to facial expressions, body language, and eye contact—your own and your patient's. These physical cues will help you and your patient to truly understand the message being sent.

Transition Tip

Anyone who has dealt with people experiencing a crisis can tell you that a smile can greatly help relieve stress. Think back to a time when you were troubled by something and someone's smile told you that everything was going to be all right. Your ability to smile can be just as valuable when you are communicating with patients.

Various physical factors also affect communication detrimentally. These factors, referred to as noise, include anything that dampens or obscures the true meaning of the message. Literal noise, or sounds in the environment, can make it difficult to hear and understand the patient.

Proxemics is the study of space and the way in which the distance between people affects communication **TABLE 3-3**. The degree to which people feel comfortable depends on the person with whom they are communicating. As a person gets closer, a greater and greater sense of trust must be established. To enter someone's intimate space, a high sense of trust must be present.

Proxemics The study of space between people and its effects on communication.

Table 3-3
Proxemics for the American Culture

Space	Distance	Description
Intimate	Less than 18"	Whispering, touching; must be invited
Personal	18" to 4'	Conversations with close friends or family
Social	4' to 10'	Conversations with acquaintances
Public	10' to 25'	Interacting with strangers

Special Situations

Communicating With Elderly Patients

A person's actual age might not be the most important factor in making him or her geriatric. It is more important to determine a person's functional age. The functional age relates to the person's ability to function in daily activities, mental status, health status, and activity pattern.

Oftentimes, elderly patients who express that they are not well or who are overly concerned about their health are at risk for a serious decline in their physical, emotional, or psychological state. **TABLE 3-4** provides guidelines for interviewing an elderly patient.

Generally, elderly people think clearly, can give a clear medical history, and are able to answer questions appropriately. Do not assume that the patient is senile or confused. Sometimes, however, communicating with an elderly patient may be extremely difficult. You may encounter hostility, irritability, and some confusion. It is important to not assume this presentation is normal behavior for an elderly patient. Instead, these signs may be caused by a lack of oxygen (hypoxia), brain injury (including a cerebrovascular accident), unintentional drug overdose, or even hypovolemia.

Table 3-4
Interviewing an Elderly Patient

In general, when interviewing an elderly patient, use the following techniques:

- **Identify yourself.** Do not assume the patient knows who you are.

- **Be aware of how you present yourself.** Frustration and impatience can be conveyed through body language.

- **Look directly at the patient.**

- **Speak slowly and distinctly.**

- **Explain what you are going to do before you do it.** Use simple terms to explain the use of medical equipment and procedures, avoiding medical jargon or slang.

- **Listen to the answer the patient gives you.**

- **Show the patient respect.** Refer to the patient as Mr., Mrs., or Miss.

- **Do not talk about the patient in front of him or her;** to do so gives the impression that the patient has no choice in his or her medical care. This is easy to forget when the patient has impaired cognitive (thought) processes or has difficulty communicating.

- **Be patient!**

Never attribute altered mental status to old age; look for another cause first.

Watch for signs of confusion, anxiety, or impaired hearing or vision. Make the patient confident that you are in charge and that everything possible is being done for him or her.

Communicating With Children

Although everyone who is thrust into an emergency situation becomes frightened to some degree, fear is probably most obvious and severe in children. Children may be frightened by your uniform, the ambulance, and the number of people who have suddenly gathered around.

Familiar faces and objects will help to reduce this fright. Let a child keep a favorite toy, doll, or security blanket to give the child some sense of control and comfort. Having a family member or friend nearby is also helpful. When possible, let the parent or a guardian hold the child during your evaluation and treatment. However, make certain this person will not upset the child or prevent the child from telling you important information. Also, keep in mind that an overly anxious parent or relative can make things worse. Explain the importance of providing calm reassurance to the child.

Respect a child's modesty. Children are often embarrassed if they have to undress or be undressed in front of strangers. This anxiety intensifies during adolescence.

Transition Tip

Children can easily see through lies or deceptions, so you must always be honest with them. Make sure to explain to the child what is happening and why. If treatment is going to hurt, such as applying a splint, tell the child ahead of time.

Speak to a child in a professional yet friendly way. A child should feel reassured that you are there to help in every way possible. Maintain eye contact with a child, as you would with an adult, to let the child know that you can be trusted. It is helpful to position yourself at the child's level so you do not tower above the child.

Communicating With Hearing-Impaired Patients

Patients who are hearing impaired are usually not ashamed or embarrassed by their disability. Rather, it is often the people around them who may have problems coping with their hearing impairment. It is important to know how to communicate with hearing-impaired patients so you can provide necessary or even lifesaving care.

Most hearing-impaired patients have normal intelligence and can usually understand what is going on around them. They can often read lips to some extent. Therefore, while talking to the patient, position yourself so the patient can see your lips. In addition, many hearing-impaired patients have hearing aids **FIGURE 3-4** .

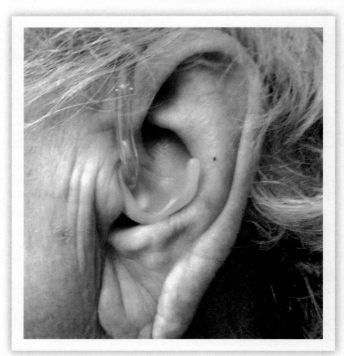

Courtesy of Catherine Parvensky Barwell
FIGURE 3-4 Hearing aids are used to amplify sounds for patients with difficulty hearing.

A.

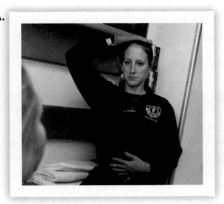

B.

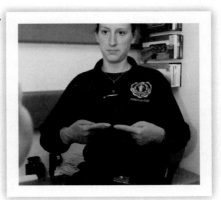

C.

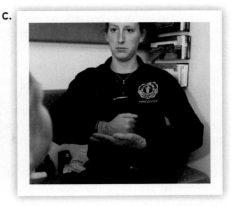

FIGURE 3-5 Learn simple phrases in sign language. **A.** Sick. **B.** Hurt. **C.** Help.

Remember the following five steps to efficiently communicate with patients who are hearing impaired:

1. Have paper and a pen available. This way, you can write down questions and the patient can write down answers as necessary. Be sure to print so that your handwriting is easy to read.
2. If the patient can read lips, face the patient and speak slowly and distinctly. Do not cover your mouth or mumble. If it is dark, consider shining a light on your face.
3. Never shout.
4. Be sure to listen carefully, ask short questions, and give short answers. Remember that although many hearing-impaired patients can speak distinctly, some cannot.
5. Learn some simple phrases in sign language. For example, knowing the signs for "sick," "hurt," and "help" may be useful if you cannot communicate in any other way **FIGURE 3-5**.

Communicating With Visually Impaired Patients

Like hearing-impaired patients, visually impaired and blind patients have usually accepted and learned to deal with their disability. Of course, visually impaired patients are not necessarily completely blind. Many can perceive light and dark and can see shadows or movement. Ask the patient whether he or she can see at all. Also remember, as with other patients who have disabilities, you should expect visually impaired patients to have normal intelligence.

As you begin caring for a visually impaired patient, explain everything you are doing in detail as you are doing it. Be sure to stay in physical contact with the patient as you begin your care. Hold your hand lightly on the patient's shoulder or arm and try to avoid sudden movements. If the patient can walk to the ambulance, begin by placing his or her hand on your arm, taking care not to rush. Transport any mobility aids, such as a cane, with the patient to the hospital. A visually impaired person may have a guide dog. Guide dogs, which are easily identified by their special harnesses, are trained not to leave their masters and not to respond to strangers. A visually impaired patient who is conscious can tell you about the dog and give instructions for handling it. The exact method for managing a patient with a guide dog (or other medical care animal) should be outlined in your local department's policies and procedures. Follow your local protocols.

Communicating With Non–English-Speaking Patients

Part of patient care includes obtaining a medical history from the patient. You cannot skip this step simply because the patient does not speak English. Most patients who do not speak English fluently will still know certain important words or phrases. In addition, pocket guides and picture boards are available that allow patients to point to pictures of key information.

Your first step is to find out how much English the patient can speak. Use short, simple questions and simple words whenever possible. Avoid difficult medical terms. You can help patients better understand if you point to specific parts of the body as you ask questions. Speaking louder will not increase a patient's ability to understand you. In fact, it may frighten him or her and increase anxiety.

In many areas, particularly large urban centers, major segments of the population do not speak English. Your job will be much easier if you learn some common words and phrases in their language, especially common medical terms. Pocket cards that show the pronunciation of these terms are available. If the patient does not speak any English, find a family member or friend to act as an interpreter. Notify personnel at the hospital of the patient's language barrier so they can arrange for an interpreter if needed.

Communicating With Difficult Patients

You may at times need to gather information from a reluctant audience. Patients may be defensive about their problems and may not want to talk about them because they are embarrassed. They may direct the conversation away from the true problem. With these patients, start the conversation as usual. Introduce yourself. Be open and compassionate. If you find yourself not getting any real answers, then consider one of the techniques in Table 3-1.

Patients can become hostile toward EMS providers. To help defuse these potentially escalating circumstances, stay calm. Talk to the patient openly and honestly. You will find that meeting hostility with calmness and confidence defuses a situation. Use open-ended questions, provide positive feedback, make sure the patient understands the questions, and continue to calmly ask them for information. Consider the safety of the scene. Decide whether you need police backup. Make sure that you have sufficient backup to provide safety for the patient and the crew. Then, with your backup clearly visible, calmly advise the patient what needs to be done. "Sir, I need you to sit on the ambulance cot now. You may proceed to the cot or we can help you to the cot." Do not threaten the patient. Discipline yourself; never respond to unpleasant insults from patients. No one should move toward the patient. In this rare circumstance, you are providing the patient with choices, while at the same time limiting those choices to ones you can accept.

Your primary responsibility is to yourself and your partner by ensuring scene safety. It is imperative to recognize the potential for violence and to react accordingly. Call for law enforcement as soon as you have reason to believe you may be encountering a difficult patient, especially if drugs or alcohol are involved. This may be en route to the call, based on information obtained by the dispatcher. Remember, it is better to have law enforcement and not need them than to wait until the situation escalates.

You may also encounter patients who are sexually aggressive. In this instance, simply changing caregivers may solve the problem. If not, firmly explain to the patient that this is not an option and that he or she will be turned over to law enforcement if the behavior continues. In most situations, simply rebuking the advancement is enough to stop the aggression.

Communicating With Other Health Care Professionals

Effective communication between the AEMT and health care professionals in the receiving facility is an essential cornerstone of efficient, effective, and appropriate patient care.

The transfer of patient care officially occurs during your oral report at the hospital. Your oral report is usually given at the same time that the staff member is providing care for the patient. For example, a nurse or physician may start assessing the patient or help you to move the patient from the stretcher to an examination table. Therefore, the report must be given in a complete and precise way. The following six components must be included in the oral report:

1. **Opening information** that includes the patient's name (if you know it), chief complaint, nature of the illness, or mechanism of injury
2. **Detailed information** that was provided during the radio report
3. **Any important history** that was not already provided
4. **The patient's response to treatment** given en route. It is especially important to report any changes in the patient's condition or the treatment provided since your initial radio report.
5. **Vital signs** assessed during transport and after the radio report
6. **Other information** you may have gathered that was not important enough to report sooner. Information that was gathered during transport, patient medications you have brought, and any other details about the patient that were provided by family members or friends may be included.

PREP KIT

Ready for Review

- The Shannon-Weaver model of communication is a valuable tool in understanding the variables involved in human communications.
- Many verbal and nonverbal factors and strategies must be taken into account to ensure effective therapeutic communication.
- Excellent communication skills are crucial in relaying pertinent information to the hospital before the patient's arrival.
- People who are sick or injured may not understand what an AEMT is doing or saying. Therefore, your body language and attitude are very important in gaining the trust of both the patient and family. You must carefully consider the special communications challenges associated with the care of children, elderly patients, hearing impaired, visually impaired, non–English-speaking, and difficult patients.
- Effective communication between the AEMT and health care professionals in the receiving facility is an essential cornerstone of efficient, effective, and appropriate patient care.

Case Study

You are dispatched to a local residence for a 75-year-old woman with chest pain and dyspnea. Upon arrival, you are directed by family members into the living room where you find an elderly female sitting on the couch. She is pale and diaphoretic and in apparent respiratory distress. The family tells you the patient only speaks Spanish and has difficulty hearing. The patient is anxious and is grasping her chest as you kneel down next to her. The family tells you the patient is visiting from Puerto Rico and has a history of angina and COPD.

1. What are some techniques that should be considered when communicating with a 75-year-old patient?

2. The family stated the patient has difficulty hearing. How can you facilitate better communication with someone who may be hearing impaired?

3. The patient in this scenario only speaks Spanish. What are some ways you can establish communications with this patient?

4. What are some techniques to avoid when interviewing a patient?

5. Compare and contrast open-ended questions with closed-ended questions.

CHAPTER 4

Life Span Development

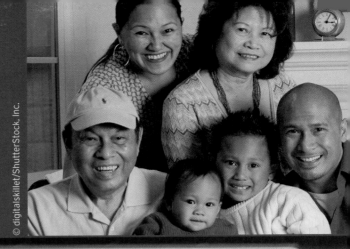

© digitalskillet/ShutterStock, Inc.

Introduction

One of the most interesting things about humans is that we evolve over our life span. For the AEMT, it is important to understand the obvious and subtle changes a person undergoes over time, both physically and mentally, and to apply this knowledge to patient care.

Infants

A *neonate* is a child from birth to 1 month of age **FIGURE 4-1**. An *infant* is age 1 month to 1 year. During the first year of life, children develop at a startling rate.

> *Neonates* Persons who are between birth and 1 month of age.
>
> *Infants* Persons who are from 1 month to 1 year of age.

Physical Changes

Vital Signs

TABLE 4-1 lists the normal ranges of vital signs for various age groups. The general rule is the younger the person,

the faster the pulse rate and respirations. At birth, a pulse rate of 90 to 180 beats/min and a respiratory rate of 30 to 60 breaths/min are considered normal. Within the first half-hour after birth, however, a neonate's pulse rate often drops to a high of 120 beats/min and the respiratory rate falls to between 30 to 40 breaths/min. By age 1 year, the respiratory rate slows to 20 to 30 breaths/min. Tidal volume in neonates starts at 6 to 8 mL/kg. By the end of the first year of life, the volume increases to 10 to 15 mL/kg.

Blood pressure directly corresponds to the patient's weight, so it typically increases with age. At birth, the average systolic blood pressure of a neonate is 50 to 70 mm Hg. By 1 year of age, it ranges between 70 and 95 mm Hg.

Weight

A neonate usually weighs 6 to 8 lb (3 to 3.5 kg) at birth. Remarkably, the head accounts for 25% of the newborn's body weight. In the first week after birth, neonates typically lose 5% to 10% of their birth weight as a result of fluid loss. By week 2, neonates begin to gain weight. Infants then grow at a rate of approximately 30 g per day, doubling their weight by 4 to 6 months and tripling it by the end of the first year of life.

Table 4-1
Vital Signs at Various Ages

Age	Pulse Rate (beats/min)	Respirations (breaths/min)	Systolic Blood Pressure (mm Hg)*	Temperature (°F)
Neonate (0 to 1 month)	90 to 180	30 to 60	50 to 70	98 to 100
Infant (1 month to 1 year)	100 to 160	25 to 50	70 to 95	96.8 to 99.6
Toddler (1 to 3 years)	90 to 150	20 to 30	80 to 100	96.8 to 99.6
Preschool age (3 to 6 years)	80 to 140	20 to 25	80 to 100	98.6
School age (6 to 12 years)	70 to 120	15 to 20	80 to 110	98.6
Adolescent (12 to 18 years)	60 to 100	12 to 20	90 to 110	98.6
Early adult (19 to 40 years)	60 to 100	12 to 20	90 to 140	98.6
Middle adult (41 to 60 years)	60 to 100	12 to 20	90 to 140	98.6
Late adult (61 and older)	Depends on health	Depends on health	Depends on health	98.6

*As a general rule, the systolic BP of a child is 80 plus 2 times the person's age. For an adult female, it is 90 plus the age to the age of 40; for an adult male, it is 100 plus the age to the age of 40.

Transition Tip

Infants often land head first when they fall because their heads account for 25% of their total body weight. Also, most infants cannot stretch out their arms in time to cushion or slow their fall. Keep this point in mind when considering spinal immobilization of an infant.

Cardiovascular System

Prior to birth, fetal circulation occurs through the placenta. During the birthing process, hormones and pressure changes help the neonate make the transition from fetal circulation to independent circulation. The neonate's heart rate will be 120 beats/min or higher.

Pulmonary System

Prior to a neonate's first breath, the lungs have never been inflated. As such, a neonate's first breath is forceful—it has to be! A neonate will usually begin breathing spontaneously within 15 to 30 seconds after birth.

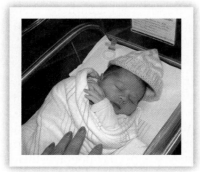

Courtesy of Catherine Parvensky Barwell

FIGURE 4-1 A neonate, or newborn, is from birth to 1 month of age.

Neonates and infants are primarily nose breathers, breathing through the nose rather than the mouth. Infants younger than 6 months, however, are particularly prone to nasal congestion, which can lead to upper respiratory viral infections. If you are called because a baby is choking, ensure that the patient's nasal passages are clear and unobstructed by mucus. If mucus is present, use a bulb syringe to clear out the nasal passage. If one is not readily available, remember that this equipment comes prepackaged in an OB delivery kit.

The rib cage of an infant is less rigid and the ribs sit horizontally, resulting in diaphragmatic breathing (belly breathing) in infants.

Two important anatomic differences relevant to the airway of an infant as compared to an adult are the proportionally large size of the tongue and the shorter and narrower airway. As a result of these factors, infants can much more easily occlude their airway than older children or adults.

Transition Tip

When you are counting respirations in an infant, count the number of times the abdomen rises instead of concentrating solely on the chest rise.

Other factors to keep in mind relative to an infant's airway and breathing include:

- An infant's lungs are fragile. Bag-valve-mask device ventilations that are too forceful can result in trauma from the pressure.
- Because of the large size of the infant's occiput (posterior portion of the head) and the increased flexibility of the trachea, the airway can be inadvertently occluded by incorrect positioning (either over-extension or over-flexion of the head).
- Infants have very little reserves available to assist with breathing. The muscles they use to breathe are immature. While they can manage normal requirements easily, they become fatigued when stressed.

- The number of alveoli in the infant's lungs is relatively small. Fortunately, the amount of oxygen the infant needs is also relatively small.
- As the infant grows and becomes more active, the need for greater amounts of oxygen triggers growth in the number of alveoli.
- In very small infants, respiratory problems can quickly turn life threatening. Infants who are struggling to breathe can quickly tire, become overheated, and become dehydrated.

Nervous System

Although the infant's nervous system is developed at birth, its evolution continues after birth. For example, when neonates are born, they tend to move their extremities together. They do not develop independent arm or leg movements until several weeks later.

A neonate is born with certain reflexes. The *moro reflex* (startle reflex) happens when a neonate is caught off guard by something or someone and opens his or her arms wide, spreads the fingers, and seems to grab at things. A *palmar grasp* occurs when an object is placed into the neonate's palm and he or she grasps it. The *rooting reflex* takes place when something touches a neonate's cheek; the neonate will instinctively turn his or her head toward the touch. This reflex is often used in conjunction with the *sucking reflex*, which occurs when a neonate starts sucking as the lips are stroked, often when feeding.

> *Moro reflex* A reflex in which, when an infant is caught off guard, the infant opens his or her arms wide, spreads the fingers, and seems to grab at things.
> *Palmar grasp* A reflex that occurs when something is placed in the infant's palm; the infant grasps the object.
> *Rooting reflex* A reflex that occurs when something touches an infant's cheek; the infant instinctively turns his or her head toward the touch.
> *Sucking reflex* A reflex in which the infant starts sucking when his or her lips are stroked.

Fontanelles allow the head to be molded—for example, when the neonate passes through the birth canal FIGURE 4-2 . These three or four bones of the skull eventually bind together and form suture joints. The posterior fontanelle normally fuses by the third month of life. The anterior fontanelle fuses between 9 and 18 months of age. If either of the fontanelles is depressed (if you feel a dip when moving your hand over the surface of the skull), the infant may be dehydrated. A bulging fontanelle is indicative of increased intracranial pressure.

> *Fontanelles* Areas in the head where the infant's skull has not fused together; they usually disappear by approximately 18 months of age.

It is interesting to watch the growth and development of a child through the first 12 months of life. At birth, the neonate is not able to do much without assistance; he or she cannot turn over or even focus his or her eyes beyond a very short distance. Sleep patterns begin to develop during this period. By 2 months of age, the infant is able to track objects with his or her eyes and should recognize familiar faces. At 6 months of age, the infant is able to sit upright and begins to say one-syllable words. By 12 months of age, the infant can walk with assistance and even knows his or her name.

Immune System

While in the womb, a fetus collects antibodies from the maternal blood. For the first year of life, the infant maintains some of the mother's immunities to certain diseases (naturally acquired passive immunity). Infants can also receive antibodies via breastmilk, further bolstering their immune system.

Psychosocial Changes

An infant's psychosocial development begins at birth and continues to evolve as the infant interacts with, and reacts to, the environment. Parents often obsess about whether their child is developing within the socially accepted norms.

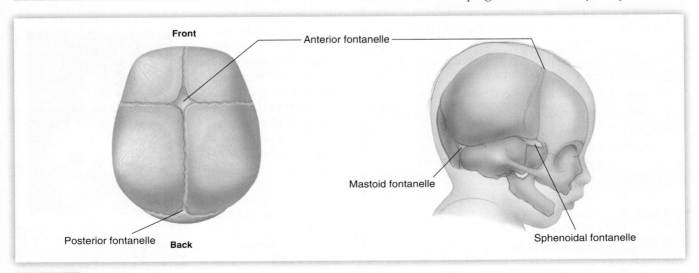

Front

Anterior fontanelle

Mastoid fontanelle

Posterior fontanelle **Back**

Sphenoidal fontanelle

FIGURE 4-2 Fontanelles.

TABLE 4-2 outlines typical ages at which major psychosocial changes are noticed.

In most infants, the primary method of communicating distress is through crying. Parents can often tell what is upsetting their child simply by listening to the tone of the child's crying—that is, they know the difference between tears for anger, frustration, pain, fear, hunger, discomfort, and sleepiness. Infants occasionally make another distinct cry—an alarming, distressed cry. This cry may be heard when an unexpected event occurs, causing a situational crisis for the infant.

The key to having a happy, healthy infant is spending time with the child. Nevertheless, infants often have their own timetable as to when they will become attached to their parents and other family members. *Bonding*, or the formation of a close, personal relationship, is usually based on a *secure attachment*. This phenomenon occurs when an infant understands that parents or caregivers will be responsive to his or her needs. Such a realization encourages a child to reach out and explore, knowing that the parents will provide a safety net.

> *Bonding* The formation of a close, personal relationship.
> *Secure attachment* A bond between an infant and his or her parent or caregiver, in which the infant understands that his or her parents or caregivers will be responsive to his or her needs and take care of him or her when help is needed.

Another type of attachment, referred to as *anxious-avoidant attachment*, is observed in infants who are repeatedly rejected. In this attachment style, children show little emotional response to their parents or caregivers and treat them as they would strangers. These children develop an isolated lifestyle where they do not have to depend on the support and care of others.

> *Anxious-avoidant attachment* A bond between an infant and his or her parent or caregiver in which the infant is repeatedly rejected and develops an isolated lifestyle that does not depend on the support and care of others.

Separation anxiety is common in older infants. This normal reaction peaks between 10 and 18 months and involves clingy behavior and fear of unfamiliar places and people. Protesting by crying is another normal reaction in older infants. As infants become accustomed to their homes and families, they begin to need the security of a predictable environment. If the infant's environment is too unpredictable, he or she may become withdrawn and develop trust issues.

Trust and mistrust refers to a stage of development from birth to approximately 18 months of age that involves an infant's needs being met by his or her parents or caregivers. When caregivers and parents provide an organized, routine environment, infant gains trust in those individuals. If the environment is not perceived as secure by the infant, a sense of mistrust will develop.

> *Trust and mistrust* A stage of development from birth to approximately 18 months of age, during which infants develop trust in their parents or caregivers if their world is planned, organized, and routine.

Table 4-2 Noticeable Characteristics at Various Ages	
Age	**Characteristics**
2 months	Can recognize familiar faces; able to track objects with the eyes
3 months	Can bring objects to the mouth; can smile and frown
4 months	Reaches out to people; drools
5 months	Sleeps through the night; can tell family from strangers
6 months	Teething begins; sits upright in a chair; one-syllable words spoken
7 months	Afraid of strangers; mood swings
8 months	Responds to "no"; can sit alone; plays peek-a-boo
9 months	Pulls himself or herself up; places objects in mouth to explore them
10 months	Responds to his or her name; crawls efficiently
11 months	Starts to walk without help; frustrated with restrictions
12 months	Knows his or her name; can walk

Toddlers and Preschoolers

Physical Changes

In *toddlers* (ages 1 to 3 years), the pulse rate is 90 to 150 beats/min and the respiratory rate is 20 to 30 breaths/min, slower than the corresponding vital signs in infants, whereas the systolic blood pressure is higher (80 to 100 mm Hg). The average temperature of children at this age is 96.8°F to 99.6°F, usually leveling off at 98.6°F by school age **FIGURE 4-3**.

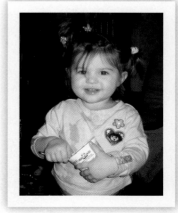

Courtesy of Catherine Parvensky Barwell
FIGURE 4-3 A toddler is from 1 to 3 years of age.

> *Toddlers* Persons who are 1 to 3 years of age.
> *Preschoolers* Persons who are 3 to 6 years of age.

In *preschoolers* (ages 3 to 6 years), the pulse rate is 80 to 140 beats/min and the respiratory rate is 20 to 25 breaths/min. The systolic blood pressure is 80 to 100 mm Hg. At the same time, weight gain should level off FIGURE 4-4 .

A toddler's cardiovascular system is not dramatically different from an adult's. Their lungs continue to develop more terminal bronchioles and alveoli. Although toddlers and preschoolers have more lung tissue, they do not have well-developed chest wall musculature. This anomaly prevents them from sustaining deep or rapid respirations for an extended period of time.

The loss of passive immunity as the effects of the mother's antibodies wear off is possibly the most obvious development at this stage of human life. Colds often develop that may manifest as gastrointestinal distress or upper respiratory tract infections. As toddlers spend more time around playmates and classmates, their bodies are exposed to various viruses and germs, and they acquire their own immunity.

Neuromuscular growth also makes considerable progress at this age. Toddlers and preschoolers spend a great deal of time finding out exactly how to use their expansive nervous system and the muscles it controls by walking, running, jumping, and playing catch. Watching children play as they age from 1 to 6 years demonstrates how they move from gross motor activities (grabbing an object with the full palm) to fine motor activities (picking up a crayon). By the end of this stage, preschoolers have a brain that weighs 90% of its final adult weight. In addition, their muscle mass and bone density increase as a result of stress on muscles and bones from increased activity and movement.

Continued development of the renal system and of elimination patterns (ie, toilet training) also occurs during this stage. Physiologically, toddlers have the neuromuscular capacity to achieve bladder control by 12 to 15 months of age. Nevertheless, the child may not be psychologically ready for toilet training until 18 to 30 months of age. The average age for completion of toilet training is 28 months, although girls tend to be trained earlier than boys.

Other developments that occur during this time include the emergence of baby teeth. Teething (ie, teeth breaking through the gums) can be painful and is sometimes accompanied by fever. In addition, toddlers (and their parents) are enthralled with sensory development activities—for example, tickling.

Psychosocial Changes

This period of development is often exciting for parents. Toddlers or preschoolers are learning to speak and express themselves, thereby taking a major step toward independence. At the same time, they are still very attached to their parents and feel safe with them. Separation anxiety peaks between 10 and 18 months of age. It is fascinating to watch a child struggle through the conflict of wanting to play, yet wanting to be protected.

At 36 months of age, most toddlers have mastered basic language. By the age of 3 or 4 years, most children can use and understand full sentences. As they progress through this stage, they will go from using language to communicate what they want to using language creatively and playfully.

This is also the time when toddlers begin to interact with other children and start to play games. Playing games teaches control, following of rules, and even competitiveness. Significant learning and development take place by the child watching his or her peers during group outings, such as play dates with other children. In addition, children learn the importance of sharing during this stage of development. By 18 to 24 months, toddlers begin to understand cause and effect. Of course, behavior observed on television and computers can also be learned, which is why some parents limit their children's viewing choices or the amount of time they devote to these activities. During this phase of development, children also learn to recognize sexual differences by observing role models.

█ School-Age Children

Physical Changes

From ages 6 to 12 years, *school-age children's* vital signs and bodies gradually approach those observed in adulthood FIGURE 4-5 . The pulse rate is approximately 70 to 120 beats/min, respiratory rate is 15 to 20 breaths/min, and systolic blood pressure is 80 to 110 mm Hg. Physical traits and body function changes become apparent as most children grow in terms of both weight—approximately 4 lb (2 kg)—and height—2½ inches (6 cm)—each year. Permanent teeth also come in during this period, and brain activity increases in both hemispheres.

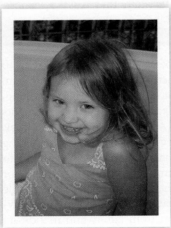
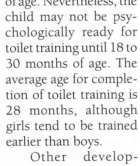

Courtesy of Catherine Parvensky Barwell

FIGURE 4-4 A preschooler is from 3 to 6 years of age.

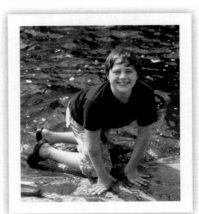

Courtesy of Catherine Parvensky Barwell

FIGURE 4-5 A school-age child is from 6 to 12 years of age.

School-age children Persons who are 6 to 12 years of age.

Psychosocial Changes

School-age children engage in a great deal of psychosocial development. Parents as a whole do not devote as much time to their children during this phase. Nevertheless, it is at this critical time in human development that children learn various types of reasoning. In *preconventional reasoning*, children act almost purely to avoid punishment and to get what they want. In *conventional reasoning*, they look for approval from their peers and society. In *postconventional reasoning*, children make decisions guided by their conscience.

Preconventional reasoning A type of reasoning in which a child acts almost purely to avoid punishment and to get what he or she wants.
Conventional reasoning A type of reasoning in which a child looks for approval from peers and society.
Postconventional reasoning A type of reasoning in which a child bases decisions on his or her conscience.

During this stage, children begin to develop a self-concept and self-esteem. Self-concept is an individual's perception of oneself; self-esteem is how one feels about oneself and how one fits in with peers.

■ Adolescents (Teenagers)

Physical Changes

In *adolescents* (ages 12 to 18 years), vital signs begin to level off to adult ranges, with a systolic blood pressure generally between 90 and 110 mm Hg, a pulse rate between 60 and 100 beats/min, and respirations in the range of 12 to 20 breaths/min **FIGURE 4-6**.

Adolescents Persons who are 12 to 18 years of age.

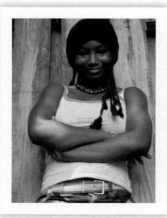

© Jamie Wilson/ShutterStock, Inc.
FIGURE 4-6 An adolescent is from 12 to 18 years of age.

Adolescence is also the time of life when humans experience a 2- to 3-year growth spurt (ie, an increase in muscle and bone growth) and body changes. Growth begins with hands and feet, then moves to the long bones of the extremities, and finishes with growth of the torso. As a whole, boys typically experience this growth spurt later in life than girls. Girls finish their growth spurt by 16 years of age and boys by 18 years of age. When this period of growth has finished, however, boys are generally taller and stronger than girls. Muscle mass and bone density at that point are nearly at adult levels.

One of the less subtle changes during adolescence is the maturation of the human reproductive system. Secondary sexual development begins, along with enlargement of the external sex organs. Pubic hair and axillary hair begin to appear. Voices start to change in range and depth. In females, the breasts and thighs increase in size as adipose (fat) tissue is deposited. Menarche, the first menstrual bleeding, occurs during this time, although it may have occurred prior to becoming a teenager.

Changes in the endocrine and reproductive systems provide the platform for reproduction. By the middle of adolescence, boys are able to produce sufficient sperm and girls are able to develop eggs to reproduce. In addition, acne may occur because of hormonal changes.

Psychosocial Changes

Adolescents and their families often deal with conflict as adolescents try to take control of their own lives. Privacy becomes an issue among adolescents, their siblings, and their parents. Self-consciousness also increases. Adolescents may struggle to create their own identity—to define themselves. For example, they may dress in a certain style of clothing to fit their personality. Adolescents use the feedback from their family and peers to help create their adult image. These youths are often caught between two worlds: They want to be treated like adults, while still wanting to be cared for like younger children.

Transition Tip

When interviewing adolescents in the presence of other family members, recognize that adolescents may not tell you the complete truth in an attempt to protect their privacy or image. It is best to ask these patients certain questions in private, where they feel they can answer without constraint.

Rebellious behavior can be part of an adolescent trying to find his or her identity. Antisocial behavior and peer pressure typically tend to peak at around age 14 to 16 years. Smoking, illicit drug use, unprotected sex, and other high-risk behaviors also peak during this period. Adolescents may try to exhibit self-control through what they eat, which can lead to eating disorders. Although these behaviors can be very troubling to parents, the adolescent is trying to determine whether he or she is ready to take control of his or her own life. This struggle toward independence may have setbacks that may be devastating. Patience and support from family and friends are essential in assisting an adolescent's transition into adulthood.

Adolescents may also show greater interest in sexual relations. Many adolescents are fixated on their public image and are terrified of being embarrassed. At this age, a code of personal ethics is developed, based partly on parents' ethics and values and partly on the influence of the adolescent's environment. During this tumultuous time, adolescents are at a higher risk than other populations for suicide and depression.

Early Adults

Physical Changes

Early adults range in age from 19 to 40 years FIGURE 4-7. Their vital signs do not vary greatly from those seen throughout adulthood. Ideally, the human pulse rate will average 70 beats/min, the respiratory rate will stay in the range of 12 to 20 breaths/min, and the systolic blood pressure will range approximately between 90 and 140 mm Hg.

> **Early adults** Persons who are 19 to 40 years of age.

From age 19 years to shortly after 25 years, the human body should be functioning at its optimal level. Lifelong habits such as eating preferences, exercise, and tobacco use are solidified during this stage of life. At the beginning of this period, the body is working at peak efficiency, but as adulthood continues, subtle erosion begins.

The disks in the spine begin to settle, and height can sometimes be affected, causing shrinking. Being able to eat anything without gaining weight becomes a thing of the past. Fatty tissue increases, which leads to weight gain. Muscle strength decreases and reflexes slow.

Psychosocial Changes

Three words best describe the world of early adulthood: work, family, stress. During this period, early adults strive to create a place for themselves in the world, and many do everything they can to settle down. Along with this natural

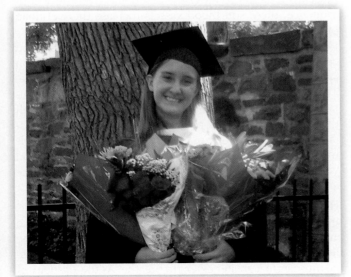

Courtesy of Catherine Parvensky Barwell

FIGURE 4-7 An early adult is from 19 to 40 years of age.

tendency to settle comes love and childbirth. Despite all of this stress and change, this age group enjoys one of the more stable periods of life.

Middle Adults

Physical Changes

Middle adults are those between the ages of 41 and 60 years FIGURE 4-8. The average pulse rate for this age remains at 70 beats/min, the respiratory rate continues at 12 to 20 breaths/min, and the blood pressure also remains between 90 and 140 mm Hg. This group is vulnerable to vision and hearing loss. Cardiovascular health also may become an issue in many of these persons, as does the greater incidence of cancer. In women, menopause—the cessation of menstruation—begins in the late 40s or early 50s. Middle adults may begin having medical problems or be unaware of problems such as diabetes and hypertension. When health care is necessary, medications or underlying conditions may affect patient response to treatments.

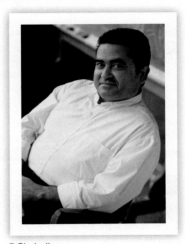

© Photodisc

FIGURE 4-8 A middle adult is from 41 to 60 years of age.

Other concerns include an increase in cholesterol levels, a decrease in the efficiency of the heart, and problems with weight control. Many of the effects of aging can be diminished, however, with exercise and a healthy diet.

> **Middle adults** Persons who are 41 to 60 years of age.

Psychosocial Changes

Middle adults tend to focus on achieving life goals, as they approach the halfway point in human life expectancy. After years of nurturing and living with children, parents must readjust their lifestyle as children leave home, commonly called the empty nest syndrome. Finances may become a worrisome issue, as people prepare for retirement while still managing everyday financial demands. During this time, people often view crises as a challenge to be overcome, rather than as a threat to be avoided. Generally, their health is stable and they have the physical, emotional, and spiritual reserves to handle life's issues.

The parents of adults in this age group are getting older, and many now need care. Most of the elderly in the United States are cared for by family members inside the home. Therefore, a person in middle adulthood may need

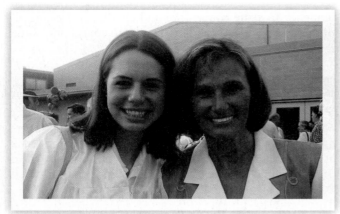

Courtesy of Catherine Parvensky Barwell

FIGURE 4-9 A person in middle adulthood may need to manage children who are leaving for college while at the same time caring for parents who require greater assistance.

to manage children who are leaving for college while at the same time caring for parents who require greater assistance. For this reason, middle adults are often referred to as the sandwich generation **FIGURE 4-9**.

Late Adults

Physical Changes
Late adults include those ages 61 and older **FIGURE 4-10**. *Life expectancy* is constantly changing. In the early 1900s, life expectancy was only 47 years. It is now approximately 78 years in the United States, with maximum life expectancy estimated at 120 years. The age to which a person will live is based on many factors. Perhaps surprisingly, the year that you were born and the country in which you live can have an effect on your life expectancy. These two factors reflect public health advances, changes in diets, attitudes regarding exercise, advances in medical care, access to medical care, and personal behaviors.

> *Late adults* Persons who are 61 years of age or older.
> *Life expectancy* The typical number of years a person can be expected to live.

Vital signs during this stage of life depend on the patient's overall health, medical conditions, and medications taken. Thanks to medical advances, today's late adults are staying active longer than their ancestors did. They are often able to overcome numerous medical problems but may need multiple medications to do so.

Cardiovascular System
Cardiac function declines with age as a result of anatomic and physiologic changes largely related to *atherosclerosis*, a buildup of cholesterol and calcium inside the walls of blood vessels. The accumulation of plaque eventually leads to partial or complete blockage of blood flow to body organs. More than 60% of people older than 65 years have atherosclerotic disease.

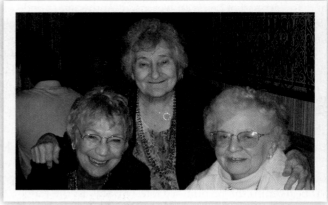

Courtesy of Catherine Parvensky Barwell

FIGURE 4-10 Late adulthood occurs after age 61.

> *Atherosclerosis* A disorder in which cholesterol and calcium build up inside the walls of the blood vessels, forming plaque, which eventually leads to partial or complete blockage of blood flow.

Other age-related changes typically include a decrease in heart rate, a decline in cardiac output (the amount of blood circulated in the body each minute), and an inability to elevate cardiac output to match the demands of the body. Collectively, these factors translate into a heart that is less able to respond to exercise or disease. In the event of a life-threatening illness, the body typically needs to increase the heart rate to ensure adequate blood pressure. Because heart muscle may be weakened with age, the increase in heart rate can actually cause damage to the heart itself.

The vascular system also becomes stiff. The diastolic blood pressure increases with age, and compensation is hampered because the vessels are less able to dilate and contract. As blood vessels become stiffer with age, the heart must work harder to move the blood effectively. As a consequence, these stiff blood vessels increase the workload of the heart.

Blood cells are also affected by aging. The body's blood cells originate from within the bone marrow. As a person ages, more of the bone marrow is replaced with fatty tissue. This replacement decreases the ability of the bones to manufacture more blood cells when needed. Although by itself this issue rarely poses a problem, if an elderly person sustains trauma, the ability of the body to produce blood cells to replace those lost is diminished. Finally, functional blood volume gradually declines over time, thereby reducing the amount of oxygen being transported to tissues.

Respiratory System
In late adults, the size of the airway increases and the surface area of the alveoli decreases. The natural elasticity of the lungs also decreases, forcing individuals to use the intercostal muscles to a greater extent to breathe. As the elasticity of the lungs decreases, the overall strength of the intercostal muscles and diaphragm also decreases. These factors make

breathing more labor intensive for the elderly. Although one might think that a rigid chest would be more protecting, this rigidity actually makes the chest more fragile. Instead of the chest being able to bend and give if struck, the calcified chest can more easily fracture. As with all of the physical changes related to aging, however, the changes in the respiratory system are often gradual and go unnoticed until a severe, life-threatening condition occurs. The older person will then have less respiratory reserves to call upon to maintain adequate breathing.

Within the mouth and nose of a late adult, there is a gradual loss of the mechanisms that protect the upper airway. This transformation leads to a decreased ability to clear secretions as well as decreased cough and gag reflexes. The cilia that line the airways diminish with age, while the innervation of the airway structures provides increasingly less sensation. Without the ability to maintain the upper airway, aspiration and obstruction become more likely.

When a younger patient inhales, the airway maintains its shape, allowing air to enter. As the smooth muscles of the lower airway weaken with age, however, strong inhalation can make the walls of the airway collapse inward and cause inspiratory wheezing. The collapsing airway results in low flow rates, because less air can move through the now smaller airway, and air trapping, which occurs when air does not completely exit the alveoli (incomplete expiration). Also, the cells of the immune system within the airway become less functional. As a result of overall decreases in the metabolic activity of the elderly body, the white blood cells found within the airway are less aggressive in fighting invading organisms, which in turn leads to an increased risk of lung infections.

By age 75 years, the vital capacity (the volume of air moved during the deepest inspiration and expiration) may amount to only 50% of the vital capacity of a young adult. Factors contributing to this decline include loss of respiratory muscle mass, increased stiffness of the thoracic cage, and decreased surface area available for the exchange of air.

Physiologically, vital capacity decreases and residual volume (the amount of air left in the lungs after expiration of the maximum possible amount of air) increases with age. A lifetime of breathing—especially breathing air with high levels of pollution—causes the accumulation of pollutants in the lungs. As a consequence, stagnant air remains in the alveoli and hampers diffusion of gases. The net effect is that the respiratory system is increasingly less able to handle the stresses of disease. This is why a simple cold, which might mean a runny nose and body aches for a 30-year-old, could mean pneumonia and possible death for an 80-year-old.

Endocrine System

As with the other systems of the body, the function of the endocrine system gradually declines as a person ages. In particular, insulin production begins to drop and metabolism decreases. As people get older, they tend to slow down their physical activity. Unfortunately, they do not decrease their food intake. When a person gains weight, more insulin is needed to control the body's metabolism and blood glucose (sugar) level. The pancreas may not be able to produce enough insulin for the person's body size, which can lead to diabetes mellitus.

The reproductive systems of both men and women also change with age. Although men are able to produce sperm long into their 80s, the rigidity of the penis tends to decrease over time. It is unclear whether this change is a result of the aging process itself or is the result of other disorders such as cardiovascular disease. Women have a decrease in the size of the uterus and vagina. In addition, hormone production for both sexes gradually decreases with age. Sexual desire may also diminish with age but certainly does not cease.

Digestive System

Changes in gastric and intestinal function may inhibit nutritional intake and utilization in older adults. For example, taste bud sensitivity to salty and sweet sensations decreases. The sense of smell can also be diminished. As a result, the elderly may find food bland and flavorless.

Saliva secretion decreases as well, which reduces the body's ability to process complex carbohydrates. Older people may have loss of teeth that hinders their ability to chew. The ability of the intestines to contract and move food along also diminishes with age, which can cause older adults to feel constipated or not hungry. Likewise, gastric acid secretion diminishes. Blood flow may drop by as much as 50%, decreasing the ability of the intestines to extract vitamins and minerals from digested food. In addition, gallstones become increasingly common with age, and anal sphincter changes reduce elasticity and can produce constipation, impaction, or fecal incontinence.

Renal Systems

In the kidneys, both structural and functional changes occur in late adulthood. The filtration function of these organs, for example, declines by 50% from age 20 to 90 years. Kidney mass decreases by 20% over the same span, caused in part by the decreased effectiveness of the blood vessels that supply blood to the *nephrons*, sophisticated capillaries in the kidney that filter the blood. One of the portions of the nephron is called the glomerulus (plural, glomeruli). The decreased blood supply causes more abnormal glomeruli to be present as the person ages. The number of nephrons also declines between the ages of 30 and 80 years. This loss of renal function means a decrease in the ability to clear wastes from the body and to conserve fluids when needed.

Nephrons The basic filtering units in the kidneys.

Nervous System

Nervous system changes can result in the most debilitating of age-related ailments. In the central nervous system, the brain may shrink 10% to 20% in weight by age 80. Motor and sensory neural networks become slower and less responsive, although the metabolic rate in the older brain does not change. Oxygen consumption remains constant throughout life.

Generally, you have fewer brain cells (neurons) today than you did yesterday. If measured strictly based on numbers of brain cells, infants are far more intelligent than the rest of us. Of course, this is not how the brain actually works. Although it is true that elderly persons have a diminished number of brain cells, there is great flexibility in the operation of the brain. Interconnections between brain cells continue to develop as people age. These new connections provide redundancy within the brain, allowing for loss of neurons without loss of knowledge or skill.

One of the consequences of the loss of neurons is a change in the sleep patterns in the elderly. Instead of sleeping through the night, older adults may take a nap during the day and stay up late at night. Their sleep cycle may move into a biphasic (two-phased) sleep cycle—sleep from 1:00 AM to 6:00 AM and then nap from 12:00 PM to 3:00 PM.

The brain, which is surrounded by the meninges, takes up almost all of the space in the skull. Cerebrospinal fluid protects the brain inside these membranes. Unfortunately, age-related shrinkage creates a void between the brain and the outermost layer of the meninges, providing room for the brain to move more when stressed **FIGURE 4-11** . If trauma moves the brain forcefully, the bridging veins can tear and bleed. Blood can empty into the void and may go unnoticed for some time.

Functioning of the peripheral nervous system also slows with age. Sensation becomes diminished and misinterpreted. The ability to know where the body is in space—proprioception—can be diminished. Increased reaction times cause longer delays between stimulation and motion. The resulting slowdown in reflexes and decreased proprioception may contribute to a higher incidence of falls and trauma. Nerve endings deteriorate, and the ability of the skin to sense the surroundings becomes hindered. Hot, cold, sharp, and wet items can all create dangerous situations because the body cannot sense them quickly enough.

Sensory Changes

It is often assumed that the elderly are hard of hearing and have difficulty seeing. Certainly, some changes diminish the effectiveness of the eyes and ears; however, most elderly individuals can hear well and are able to see clearly. They may need glasses or hearing aids, but do not assume that an older patient is deaf or nearly blind. However, pupillary reaction and ocular movements do become more restricted with age. The pupils are generally smaller in older patients, while the opacity of the eye's lens diminishes visual acuity and makes the pupils sluggish when responding to light. Visual distortions are also common in older people. Thickening of the lens makes it harder for the eye to focus, especially at close range. Peripheral fields of vision become

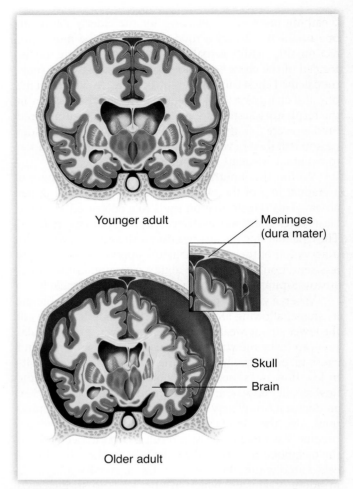

FIGURE 4-11 Age-related atrophy or shrinkage of the brain results in a space between the brain and its cover, the dura mater. Bleeding into this area can occur because veins are stretched.

narrower and a greater sensitivity to glare constricts the visual field.

Loss of hearing is approximately four times more common than loss of vision in late adulthood. Changes in several hearing-related structures may lead to a loss of high-frequency hearing or even deafness.

Psychosocial Changes

EMTs should treasure opportunities to spend time with and communicate with the elderly. Many of them have amazing stories and experiences to share with us, yet we often take them for granted. They can share with us a great amount of wisdom, and we need to remind them of their self-worth. Until approximately 5 years before death, most late-stage adults retain high brain function. In the 5 years preceding death, however, mental function is presumed to decline, a concept referred to as the *terminal drop hypothesis*.

Terminal drop hypothesis The theory that a person's mental function declines in the last 5 years of life.

As the elderly population continues to grow in the United States, it is becoming increasingly necessary to find ways to accommodate their needs during the last 20 to 40 years of life. Statistics indicate that 95% of the elderly live at home. They may have the assistance of family, friends, or home health care, but they remain relatively healthy, active, and independent.

Throughout the past decade, the increasing number of elderly persons in the United States as a result of the baby boom of the 1940s and 1950s has produced a need for additional assisted-living facilities. These facilities allow older adults to live in campus-based communities with people their own age while enjoying the privacy of their own apartment and the security of nursing care, maintenance, and food preparation, if desired. Unfortunately, these facilities can be very expensive. As such, the government provides many services for the aging to keep them in their homes and out of nursing homes for as long as possible.

Most people deal with financial issues throughout their lives. Indeed, few things in life produce more worry and stress than money problems. Late adults, in particular, may constantly worry about the rising cost of health care and are often forced to make decisions such as whether to pay for groceries or medication. Modern families often take less responsibility for elderly family members than earlier generations did. Today, more than 50% of all single women in the United States who are 60 years of age or older are living at or below the poverty level. This problem remains unresolved.

One of the important issues that the elderly need to face is their own mortality. Ultimately, everyone dies. Elderly persons often witness their friends and loved ones, including some people with whom they have shared their life journey for half a century or more, die. Consequently, isolation and depression are challenges for the elderly.

Many elderly persons are happy and actively participating in life. With good financial resources and a good support system of family and friends, individuals well in their 80s and 90s can enjoy life and continue to feel productive.

Transition Tip

Be patient when interviewing older persons. Some elderly patients may have physical, intellectual, and psychological barriers that may slow or interfere with effective communication.

PREP KIT

Ready for Review

- Whereas each developmental stage is marked by different physical and psychosocial changes and characteristics, infants (1 month to 1 year) develop at a startling rate.
- The vital signs of toddlers (ages 1 to 3 years) and preschoolers (ages 3 to 6 years) differ somewhat from those of an infant. During the toddler/preschooler stage, children learn to speak and express themselves.
- From ages 6 to 12 years, the school-age child's vital signs and body gradually approach those observed in adulthood. Children develop self-esteem during this stage.
- The vital signs of adolescents (ages 12 to 18 years) begin to level off within the adult ranges. Adolescents focus on creating their self-image.
- Early adults are those who are age 19 to 40 years. This age group focuses primarily on work and family.
- Middle adults are those who are between the ages of 41 and 60 years. The main focus of middle adults is achieving life goals.
- Late adults are those who are age 61 years and older. As individuals age (in their 80s and 90s), they often tend to focus on their own mortality and the mortality of friends and loved ones.
- Vital signs do not vary greatly throughout adulthood.

Case Study

You respond to a motor vehicle crash where a van hydroplaned and left the roadway, striking a culvert. There is minimal damage to the center front of the vehicle, and driver and passenger airbags were deployed. All five of the occupants were appropriately restrained. A 44-year-old male was driving and his 78-year-old mother was in the passenger seat. Two children ages 3 months and 7 years were in the middle section and a 13-year-old was in the rear. Upon EMS arrival, the grandmother is sitting in the front passenger seat holding the infant. The other children and the father are walking around. All patients appear to have no injuries, but the father wants everyone evaluated.

1. What are the expected vital sign ranges when examining a 7-year-old patient?

2. What differences might be found in the cardiovascular system of the 78-year-old grandmother as compared with the 44-year-old father?

3. As you approach to examine the infant, which type of reaction do you expect from him or her?

4. Which phenomenon occurs when an infant understands that parents or caregivers will be responsive to his or her needs?
   A. Bonding
   B. Secure attachment
   C. Trust
   D. Anxious-avoidant attachment

5. Briefly explain the reflexes typically found in a neonate.

CHAPTER 5

Patient Assessment

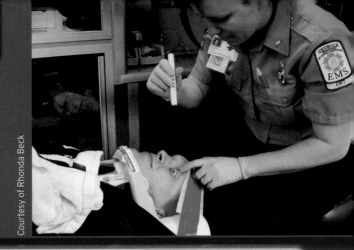

Courtesy of Rhonda Beck

▌Introduction

The importance of patient assessment cannot be overemphasized. Patient assessment is used in every patient encounter. Although the steps of the assessment process represent a logical approach to evaluation of a patient, the order in which the steps are performed is dictated by the patient's condition.

The new assessment process is divided into five main parts **FIGURE 5-1**:

1. Scene size-up
2. Primary assessment
3. History taking
4. Secondary assessment
5. Reassessment

▌Scene Size-up

Scene size-up is how you prepare for a specific situation; it includes analysis of the dispatch information combined with an inspection of the scene on arrival. Numerous issues must be considered from the moment the call comes in to the moment you reach the scene. During scene size-up, the primary emphasis is always on safety **FIGURE 5-2**:

- Ensure scene safety.
- Determine the mechanism of injury (MOI) or nature of illness (NOI).
- Take standard precautions (formerly known as body substan6ce isolation).
- Determine the number of patients.
- Consider the need for additional or specialized resources.

> *Scene size-up* A step within the patient assessment process that involves a quick assessment of the scene and its surroundings to provide information about scene safety and the mechanism of injury or nature of illness before you enter and begin patient care.

47

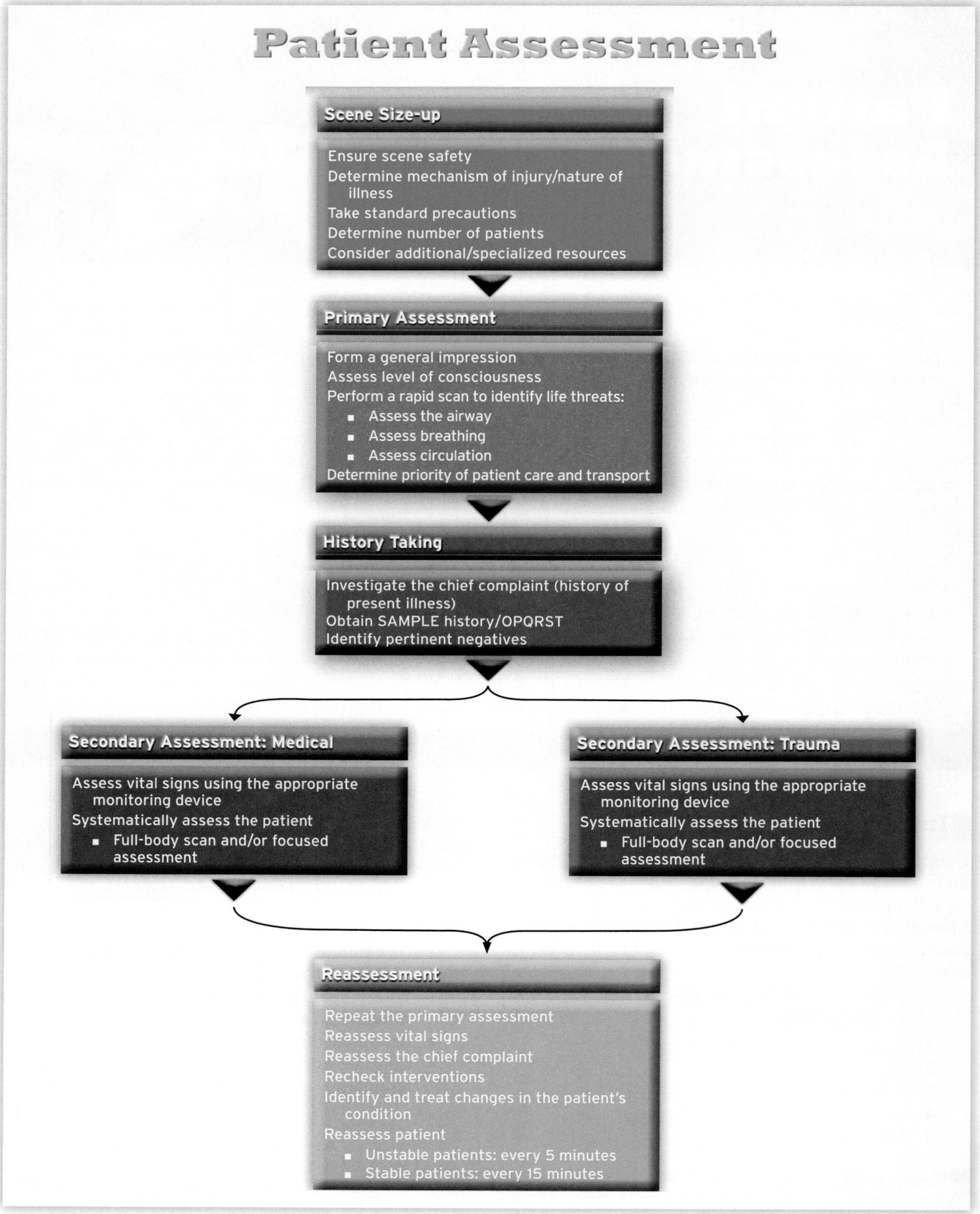

Patient Assessment

Scene Size-up

Ensure scene safety
Determine mechanism of injury/nature of illness
Take standard precautions
Determine number of patients
Consider additional/specialized resources

Primary Assessment

Form a general impression
Assess level of consciousness
Perform a rapid scan to identify life threats:
- Assess the airway
- Assess breathing
- Assess circulation

Determine priority of patient care and transport

History Taking

Investigate the chief complaint (history of present illness)
Obtain SAMPLE history/OPQRST
Identify pertinent negatives

Secondary Assessment: Medical

Assess vital signs using the appropriate monitoring device
Systematically assess the patient
- Full-body scan and/or focused assessment

Secondary Assessment: Trauma

Assess vital signs using the appropriate monitoring device
Systematically assess the patient
- Full-body scan and/or focused assessment

Reassessment

Repeat the primary assessment
Reassess vital signs
Reassess the chief complaint
Recheck interventions
Identify and treat changes in the patient's condition
Reassess patient
- Unstable patients: every 5 minutes
- Stable patients: every 15 minutes

FIGURE 5-1 The patient assessment process.

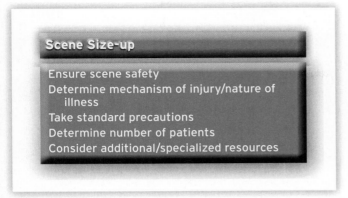

Scene Size-up

Ensure scene safety
Determine mechanism of injury/nature of illness
Take standard precautions
Determine number of patients
Consider additional/specialized resources

FIGURE 5-2 Scene size-up process.

Transition Tip

The following is a comparison between the old and the new standard as it relates to the patient assessment process:

OLD STANDARD	NEW STANDARD
Scene size-up	Scene size-up
Initial assessment (A-B-C)	Primary assessment (A-B-C or C-A-B)
Focused history and physical examination—rapid trauma/medical assessment—focused physical examination—SAMPLE/OPQRST	History taking and secondary assessment
Detailed physical exam	Secondary assessment
Ongoing assessment	Reassessment

Scene Safety

To ensure your safety at the incident scene, consider traffic safety issues. Wear an American National Standards Institute 207 certified high-visibility public safety vest and park your vehicle in a safe location that allows access to equipment and to your patient. Hazards at the scene should be identified and addressed as you approach the scene and as a part of ongoing scene management. They include environmental considerations such as weather, extreme temperatures, toxins and gases, secondary collapse of structures or potential falls, rough terrain, or other unstable conditions. If the environment is not safe for the patient or bystanders, minimize the hazards or move the patient and bystanders to a safe location. Always ensure your safety and that of your crew first and the safety of patients or bystanders second. However, any actions you take to protect yourself should also be considered for others. Many bystanders attempt to help during an emergency; always remember that they

are not trained to handle complicated EMS equipment, illnesses, or injury.

Transition Tip

There is no change in the components of scene size-up with the new National EMS Education Standards. Priority remains with ensuring scene safety and identifying potential hazards.

Mechanism of Injury or Nature of Illness

As you are aware, traumatic injuries are the result of physical forces applied to the body. To care for trauma patients properly, you must understand how their traumatic injuries occurred, or the MOI. Use the MOI as a guide to predict the potential for serious injury by evaluating three factors: the amount of force applied to the body, the length of time the force was applied, and the areas of the body involved.

For medical patients, assess the general type of illness the patient is experiencing, or the NOI. The NOI and MOI share some similarities. Specifically, both require you to search for clues regarding how the incident occurred. For a medical patient, you must make an effort to determine the general type of illness, which is often best described by the patient's chief complaint—that is, the reason EMS was called. To quickly determine the NOI, talk with the patient, family, or bystanders about the problem. At the same time, use your senses to check the scene for clues as to the possible problem. You may see open or spilled medication containers, poisonous substances, or unsanitary living conditions. You may smell an unusual or strong odor, such as the odor of fresh paint in a closed room. You may hear a hissing sound, such as a leak from a home oxygen system. Keep these observations of the scene in mind as you begin to assess the medical patient.

An understanding of the MOI or NOI should guide you during the assessment, providing a clue as to what might be wrong with a patient and which signs and symptoms to look for. For example, if the MOI is a fall, you would look for possible head, neck, and spine injuries. If the NOI is altered mental status, look for signs of stroke, hypoxia, seizure, poisoning, overdose, trauma, medication reaction, or diabetes. Knowing the MOI or NOI simply gives you a starting point for patient care.

Standard Precautions

Standard precautions and personal protective equipment (PPE) need to be considered and adapted to the prehospital task at hand.

Standard precautions are protective measures that have traditionally been developed by the Centers for Disease Control and Prevention for use in dealing with objects, blood, body fluids, and other potential exposure risks of communicable disease. The concept underlying these guidelines is an assumption that all blood, body fluids (except sweat), nonintact skin, and mucous membranes may pose a substantial risk of infection. When dealing with body fluids and patients, "If it's wet, it's infectious."

> *Standard precautions* Protective measures that have traditionally been developed by the Centers for Disease Control and Prevention for use in dealing with objects, blood, body fluids, and other potential exposure risks of communicable disease.

PPE includes clothing or specialized equipment that provides protection to the wearer. The type of PPE used will depend on the specific job duties required during a patient care interaction. For example, firefighters may wear PPE such as steel-toe boots, helmets, turnout gear, gloves, heat-resistant outerwear, and self-contained breathing apparatus (SCBA) designed to protect them from injury when performing a forced entry. Hazardous materials technicians may don a protective, encapsulated suit designed to prevent contamination by potentially lethal hazardous materials.

> **Transition Tip**
>
> The term "standard precautions" has replaced the term "body substance isolation" in EMS practices. This concept is described in more detail in the chapter on Infectious Diseases.

Number of Patients

It is important to identify the number of patients on the scene so as to determine the resources needed to manage an incident.

The incident command system may be used for incidents where multiple patients require care.

Additional and Specialized Resources

An important action during the scene size-up is to quickly identify the need for additional resources. Additional resources may include additional ambulances for multiple patients; advanced life support (ALS); the fire department for fire hazards or assistance with lifting as needed; rescue personnel for gaining access to a patient; and law enforcement personnel for traffic control, potential violence, or if something at the scene leads you to believe a criminal or reportable activity has occurred. Bystanders can also be used for certain tasks.

■ Primary Assessment

The *primary assessment* has a single, critical goal: to identify and initiate treatment of immediate or potential life threats. The patient's level of consciousness (LOC), airway, breathing, and circulation, will determine the extent of treatment at the scene. The primary assessment begins with forming a general impression of the patient **FIGURE 5-3**.

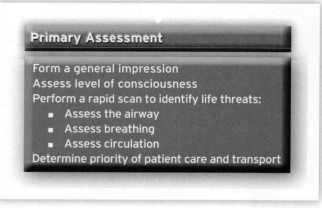

Primary Assessment

Form a general impression
Assess level of consciousness
Perform a rapid scan to identify life threats:
- Assess the airway
- Assess breathing
- Assess circulation
Determine priority of patient care and transport

FIGURE 5-3 Primary assessment process.

> *Primary assessment* A step within the patient assessment process in which the health care provider identifies and initiates treatment of immediate or potential life threats.

Form a General Impression

The initial *general impression* is formed to determine the priority of care based on immediate assessment of the patient. It includes noting the patient's age, sex, race, level of distress, and overall appearance. It is important to take notes while gathering your initial general impression. While approaching the patient, remember the following:

- Avoid surprising the patient. Make sure he or she sees you coming.
- Note the patient's position: Is the patient moving or still?
- Refer to the patient by name and introduce yourself.
- Ask the patient about the chief complaint.
- Determine whether the patient's condition is stable, stable but potentially unstable, or unstable.

If a life-threatening problem is found while obtaining an initial general impression, it should be treated immediately.

> *General impression* The overall initial impression that determines the priority for patient care; based on the patient's surroundings, the mechanism of injury, signs and symptoms, and the chief complaint.

Assess the Level of Consciousness

Assess the patient's LOC to determine the patient's neurologic and mental status. Is the patient conscious with an unaltered mentation, conscious with an altered mentation, or unconscious?

Assess responsiveness by using the AVPU scale (Awake and alert, responsive to Verbal stimuli, responsive to Pain, Unresponsive). Choose from one of the following options to describe the patient:

- *A*lert: The patient's eyes open spontaneously when you approach and the patient appears to follow commands.

- **V**erbal: The patient's eyes do not open spontaneously; however, the patient does respond when spoken to.
- **P**ain: The patient only responds to a painful stimulus such as rubbing the sternum, pinching an earlobe, or pressing down on the bone above the eye.
- **U**nresponsive: The patient does not respond to any stimulus.

Orientation tests mental status by checking a patient's memory and thinking ability. To assess mental status, evaluate the patient's ability to remember the following:

- **Person:** The patient is able to remember his or her name.
- **Place:** The patient is able to identify his or her current location.
- **Time:** The patient is able to tell you the current year, month, and approximate date.
- **Event:** The patient is able to describe what happened (MOI or NOI).

These questions evaluate long-term memory (person and place—if at home), intermediate memory (place and time—asking the month or year), and short-term memory (time—asking the approximate date and event). If the patient knows all facts, he or she is said to be "alert and oriented × 4."

Transition Tip

In October 2010, the CPR and emergency cardiac care (ECC) guidelines changed for CPR. In cases of cardiac arrest, the emphasis has changed from addressing life threats in the order ABC (airway, breathing, circulation) to following a CAB (chest compressions, airway, breathing) system. It is believed that early chest compressions and early defibrillation are key to successful resuscitations for adults, children, and infants (excluding newborns). The 2010 *Handbook for Emergency Cardiovascular Care* recommends a 10-second maximum pulse check for health care providers prior to initiating chest compressions.

On the basis of the 2010 CPR guidelines, if the patient does not show signs of life (ie, is unresponsive, with no normal breathing), follow the C-A-B approach to patient care. If the patient has signs of life (breathing is noted), follow an A-B-C approach. The C-A-B approach is described in the chapter on *Shock and BLS Resuscitation*.

Assess the Airway: Identify and Treat Life Threats

Determine if the airway is patent. Assess the patient for sounds of stridor, a brassy, crowing sound that is prominent on inspiration, which suggests a mild obstruction caused by swelling. High-pitched crowing sounds may indicate a mild airway obstruction from a foreign body. A responsive patient who cannot speak or cry is most likely suffering from a severe or complete airway obstruction.

If the patient is unresponsive or has a decreased LOC, look for signs of airway obstruction including obvious trauma or blood near the airway; noisy breathing including gurgling, bubbling, crowing, or snoring; or extremely shallow or absent breathing.

Unresponsive patients should be considered to have experienced a traumatic event. If a trauma MOI may be involved, use the modified jaw-thrust technique to open the patient's airway and insert an oropharyngeal airway. If it can be confirmed that the patient did not experience a traumatic event, apply the head tilt-chin lift technique to open and maintain a patent airway. If the patient is unresponsive, the obstruction may be caused by relaxation of the tongue or by the presence of broken teeth or dentures, blood, vomitus, mucus, food, or other foreign objects.

Assess Breathing: Identify and Treat Life Threats

Assess the adequacy of the patient's breathing. A single breath consists of two distinct phases: inspiration and expiration. Whereas normal breathing is silent, abnormal breath sounds may be heard in one or both phases of respiration. A patient who is breathing without assistance is said to have spontaneous respirations. Breathing should be an automatic process that occurs without thought, visible effort, marked sounds, or pain. When assessing breathing, identify the following elements:

- Respiratory rate **TABLE 5-1**
- Rhythm (regular or irregular)
- Quality of breathing (adequate or inadequate; labored or unlabored; diminished or absent lung sounds on one side)
- Depth of breathing (deep or shallow)

Determine if respirations are too fast, slow, shallow, or deep. Is the patient cyanotic? Do you hear abnormal lung sounds? Is there equal lung expansion on both sides?

Observe how much effort is required for the patient to breathe. Normal respirations are neither shallow nor excessively deep. Look for the presence of retractions, which will present as indentations above the clavicles and in the spaces between the ribs, or the use of accessory muscles. Nasal flaring, "see-saw" breathing, and grunting in pediatric patients indicate inadequate breathing.

Table 5-1 Normal Ranges for Respirations	
Age	**Range (breaths/min)**
Adults and adolescents	12 to 20
Children (1 to 12 years)	15 to 30
Infants	25 to 50

Look at the positioning of the patient. Patients who are having marked difficulty breathing will instinctively assume a posture in which it is easier to breathe. A patient sitting upright and leaning forward on outstretched arms with the head and chin thrust slightly forward, making a conscious effort to breathe, is in the tripod position **FIGURE 5-4**. A child with difficulty breathing may assume a sniffing position in which the child sits upright with the head and chin thrust slightly forward, appearing to be sniffing **FIGURE 5-5**.

Listen to the patient talk. A patient who can speak smoothly without unusual pauses is breathing normally. In contrast, a patient who can speak only one word or must stop every two to three words to catch his or her breath (a condition known as two-word dyspnea) has a serious breathing problem.

Auscultate breath sounds. Normal breath sounds include only the sound of air movement during inspiration and expiration. Abnormal lung sounds indicate the following significant respiratory problems:

- Wheezing is a high-pitched whistling sound, most prominent on expiration, which suggests an obstruction of the lower airways.
- Rales are moist, crackling sounds, also known as crackles, heard on both inspiration and expiration. This sound is usually associated with fluid in the lungs and sounds similar to blowing bubbles into a cup of water through a straw.
- Rhonchi are low-pitched, noisy sounds most prominent on expiration, suggesting the presence of

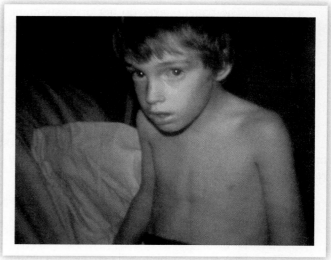

Courtesy of Health Resources and Services Administration, Maternal and Child Health Bureau, Emergency Medical Service for Children Program

FIGURE 5-5 Child in a sniffing position.

mucus in the lungs. Patients often report a productive cough associated with these sounds because of chest congestion.

- Stridor is often heard without a stethoscope and may indicate the patient has an upper airway obstruction. Stridor is a brassy, crowing sound that is most prominent on inspiration.

Always administer oxygen to patients who are experiencing difficulty breathing. Patients with a significant MOI or NOI should also receive oxygen. Positive-pressure ventilation should be applied to apneic patients or those with shallow or slow respirations.

Assess Circulation: Identify and Treat Life Threats

During the primary assessment, it is important to assess circulation to determine perfusion. Evaluate circulation by assessing the pulse as well as the skin.

If the patient has a pulse but is not breathing, provide ventilations at a rate of 12 breaths/min for adults and 20 breaths/min for an infant or child. Continue to monitor the pulse to evaluate ventilation effectiveness. If at any time the pulse is lost, begin CPR. The apparent absence of a palpable pulse in a responsive patient is not caused by cardiac arrest, so you should never begin CPR or use an AED on a responsive patient.

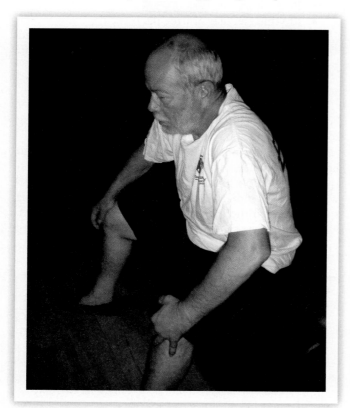

Courtesy of Catherine Parvensky Barwell

FIGURE 5-4 Person in a tripod position.

Transition Tip

Patients with no signs of life: Assess pulse. If you are unable to detect a pulse within 10 seconds, begin CPR starting with 30 chest compressions at a rate of at least 100/min. Then, open the airway and administer two breaths. Refer to the chapter *Shock and BLS Resuscitation* for more detail.

Patients with signs of life: You should spend no more than 10 seconds checking for a pulse. If a pulse is definitely not felt within 10 seconds, begin CPR and use the AED if available. Once you have determined that the patient has a pulse, check its adequacy by assessing the pulse rate, quality, and rhythm. Is the pulse rate normal for an adult (between 60 and 100 beats/min), tachycardic (more than 100 beats/min), or bradycardic (fewer than 60 beats/min) **TABLE 5-2**? If the pulse rate is weak and difficult to palpate, irregular, or extremely slow, it should be counted for one full minute. Is the quality of the pulse normal, bounding, weak, or thready? Is the rhythm regular or irregular?

Evaluate the patient's skin to determine the adequacy of tissue perfusion. Assess color, temperature, and moisture to identify any circulatory compromise. Changes in perfusion may indicate more serious cardiac compromise. For example, poor peripheral circulation will cause skin to appear pale, white, ashen, or gray. Abnormally cold skin will also have such an appearance. When the blood is not properly saturated with oxygen, it appears bluish. Therefore, in a patient with insufficient air exchange and low levels of oxygen in the blood, the blood and vessels become bluish, and the lips, mucous membranes, nail beds, and skin over the blood vessels appear blue or gray (cyanotic). In contrast, high blood pressure may cause the skin to appear abnormally flushed or red. A patient with carbon monoxide poisoning or a significant fever, heatstroke, or sunburn will have red skin. Yellow skin or sclera, also known as jaundice, may be the result of a chronic disease such as a liver disease or dysfunction.

Skin that is wet (diaphoretic), moist (clammy), or excessively dry and hot indicates a problem as well. Skin temperature should be 98.6°F and is normally warm to the touch. Cool, pale, clammy skin may be an indication of hypoperfusion or shock. If the patient is younger than 6 years, assess capillary refill. When you are reporting on or describing the skin, identify the color, temperature, and moisture level.

Finally, perform a quick scan of the body to identify and control any major bleeding or any significant edema in the extremities. If severe bleeding is identified, use direct pressure to control it and bandage the wound appropriately. Use direct pressure and elevation for extremities. If this effort is not immediately successful in controlling the bleeding, move to the use of a tourniquet.

Transition Tip

If a patient experiences difficulty breathing after you have completed the primary assessment, immediately reevaluate the airway. If respirations are fewer than 8 breaths/min or more than 24 breaths/min, consider assisting ventilation with a bag-mask device. Remember, however, that air exchange is the critical issue, not the number of breaths. If respirations are not adequate, as identified by signs of poor tissue perfusion, the patient needs assistance.

Determine the Priority of Patient Care and Transport

At this stage, it is time to make decisions about treatment and transport based on your rapid scan and assessment of vital signs (ABCs). Priority designation is used to determine whether your patient needs immediate transport or will tolerate a few more minutes on scene. Patients with any of the following conditions should be transported immediately:

- Difficulty breathing
- Poor general impression
- Unresponsive with no gag or cough reflex
- Severe chest pain
- Pale skin or other signs of poor perfusion
- Complicated childbirth
- Uncontrolled bleeding
- Responsive but unable to follow commands
- Severe pain in any area of the body
- Inability to move any part of the body

Your decision to stay on scene to continue the assessment process or to transport immediately should be based on the patient's condition, the availability of more advanced help, the distance you must transport, and your local protocols.

The patient's condition should fall into one of three groups:

- Stable
- Potentially unstable
- Unstable

Golden Period The time from injury to definitive care, during which treatment of shock or traumatic injuries should occur because survival potential is best when care is delivered in this time span.
History taking A step within the patient assessment process that provides detail about the patient's chief complaint and an account of the patient's signs and symptoms.

Table 5-2 Normal Ranges for Pulse Rate	
Age	**Range (beats/min)**
Infant: 1 month to 1 year	100 to 160
Toddler: 1 to 3 years	90 to 150
Preschool-age child: 3 to 6 years	80 to 140
School-age child: 6 to 12 years	70 to 120
Adolescent: 12 to 18 years	60 to 100
Adult	60 to 100

Transition Tip

Some people now use the term *Golden Period* instead of the term Golden Hour. Many injured patients require definitive care in less than an hour. Others may be critically ill, but tolerate intervention after more prolonged delay. Thus some people prefer the term Golden Period. Both terms, Golden Period and Golden Hour, are commonly used.

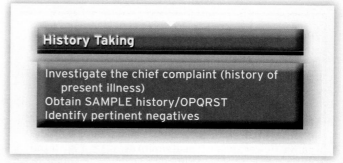

History Taking

Investigate the chief complaint (history of present illness)
Obtain SAMPLE history/OPQRST
Identify pertinent negatives

FIGURE 5-6 History-taking process.

History Taking

Although history taking is listed after the primary assessment, it is an integral part of the assessment process and should be initiated, if possible, on scene simultaneously with other tasks **FIGURE 5-6**. For example, one AEMT can manage a life-threatening wound during the primary assessment while another AEMT begins to gather a history from the patient. It is important to get as much history as possible from family, friends, and bystanders; such information may be essential to determine the underlying illness or injury.

History taking provides details about the patient's chief complaint and an account of the patient's signs and symptoms. It is important to document all of the information gathered during this phase of the assessment process, including any demographics, past medical history, and the current health status of the patient.

The use of the SAMPLE and OPQRST mnemonics are not new skills. The SAMPLE mnemonic is used to gather a general past medical or trauma history and to obtain the following information:

S Signs and symptoms
A Allergies
M Medications
P Pertinent past medical history
L Last oral intake
E Events leading up to the injury or illness

The OPQRST mnemonic is used to assess the level of pain or distress:

O Onset
P Provocation or palliation
Q Quality
R Region/radiation
S Severity
T Timing

All pertinent negatives should be documented; pertinent negatives are findings to rule out a specific condition because a strong indicator that should be present in a condition is absent. For example, you would expect a patient having a heart attack (acute myocardial infarction, or AMI) to have chest pain that radiates up to the neck or down the left arm. If the patient denies this symptom, it is a pertinent negative, which would make it more likely that the patient is suffering from angina than an AMI. The pages that follow contain information intended to help you identify techniques for obtaining a history on difficult patients. In addition, specific assessment techniques associated with various disease processes are described in each chapter of this textbook. For additional general information on how to obtain these histories, refer back to your EMT-I textbook.

History Taking on Sensitive Topics

Alcohol and Drug Use

Presenting signs and symptoms of a patient under the influence of alcohol or drugs may be confusing, hidden, or disguised. Many patients who abuse alcohol and/or drugs deny having any problems. In addition, families, friends, and coworkers may be unaware that a patient has any drug or alcohol troubles because those who engage in substance abuse often hide their dependency. Patients may deny using alcohol or drugs out of fear of losing their employment or driver's license, worry about what friends may think about them, and exhibit embarrassment or insecurity about their dependency.

The history gathered from chemically dependent patients may be unreliable. If these individuals are unwilling to tell the people closest to them that they have a problem, they may be even less likely to tell you, a stranger. Furthermore, signs and symptoms of alcohol or drug use may be masked by the patient's presentation. For these reasons, it is important to use all of your senses when assessing a patient.

Establish a strong rapport with your patient. Do not judge someone who may have a chemical dependency. Be professional in your approach, and be honest and open. Most importantly, impress on the patient that information received will be kept in confidence. Stress to the patient that this information is vital for the assessment and treatment of his or her current condition.

Physical Abuse or Violence

All cases of suspected physical abuse or domestic violence must be reported to the appropriate authorities. Follow local protocols when dealing with such cases. If you suspect a patient is a victim of physical abuse or domestic violence, do not accuse any person of being responsible for the situation. Instead, immediately involve law enforcement.

Because abuse and physical violence are very sensitive situations that often remain well hidden, you will need to look for clues that such a situation exists. Information gathered at the scene, during the assessment process, and while transporting a patient may indicate violence or abuse.

While gathering a patient's history, determine whether the information provided by the patient and others present at the scene is inconsistent. Do you observe multiple injuries in various stages of healing? Are some bruises red, black, brown, or even green? These findings may lead you to suspect abuse. In some cases, a victim of abuse or violence will not tell you what happened because of fear of further violence when EMS personnel are not present. Victims may not answer your questions because the physical aggressor is still present and is answering questions for the patient. They may be vague in responses and avoid eye contact. If possible, separate the people present and interview each party individually about the situation.

Transition Tip

Prehospital calls involving domestic violence will occasionally end up in court proceedings. As the responding AEMT, you may be summoned at a later date to provide objective and truthful testimony regarding what may have happened. If you suspect that the emergency response is part of a domestic abuse situation, call law enforcement personnel immediately and complete an accurate and thorough documentation of your response.

When physical abuse is potentially present, be very observant and open-minded. Maintain a high index of suspicion and remain nonjudgmental. Documentation is very important in cases of abuse and domestic violence and should consist of an objective report of the facts. Avoid subjective or judgmental statements. Include any pertinent statements made by the patient or others present, in their own words, using quotation marks to indicate direct quotes.

Sexual History

Obtaining information about a patient's sexual history may be difficult. Religious beliefs, cultural stereotypes, and society's expectations may cause the patient to be reluctant to reveal information about this very personal side of his or her life, including practices considered by some people to be bizarre or exotic. In additional, some patients find sharing information regarding their sexual history with others very uncomfortable.

Information about a patient's sexual history is especially important when caring for female patients. Consider all females of childbearing years who are complaining of lower abdominal pain to be pregnant unless that assumption is ruled out by history or other information. When you are treating a female patient with abdominal pain, ask the following questions:

- When was your last menstrual period?
- Are your periods normal? (Is there any vaginal discharge or bleeding not associated with a menstrual period?)
- Do you have urinary frequency or burning?
- What is the severity of cramping, and are there any foul odors?
- Is there a possibility you may be pregnant?
- Are you taking birth control pills?
- Have you had recent sexual encounters?

When you are treating a male patient, it may be necessary to inquire about urinary symptoms as follows:

- Is there pain associated with urination?
- Do you have any discharge, sores, or an increase in urination?
- Do you have burning or difficulty voiding?
- Has there been any trauma?
- Have you had recent sexual encounters?

In obtaining a history in all patients, ask about the potential for sexually transmitted diseases. The process of gathering this information may be difficult and uncomfortable for the patient. Do not be judgmental once this information is gathered. All patients should be, and expect to be, treated with compassion and respect, with all information gathered kept strictly confidential. A quiet setting and an EMS provider who is the same gender as the patient will likely be beneficial for these discussions.

Special Challenges in Obtaining a Patient's History

You may face a number of challenges when obtaining a history from certain patients. This section identifies some helpful techniques for handling various types of situations.

Silence

Dealing with patients who say very little or say nothing at all can be difficult and frustrating for an AEMT. Patience is extremely important when dealing with these patients and their emergency crises. The patient may be thinking about how to answer you, getting facts straight, or assessing your crew to determine if he or she feels comfortable providing answers. A closed-ended question that requires a simple yes-or-no answer may work best. Consider whether the silence is a clue to the patient's chief complaint.

Always look for visual signs in the patient's environment that may indicate why a patient is not communicating. Look for nonverbal clues, including facial expressions or body language that may show pain or fear. Is the patient distressed or intimidated by your presence or the presence of someone else? How is the patient sitting or standing? Is there a communication problem? Is there a language problem? The number of reasons why a patient might remain silent during the prehospital encounter is endless. A good

AEMT will continue to assess the situation and identify a way to communicate with the patient.

Overly Talkative

At the other end of the communication spectrum is the patient who is extremely talkative. Gathering details about his or her medical condition may be difficult if the person talks around your question or you have a difficult time refocusing the conversation. While some people are just normally talkative, possible causes as to why a patient might be overly talkative could include excessive caffeine consumption; nervousness; and ingestion of cocaine, crack, or methamphetamines.

Once you have allowed a talkative patient a chance to express himself or herself, you must keep the patient focused on your questions. Redirect the patient. Instruct him or her to stick to the facts. Clarify statements for the purpose of making sure the information you are gathering is correct.

Multiple Symptoms

Geriatric patients often present with multiple symptoms during a single patient encounter. Prioritize the patient's complaints as you would in triage, starting with the most serious and ending with the least serious. Always ask for specific information to determine why EMS was called.

Keep an open mind. Do not focus on one complaint or detail to determine a treatment plan. Always remember there may be a number of possible medical or traumatic causes for a patient's chief complaint.

Anxiety

When involved in an emergency situation, it is natural for a person to be excited or anxious. When faced with a true emergency, the reactions of individuals may be unpredictable. The patient or bystander may be nervous, pacing, vocal, panicked, or, in some extreme cases, experiencing complete hysteria. It is your responsibility to deal not only with the emergency crisis at hand, but also with the people present who are having difficulties coping with the situation. Frequently, anxious patients can be observed in emergency scenes involving a large number of patients, such as during a disaster. Anxiety may also be observed or encountered during a routine EMS call when family members or patients cannot cope with the stress of the situation.

Anxious patients may exhibit signs of psychogenic shock, such as pallor, diaphoresis, shortness of breath, numbness in the hands and feet, dizziness or light-headedness, and even loss of consciousness. Some anxious patients may have no real medical complaint but may be hiding or concealing something, such as trying to keep a family member, friend, or employer from discovering the individual's dependency on alcohol or drugs. In some cases, the patient may have been involved in a physical abuse or domestic situation that he or she wants to keep quiet. Anxiety may also have a medical cause. In any situation involving an anxious patient, you must be aware of verbal and nonverbal clues. Is the patient making sense during a verbal conversation? Can the patient be calmed down, or might the patient potentially need to be restrained?

During a crisis situation, reassure the patient that any nervous or anxious response is normal and can be overcome. It may be possible for you to control an anxious patient by simply smiling or using a delicate touch. Be confident in your approach, and have a positive demeanor. In many patient care interactions, your presence may be all that is necessary to calm the patient.

As in every response, safety is a paramount concern when dealing with anxiety-laden situations. Be aware that emergency responses involving anxious and possibly hysterical patients can turn violent. A confident but cautious EMT can prevent a bad situation from getting worse. Be professional and calm while controlling anxious patients, friends, and family members.

Anger and Hostility

Every patient encounter has the potential for violence and hostility, from a situation involving a 9-year-old boy who was hit by a vehicle to a 90-year-old grandmother experiencing chest pain. These emergency calls have a high potential for unexpected violence because friends, family, or bystanders may direct their anger and rage toward you. Do not take this anger and frustration personally. Even more importantly, do not become angry yourself because anger feeds anger. Instead, use the opportunity to reinforce professional behavior.

In handling potentially violent situations, remain calm, reassuring, and gentle **FIGURE 5-7**. Call for law enforcement and be observant. Be aware of nonverbal clues, such as posture, position, and facial expressions. Look at the patient and be aware of how he or she is positioned. Is the patient stiff, with hands clenched and feet wide apart? Is his or her body weight all on one leg? These stances may indicate the patient has assumed a position to allow him or her to kick.

It is not unusual for a patient, family member, or friend to vent hostility toward EMS responders. If the scene is not

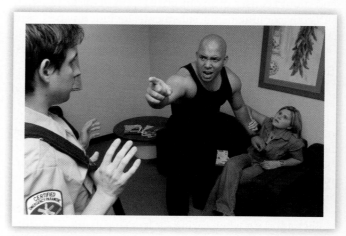

FIGURE 5-7 Do not handle potentially violent calls on your own. Remain calm, reassuring, and gentle, and call for law enforcement.

safe or secured, get it secured. Never let a potentially violent or hostile patient leave the room alone. Understand that everything in reach of a patient has the potential to be used as a weapon.

Intoxication

The number of EMS calls dealing with an intoxicated patient has increased over the years. When gathering a history from an intoxicated patient, be aware the information may be difficult to obtain and unreliable. An intoxicated patient may become very impatient when providing information. As the patient's impatience increases, so does his or her anger level. Do not put an intoxicated patient in a position where he or she feels threatened. At all times, be aware that the potential for violence and physical confrontation is high when a patient is intoxicated.

During the assessment and treatment of a patient who has consumed alcohol, be accepting, diplomatic, objective, and nonjudgmental. An intoxicated patient may be unable to reveal everything about how he or she feels. Alcohol dulls a patient's senses, which makes it difficult to tell you about any pain or discomfort. Remember to treat an intoxicated patient as you do all patients, with dignity and respect. Never assume the patient's condition is the result of alcohol consumption when there may be an underlying medical or traumatic cause for the patient's presentation.

Crying

A crying patient is a breathing patient. Regardless of the reason a patient is crying, you need to remain calm; be patient, reassuring, and confident and maintain a soft voice.

Your presence may make a crying patient feel more secure. In some extreme cases, additional diplomacy and verbal intervention will help. Be sympathetic and treat the patient with respect and dignity.

Depression

Depression is a common reason why patients call EMS. In fact, according to the World Health Organization, depression is among the leading causes of disability worldwide. Symptoms associated with depression include sadness, a feeling of hopelessness, restlessness, and irritability. The patient may also have sleeping and eating disorders and exhibit a decreased energy level. Although depression is a normal human response, it can sometimes lead to harmful behavior. In the treatment of depression, be nonjudgmental and compassionate toward the patient's feelings. The most effective treatment in handling a patient's depression is being a good listener. Often, the patient just needs someone to talk to and someone to listen. Report all findings during the transfer of care—this information could be lifesaving.

Confusing Behavior or History

Sometimes the history obtained from a patient is confusing. Numerous conditions, such as hypoxia, stroke, diabetes, trauma, some medications, and other drugs, have the potential to alter a patient's explanation of events, causing confusion. One of the most common causes of confusion is hypoxia. When caring for geriatric patients, it is not uncommon to encounter a patient with dementia, delirium, or Alzheimer disease, where confusion is the norm. For all these reasons, it is important to verify the normal mental status of each patient before determining the cause of the confusion. Talk with family members, bystanders, or others who know the patient. Do not assume that just because a patient is elderly, he or she suffers from dementia, delirium, or Alzheimer disease.

Confusing behavior is not a normal response. After you have properly assessed and treated any life threats, attempt to ask the patient again about the chief complaint. Ask family members or friends for additional information to clarify confusing details.

Limited Cognitive Abilities

Patients with limited cognitive abilities may be developmentally disabled. These disabilities can range from barely recognizable to very severe. Develop a habitual method for dealing with a patient who has limited cognitive abilities. First, assume that you can get an adequate history. Keep your questions simple and limit the use of medical terms. Be alert for partial answers, and reword the question to elicit more details. In cases of patients with severely limited cognitive function, rely on the presence of family, caregivers, and friends to supply answers to your questions.

Language Barriers

The United States is, quite famously, a melting pot of people with diverse nationalities. Given that not everyone speaks the native language, you may encounter patients who do not speak English. What happens if you ask a patient what happened to him or her, and the person answers in French? Or if the patient can tell you his or her name and address, but that is the only English the individual knows? How will you ask the patient to describe what happened and what hurts?

The best answer is to find an interpreter, but one is not always available and finding such assistance takes time. In such a case, first determine whether the patient speaks or understands any English by asking the patient or others who may be present. Introduce yourself and state your name, and determine whether the patient understands who you are. If the patient is able to respond by giving you his or her name, the patient has the ability to understand some English; even more important, the patient has cognitive ability, or the ability to understand. Remember that increasing the volume of your questions will not increase the patient's understanding of what you are asking him or her. Keep questions straightforward and brief: Simple is best in these patient encounters. Use of hand gestures may be helpful.

Pocket resource guides for translating medical terms into different languages are available and should be kept in the ambulance for reference. In addition, translation applications can be downloaded to smart phones.

Be aware of the language diversity in your community. Most hospitals have set up programs within the institution that identify various employees who can speak different languages. Provide the hospital with advance notice that a non–English-speaking patient will be arriving. This will allow the hospital the opportunity to make arrangements for an interpreter.

Hearing Problems

Hearing disabilities in patients range from very slight to total deafness. Hearing problems can make the process of obtaining an in-depth history difficult. When treating a patient with hearing loss, ask questions slowly and clearly. Determine from family members if the patient has a hearing aid. If so, it may not be turned on or may need new batteries. Use a stethoscope to function like a hearing aid. Have the patient place the stethoscope in his or her ears and speak into the stethoscope bell to amplify the sound. Changing the pitch of your voice may also help the patient hear you better.

Often, a patient who has had a hearing disability for some time will have mastered the technique of reading lips. Speak slowly and in a face-to-face orientation toward the patient. Some deaf patients will attempt to use sign language for communication, which can be difficult for others to understand; learning simple sign language can be of help in this situation. Probably the simplest way to communicate with a patient who has a hearing deficit is to use a pencil and paper. Write uncomplicated questions that require simple yes-or-no answers where the patient can shake his or her head in response (assuming there is no traumatic injury), or have the individual write responses to your queries.

Visual Impairments

When you are entering the home or room of a visually impaired patient who has called for help, identify yourself verbally. By announcing yourself when you enter a residence, you let the patient know that help has arrived; any response from the patient may help you locate his or her whereabouts. It is also a safe thing to do, so that patient and family members are not surprised when a stranger appears in their home.

During assessment and subsequent treatment of a patient who is significantly visually impaired, it is important that you put any items that have been moved back into their previous position. Many visually impaired patients can move freely about their homes because they know exactly where everything is placed.

During the assessment and history-taking process, explain to the patient what is happening. Explain that you will be checking vital signs by feeling for the pulse, listening to breath sounds, and applying a blood pressure cuff to the patient's arm. Remember, you are a stranger to the patient, and an EMS vehicle is a foreign and sometimes scary environment. A little communication can go a long way in easing uncertainty in a visually impaired patient.

Secondary Assessment

A *secondary assessment* is a systematic physical examination of the patient. This physical examination may be a full-body scan (head-to-toe) or an assessment that focuses on a certain area or region of the body (focused assessment), usually determined by the chief complaint. The circumstances of the call will dictate which aspects of the physical examination are appropriate **FIGURE 5-8**.

> *Secondary assessment* A step within the patient assessment process in which a systematic physical examination of the patient is performed. This examination may be a systematic full-body scan or a systematic assessment that focuses on a certain area or region of the body, often determined through the chief complaint.

If the patient is in stable condition and has an isolated complaint, the secondary assessment may occur at the scene. If it is not performed at the scene, it may be performed in the back of the ambulance en route to the hospital. However, if you are continually managing life threats identified during the primary assessment or if the patient's condition worsens, you might not have time to perform a secondary assessment at all, unless additional personnel are available.

Use a systematic approach to examine the patient. Place special emphasis on areas suggested by the chief complaint and history of the present illness. If the patient's condition worsens during the physical exam, repeat the primary assessment.

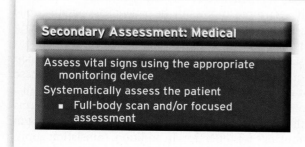

Secondary Assessment: Medical

Assess vital signs using the appropriate monitoring device
Systematically assess the patient
- Full-body scan and/or focused assessment

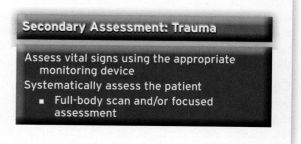

Secondary Assessment: Trauma

Assess vital signs using the appropriate monitoring device
Systematically assess the patient
- Full-body scan and/or focused assessment

FIGURE 5-8 Secondary assessment process is similar for medical and trauma patients.

Assess Vital Signs Using Monitoring Equipment

The use of monitoring equipment in the prehospital setting continues to expand. Today, EMTs at all levels use a wide variety of devices in the continuous monitoring of patients. Of course, it is important to remember that such devices are manufactured items subject to limitations and failures. They should never be used to replace the comprehensive assessment of your patient. Rather, they should be used as complementary tools in the assessment and treatment. Information that can be obtained from patient monitoring devices includes, but is not limited to, data from pulse oximetry and noninvasive blood pressure monitoring.

Pulse Oximetry

Pulse oximetry is an assessment tool used to evaluate the effectiveness of oxygenation. The *pulse oximeter* is a photoelectric device that monitors the oxygen saturation of hemoglobin (the iron-containing portion of the red blood cell to which oxygen attaches) in the capillary beds **FIGURE 5-9**. The parts that make up the pulse oximeter include a monitor and a sensing probe. The sensing probe clips onto a finger or earlobe. The light source must have unobstructed access to a capillary bed, so fingernail polish should be removed before the probe is applied. If nail polish removal is not practical, rotate the pulse oximeter sideways when placing it on the patient's finger. Results appear as a percentage on the display screen. Normally, pulse oximetry values in ambient air will vary depending on the altitude, with the majority of values falling between 95% and 100%.

> *Pulse oximeter* An assessment tool that measures oxygen saturation of hemoglobin in the capillary beds.

The goal of any oxygen therapy is to increase oxygen saturation to a normal level. Thus, pulse oximetry is a useful assessment tool to determine the effectiveness of oxygen therapy, bronchodilator therapy, and the bag-mask device in

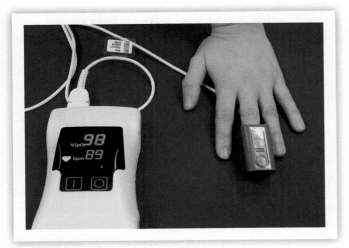

FIGURE 5-9 A pulse oximeter measures the saturation of oxygen in the blood as a percentage.

certain conditions. Nevertheless, use of the pulse oximeter does not take the place of good assessment skills, and its application should not prevent the administration of oxygen to any patient who reports difficulty breathing, regardless of the pulse oximetry value seen on the monitor.

Because the pulse oximeter assumes that the patient has adequate perfusion and numbers of red blood cells, any situation that causes vasoconstriction or loss of red blood cells (such as bleeding or anemia) will result in inaccurate or misleading values. The device also assumes that oxygen is saturating the hemoglobin. Thus the presence of any chemical that displaces oxygen (such as carbon monoxide) will also cause misleading values.

The pulse oximeter will also display the patient's pulse rate. Always verify the accuracy of the device by assessing the pulse manually first.

The pulse oximeter is a useful tool as long as you remember that it is only a tool, not a substitute for a good assessment. This device should not be used when hypoperfusion or known anemia is present, carbon monoxide or exposure to other toxic inhalants has occurred, or the patient's extremities are cold. Follow the steps in **SKILL DRILL 5-1** to measure pulse oximetry:

1 Remove any nail polish if possible. Place the index or middle finger into the pulse oximeter probe. Turn on the pulse oximeter and note the LED reading of the SpO_2 (**Step 1**).

2 Palpate the radial pulse to ensure that it correlates with the LED display on the pulse oximeter (**Step 2**).

End-Tidal Carbon Dioxide

Pulse oximetry cannot measure the amount of oxygen being consumed by a patient's cells during cellular metabolism. Metabolism refers to the chemical reactions that occur in the body or cells to maintain life. To determine oxygen consumption, you will need to measure carbon dioxide (CO_2) levels. CO_2 is the by-product of aerobic cellular metabolism, and its concentration in the body reflects the amount of oxygen being consumed during the metabolic process. Capnography is a noninvasive method that can quickly and efficiently provide information on a patient's ventilatory status, circulation, and metabolism. It can be used as a secondary tool during the confirmation of endotracheal intubation or to assess the effectiveness of ongoing CPR.

End-tidal CO_2 is the partial pressure or maximum concentration of CO_2 at the end of an exhaled breath, which is expressed as a percentage of CO_2, or millimeters of mercury. The normal range is 35 to 45 mm Hg, or 5% to 6% CO_2. When the CO_2 value is absent from the capnography results, it may indicate the endotracheal tube is in the wrong position or there is an absence or decrease in the level of CO_2 in the lungs, possibly from cardiac arrest, ineffective CPR, or shock. When cardiac output increases, the end-tidal CO_2 measurement will provide information on the adequacy of ventilations and circulation.

SKILL DRILL 5-1

Performing Pulse Oximetry

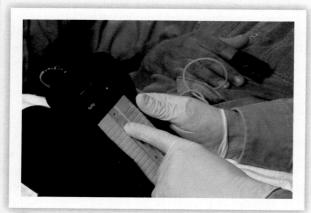

1 Place the index or middle finger into the pulse oximeter probe. Turn on the pulse oximeter and note the LED reading of the Spo_2.

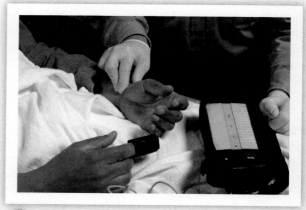

2 Palpate the radial pulse to ensure that it correlates with the LED display on the pulse oximeter.

End-tidal CO_2 is measured or detected by colorimetry, capnometry, and capnography devices. Colorimetric devices come in different shapes and sizes but provide continuous end-tidal monitoring by displaying one of three colors. Purple indicates a CO_2 level of less than 0.5%, tan indicates a range of 0.5% to 2%, and yellow indicates a level of greater than 2%. A reading of yellow indicates adequate circulation. Remember to check these devices regularly for damage, cracks, and blockages caused by gastric secretions, because such problems will affect the accuracy of the readings.

Capnometry and capnography provide a digital reading and waveform of end-tidal CO_2, expressed in millimeters of mercury or as a percentage of exhaled gas. Normal values should be in the range of 35 to 45 mm Hg. Capnometry and capnography devices are typically used in the prehospital setting as a secondary means to determine endotracheal placement, to maximize a patient's ventilatory status, and to avoid inadvertent hyperventilation of head-injured patients, as this problem has been linked to poor outcomes. Follow local protocols regarding the use of this device because it may be an ALS skill.

Blood Glucose Determination

The glucometer is used to assess blood glucose levels. Repeated checks allow an AEMT to assess the impact of interventions, such as the administration of 50% dextrose. While determining glucose levels is largely a routine part of the patient assessment, indications include known diabetes in patients with a decreased LOC and a decreased LOC of unknown origin in any patient.

Most glucometers operate in much the same manner; however, refer to the manufacturer's instructions for the device being used. Clean the site (typically the pad of any finger) with alcohol and allow to dry. Use a lancet or needle to stick the finger and place a drop of blood on the test strip. Promptly dispose of sharps in an appropriate container. There is only a small difference in the blood glucose results when samples are taken from capillary or venous sources. Samples may be obtained when inserting an intravenous catheter rather than sticking the patient's finger. A normal glucose reading is 80 to 120 mg/dL.

Like most mechanical devices, the glucometer may fail. Lack of calibration is a common problem for incorrect readings or failure of the device to work. Glucometers also have a set limit and will just read "Hi" above certain levels. Refer to the user manual as needed.

Noninvasive Blood Pressure Measurement

The sphygmomanometer, or blood pressure cuff, is used in the measurement of the patient's blood pressure. This device consists of an inflatable cuff that occludes blood flow and a manometer (pressure meter) used to determine the pressure in the artery at various points in the physical examination. These two components are connected via tubing. In manual cuffs, a separate tube connects to an inflation bulb. The auscultatory method (listening) is the most widely used means of measuring a patient's blood pressure using a sphygmomanometer.

As an AEMT, you should be expert to take manual blood pressures to establish a baseline value. Oscillometric measurement, or electronic measurement, is another method of obtaining blood pressure readings on patients **FIGURE 5-10**. An electronic device measures changes in pressure oscillations that occur during cuff deflation and are related to

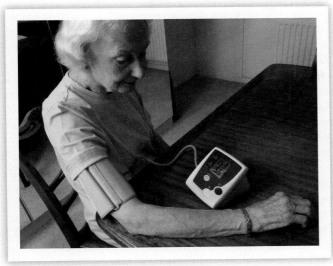

© Steve Horrell/Photo Researchers, Inc.

FIGURE 5-10 Oscillometric measurement (electronic measurement) is one method of obtaining blood pressure readings on patients.

systolic, mean, and diastolic pressures. Two different types of electronic devices are used in the prehospital setting, with the blood pressure cuff being deflated differently in each device.

The first device measures blood pressure using linear deflation, and the second type takes readings by using stepped deflation. An electronic blood pressure cuff that uses linear deflation allows for a uniform decline in pressure in the cuff during deflation. Conversely, stepped deflation allows the cuff to be deflated in small steps or intervals. Although both devices are accurate in the prehospital setting, stepped deflation tends to be more accurate in patients who are moving and in patients who may be hypotensive. Stepped deflation can release the pressure in the cuff in intervals at variable lengths, allowing the system to better detect oscillations.

Systematically Assess the Patient: Full-Body Scan

The full-body scan is a systematic, head-to-toe examination of the patient. The goal of this process is to identify hidden injuries or identify possible causes of patient symptoms. Any patient who has sustained a significant MOI, is unconscious or has an altered mental status, or is in critical condition should receive this examination, although it should never delay transport to the hospital or your interventions for any immediate life threats.

To perform a full-body secondary assessment, complete a head-to-toe examination. Inspect, palpate, and auscultate the body for any abnormalities using the mnemonic DCAP-BTLS. Assess all anatomic regions, including the following:

- Head and face
- Neck
- Chest

- Abdomen
- Pelvis
- Extremities
- Posterior body

If problem areas are identified during the full-body scan, perform a focused examination on the anatomical region/body system involved.

> **Transition Tip**
>
> Assessment using the mnemonic DCAP-BTLS has not changed. Inspect, palpate, and auscultate body systems for the following abnormalities:
> - **D**eformities
> - **C**ontusions
> - **A**brasions
> - **P**unctures/penetrations
> - **B**urns
> - **T**enderness
> - **L**acerations
> - **S**welling

Focused Assessment

A focused assessment is generally performed on patients who have not sustained a significant MOI or on medical patients who are alert and oriented. This type of examination is based on the chief complaint and MOI. For example, if the patient complains of a headache, carefully and systematically assess the head and/or the neurologic system. A person with a laceration to the arm may need to have only that arm evaluated. The goal of a focused assessment is to focus attention on the immediate problem after all life threats have been addressed.

On the basis of the information found during the focused assessment, you can develop a treatment plan and prioritize transport procedures.

Respiratory System

When the patient's chief complaint focuses on the respiratory system, you should have identified and managed life threats during the primary assessment. During the secondary assessment, perform an examination directed at obtaining clues about the cause of the respiratory symptoms.

Assess the chest for shape and symmetry; determine the level of respiratory effort by identifying nasal flaring, retractions, or the use of accessory muscles; and auscultate breath sounds. Expose the patient's chest. Look again for signs of trauma to the neck or chest. Inspect the chest for overall symmetry. Does the right side look like the left side? Listen carefully to breath sounds, noting any abnormalities. Determine the respiratory rate, chest rise and fall (for tidal volume), and effort. Look for retractions. Is the patient using accessory muscles to help with breathing, and is increased work of breathing evident? Is there equal lung expansion?

Inspect and palpate from the clavicles to the shoulder to the abdomen. Assess breath sounds. Note any abnormalities and document those findings on the patient care report. With this information, you can develop a treatment plan and prioritize transport procedures.

Cardiovascular System

When the patient's chief complaint is associated with chest pain, look, listen, and feel for abnormalities in the patient's thoracic region. Inspect the chest to rule out trauma. Inspect and palpate from the clavicles to the shoulder to the abdomen and assess breath sounds. Check and compare distal pulses in all extremities to determine any differences between the right and left sides. Always remember that a patient's chief complaint may have a medical cause or may be the result of trauma.

Reevaluate the pulse, respiratory rate, and blood pressure. Determine the rate, rhythm, and strength of the pulse. Assessment of these functions will allow you to determine how well the cardiovascular and respiratory systems are functioning.

Determine the patient's level of perfusion by obtaining a blood pressure reading and by assessing the color, temperature, and condition of the patient's skin. Blood pressure comprises the pressure of circulating blood against the walls of the arteries. **TABLE 5-3** serves as a guideline for normal blood pressure ranges.

Transition Tip

The new full-body scan and/or focused assessment should be conducted in the same manner as the old rapid trauma/rapid medical examination and should take no more than 90 seconds to complete.

Neurologic System

Assessment of a patient's neurologic system can be time consuming. Nevertheless, a neurologic assessment should be performed whenever you are confronted with a patient with altered mental status, possible head injury, stupor, dizziness, drowsiness, or syncope. A neurologic assessment

begins without even touching the patient. It can be as simple as talking with the patient, asking questions, and receiving an appropriate reply from the patient—all of which may take place during the primary assessment.

As part of the neurologic review, assess the patient's mental status for appearance and behavior. Determine the LOC and orientation using the AVPU scale. Check the patient's mental status. Is he or she alert and oriented to person, place, time, and events? Observe the patient's posture, motor behavior, and facial expression.

Also assess the patient's speech and language for rate and appropriateness. Does he or she appear drowsy or in a state of lethargy? Is the patient aware of his or her surroundings? Determine if speech is slurred, garbled, or nonexistent. Aphasia is the inability to speak. If the patient cannot speak, determine if this is a new symptom. When you are evaluating speech, assess the patient's thought process and determine if he or she may be delusional or has unusual reasoning.

Assess the patient's mood to determine its nature and intensity. Does the patient appear to have suicidal ideation? Assess thought process and perceptions. Do they appear logical and organized? Does the patient have unusual or unpleasant thoughts, or are his or her perceptions altered? Is the patient hearing or seeing things?

What do the patient's facial expressions tell you? Is he or she angry, fearful, depressed, anxious, or restless? Does the patient appear uncomfortable? Does he or she make incomprehensible or understandable statements? Is the patient's memory affected? Does the patient remember who family members are? What is his or her perception or view on what is happening? These are all important considerations when assessing the neurologic system.

Inspect the head for trauma. Pulse, blood pressure, and skin changes may indicate hypoperfusion of the brain. Use a penlight to check the patient's eyes. Are the pupils equal and reactive to light (PEARL)?

Perform a hands-on assessment to determine PMS (presence of equal pulses [P], equal motor skills [M], and sensation on all extremities [S]). Perform a stroke assessment. Assess for symmetry, facial droop, and arm lift.

Musculoskeletal System

If the patient's chief complaint is caused by traumatic injury, assessment of the patient's musculoskeletal system is necessary. Do all extremities appear to be properly positioned and functioning normally? Assess the patient's posture if he or she is standing. Also, look at the joints, checking for range of motion (ROM) by asking the patient how much he or she can move the extremity or joint. Ask if any ROM limitations are a new sign or chronic condition. Never force a painful joint to move. Always compare the right side with the left side, looking for weakness or atrophy, and assess equality of grip strength. Expose the site of injury, and evaluate the pulse and motor and sensory function adjacent to and below the affected area.

Table 5-3 Normal Range for Blood Pressure	
Age	**Range (mm g)**
Adults	90 to 140 (systolic)
Children (ages 1 to 8 years)	80 to 110 (systolic)
Infants (newborn to age 1 year)	50 to 95 (systolic)

Anatomic Regions

Inspect for abnormalities of the head, neck, and cervical spine. Gently palpate the scalp and skull for any pain, deformity, tenderness, crepitus, and bleeding. Ask a responsive patient if he or she feels any pain or tenderness.

Look at the patient's face. Check his or her eyes and assess pupillary function, shape, and response. Assess the color of the sclera and check the patient's cheekbones (zygomas) for possible injury. Inspect the patient's ears and nose for fluid.

Next, before opening the patient's mouth, check the upper (maxillae) and lower (mandible) jaw. Open the patient's mouth, looking for any broken or missing teeth. Note the presence of any unusual odors that may be present in the patient's mouth; this may give an indication of which type of emergency you are dealing with.

Check the neck for signs of swelling or bleeding. Palpate for signs of trauma, such as deformities, bumps, swelling, bruising, or bleeding as well as a crackling sound produced by air bubbles under the skin. Also, in patients where spinal injury is not suspected, inspect for pronounced or distended jugular veins with the patient sitting at a 45° angle. This is a normal finding in a person who is lying down; in contrast, jugular vein distention in a patient who is sitting up suggests a problem with blood returning to the heart. If spinal injury is suspected, apply a cervical collar at this time. Report and record your findings carefully.

When you are assessing the chest, inspect, visualize, and palpate over the chest area for injury or signs of trauma, including bruising, tenderness, or swelling. Watch for both sides of the chest to rise and fall together with normal breathing. Observe for abnormal breathing signs, including retractions or paradoxical motion. Retractions indicate the patient has some condition, usually medical, that impairs the flow of air into and out of the lungs. Paradoxical motion is associated with a fracture of several ribs (flail chest), which causes a section of the chest to move independently from the rest of the chest wall. Feel for grating of the bones as the patient breathes. Crepitus is often associated with rib fractures. Palpate the chest for subcutaneous emphysema, especially in cases of severe blunt chest trauma.

If the patient reports difficulty breathing or has evidence of trauma to the chest, auscultate breath and lung sounds. This step helps you evaluate air movement in and out of the lungs. During this assessment, it is important to compare one side to the other. If the patient's breathing is abnormal, reassess breathing, apply oxygen and, if necessary, assist with ventilations using positive pressure with a bag-mask device.

Inspect and palpate the abdomen for any obvious injuries, bruising, and bleeding. Be sure to palpate all four quadrants of the abdomen, evaluating for symmetry, masses, tenderness, and bleeding. Ask about pain as you perform the examination. Always start the palpation of the abdomen in the quadrant farthest from the patient's pain, palpating the painful quadrant last. Consider the anatomy underlying the quadrant of the abdomen being examined; this may suggest the possible cause of the problem or the area that is likely to be injured.

Reassessment

Reassessment should be performed at regular intervals during the assessment process to identify and treat changes in the patient's condition **FIGURE 5-11**. For a stable patient, reassessment should occur at least every 15 minutes; an unstable patient should be reassessed every 5 minutes. Reassessment may involve the following steps:

1. Repeat the primary assessment.
2. Reassess and record vital signs and identify trends.
3. Reassess the chief complaint. Determine whether the pain or discomfort remains the same or whether it is getting better or worse. Identify any new or previously undisclosed complaints.
4. Reassess previously applied interventions to monitor their effectiveness and determine the need for new interventions.
5. Identify and treat any new life threats or changes in the patient's condition.
6. Reassess unstable patients every 5 minutes (or as often as practical depending on the patient's condition) and stable patients every 15 minutes (or as deemed appropriate by the patient's condition).

Reassessment A step within the patient assessment process that is performed at regular intervals during the assessment process. Its purpose is to identify and treat changes in a patient's condition. An unstable patient should be reassessed every 5 minutes, whereas a stable patient should be reassessed every 15 minutes.

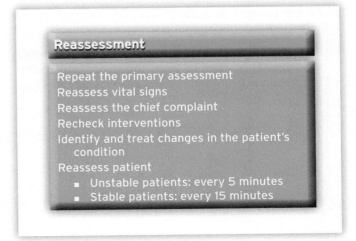

FIGURE 5-11 Reassessment process.

Clinical Decision Making and Critical Thinking

Effective clinical decision making is dependent on an AEMT's ability to gather and evaluate patient information, develop an idea of the patient's problem based on gathered information and the patient's presentation, and formulate a field impression on which an appropriate patient treatment plan will be based.

The prehospital setting may be one of controlled chaos; your sources of information can be overwhelming or severely limited. You must be able to mentally triage this information in a very short time, separate relevant from irrelevant data, and provide the most appropriate care for the patient. These are the cornerstones of being an effective EMS provider.

Gathering, analyzing, and correctly synthesizing patient information will culminate in an appropriate treatment plan. This process requires an understanding of the patient's injury or illness and the impact that your care will have on it. You will develop needed critical thinking skills through field experience in dealing with multiple patients with varying problems. In every assessment you perform, practice the following critical thinking skills:

- Ensure that you have an adequate fund of knowledge. This refers to your knowledge and understanding of how injuries and illnesses may affect the patient. Knowledge is acquired from initial training, continuing education, and experience.
- Focus on specific and multiple elements of data. Multiple amounts of specific, crucial data, often from multiple sources, must be obtained to direct your assessment and subsequent treatment.
- Identify and organize data and form concepts. Your overall understanding of the situation and the treatment you provide to the patient are only as good as the quality and quantity of data you obtain.
- Differentiate between relevant and irrelevant data. You must be able to determine which data are relevant to your assessment and care of the patient. Irrelevant or extraneous data can skew your interpretation of the overall situation, potentially leading to inappropriate care.
- Analyze and compare similar situations. Although no two patients present in the exact same manner, you must be able to integrate the information obtained regarding the current incident with similar situations and experiences. This will enhance your overall understanding of the current situation and will prepare you to deal with future situations.
- Recall contrary situations. Recalling and learning from bad experiences enhances your ability to manage the current situation.
- Articulate assessment-based decisions and construct arguments. You must be able to defend your actions and justify the decisions on which you based your treatment.
- The performance of your duties will constantly be challenged by the environment in which you must function. Time is perhaps your biggest challenge, especially when managing a critically ill or injured patient. Factors that can hamper your ability to perform patient care—crowds of people, volatile scenes, poor lighting, weather extremes, bumpy ambulances—usually do not exist in other medical settings. Your ability to improvise, adapt, and overcome these unique obstacles—and still provide appropriate patient care—will make you an effective clinical decision maker and a true prehospital professional. Always base your treatment or transport decisions on a complete assessment.

PREP KIT

Ready for Review

- The assessment process begins with the scene size-up, which identifies real or potential hazards. The patient should not be approached until these hazards have been dealt with in such a way that eliminates or minimizes risk to the AEMTs, the patient(s), and any bystanders.
- A primary assessment is performed on all patients. It includes forming an initial general impression of the patient, including the LOC, and identifies any life-threatening conditions to the patient's airway, breathing, and circulation. Any life threats identified must be treated before moving on to the next step of the assessment.
- History taking includes an investigation of the patient's chief complaint or history of present illness. A SAMPLE history is generally taken during this step of the assessment process, with the necessary information being obtained from the patient, family, friends, or bystanders.
- The secondary assessment is a physical examination of the patient. The physical examination may be a systematic head-to-toe, full-body scan or one that focuses on a certain area or region of the body; this is often determined on the basis of the chief complaint.
- The secondary assessment is performed on scene or in the back of the ambulance en route to the hospital. If the patient has uncontrolled problems identified during the primary assessment, the AEMT may not have time to perform a secondary assessment.
- Reassessment of a patient includes re-evaluation of the chief complaint, patient status including the ABCs, and interventions to ensure that they are still being delivered correctly. Information from this reassessment is used to identify and treat changes in the patient's condition.
- A patient in stable condition should be reassessed every 15 minutes, whereas a patient in unstable condition should be reassessed every 5 minutes.
- The assessment process is systematic and dynamic. Each assessment performed will be slightly different, depending on the condition of the patient and the MOI or NOI, or both. This process enables the AEMT to quickly identify and treat the individual needs of all patients.

Case Study

You and your partner arrive at the residence of a 43-year-old non–English-speaking woman who complains of abdominal pain. Her husband explains that her pain began last evening and has gotten progressively worse. He tells you the pain is "sharp" and reports it has localized to the right upper quadrant of his wife's abdomen. The pain is accompanied with several episodes of vomiting, and her husband reports that his wife's eyes are turning yellow. Her vital signs are a blood pressure of 138/82 mm Hg, a pulse of 102 beats/min, a respiratory rate of 20 breaths/min, a temperature of 101.8°F, and a pulse oximetry of 98% on room air. The patient has a past medical history of asthma and takes albuterol as needed. The husband denies any allergies.

1. Explain the difference between primary assessment and secondary assessment.

2. This patient's eyes would be described as:
   A. erythematous.
   B. cyanotic.
   C. jaundiced.
   D. pallor.

3. The patient in this scenario has a pulse oximetry reading of 98%. In which situations would a pulse oximetry reading be considered inaccurate?

4. This patient presents with a language barrier. How can you best manage this situation?

5. What is a pertinent negative?
   A. A negative finding that requires further care and/or intervention
   B. A negative finding that requires ALS
   C. A negative finding that implies another condition may be present
   D. A negative finding that requires no further care or intervention

CHAPTER 6

Pharmacology

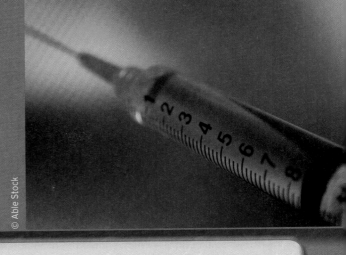

© Able Stock

National EMS Education Standard

Pharmacology
Applies to patient assessment and management fundamental knowledge of the medications carried by AEMTs that may be administered to a patient during an emergency.

Review

During your EMT-I training you learned about medication names, classifications of drugs, indications and contraindications of medication administration, and how medications are supplied. This chapter takes a close look at each of the forms of medications you may be called on to administer or help patients to self-administer.

What's New

As an AEMT, there are more medications that you may administer based on protocols or with permission from medical control. You must have an understanding of how these medications work and the correct dosage and administration for specific patients. The *National EMS Education Standards* include more in-depth information regarding medication safety and legislation, as well as autonomic pharmacology, metabolism and excretion, mechanism of drug action, and much more.

▌Introduction

All medications are poisons if they are given to the wrong patient or in toxic quantities. As an AEMT, you will be responsible for administering certain medications to patients and helping them to self-administer others. You will ask patients about their medication allergies and you will report this information to hospital personnel. To act without understanding how medications work will place patients and you in danger.

Before you administer any medication to a patient, you must have a thorough understanding of how the medication will affect the body—both negatively and positively. This includes familiarity with the medication's mechanism of action, indications, contraindications, route(s) of administration, dose, adverse reactions, and what to do in the event of an adverse reaction. This also is true of the patient's current medications that you may assist him or her in taking.

Disastrous results, including death, may occur if you administer an inappropriate drug or dose, give a drug by the wrong route, or give the medication too rapidly or too slowly.

▌Drug Terminology

Pharmacology is the study of the properties (characteristics) and effects of drugs and medications on the body. *Drugs* are chemical agents used in the diagnosis, treatment, and prevention of disease. Although the terms drugs and medications are often used interchangeably, the word drugs may make some people think of narcotics or illegal substances. For this reason, you should try to use the word medications, especially when interviewing patients and families. In general terms, a *medication* is a chemical substance that is used to treat or prevent disease or relieve pain.

> *Pharmacology* The study of the properties (characteristics) and effects of drugs and medications on the body.
> *Drugs* Chemical agents used in the diagnosis, treatment, and prevention of disease.
> *Medication* A chemical substance that is used to treat or prevent disease or relieve pain.

Table 6-1
Components of a Drug Profile
Drug names—This includes the generic name, trade name, and chemical name.
Classification—What type of drug is this? What is it used for?
Mechanisms of action—How does it work? What is its intended purpose?
Indications—What are the reasons for taking this drug?
Contraindications—When should the drug not be given? Does it affect certain medical conditions or react with other medications adversely?
Pharmacokinetics—How is it absorbed, metabolized, and so forth? What is its *half-life*?
Side and adverse effects—Are there any side effects? What are the adverse effects?
Routes of administration—How is it given?
How supplied—What is the total quantity of the medication? What form?
Dosages—This generally includes proper dosages for adult, pediatric, and special considerations, such as when to modify the dosage based on the patient's history.
Special considerations—These are considerations for certain groups such as pediatric, geriatric, and pregnant patients, and other special patient groups.
Other—The drug profile may include any other information that is vital to the user.

A drug profile gives all of the specifics about the drug. This is the information included on the package insert and listed in various pharmaceutical publications. **TABLE 6-1** lists components of a drug profile.

Half-life The time required by the body, tissue, or organ to metabolize or inactivate half the amount of a substance taken in—an important consideration in determining the proper dose of drug and frequency of administration.

US Regulation of Pharmaceuticals

The manufacture of pharmaceuticals in the United States and most other countries is subject to a variety of laws and regulations. The goal of these laws and regulations is to protect consumers. In particular, they prohibit manufacturers from making false claims about the benefits of their drugs and prohibit advising patients on the administration of the drugs, which may be incorrect. These laws also seek to protect patients from drugs that might cause harm and require

drug manufacturers to publish information about side effects and known potential harmful effects of their products.

Laws and regulations also outline standards for drug manufacture to ensure that drugs produced by different manufacturers are uniform in strength and purity. In the United States, these drug standards are published in the *USP* and the *National Formulary*. In addition, several federal laws have been enacted to protect consumers (patients) from unsafe substances and unscrupulous manufacturers and distributors.

In 1970, Congress enacted the Controlled Substances Act, comprehensive legislation dealing with narcotic and nonnarcotic drugs that have a potential for abuse. This act specifies requirements for registration, procurement, storage, distribution, and record keeping for these drugs as well as penalties for failure to comply with these requirements. The drugs covered by the Controlled Substances Act are classified into five categories, or *schedules*, according to their abuse potential **TABLE 6-2**. Schedule I includes drugs with the highest abuse potential, and Schedule V includes drugs with the lowest abuse potential.

Manufacturing-Related Regulations

Federal legislation also focuses on guaranteeing standardization of doses. Standardization assures patients that when they take a medication with a stated amount of the active ingredient, they will, in fact, receive that amount of the drug. Clearly, no one would want to be prescribed a certain dose of a drug and find that the actual medication contained twice (or half) the amount of active ingredient stated on the drug's label. For a drug to carry the USP label, the amount of active ingredients must be within 95% to 105% of that stated on the label. For example, if the label says "300 mg of amiodarone," the medication must contain between 285 mg and 315 mg of the drug.

Government Agencies That Regulate Drugs

Today, regulation of drugs in the United States falls under the jurisdiction of several agencies:

- The FDA enforces the Food, Drug, and Cosmetic Act. As part of its responsibilities, the FDA is charged with determining the safety and efficacy of drugs before they are allowed to enter the US market.
- The Drug Enforcement Agency (DEA), formerly the Bureau of Narcotics and Dangerous Drugs, was created by the Federal Controlled Substances Act of 1970. The DEA, which is a division of the Justice Department, is responsible for executing the provisions of the Controlled Substances Act, including the registration of physicians who are permitted to dispense controlled substances.
- The Public Health Service regulates biologic products—that is, medications made from living organisms such as antitoxins and vaccines.

Table 6-2
Drug Schedules According to the Controlled Substances Act*

- Schedule I. These drugs generally have high abuse potential and a propensity for severe dependence; many of them have no accepted medical application. In general, Schedule I drugs are outlawed under federal law, although certain states may actually have less control on certain drugs within this category. On rare occasions, and under the strictest control by the FDA and DEA, these drugs may be used for research, analysis, and instruction only. Examples are heroin, lysergic acid diethylamide (LSD), marijuana, methylenedioxymethamphetamine (MDMA), psilocybin, and mescaline.

- Schedule II. These drugs have a very high abuse potential and may lead to severe addiction, but some have a lower propensity for addiction than Schedule I drugs. Examples are amphetamines, opiates, cocaine, meperidine-hydrochloride (Demerol), and short-acting barbiturates.

- Schedule III. The narcotics listed in Schedule III (limited opioids combined with noncontrolled substances such as hydrocodone-acetaminophen combination [Vicodin] and acetaminophen [Tylenol] with codeine) have a lower potential for abuse than Schedule I and II drugs. These drugs may lead to low or moderate physical dependence or high psychological dependence.

- Schedule IV. These drugs have a low abuse potential compared with Schedule III drugs and have limited dependence potential. Examples are phenobarbital, chloral hydrate, diazepam (Valium), and lorazepam (Ativan).

- Schedule V. Schedule V drugs (which include some opioids) have the lowest potential for abuse of all controlled substances, although they may lead to limited dependence. Examples include cough syrups containing codeine.

*Some states have enacted their own laws or regulations related to the use, storage, and handling of controlled substances, including medical marijuana, and individual state requirements may vary. If the state law is more stringent than the federal law, the state law takes precedence.

Table 6-3
Four Phases of a Clinical Trial

- Phase I. The new drug is tested in healthy volunteers to compare human data with those in animals to determine safe doses of the drug and to assess its safety.

- Phase II. These trials are performed in homogeneous populations of patients (50 to 300 patients). In double-blind studies, one group receives the drug and the other group receives a placebo. These studies are designed to evaluate the efficacy and safety of the drug and to establish which form is the most effective dose.

- Phase III. In these clinical trials, the drug is made available to a larger group of patients (several thousand). These studies, which usually last several years, definitively establish the efficacy of the drug and monitor the nature and incidence of side effects.

- Phase IV. After successful completion of Phase III clinical trials, the drug company can apply to the FDA for approval to market the drug. Phase IV trials compare the new drug with others on the market and examine the drug's long-term efficacy and cost-effectiveness.

The Drug-Approval Process

New drugs are constantly being developed. The commercialization process, however, takes years—the average time for a drug to be developed, tested, and approved is about 9 years. In some cases, manufacturers spend most of those 9 years developing a drug, only to find out that the drug does not work as envisioned or is too dangerous for human consumption.

All new drugs must go through animal studies and clinical trials in humans before they are approved for distribution. Animal studies are designed to learn more about the properties of a drug and to identify tissues and organs that are sensitive to the actions of the drug. Testing in at least two animal species is required by law. After successful completion of animal studies, an investigational new drug may enter clinical trials in humans. Clinical trials proceed in four phases, as described in TABLE 6-3 .

FDA Classification of Newly Approved Drugs

In an effort to effectively and accurately categorize medications, the Center for Drug Evaluation and Research (CDER) at the FDA uses a streamlined process to assign a numeric and letter classification to aid in the approval process. The classifications used by CDER reflect the type of drug being submitted and its intended uses.

Numeric classifications are as follows:

1. A new molecular drug: A completely new medication that is not derived from an existing drug

- The Federal Trade Commission (FTC) monitors drug advertising and ensures that it is not misleading or inappropriate. The FTC has become involved in making recommendations to the FDA regarding direct-to-consumer (DTC) advertisements. The FTC found that DTC advertisements "generally benefit consumers" but stated that DTC ads should contain a major statement of drug risks along with adequate provision for more complete risk information.

2. A new salt of a previously approved drug (not a new molecular drug): A new medication that is derived from an existing drug

3. A new formulation of a previously approved drug (not a new salt *or* a new molecular drug): Manufacturer changes made to a drug that has already been created and approved

4. A new combination of two or more drugs: Two or more medications that have been combined to make administration easier by reducing the number of pills needed

5. An already marketed drug product (for example, a duplication, a new manufacturer): Often seen when a manufacturer's patent is expired and generic versions are produced

6. A new indication or claim for a drug that is already being marketed (including drugs that switch from prescription to over-the-counter [OTC]): Additional benefits of a drug that have been found beyond those originally stated

7. A drug that is already marketed with no new drug application: Classification of medications that are already in use but not classified according to this system

Special Considerations in Drug Therapy

Pregnant Patients

Before you administer any medications to a female of childbearing age, the patient should be asked whether she could possibly be pregnant. In an emergency situation, the health of the woman is the priority. However, before using any drug during pregnancy, the expected benefits should be considered against the possible risk to the fetus. Drugs, whether prescription or OTC, have the potential to harm the fetus by crossing the placental barrier, as well as through lactation. A *teratogenic* drug is one that poses a risk to the normal development or health of the unborn fetus.

> *Teratogenic* Poses a risk to the normal development or health of the unborn fetus.

Changes in a pregnant woman's body also affect the way drugs are processed and may increase the chance of harm to the fetus. Metabolism of drugs in the liver is decreased during pregnancy, along with an increased rate of excretion because of increased cardiac output.

The FDA has established a scale with the categories A, B, C, D, and X to indicate drugs that have documented problems in animals and/or humans during pregnancy **TABLE 6-4**. Category A drugs pose the least risk, whereas Category X drugs pose the greatest risk to the fetus.

There are still many drugs used with unknown effects during pregnancy. For this reason, it is better to delay

Table 6-4
FDA Categories of Drugs That May Pose Risk to the Fetus

- Category A. No documented risk to the human fetus at any point throughout the pregnancy has been shown.

- Category B. Studies in animals have not demonstrated a risk to the fetus; however, adequate studies have not been performed in humans. Drugs in this category also include those in which human studies have not demonstrated adverse effects in the first or third trimester of pregnancy; however, studies in animals have demonstrated adverse effects during these same time periods.

- Category C. Studies in animals have demonstrated adverse effects; however, studies have not been conducted in humans. Drugs in this category also include those in which adequate studies have not been conducted in animals or humans.

- Category D. Risk to the human fetus has been demonstrated; however, administration of the drug may outweigh the risk of potential adverse effects in certain circumstances.

- Category X. Risk of adverse effects has clearly been demonstrated in humans; therefore, these drugs should not be administered to pregnant women or women who could potentially be pregnant.

pharmacologic treatments for pregnant patients until they reach the hospital except in life-threatening situations.

In the field, you must be able to quickly evaluate the risks versus the benefits of drug administration. Does the potential benefit to the pregnant woman outweigh the risk to the fetus? If the drug is the only option for saving the woman's life, then that consideration would be paramount. When in doubt, contact medical control to discuss the situation.

Pediatric Patients

Medications have much different effects in adults than they do in children—whether the pediatric patient is a newborn, a neonate, an infant, or a toddler. Young infants have a sharply reduced metabolic capacity. The incomplete development of the gastrointestinal tract in young infants slows absorption of oral medications and delays elimination, so the same medication may be more potent in an infant than in an adult.

However, children can metabolize some medications much more quickly than adults do, so they may require relatively higher doses or more frequent administration of some medications. Also, the products of metabolism in children can vary from those seen in adults, which may sometimes result in unexpected responses.

Transition Tip

When you are treating pediatric patients, it is imperative to remember that they are not little adults. Medication dosage is usually based on a child's weight or body surface area as opposed to age because size varies greatly from child to child. If possible, determine the exact weight of the child by asking the parent or guardian. With infants and toddlers, a length-based resuscitation tape works well for estimating and also gives accurate dosage information for most emergency drugs and sizes for endotracheal tubes and IV catheters.

When you are treating neonates, it is important to remember that they have immature body systems and are unable to metabolize drugs as quickly as an older child or adult can. Medications tend to remain in the system for longer periods, resulting in lengthened times of drug effect. Dosages may need to be altered to prevent inadvertent overdose.

Table 6-5
Guidelines for Providing Drug Therapy

Understand pharmacology.
Use correct precautions and techniques.
Observe and document the effects of drugs, good or bad.
Obtain a drug history from patients, including prescribed medications (name, strength, and daily dosage), OTC medications, vitamins, herbal preparations, and drug reactions. If possible, gather all medications to take along to the hospital with the patient.
Perform an evaluation to identify drug indications and contraindications.
Establish and maintain professional relationships.
Keep your knowledge base current for changes and trends in pharmacology.
Seek drug reference literature.
Consult with medical direction.

Geriatric Patients

The changes in pharmacokinetics in geriatric patients are comparable to those observed in young children. In elderly people, hepatic functions and gastrointestinal activity slow, which in turn delays absorption and elimination. In addition, geriatric patients are often taking several medications; these concomitant therapies may interact and modify the effects of each medication. Furthermore, because geriatric patients may take a large number of medications and may have alterations in their normal mental status, geriatric patients may unintentionally overdose on a particular drug or forget to take it.

■ Scope of Practice

As an AEMT, you are legally, morally, and ethically responsible for each drug you administer. You must have a good foundation of knowledge of OTC and prescription medications that may interact with drugs you may give, and you must have enough knowledge to obtain a medical history for patients who are unable to communicate.

Drug administration must be safe and therapeutically effective. You should always keep a field guide or other medication reference handy to look up medications that are unfamiliar to you. Follow the standardized national guidelines listed in **TABLE 6-5** when providing drug therapy.

■ Methods of Drug Classification

Classifications of drugs are based on the effect the drugs will have on a particular part of the body or on a specific condition. Antiemetic medications, for example, suppress the sensation of nausea. Many medications fall into more than one classification. For example, promethazine (Phenergan) is an antiemetic and an antihistamine. This section discusses a few of the classifications of drugs and their subcategories.

Drugs or medications can be classified into the following three categories:

- By body system: Classification by body system is simply categorizing by the system affected by that drug. Nitroglycerin is a vasodilator that is used predominantly for cardiac ischemia; therefore, it is classified as a cardiac drug. Understanding which systems are affected by which drugs will help you make the appropriate decisions for patient care.
- Class of agent: The class of a medication tells how it affects the system. For example, an antipyretic is given to reduce fever and an antiemetic is used to control vomiting.
- Mechanism of action: The mechanism of action is the particular action by which the drug creates its desired effect on an organism. Again using the example of nitroglycerin, it is a potent vasodilator given for cardiac ischemia because it opens the vessels to allow oxygenated blood to pass through.

Nervous System Classifications

The nervous system is the body's principal control system. It is composed of the central nervous system (CNS), made up of the brain and spinal cord, and the peripheral nervous system, which includes all of the nervous tissue outside the CNS.

Recall that the peripheral nervous system contains the *autonomic nervous system (ANS)*, which controls all of the automatic, or involuntary, functions. The ANS is divided into the sympathetic nervous system and the parasympathetic nervous system. The *sympathetic nervous system* is responsible for the body's response to shock and stress and is known as the "fight-or-flight" division. This response is associated with the release of adrenaline from the adrenal glands. The sympathetic nervous system response is called *adrenergic* because special adrenergic nerve fibers ultimately cause the release of the hormones epinephrine (adrenaline) and norepinephrine (noradrenaline). Sympathetic responses include shunting of blood from the extremities to the vital core organs, increasing the heart rate and respirations, increasing blood pressure, dilation of the pupils, and reduction of digestive system activity.

The *parasympathetic nervous system* relaxes the body. It controls automatic functions during nonstressful times and is referred to as the "rest and relax" division. Stimulation of the parasympathetic nervous system results in effects opposite from those of the sympathetic nervous system. Heart and respiratory rates decrease, lowering the blood pressure, constricting the pupils, and increasing digestive system activity.

> *Autonomic nervous system (ANS)* The part of the nervous system that regulates functions not controlled consciously, such as digestion and sweating.
> *Sympathetic nervous system* Subdivision of the autonomic nervous system that governs the body's fight-or-flight reactions by inducing smooth muscle contraction or relaxation of the blood vessels and bronchioles.
> *Adrenergic* Pertaining to nerves that release the neurotransmitter norepinephrine or noradrenaline; also pertains to the receptors acted on by norepinephrine.
> *Parasympathetic nervous system* A subdivision of the autonomic nervous system, involved in control of involuntary, vegetative functions, mediated largely by the vagus nerve through the chemical acetylcholine.

The sympathetic and parasympathetic divisions work in constant opposition to each other to maintain basic harmony in the body, with each division taking more precedence in the proper circumstances.

The hormones released by sympathetic system stimulation are carried throughout the body, where they cause their intended effects by acting directly on hormone receptors. This stimulates tissues that are not innervated by sympathetic nerves and also prolongs the effects of direct sympathetic stimulation. Adrenergic receptors are located throughout the body and, once stimulated by the appropriate hormone, they cause a response in the target organ. Adrenergic receptors are generally divided into four types **TABLE 6-6**.

Drugs Affecting the Sympathetic Nervous System

To give the best patient care, it is imperative for the AEMT to recognize how certain medications affect the body. Drugs can be given that produce the same effects on a body system as the hormones of the sympathetic nervous system that are released naturally in the body. These drugs are known as *sympathomimetics* because they mimic the effects of the sympathetic nervous system. Medications that have the opposite effect, or inhibit the sympathetic nervous system, are known as *sympatholytics* (also known as antiadrenergics), which antagonize, or fight against the effects of the sympathetic nervous system. Drugs that counteract the action of something else are called *antagonists*, while drugs that bind to a receptor and cause a response are called *agonists*.

> *Sympathomimetics* Drugs that produce the same effects as the hormones of the sympathetic nervous system.
> *Sympatholytics* Drugs that block the actions of the sympathetic nervous system.
> *Antagonists* Molecules that block the ability of a given chemical to bind to its receptor, preventing a biologic response; in the pharmacologic sense, drugs that counteract the action of something else.
> *Agonists* Substances that mimic the actions of a specific neurotransmitter or hormone by binding to the specific receptor of the naturally occurring substance.

Transition Tip

Imagine beta blockers as the plastic plugs placed in electric sockets to prevent children from sticking things into them. The plugs do not do anything; they only plug up the holes. Beta blockers work the same way. They have no effect on the body; they only plug up the receptor sites, preventing beta agonists from binding.

Transition Tip

Think of the hormones of the sympathetic nervous system as a key that starts a car. When the key is placed in the ignition (or the hormone is placed in the receptor site) and the key is turned, a certain sequence of events occurs to start the car. If you have a duplicate key made and use it to start the car, the same sequence of events takes place. This is exactly what happens when a sympathomimetic drug (the duplicate key) is introduced into the body. The same sequence of events takes place when the duplicate is joined with the receptor site.

Some medications stimulate alpha and beta receptors, whereas others are selective to specific receptors. A medication that agonizes (stimulates) the alpha-1 receptors causes vasoconstriction of the vessels, thereby increasing blood pressure, cardiac preload, and afterload. When these receptors are antagonized (suppressed), the blood pressure is lowered by preventing vasoconstriction.

Many patients take medications that belong to the *beta blocker* class. These are used to control blood pressure in some patients and heart rhythm disturbances in others. Beta blockers work by filling a portion of the beta receptor sites—the portion to which beta stimulators would normally bind. In this way, beta effects are prevented.

Beta blocker A common class of cardiac drugs that blocks beta effects, causing a decrease in the workload of the heart by reducing the speed of contraction and reducing blood pressure.

In the prehospital setting, you will often administer drugs that agonize the beta-1 receptors in an attempt to treat cardiac arrest and hypotension. Stimulation of these receptors increases myocardial contractility. In contrast, antagonizing the beta-1 receptors lowers the blood pressure by limiting the myocardial contractility and the heart rate. It also decreases impulse generation in the heart and slows the conduction at the atrioventricular node, thereby treating tachycardia.

Beta-2 selective drugs cause bronchodilation with little effect on the heart, which only has beta-1 receptor sites. Stimulation of the beta-2 receptors allows you to treat asthma and other diseases that cause excessive narrowing of the bronchioles.

Drugs Affecting the Parasympathetic Nervous System

Like the sympathetic division, agonists to the parasympathetic nervous system are known as *parasympathomimetics* and antagonists are known as *parasympatholytics*. One of the most commonly used parasympatholytics is the drug atropine, which is used for symptomatic bradycardia as well as exposure to organophosphates and certain chemical nerve agents.

Parasympathomimetics Drugs that produce the same effects as those of the parasympathetic nervous system; also known as cholinergics.
Parasympatholytics Drugs that block the actions of the parasympathetic nervous system; also known as anticholinergics.

Transition Tip

Atropine is a potent *parasympatholytic* used to increase the heart rate in symptomatic bradycardia. Because increasing the heart rate is an effect of the sympathetic nervous system, you might think that atropine is classified as a sympathomimetic. However, atropine has no effect on the heart itself. Instead, it acts as a roadblock to the vagus nerve and prevents innervation by acetylcholine. It does not directly affect the target organ, in this case the heart, but prevents anything from passing through. Because it decreases the effects of the parasympathetic nervous system (which slows the heart rate), it is an antagonist to the parasympathetic division, or a parasympatholytic.

Parasympathomimetics are also called *cholinergic* medications because they stimulate the cholinergic receptors, to which acetylcholine (ACh) normally binds. ACh is an

Table 6-6 Alpha and Beta Responses	
Alpha-1 (α_1)	Peripheral vasoconstriction
Alpha-2 (α_2)	Peripheral vasodilation Little or no bronchoconstriction
Beta-1 (β_1)	Increased heart rate Increased automaticity Increased contractility Increased conductivity
Beta-2 (β_2)	Bronchodilation Vasodilation

important neurotransmitter in the parasympathetic nervous system. Cholinergic medications may act directly or indirectly on cholinergic receptors. A drug that has direct action binds with cholinergic receptors, thereby blocking ACh. A drug that has indirect action interacts with acetylcholinesterase (AChE), which normally deactivates ACh.

Cholinergic Fibers in the parasympathetic nervous system that release a chemical called acetylcholine.

When a drug interacts with AChE, deactivation of ACh does not occur. If excessive cholinergics are present, the patient may exhibit the SLUDGE phenomena: increased Salivation/sweating, Lacrimation, Urination, Defecation/drooling/diarrhea, Gastric upset/cramps, and Emesis. Patients exposed to certain fertilizers, insecticides, VX (a nerve agent), and sarin gas exhibit SLUDGE symptoms because all of these substances have cholinergic properties.

Parasympatholytics are also called *anticholinergic* medications; they block the two types of cholinergic receptors (muscarinic and nicotinic). *Muscarinic cholinergic antagonists* block ACh exclusively at the muscarinic receptors. Atropine, for example, is a muscarinic cholinergic antagonist; it decreases secretions, increases the heart rate, dilates the pupils, and decreases gastrointestinal system activity. On the other hand, nicotinic cholinergic antagonists block ACh exclusively at the nicotinic receptors. This inhibition effectively disables the ANS, so it is virtually never used.

Anticholinergic Of or pertaining to blockage of acetylcholine receptors, resulting in inhibition of transmission of parasympathetic nerve impulses.
Muscarinic cholinergic antagonists Medications that block acetylcholine exclusively at the muscarinic receptors; an example is atropine.

Analgesics and Antagonists

Analgesics include medications that relieve pain—that is, induce analgesia (the absence of the sensation of pain). Sometimes the analgesic itself is not sufficient to relieve pain, in which case an adjunct medication may be given to enhance the effects of the analgesic.

The most common class of medications used for analgesia in the prehospital setting is opioid agonists. *Opioid agonists*, which are similar to or derived from the opium plant, bind to opiate receptors. By blocking these receptors, they prevent the neurons from sending pain signals. These medications are also CNS depressants. Fentanyl (Sublimaze) is a popular opioid agonist because it is rapid acting, very potent, and has a relatively short duration of action. The patient will experience analgesia within about 90 seconds, and the drug's effective duration lasts approximately 30 minutes.

Morphine is a popular option for prehospital analgesia. In addition to analgesia, morphine has a tendency to cause a euphoric feeling. Morphine has direct applications in cardiac emergencies because it decreases the workload on the heart (that is, cardiac preload and afterload) and, thereby, decreases the heart's consumption of oxygen.

Several *nonopioid analgesics* exist, many of which are available as OTC drugs. Many of these nonopioid analgesics have antipyretic properties as well, meaning they can reduce the patient's fever. All of them alter the production of prostaglandins and cyclooxygenase (Cox) to produce their effects. Three forms of nonopioid analgesics are particularly popular: salicylates (such as aspirin); *nonsteroidal anti-inflammatory drugs (NSAIDs)*, such as ibuprofen; and para-aminophenol derivatives (such as acetaminophen [Tylenol]).

> *Analgesics* A classification for medications that relieve pain, or induce analgesia.
> *Opioid agonists* Chemicals similar to or derived from the opium plant.
> *Nonopioid analgesics* Medications designed to relieve pain without the side effects of opioids.
> *Nonsteroidal anti-inflammatory drugs (NSAIDs)* Medications with analgesic, anti-inflammatory, and fever-reducing properties.

The NSAIDs are designed to reduce pain, inflammation, and fever. They work by inhibiting the Cox enzymes, which produce the chemical prostaglandin; prostaglandin, in turn, promotes pain, inflammation, and fever. Aspirin differs slightly from other NSAIDs in that it targets the Cox-1 enzymes to reduce platelet aggregation, which provides great benefit in patients who are suspected of having a myocardial infarction. This also explains why you cannot substitute another NSAID such as ibuprofen, which lacks the same anti-platelet aggregation effects for aspirin in this situation.

Opioid antagonists reverse the effects of opioid drugs. They bind with the opiate receptors in an antagonistic manner; as a result of this binding, the opioid molecules cannot get to the receptor, and the receptor cannot initiate its action. The most common opioid antagonist used in the prehospital setting is naloxone (Narcan).

Finally, *opioid agonist-antagonists* have agonistic and antagonistic properties. They are often preferred because they can decrease pain but do not diminish the function of the respiratory system or lead to dependence or addiction, unlike some other analgesics.

> *Opioid antagonists* A classification of medications that reverse the effects of opioid drugs.
> *Opioid agonist-antagonists* Medications designed to relieve pain without the side effects of opioids.

Antianxiety, Sedative, and Hypnotic Drugs

Drugs that produce sedation are used to help a patient sleep through a medical procedure. To ensure that the patient sleeps through the event, he or she also receives drugs that produce hypnosis. Drugs that create sedation and hypnosis include benzodiazepines, barbiturates, opioid agonists, and nonbarbiturate hypnotics. There are currently no drugs in these categories that are within the scope of practice of the AEMT.

Benzodiazepines are the sedatives most commonly used to prepare patients for invasive procedures. Although their exact mechanism of action is not fully understood, these drugs are believed to affect the neurotransmitter gamma-aminobutyric acid (GABA) in the brain. Benzodiazepine molecules bind to a receptor near GABA binding sites, which is thought to enhance their affinity for GABA. This increased affinity causes brain activity to slow. *Barbiturates* are believed to work very similarly to benzodiazepines by increasing the affinity between receptor sites and the neurotransmitter GABA.

> *Benzodiazepines* Sedative-hypnotic drugs that provide muscle relaxation and mild sedation; includes drugs such as diazepam (Valium) and midazolam (Versed).
> *Barbiturates* Potent sedative-hypnotics historically used as sleep aids, antianxiety drugs, and as part of the regimen for seizure control.

The *nonbarbiturate hypnotics* have almost identical properties to benzodiazepines and barbiturates in terms of how they affect GABA receptors. The difference is that nonbarbiturate hypnotics tend to have comparatively fewer side effects, particularly in terms of cardiovascular compromise.

> *Nonbarbiturate hypnotics* Medications designed to sedate without the side effects of a barbiturate.

Anticonvulsants

A seizure, in general terms, is a state of neurologic hyperactivity. Active seizures generally require treatment in the prehospital setting because of the complications associated with them. Although the exact mechanism behind *anticonvulsant medications* is not completely clear, these drugs are believed to work by inhibiting the influx of sodium into cells. This halt of sodium transport decreases the cells' ability to depolarize and propagate the seizures. Several other types of drugs are used as anticonvulsants, including benzodiazepines, barbiturates, hydantoins, and valproic acids.

> *Anticonvulsant medications* The medications used to treat seizures; believed to work by inhibiting the influx of sodium into cells.

Stimulants

A common group of CNS agents is *stimulants*, which exert their action by excitation of the CNS. Stimulation of the CNS can be accomplished one of two ways: by increasing excitatory neurotransmitters or by decreasing inhibitory neurotransmitters. Caffeine, cocaine, and amphetamines (prescription and illicit) are examples of CNS stimulants. They increase the release of dopamine and norepinephrine to increase wakefulness and awareness and reduce drowsiness and fatigue. They also increase tachycardia and hypertension and can cause seizures and psychosis. High doses of these agents can cause increased nervousness, irritability, tremors, and headache. Some people may also experience withdrawal symptoms when they stop taking stimulants.

> *Stimulants* An agent that increases the level of body activity.

Depressants

In other cases, patients may be prescribed CNS *depressants*. These agents are used to slow brain activity. They may be prescribed to treat anxiety, muscle tension, pain, insomnia, stress, panic attacks, and, in some cases, seizures. Some other CNS depressants are used as anesthetics. Examples of CNS depressants include lorazepam (Ativan), triazolam (Halcion), chlordiazepoxide (Librium), diazepam (Valium), alprazolam (Xanax), and zolpidem tartrate (Ambien).

> *Depressants* Agents used to slow brain activity.

Psychotherapeutic Drugs

Most psychotherapeutic drugs work by blocking dopamine receptors in the brain. Schizophrenia is often treated with medications that fit into the phenothiazine and butyrophenone classifications. These medications are associated with a host of side effects, which may include extrapyramidal symptoms, orthostatic hypotension, and sedation. They also have a tendency to cause sexual dysfunction. *Extrapyramidal symptoms* include a wide array of symptoms such as involuntary movements, tremors, rigidity, muscle contractions, restlessness, and changes in breathing and heart rate.

Depression is a common disorder for which many treatments are available. In particular, it is often treated with selective serotonin reuptake inhibitors (SSRIs) and monoamine oxidase inhibitors (MAOIs), which block the metabolism of monoamines in the brain. Although their popularity is waning, tricyclic antidepressants (TCAs) are still occasionally used as antidepressants.

> *Extrapyramidal symptoms* A wide array of symptoms such as involuntary movements, tremors, rigidity, muscle contractions, restlessness, and changes in breathing and heart rate; usually as a result of taking antipsychotic drugs.

Drugs Affecting the Cardiovascular System

The walls of the heart are composed of many interconnected cells. These cells are specialized to serve particular functions: Some conduct electrical impulses; others cause the heart to contract. Medications targeting the cardiovascular system are classified according to their effects on these specialized cells.

The various effects on the heart are categorized as follows. A *chronotropic* effect is one that affects the heart rate. An *inotropic* effect changes the force of contraction. A *dromotropic* effect is when a drug alters the velocity of the conduction of electricity through the heart. All three types of effects can be positive or negative. In other words, if there is a positive chronotropic effect, the heart rate has increased. If there is a negative inotropic effect, the heart is not squeezing as forcefully.

> *Chronotropic* Affecting the rate of contraction of the heart.
> *Inotropic* Affecting the contractility of the heart muscle.
> *Dromotropic* Affecting the velocity of conduction in the heart.

Cardiac Glycosides

Cardiac glycosides are a class of medications that are derived from plants. These drugs block certain ionic pumps in the membranes of the heart cells, which indirectly increases calcium concentrations. Cardiac glycosides in general have a small therapeutic index (margin of safety), however, and are associated with numerous side effects.

> *Cardiac glycosides* A classification of medications that naturally occur in plant substances and that block certain ionic pumps in the membranes of heart cells, which indirectly increases calcium concentrations; an example is digoxin.

Antiarrhythmic Medications

Antiarrhythmic medications have long been used in the prehospital setting to treat and prevent cardiac rhythm disorders. These medications can have direct and indirect effects on cardiac tissue. Antiarrhythmics are further classified into the following four groups according to their fundamental mode of action on the heart:

- Sodium channel blockers slow the conduction through the heart; in other words, they have a negative dromotropic effect.

- Beta blockers reduce the adrenergic stimulation of the beta receptors.
- Potassium channel blockers increase the heart's contractility (positive inotropy) and work against the reentry of blocked impulses.
- Calcium channel blockers block the inflow of calcium into the cardiac cells, thereby decreasing the force of contraction and automaticity. They may also decrease the negative conduction velocity (negative dromotropic effect).

> *Antiarrhythmic medications* The medications used to treat and prevent cardiac rhythm disorders.

Antihypertensive Medications

As many as 65 million people in the United States have hypertension or prehypertension. Medications administered to treat hypertension, known as *antihypertensives*, have the following treatment goals: keep blood pressure within normal limits, maintain or improve blood flow, and reduce the stress placed on the heart.

Diuretic medications cause the kidneys to remove excess amounts of salt and water in the body. By lowering the total fluid volume, they reduce the level of stress placed on the cardiovascular system. In particular, they lower the preload on the heart and decrease the stroke volume. *Vasodilator medications* act on the smooth muscles of the arterioles and veins. This property explains why nitroglycerin, a vasodilator, is so beneficial in treating myocardial ischemia. Unfortunately, the dilation of these vessels prompts a response from the sympathetic nervous system. As a consequence, when vasodilators are used to lower blood pressure, the patient must also take medications that inhibit the sympathetic nervous system.

> *Antihypertensives* Medications used to control blood pressure.
> *Diuretic medications* Medications designed to promote elimination of excess salt and water by the kidneys.
> *Vasodilator medications* Medications that work on the smooth muscles of the arterioles and/or the veins.

Sympathetic blocking agents include beta blockers and adrenergic inhibitors. Beta blockers, mentioned earlier, compete with epinephrine to bind with available receptor sites, thereby diminishing the effects of beta stimulation.

Angiotensin-converting enzyme (ACE) inhibitors target the renin-angiotensin-aldosterone system, which partially controls blood pressure. ACE inhibitors suppress the conversion of angiotensin I to angiotensin II, thereby decreasing blood pressure. Angiotensin II is a potent vasoconstrictor that promotes smooth muscle contraction in the arterioles throughout the body. This constriction raises the blood pressure by increasing peripheral resistance.

Calcium channel blockers, mentioned earlier, have antiarrhythmic and antihypertensive properties. By causing the dilation of coronary arteries, they enable more oxygen to reach the heart via coronary artery dilation. In addition, they prevent the contraction of smooth vascular muscle, which reduces resistance in the peripheral vascular system.

> *Sympathetic blocking agents* Antihypertensive medications that decrease cardiac output and renin secretions.
> *Angiotensin-converting enzyme (ACE) inhibitors* Medications that suppress the conversion of angiotensin I to angiotensin II.

Anticoagulants, Fibrinolytics, and Blood Components

Platelets repair damage in the blood vessels. This function is critical because defects in blood vessels can cause blood flow to slow, sometimes enough to result in the formation of a blood clot (also known as a thrombus). Abnormal thrombi may cause a life-threatening crisis such as acute coronary syndrome or stroke. A variety of medications are used to prevent or minimize the detrimental effects of thrombi.

Antiplatelet agents interfere with the aggregation, or collection, of platelets. They do not break down aggregated platelets but simply prevent further buildup of these blood cells. Notably, salicylic acid (aspirin) has significant antiplatelet properties and has proved important in the prehospital setting thanks to its ability to minimize the damage to the myocardium in acute coronary syndrome.

Anticoagulant drugs, as their name suggests, work against coagulation, thereby preventing thrombi from forming. Some patients can be prescribed anticoagulants on a long-term basis as a preventive measure, thereby avoiding the formation of thrombi associated with surgeries and certain cardiovascular conditions. You need to be aware of anticoagulant use, particularly when patients have sustained a traumatic injury. Just as anticoagulants prevent blood coagulation in the vascular system, they can also prevent the lifesaving coagulation needed to prevent blood loss.

> *Antiplatelet agents* The medications that interfere with the collection of platelets.
> *Anticoagulant drugs* The medications used to prevent intravascular thrombosis by preventing blood coagulation in the vascular system.

Once a blood clot has formed, a *fibrinolytic agent* may be administered to dissolve the thrombus and prevent it from breaking off and entering the bloodstream, where it might do further damage. Fibrinolytic agents actually promote the digestion of fibrin (the protein involved in forming a blood clot). The use of fibrinolytic medications in the prehospital setting remains controversial and, in some circumstances, other forms of reperfusion therapy may be indicated.

> *Fibrinolytic agent* A medication that dissolves blood clots after they have already formed; promotes the digestion of fibrin.

Drugs Affecting the Respiratory System

Oxygen is the most commonly used medication in the pre-hospital setting. And it is, in fact, a medication—which means it has appropriate and inappropriate uses and some side effects. Supplementary oxygen therapy is reviewed in the chapter, *Airway Management and Oxygenation.*

Patients may be taking a gamut of medications to treat respiratory problems, depending on their symptoms. Especially during the cold and influenza seasons, use of OTC decongestant medications is common. Patients may also take antihistamines during allergy season. Try to find out which medications your patient is taking, and know the effects that these drugs may have on other medications as well as the signs and symptoms they can produce. Although each decongestant varies slightly in terms of its mechanism of action, all such medications seek to reduce tissue edema, facilitate drainage, and maintain the patency of the sinuses.

Unfortunately, the fact that these and other medications are readily available sometimes leads to their illicit use. People looking for a high have been known to overdose on pseudoephedrine (a decongestant), dextromethorphan (an antitussive), or diphenhydramine (an antihistamine).

Serious respiratory emergencies often arise from severe narrowing of any portion of the respiratory tract. The respiratory tract is lined by smooth muscle fibers that influence the diameter of the airway. Control of the smooth muscles is maintained by the autonomic nervous system.

Many respiratory emergency treatments attempt to expand the respiratory tract by using sympathomimetic medications. Complications arise when patients with respiratory emergencies eventually experience decreased amounts of oxygen to the vital organs, including the heart. Increased heart rate and greater force of contraction lead to a higher demand for oxygen—but, of course, oxygen is already in short supply in a respiratory emergency. Therefore, stimulation of the beta-2 receptors, which produces bronchodilation and vasodilation, is very beneficial to patients with respiratory emergencies. These drugs produce smaller increases in heart rate and force of contraction and, thereby, dramatically decrease the body's rate of oxygen consumption.

A second-line treatment in a respiratory emergency is from *xanthines*. This class of drugs relieves airway constriction by relaxing the smooth muscles of the bronchioles and stimulating cardiac muscles to work harder, thereby increasing blood flow. These drugs also stimulate the CNS—in fact, one notable xanthine is the well-known CNS stimulant caffeine.

> *Xanthines* A classification of medications that affect the respiratory smooth muscle and that relax bronchiole smooth muscles, stimulate cardiac muscle, and stimulate the central nervous system.

Other respiratory medications suppress the inflammatory response that typically causes acute distress for patients with restrictive airway diseases. In the acute care setting, corticosteroids—including methylprednisolone (Solu-Medrol) and dexamethasone (Decadron)—can be administered for this purpose.

Drugs Affecting the Pancreas

A variety of hypoglycemic medications are available that affect the pancreas. Still others may not act on the pancreas directly, but rather alter the way insulin (produced by the pancreas) is used by the body. In the absence of pancreatic function, patients may take insulin injections.

To directly affect the pancreas, sulfonylureas increase insulin secretion from the pancreatic beta cells. This medication is effective only if patients have residual beta cell function. Insulin sensitivity is increased by thiazolidinediones and biguanides, which are oral hypoglycemic agents.

Drugs Affecting the Immunologic System

Patients who undergo organ transplantation or have an autoimmune disease are often prescribed *immunosuppressant medications*. Immunosuppressants are intended to inhibit the body's ability to attack the "foreign" organ, or, in the case of autoimmune diseases, the medications inhibit the body's attack on itself. These drugs are generally derived from fungi or bacteria and tend to have a complicated mechanism of action. Put succinctly, they inhibit lymphocytes and T cells from carrying out their immune functions.

> *Immunosuppressant medications* The medications intended to inhibit the body's ability to attack the "foreign" organ or, in the case of autoimmune diseases, the medications that inhibit the body's attack on itself.

Vitamins and Minerals

Vitamins and minerals are necessary substances that allow for normal metabolism, growth and development, and cellular function. Patients may be taking vitamin and mineral supplements to replace deficient items or as a preventive measure. Vitamins affect a wide variety of functions, but one particular focus in the prehospital setting is thiamine (vitamin B_1). Thiamine aids in converting carbohydrates into energy. People with alcoholism, among others, have a propensity to be deficient in this vitamin.

Pharmacokinetics: Movement of Drugs Through the Body

The effectiveness of a drug relates to its pharmaceutical properties, pharmacokinetics, and pharmacodynamics. Pharmaceutical properties determine a drug's concentration at its site of action.

Drugs modify existing functions of tissues and organs. They do not give new functions to tissues or organs. Also, drugs in general cause multiple actions rather than a single effect. A drug action, as previously discussed, is the result

Transition Tip

Geriatric patients often take many medications. They might also save medications left over from previous medical conditions to use if they need them in the future. Make every effort to identify which medications are current and what conditions they are being used to treat. Ask family members to help distinguish current from outdated medications, or look at the expiration dates on the medication labels. Take a list of the current medications or the drugs themselves with you to the emergency department.

Elderly patients can become confused about their medication regimen. Uncertainty about whether they missed a dose may cause them to repeat the medication, possibly leading to an overdose. If you think an overdose has occurred, contact medical control.

Along with the potential for overdosing, the physiologic effects of aging can lead to altered pharmacodynamics and pharmacokinetics. As the body ages and organs (such as the liver and kidneys) function less effectively, medications are not processed and filtered out of the system as quickly as in a younger person. Each time a dose of a particular drug is taken, it results in overaccumulation of that drug in the body. Decreased gastric motility can result in greater absorption time, and a decrease in total body water along with an increase in fat can lead to a greater concentration of drugs with weight-based dosages.

Medications can interact with each other, creating potentially harmful conditions for the patient. Even though a medication may be indicated for a certain condition, it might be contraindicated in the presence of another medication. For example, if the patient is taking the heart medication propranolol (Inderal), a beta blocker, and has an acute episode of shortness of breath, any asthma remedy might be rendered ineffective. Bronchodilation is a beta effect of most emergency asthma medications.

Medications such as sildenafil (Viagra), tadalafil (Cialis), and vardenafil (Levitra)—medications used to treat erectile dysfunction—can have potentially fatal interactions with common heart medications, specifically nitroglycerin. If used in combination with any of these medications, nitroglycerin can cause life-threatening hypotension as a result of severe vasodilation. Ask a patient who has been prescribed nitroglycerin if he or she has used Viagra, Cialis, or Levitra within the previous 24 to 36 hours. Report this to medical control.

While medications help people recover from acute conditions and adjust to chronic diseases, they can pose serious problems for geriatric patients. You should distinguish current from previous medications, suspect accidental or intentional overdoses, and be prepared for potentially lethal medication interactions. Document all findings and inform medical control.

---

of a physiochemical interaction between the drug and a molecule in the body, such as a receptor.

Once administered, drugs go through four stages: absorption, distribution, metabolism, and excretion. The study of these four stages and the metabolism and action of drugs is *pharmacokinetics*.

> *Pharmacokinetics* The study of the metabolism and action of drugs with a particular emphasis on the time required for absorption, duration of action, distribution in the body, and method of excretion.

Drug Absorption

The passage of a substance through some surface of the body into body fluids and tissues is known as absorption. Numerous variables affect drug absorption, including the nature of the absorbing surface, blood flow to the site of administration, solubility of the drug, pH, drug concentration, dosage form, route of administration **TABLE 6-7**, bioavailability, diffusion, osmosis, and filtration. **TABLE 6-8** describes these primary factors.

Drug Distribution

Drugs pass freely and quickly out of the vascular space and into the interstitial fluid. Therefore, blood flow to the area determines the amount of a drug reaching a particular part of the body. Most drugs tend to pass fairly easily from the intravascular compartment, through the interstitial spaces, and on to their target tissue. These drugs tend to have a rapid onset and a short duration of action. Other drugs become bound to serum proteins in the blood and are not immediately available to act on receptor sites. With the drug bound to the protein, it cannot produce an effect in a receptor site or diffuse through the tissues.

Some areas of the body, such as the brain and placenta, are less accessible to certain drugs than others. Drugs that are protein-bound or in an ionized form are weak penetrators of the blood-brain barrier. The blood-brain barrier and the placental barrier are both less permeable to provide protection to the brain and fetus, respectively.

Biotransformation

Many drugs are inactive when administered and only become active once they have been absorbed and converted into an active form in the blood or by the target tissue. The chemical alteration that a substance undergoes in the body is known as *biotransformation*. The primary organ for biotransformation is the liver. If the liver is diseased, inactivation (detoxification) of drugs may be impaired. This will also increase elimination time of the drug from the body, possibly resulting in toxic blood levels. The liver performs synthetic reactions that yield inactive products (metabolites) that can be secreted by the kidneys and nonsynthetic reactions, which may result in products

Table 6-7
Routes of Administration: Words and Their Meanings

This Word ...	From These Latin Words ...	Means
Inhalation	*inhalatio* (drawing air into the lungs)	inhaling or breathing in
Intramuscular (IM)	*intra* (into) and *muscularis* (of the muscles)	into muscle
Intraosseous (IO)	*intra* (into) and *osse* (bone)	into bone
Intravenous (IV)	*intra* (into) and *venosus* (of the veins)	into vein
Per os (PO)	*per* (by) and *os* (mouth)	by mouth
Per rectum (PR)	*per* (by) and *rectum* (rectum)	by rectum
Subcutaneous (SC)	*sub* (under) and *cutis* (skin)	under the skin
Sublingual (SL)	*sub* (under) and *lingua* (relating to the tongue)	under the tongue
Transcutaneous	(transdermal) *trans* (through) and *cutis* (skin)	through the skin
Intranasal	*intra* (into) and *nasal* (nose)	into the nose

Table 6-8
Primary Factors of Drug Absorption

Factor	Discussion
Nature of the absorbing surface	Some surfaces are highly permeable. It is much easier for a drug to travel through a single layer of cells than through multiple layers. The greater the surface area exposed to the substance, the greater the absorption.
Blood flow to the site of administration	Blood flow to a particular area regulates how fast the medication is absorbed into the central circulation. This is why administering medications intramuscularly to a patient having a seizure produces a minimal effect. Because of the seizure activity, blood flow to the extremities is diminished. Medications introduced intramuscularly tend to stay in the tissues until the seizure activity stops. When blood flow resumes, the patient may experience the effects of an overdose if multiple doses were given.
Solubility of the drug	The more soluble the drug, the faster it enters the circulatory system.
pH	The pH of the body and that of the drug can affect the rate of absorption. Some medications are coated to keep them from being absorbed before they reach the small intestine because the acid environment of the stomach can destroy the drug.
Drug concentration	The more of a drug available for absorption, the more that will be absorbed and the more that will remain in the system. Often a loading dose (bolus) of a medication is given, followed by a continuous infusion to maintain a constant therapeutic level.
Dosage form	Form has a lot to do with the speed of absorption. A liquid will be absorbed much more quickly than a pill, which must be dissolved before it is absorbed.
Routes of administration	IV administration frequently is the most rapid route for delivering drugs in the prehospital environment. The medication bypasses the absorption process because it is introduced directly into the vascular system. Intramuscular and subcutaneous routes are much slower because they depend on blood flow to the area in which the medication is administered.
Bioavailability	Bioavailability is the rate and extent to which an active drug enters the general circulation, permitting access to the site of action. It is determined by measurement of the concentration of the drug in body fluids or by the magnitude of the pharmacologic response.
Diffusion	Diffusion is the movement of solutes (molecules) from an area of higher concentration to an area of lower concentration.
Osmosis	Osmosis is the movement of a solvent (fluid) from an area of lower solute concentration to an area of higher solute concentration.
Filtration	Filtration is the removal of particles from a solution by allowing the liquid portion to pass through a membrane or other partial barrier. The semipermeability of the membrane allows fluid to pass through, but the openings are too small for solid particles.

that are more active, charged in activity, or less active. The drugs that are biotransformed to an inactive metabolite very quickly have limited effects on the body and must be administered frequently to continue the effect. Epinephrine during cardiac arrest is an example of a drug that is rendered inactive very quickly and must be administered every 3 to 5 minutes as needed.

> **Biotransformation** A chemical alteration that a substance undergoes in the body.

Drug Elimination

Excretion is the elimination of waste products from the body. Drugs are eliminated in their original forms or as metabolites. Organs of excretion include the kidneys via the urine, the intestines through the feces, the lungs via respiration, sweat through the salivary glands, and the mammary glands through breast milk. The rate of elimination varies with the amount of drug in the body and the underlying condition of the excretion organs. During shock, when the kidneys are poorly perfused, drugs will remain in the body for longer periods. This also holds true for geriatric patients whose kidneys may not function as well because of the normal deterioration associated with aging and for patients with chronic renal impairment. A patient's poor ability to eliminate a drug may lead to an accumulation of it in the body if subsequent doses are given, resulting in toxic effects.

■ Pharmacodynamics

Pharmacodynamics is the way in which a medication produces the response we intended, also known as the *mechanism of action*. A medication's pharmacodynamics also includes factors that may alter the intended response and any side effects or unexpected effects.

> *Pharmacodynamics* The study of drugs and their actions on living organisms.
> *Mechanism of action* The way in which a medication produces the intended response.

Mechanism of Action

To produce optimal desired or therapeutic effects, a drug must reach appropriate concentrations at its site of action. Molecules of the chemical compound must proceed from the point of entry into the body to the tissues with which they react. The magnitude of the response depends on the dose and the time that it takes the drug to travel in the body.

Drugs may produce their effects locally, systemically, or both. Local effects are those that result from the direct application of a drug to a tissue. An example of a local effect would be when cortisone cream is applied to the skin to relieve itching. Systemic effects occur after the drug is absorbed by any route and distributed by the bloodstream. Systemic effects almost always involve more than

one organ, although the response of one or another organ may predominate.

Medications cause their action on the body by the following four mechanisms:

- They may bind to a receptor site.
- They may change the physical properties of cells (typically, by changing the osmotic balance).
- They may chemically combine with other chemicals (such as with the goal of turning the substance into a nonproblematic chemical).
- They may alter a normal metabolic pathway (such as by interrupting the normal growth process of cells).

Medications that bind to a receptor site are the most prevalent, particularly in the prehospital setting. Cellular responses can be wide-ranging depending on the chemical mediator and the cells being stimulated. The medication molecule must compete with the naturally occurring chemical mediator. To win this battle, the medication molecule must have a higher affinity for the receptor than the chemical mediator does. In addition, more than one medication may vie for the same receptor.

Once the medication is bound to the receptor site, it initiates a chemical change that produces the expected effect. In some cases, this chemical change *is* the intended effect. In other cases, the initial chemical change releases a second compound (known as a second messenger) that causes the intended effect.

Drug-Response Relationship

Once the medication finds the target tissue, it needs to accumulate to a sufficient concentration to produce its desired effect. The drug-response relationship correlates the amount of medication given and the response it causes.

When administering a medication, you need to know how long it will take for the concentration of the medication at the target tissue to reach the minimum effective level—that is, the *onset of action*. You also need to know how long the medication can be expected to remain above that minimum level to provide the intended action—that is, the *duration of action*. The *termination of action* is the amount of time after the concentration level falls below the minimum level to the time it is eliminated from the body. All of these factors affect the *therapeutic index*—the ratio of a drug's lethal dose for 50% of the population (LD_{50}) to its effective dose for 50% of the population (ED_{50}). In other words, the therapeutic index gives an indication of a medication's margin of safety. Each medication also has a biologic half-life—that is, the time it takes the body to eliminate half of the drug. For example, the half-life of naloxone is typically 45 minutes.

The minimal concentration required to produce the desired response is referred to as the *therapeutic threshold* or the minimum effective concentration. A concentration lower than the therapeutic threshold will not induce

Table 6-9
Factors Altering Drug Responses

Factor	Description
Age	As the body ages, metabolism slows and the organs of excretion do not always function as well as those in younger patients. This can cause a toxic level of drugs in the system if not taken into account when administering multiple doses. Likewise, infants and small children have immature organs and systems and cannot metabolize the same amount of drug as an adult.
Body mass	Many medications are given based on the patient's weight. This is especially true of children. To have a therapeutic dose, concentrations within the tissues must meet the desired level.
Sex	Owing to different body compositions of fat, water, and hormones, certain medications affect males and females differently and must be adjusted accordingly.
Environmental conditions and time of administration	Factors such as time of day, temperature, altitude, and even noise may alter the body's response to a drug.
Genetic factors	Patients who may already have some compromise in function because of an existing condition may not be adversely affected by certain medications as a result of changes in absorption, distribution, metabolism, and excretion.
Psychologic factors	Mental stresses can have negative effects on the entire system, resulting in an inability to properly metabolize medications.

a clinical response. A concentration higher than the therapeutic threshold can be detrimental and possibly fatal. The goal of drug therapy is to give the minimum concentration of a drug that will produce the desired effect. **TABLE 6-9** lists factors that alter drug responses.

Onset of action The time needed for the concentration of the medication at the target tissue to reach the minimum effective level.

Duration of action The amount of time a medication concentration can be expected to remain above the minimum level needed to provide the intended action.

Termination of action The amount of time after the concentration of a medication falls below the minimum effective level until it is eliminated from the body.

Therapeutic index The difference between the minimum effective concentration and the toxic level of a drug.

Therapeutic threshold The minimal concentration of a drug necessary to cause the desired response.

Factors Influencing Drug Interactions

There are many variables that influence drug interactions. When you are administering medications, it is important to know not only how they affect the patient, but also how they may affect other medications that were previously administered. An interaction between drugs occurs whenever the actions of one drug on the body are in some way modified by another chemical substance. This chemical substance may be another prescription medication, herbal or OTC medication, or something like nicotine from cigarette smoking, something in the diet, or anything to which the person is exposed. An example of this would be the use of bronchodilators that may be exacerbated by ingesting caffeine. The caffeine stimulates the CNS and may produce adverse effects.

It is important to be aware of the potential interactions of drugs that are prescribed and those that the patient may be self-administering. Many patients, especially elderly patients, may take several medications each day (*polypharmacy*). The chance of developing an undesired drug interaction increases rapidly with the number of drugs used. This also holds true when patients take medications that may interact with other substances such as particular foods and alcohol. Warning labels on prescription bottles serve to warn against the substances that may cause interactions. Unfortunately, however, many people do not read the warning labels.

Polypharmacy The use of many drugs by the same patient.

Predictable Responses

Because of the extensive research that goes into developing and testing a medication before it is approved, generally there is common knowledge about what a particular drug will do to the patient. Obviously, an AEMT expects to see the desired response after administering the medication. At the same time, you should anticipate responses beyond the desired effect. *Side effects* are any actions of a medication other than the desired ones. Side effects may occur even when a medication is administered properly and under the appropriate circumstances. For example, giving epinephrine to a patient who is having an allergic reaction should dilate the bronchioles and decrease wheezing. However, two side effects of epinephrine are cardiac stimulation and constriction of the arteries, which may elevate the patient's heart rate and blood pressure. These side effects are predictable.

Iatrogenic Responses

An *iatrogenic response* is an adverse condition inadvertently induced in a patient by the treatment given. An example is a urinary tract infection that develops in a patient after insertion of an indwelling (for example, Foley) catheter. When the administration of drugs leads to symptoms that mimic naturally occurring disease states, it is known as an iatrogenic drug response.

> **Side effects** Any effects of a medication other than the desired ones.
> **Iatrogenic response** An adverse condition induced in a patient by the treatment given.

Unpredictable Responses

Some patients may have unanticipated adverse effects. The most common unpredictable response encountered in the prehospital setting is an allergic reaction. An allergy develops when a person has previously been exposed to a particular antigen and develops antibodies against that substance (sensitization). After a person has become sensitized, subsequent exposure to that same substance results in *hypersensitivity*. Because the patient is hypersensitive, the drug activates the immune system. Allergic reactions are unpredictable, unless the patient has had an allergic reaction to the same drug in the past, and may lead to life-threatening anaphylaxis. Anaphylaxis is an acute systemic reaction that is potentially life threatening. An allergic reaction may be immediate or delayed. Before administering any medication, if possible, question the patient carefully about any known drug allergies. The AEMT should remain alert for an allergic reaction after administering *any* drug.

> **Hypersensitivity** Abnormal sensitivity; a condition in which there is an exaggerated response by the body to the stimulus of a foreign agent.

A delayed reaction is known as *serum sickness*. This type of reaction is a hypersensitivity similar to an allergy and occurs a considerable time after a stimulus, such as a skin inflammation occurring hours or days after exposure to the allergen. Unlike other allergic reactions to drugs that occur soon after administration, serum sickness can develop 4–7 days after the first exposure to a medication.

In rare cases, the patient may experience a completely unique response specific to that person; it is not seen in other patients. This situation is known as an *idiosyncrasy*. An *idiosyncratic reaction* is a peculiar or individual reaction

to a drug. For example, if a patient were administered nitroglycerin and then experienced a seizure, this would be an idiosyncratic reaction because seizure is not an expected reaction when administering nitroglycerin.

> **Serum sickness** A condition in which antigen antibody complexes formed in the bloodstream deposit in sites around the body, most notably in the kidney, with resultant inflammatory reactions.
> **Idiosyncrasy** An abnormal sensitivity or reaction to a drug or other substance peculiar to a specific individual.
> **Idiosyncratic reaction** A peculiar or individual response to a drug or medication through unusual susceptibility.

Patients who take a particular medication for an extended period can build up *tolerance* to it. In these cases, the patient will have a decreased response to the same amount of medication, often requiring higher doses than normal. Also, a patient can develop a tolerance to other drugs in a certain class as a result of prolonged administration of another medication in that same class. Known as *cross-tolerance*, this phenomenon is often seen in patients who take many pain medications. When patients are taking a medication such as oxycodone, they become tolerant to other opiate-based medications. If morphine is administered for pain, the patient may not have the same response as other patients because of cross-tolerance. A disease or condition that does not respond to treatment is known as *refractory*.

Any medication needs to reach a minimum concentration in the target tissue before it becomes effective; that concentration is reached by providing a specific dose. If several doses are given in a relatively short time, the patient may experience a cumulative effect. A *cumulative effect* is the increased effect when a medication is given in several successive doses, which might result in therapeutic or nontherapeutic effects.

> **Tolerance** Physiologic adaptation to the effects of a drug such that increasingly larger doses of the drug are required to achieve the same effect.
> **Cross-tolerance** A tolerance to a particular drug that crosses over to other drugs in the same class.
> **Refractory** A disease or condition that does not respond to treatment.
> **Cumulative effect** Action of increased intensity after administration of several doses of a drug.

With prolonged administration of a medication, a patient can become drug-dependent. *Drug dependence* is a psychological and sometimes physical state resulting from continued use of a substance. Characteristic behavioral response includes a compulsion to take the drug on a continuous or periodic basis to experience its effects or to avoid the discomfort of its absence. A person will have significant symptoms if he or she stops using the medication. *Habituation* is the term for physical tolerance and psychological dependence on a drug or drugs.

> *Drug dependence* A psychological and sometimes physical state resulting from continued use of a substance, characterized by a compulsion to take the drug on a continuous or periodic basis to experience its effects or to avoid the discomfort of its absence.
>
> *Habituation* The situation in which there is a physical tolerance and psychological dependence on a drug or drugs.

Many patients take multiple medications at one time. It is possible for the effects of one medication to alter the response of another medication, a phenomenon known as a *drug interaction*. Drug interaction can be fatal. The interaction may not always be anticipated. Even if two medications are sympathomimetics, for example, it does not necessarily mean the patient will experience a more dramatic sympathetic response. It is possible to see the opposite response or a completely unrelated response. When a patient is taking more than one medication, one medication could block the body's response to another medication (*drug antagonism*). You can use this fact as an advantage. For example, if the patient has taken an opiate-based drug such as morphine, you have the ability to administer another medication, naloxone, to block the response to the morphine.

> *Drug interaction* A situation in which the effects of one medication alter the response of another medication.
>
> *Drug antagonism* A decrease in the action of a drug by the administration of another drug.

A *summation effect* is an additive effect—that is, two drugs that have the same or similar effect increase the patient's response when both are administered to the patient. When the patient receives two drugs that have the same effect but produce a response greater than the sum of their individual responses, the result is known as *synergism*. At times, the interaction between two medications can cause one drug to enhance the effect of another, known as *potentiation*. For example, acetaminophen (Tylenol) and alcohol interact. In this case, it is well known that high doses of acetaminophen are damaging to the liver. When alcohol is ingested along with acetaminophen, more of the medication is taken up into the liver and may result in acute liver failure. Some potentiation effects are known and can be exploited to achieve a desired effect; in other cases, potentiation may occur unexpectedly. A direct biochemical interaction that takes place between two drugs is referred to as *interference*.

> *Summation effect* Increased effect that may occur when two drugs that have the same or similar action are given together.
>
> *Synergism* Combined effect of two drugs that is greater than the sum of their individual effects.
>
> *Potentiation* Enhancement of the effect of one drug by another drug.
>
> *Interference* A direct biochemical interaction between two drugs.

Drug Storage and Security of Controlled Substances

All drug containers or boxes should be carefully guarded against possible theft. This requires that the boxes not only be locked, but also secured within the ambulance. Certain precepts should guide the manner in which drugs are secured, stored, distributed, and accounted for. Your local protocols will dictate the manner in which the drugs are maintained.

If controlled substances such as narcotics are administered, the records must be kept separate from other paperwork. As mentioned earlier, the DEA strictly regulates these substances. If drugs are lost or stolen, the supervisor and law enforcement personnel must be notified immediately.

All medications should be stored in an environment with a constant temperature if possible. Temperature, light, moisture, shelf life, and exposure to air all affect the potency of medications. If controlled medications are not used before their expiration dates, they must be destroyed. The destruction must be witnessed by two employees and documented on the proper forms.

Specific Medications

A certified AEMT is allowed to administer or help patients self-administer numerous medications. Details about each of these are provided in Appendix A, *Drugs Used at the AEMT Level*. As an AEMT, you may administer the following:

- Oxygen
- Oral glucose
- Glucagon
- 50% dextrose ($D_{50}W$)
- Intravenous fluids—D_5W (5% dextrose), normal saline, lactated Ringer's
- Epinephrine (IM or SC)
- Metered dose inhaler (MDI) medications—albuterol
- Nebulized medications—albuterol
- Nitroglycerin—spray, tablets, paste
- Nitrous oxide
- Naloxone
- Aspirin
- Others based on local protocols

However, you may administer or help to administer these medications only under the following conditions:

- A licensed physician gives you a direct order to administer a medication and/or the local medical protocols under which you are working permit you to administer that medication. Some local protocols exclude one or more of the medications in the preceding list.
- The local medical protocols under which you are working include standing orders for the use of a medication in defined situations. It is imperative that you do not give or help patients take any other medications under any circumstances.

Ready for Review

- Pharmacology is the study of the properties (characteristics) and effects of drugs and medications on the body.
- There are indications and contraindications for each medication. Indications are the therapeutic uses for a particular medication. Contraindications are cases in which you should not give a patient medication.
- As an AEMT, you are held responsible for safe and therapeutically effective drug administration. This includes legal, moral, and ethical considerations.
- You should also know the various routes of medication administration and which routes are used for the drugs you may administer in the prehospital setting.
- Overall, it is important to learn as much as you can about the drugs you may be allowed to administer in your area. Carry a pharmacologic reference to look up drugs that may be unfamiliar.
- You should also be aware of proper drug storage and security. Follow local protocols for drug administration, and review pharmacology often.

Case Study

You arrive at the home of an elderly woman who complains of generalized weakness and respiratory distress. Her husband tells you that she was at her doctor's office a few days ago for a routine visit. At the visit, her physician added two new medications and changed the dose of another medication. Since the patient began taking this new regimen, she has experienced increasing shortness of breath and generalized weakness to the point where she has difficulty ambulating. When you ask to see the patient's medications, her husband hands you a shoebox full of prescription bottles. You notice that some of the bottles are full and some contain only one or two pills. In addition, you note various cardiac and diabetic medications as well as several antibiotics. The husband tells you that the patient does not take all of these medications; some of the medicines were stopped by her doctor. When you asked why he still has the discontinued medicines, the husband replies by telling you that he did not want to throw them away in case his wife needed them

in the future. Your partner obtains vital signs and you continue with your history and exam. The patient is transported to a local hospital without incident.

1. Explain the concept of polypharmacy and how this may affect patients.

2. Explain a summation effect in a patient.

3. Explain how the age of the patient may alter how the body responds to medication.

4. A psychological and sometimes physical state resulting from continued use of a substance is known as:
   A. tolerance.
   B. drug dependence.
   C. habituation.
   D. idiosyncratic reaction.

5. _____ is the way in which a medication produces an intended response, also known as the mechanism of action.
   A. Biotransformation
   B. Pharmacokinetics
   C. Pharmacodynamics
   D. Absorption

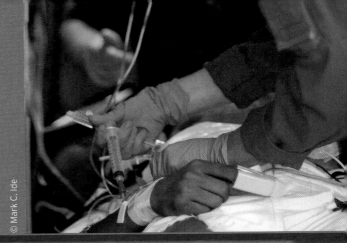
© Mark C. Ide

CHAPTER 7

Vascular Access and Medication Administration

Introduction

Before you administer any medication to a patient or assist a patient taking any medication, you must have a thorough understanding of how the medication will affect the body—both negatively and positively. You must also perform a thorough patient assessment to ensure that only beneficial medications are administered.

Drug doses and flow rate calculations are common areas of confusion for many prehospital personnel, yet they are skills you will need to perform frequently in the field. Disastrous results, including death, may occur if you administer an inappropriate drug or dose, give a drug by the wrong route, or give the medication too rapidly or too slowly.

Medical Direction

Medication administration is governed by your local protocols and online medical direction. The medical director for your service may allow the administration of certain medications as long as the patient meets certain criteria. Local policies and procedures are designed to guide you in specific situations. When questions or unusual situations arise—even if you function primarily by standing orders—contact medical control for direction. *If you have any doubt as to the correct action, consult with medical control!*

An AEMT's Responsibility Associated With Drug Orders

The danger of something going wrong when administering a drug—for example, administering the wrong drug or the wrong dose of a drug—can be minimized by confirming the "six rights" of medication administration.

Transition Tip

When requesting orders to give a particular medication, the AEMT has the responsibility to make sure that the medication is indicated for the patient's condition. Before you administer any medication, review the "six rights" of medication administration:

- Right patient
- Right drug
- Right dose
- Right route
- Right time
- Right documentation

These principles are included in the following set procedure for administering any medication. These steps also incorporate a number of safety precautions:

1. **Obtain an order from medical control.** This order may be given to you directly from online medical control via telephone or radio. Or it may be indirect, through protocols that contain standing orders for the administration of certain medications.

   When you are communicating with medical control about administering a particular medication, make sure that the medication is indicated for the patient's condition. Knowledge of the indications, contraindications, therapeutic effects, side effects, and appropriate doses for each of the drugs that you carry on your ambulance is critical to safe patient care. On the basis of the patient's clinical presentation, you must know the *right time* to administer a medication (that is, when the medication is indicated). Of equal if not greater importance is knowing when *not* to administer a medication (that is, when the medication is contraindicated). Furthermore, some of the medications you carry on the ambulance have specific intervals for repeated doses; you must be aware of these drugs and the appropriate intervals at which they are administered.

   Make sure medical control understands the situation. The decision to order the administration of any given drug is complex, involving such considerations as the patient's age, weight, clinical status, allergy history, concomitant medical problems, and other drugs he or she may be taking.

   Verify that your patient is indeed the *right patient*. In situations in which there are multiple patients, reconfirm the patient's name and compare it with the wrist band or triage tag. If you are assisting a patient with his or her medication, be sure it is prescribed for that patient.

2. **Make sure you understand the physician's orders.** If the orders are unclear or seem inappropriate for the patient's condition (for example, the dosage is more than the usual range or an unusual route of administration is requested), *ask the physician to repeat the order*. Do not assume that the physician is infallible.

3. **Repeat any orders, word for word, for verification.** This will help ensure that you understand the order and that the physician did not inadvertently give you an incorrect dosage order. In the repetition, state the *name of the drug*, the *dose*, and the *route* by which it is to be given.

4. **Inquire about any medication allergies the patient may have.** If the patient is unresponsive, try to obtain this information from another reliable source of information. Check for medical alert jewelry or tags as well.

5. **Verify the proper medication and prescription.** Read the label carefully. If it is the patient's own prescription, the bottle may show the trade name or the generic name. If you have any questions at all, contact online medical control. Examine the label to confirm that the medication is prescribed for the patient and not to a family member or friend. Note the *drug concentration* printed on the label.

6. **Verify the form, dose, and route of the medication.** You must make sure that the form of the medication, the dose, and the route are all consistent with the order you received. You are responsible for knowing the appropriate doses for the medications you carry on your ambulance. You are also responsible for accurately calculating the appropriate dose of the drug. Always recheck your drug calculations before administration to ensure that you are administering the *right dose*.

   It is imperative that you know the *right route* for the drug or drugs you are about to administer. A drug given by an inappropriate route—even if it is the right drug—could have disastrous and possibly fatal consequences.

7. **Check the expiration date and condition of the medication.** The last step before administering a medication is to make sure the expiration date has not passed. If no date can be found, you should examine the medication with suspicion. Check for defects in the vial, preloaded syringe, or ampule, noting whether the container appears to be cracked

or damaged. If the medication looks suspicious in any way, do *not* use it. In addition, if you find discoloration, cloudiness, or particles in a liquid medication, you should not administer it.

8. **Confirm medication compatibility.** If you have orders to administer more than one drug, make sure that the drugs are compatible. Some drugs will not mix with others, which could cause a precipitate to form in the solution. Should any cloudiness occur after a drug has been injected into IV tubing, *clamp the tubing immediately* and replace it with a new administration set.

9. **Dispose of any syringes and needles safely.** Do *not* try to recap a needle. Immediately dispose of the needle and syringe in a sharps container.

10. **Notify the physician** when the medication has been administered and advise the physician of any changes, whether positive or negative.

11. **Monitor the patient for possible adverse side effects.** Reassess the vital signs, especially heart rate and blood pressure, at least every 5 minutes or as the patient's condition warrants.

12. **Document.** Always document your actions and the patient's response on the patient care report after administering a medication. This includes:
    - Name of the drug
    - Dose of the drug
    - Time you administered the drug
    - Route of administration
    - Your name or the name of the person who administered the drug
    - Patient's response to the medication, whether positive or negative
      Did the patient's condition improve, get worse, or not change at all? Were there any side effects? If your performance should ever be questioned, documentation is your best defense.

◼ IV Technique and Administration

The most important point to remember about IV techniques and fluid administration is to keep the IV equipment sterile. Thinking ahead will help prevent mental and procedural errors while starting an IV.

One way to ensure proper technique is to develop a routine to follow as you assemble the appropriate equipment. A routine will help you keep track of your equipment and the steps necessary to complete a successful IV **TABLE 7-1**.

Alternative IV Sites and Techniques

Some additional IV sites and techniques available to prehospital providers require training beyond the scope of this chapter. However, because you may need to assist in these types of IV administration, you can benefit from understanding how they work.

Table 7-1 Preparing for a Successful IV
◼ Choose an IV solution.
◼ Choose an administration set.
◼ Assemble your equipment.
◼ Choose an IV site.
◼ Choose a catheter.
◼ Insert the IV catheter.
◼ Draw blood.
◼ Secure the line.
◼ Discontinue the IV line.

Saline Locks

Saline locks can maintain an active IV site without having to run fluids through the vein. These access devices are used primarily for patients who do not need additional fluids but may need rapid medication delivery. Saline locks are access ports commonly used with patients who have disorders such as congestive heart failure or pulmonary edema. A saline lock is attached to the end of an IV catheter and filled with approximately 2 mL of normal saline to keep blood from clotting at the end of the catheter **FIGURE 7-1**. Because this is a sealed-access site, the saline remains in the port without entering the vein, thus preventing clotting. These are also known as intermittent (INT) sites because they eliminate the need to completely reestablish an IV each time the patient needs medication or fluid.

> *Saline locks* A type of IV access device that allows an active IV site to be maintained without having to run fluids through the vein; also called a buff cap or intermittent site.

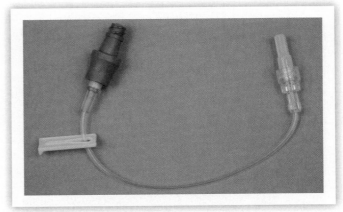

FIGURE 7-1 A saline lock is attached to the end of an IV catheter and filled with approximately 2 mL of normal saline in order to keep blood from clotting at the end of the catheter.

Intraosseous Lines

Intraosseous (IO) lines are used for emergency venous access in pediatric patients as defined by protocol when immediate IV access is difficult or impossible. They may also be used in adults in specific circumstances guided by local protocols. Use IO lines when you are unable to gain IV access in three tries or 90 seconds in a critical pediatric patient. Often these children are experiencing a life-threatening situation such as cardiac arrest, status epilepticus, or progressive shock. IO lines are contraindicated with a fractured tibia.

> *Intraosseous (IO) lines* A method of delivering fluids or medications into the medullary canal of the bone; used when IV access cannot be quickly obtained.

IO lines are usually established in the proximal tibia of pediatric patients with a rigid boring catheter. Common IO needles include the Jamshidi needle and the Cook catheter **FIGURE 7-2**. This double needle, consisting of a solid boring needle inside a sharpened hollow needle, is pushed into the bone with a screwing, twisting action. Once the needle pops through the bone, the solid needle is removed, leaving the hollow steel needle in place. The IV tubing is attached to this catheter. Once established, these lines work as well as peripheral IV lines. IO lines require full and careful immobilization because they rest at a 90° angle to the bone and are easily dislodged. Stabilization is critical for maintaining adequate flow.

Any fluid or medication that may be given through an IV line can also be given by the IO route. Shock and status epilepticus are only two of the reasons for establishing IO access. Unlike an IV line, fluid does not flow well into the bone because of resistance; therefore, it is necessary to use a large syringe to infuse the fluid.

Complications of using the IO route are similar to those of the IV route. Along with the complications discussed in the previous section, there is also the potential for compartment syndrome if fluid leaks outside of the bone and into the osteofascial compartment, fracture of the tibia from

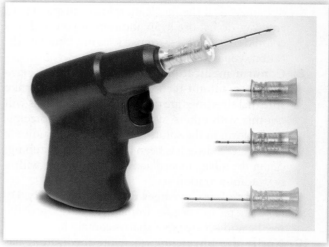

Courtesy of VidaCare Corporation

FIGURE 7-3 The EZ-IO insertion device features a hand-held battery-powered driver to which a special intraosseous needle is attached. The driver of the EZ-IO is universal, but different sizes of needles are available for adults and children.

improper technique, and pulmonary embolism of bone and fat particles.

As discussed, manually inserted IO needles are often used to access the IO space. Other products that may be used include the F.A.S.T.1, the EZ-IO, and the Bone Injection Gun (BIG) **FIGURE 7-3**. Use of all IO insertion devices requires specialized training and thorough familiarity with the features of each device, its functionality, and clinical application. If your EMS system uses any of these devices, follow local protocols regarding their use.

External Jugular IVs

External jugular IVs provide venous access through the external jugular veins of the neck, the same veins used to assess jugular vein distention. The vein is tamponaded by placing a finger or the edge of a tongue depressor on the vein just above the clavicle, causing it to fill. If the vein is difficult to find, place the patient in the Trendelenburg position to facilitate venous return. The catheter is inserted into the vein in the same manner as a normal IV, except the insertion point is very specific. The catheter is inserted midway between the angle of the jaw and the midclavicular line with the catheter pointed toward the shoulder on the same side as the puncture site **FIGURE 7-4**. These punctures are difficult because of a very tough fibrous sheath surrounding these veins that makes access difficult.

> *External jugular IVs* IV access established in the jugular veins of the neck.

These techniques require more advanced education and training than this chapter will provide. Understanding their application and use is important because you may need to perform these procedures.

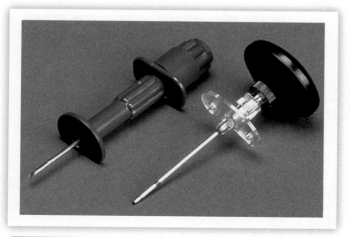

FIGURE 7-2 Manually inserted intraosseous needles.

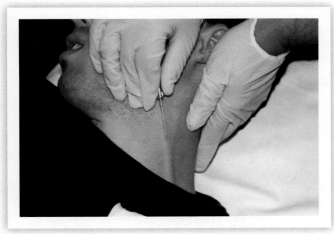

Courtesy of Rhonda Beck

FIGURE 7-4 The external jugular IV requires a very specific insertion site midway between the angle of the jaw and the midclavicular line with the catheter pointed toward the shoulder on the same side as the puncture.

Transition Tip

ALWAYS feel very carefully for a pulse prior to cannulating an external jugular vein. It is imperative not to pierce the carotid artery.

Transition Tip

To document IV administration, you need to include four things:

- The gauge of the needle
- The site
- The type of fluid you are administering
- The rate the fluid is running

Troubleshooting IV Therapy

Several factors can influence the flow rate of an IV line. For example, if the IV bag is not hung high enough, the flow rate will not be sufficient. It is always helpful to perform the following checks after completing IV administration. Also, if there is a flow problem, rechecking these items will help determine the cause of the problem.

- Check your IV fluid. Thick, viscous fluids such as blood products and colloid solutions infuse slowly and may be diluted if needed to help speed delivery. Cold fluids run slower than warm fluids. If you can, warm IV fluids before administering them in cold weather.
- Check your administration set. Macrodrips are used for rapid fluid delivery, whereas microdrips are designed to deliver a more controlled flow.

- Check the height of your IV bag. The IV bag must be hung high enough to overcome the patient's own blood pressure. Hang the bag as high as possible.
- Check the type of catheter used. The wider the catheter (the smaller the gauge), the more fluid can be delivered—14-gauge is the widest, 27-gauge the narrowest.
- Check the IV site for infiltration or extravasation of the fluid. The catheter may also be kinked or may need to be adjusted if the end is against a valve. This is known as a positional IV.
- Check your constricting band. One of the most overlooked factors is leaving the constricting band on the patient's arm after establishing the IV line.

Mathematical Principles Used in Pharmacology

It is important to administer the appropriate dose of medication to your patients. As an AEMT, you will need to be able to calculate the amount of medication to administer. Appendix B, *Mathematical Principles Used in Pharmacology*, reviews some of the basic mathematical principles in order to convert accurate medication dosages.

Steps for Administering by Specific Routes

This section will discuss steps for administering medications by the specific routes.

Administering Enteral Medications

Enteral medications are those given through some portion of the digestive or intestinal tract. This includes medications administered orally, through a feeding tube, or rectally.

Oral Administration

Forms of solid and liquid oral medications include capsules, timed-release capsules, lozenges, pills, tablets, elixirs, emulsions, suspensions, and syrups. Oral medications are used when the desired effect is systemic and the medications are taken up by the intestines. Oral medications may not be as effective if the uptake of drugs occurs in the stomach without reaching the intestines. To give oral medications, you may use a small medicine cup, a medicine dropper, a teaspoon, an oral syringe, or a nipple. Gather the appropriate equipment for the form of medication you are administering. As with any drug, check for indications, contraindications, precautions, and the six rights before administering an oral medication. Medications administered by AEMTs using the oral route include aspirin and oral glucose.

Follow these steps when administering an oral medication **FIGURE 7-5** :

1. Take standard precautions.
2. Determine the need for the medication based on patient presentation.

3. Obtain a history, including any drug allergies.
4. Follow standing orders or contact medical control for permission.
5. Check the medication to be sure it is the right medication, that it is not cloudy or discolored, and that its expiration date has not passed. Check the six rights.
6. Determine the appropriate dose. If the medication is liquid, pour the desired amount into a calibrated cup.
7. If giving a pill or tablet, instruct the patient to swallow the medication with water.
8. Monitor the patient's condition and document the medication given, route, time of administration, and patient response.

> *Enteral medications* Medications that are given through a portion of the gastrointestinal tract.

Transition Tip

Standard precautions should be used any time you are administering a medication.

Rectal Administration

Some AEMTs may be allowed to administer D_{50}, but whether this route is allowed depends on local protocols. If it is allowed, administering D_{50} by this route is a last resort, when a patient is hypoglycemic and no other route is an option (IV access cannot be established). Check for indications, contraindications, and precautions before giving D_{50} rectally **FIGURE 7-6**.

Follow these steps to administer a drug rectally:

1. Take standard precautions.
2. Determine the need for the medication based on patient presentation.

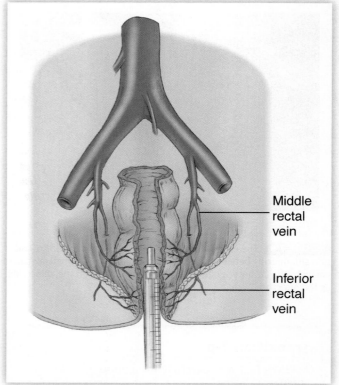

Used with permission of the American Academy of Pediatrics, Pediatric Education for Prehospital Professionals, © American Academy of Pediatrics, 2000.

FIGURE 7-6 The rectal mucosa is highly vascular and rapidly absorbs medications.

3. Obtain a history including any drug allergies.
4. Follow standing orders or contact medical control for permission.
5. Determine the appropriate dose and check that the medication is the right medication, there is no cloudiness or discoloration, and the expiration date has not passed.

A.

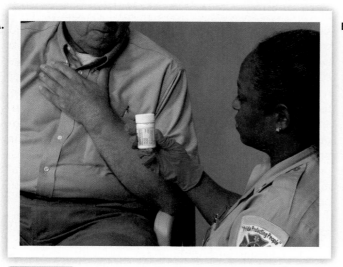

B.

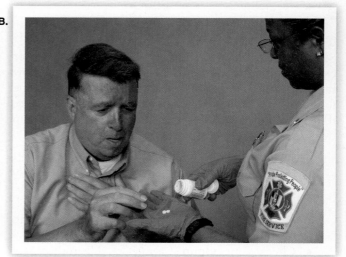

FIGURE 7-5 Administering an oral medication. **A.** Check the medication and its expiration date. **B.** Have the patient take the medication. Administer a cup of water if necessary.

6. When inserting a suppository, use a water-soluble gel for lubrication. Insert the suppository into the rectum approximately 1 to 1½ inches while instructing the patient to relax and not to bear down.

7. For medications in liquid form, some modifications are needed. You may use a nasopharyngeal airway or a small endotracheal tube as your delivery route.

   a. Lubricate the end of the nasal airway or endotracheal tube with a water-soluble gel and gently insert it approximately 1 to 1½ inches into the rectum. Instruct the patient to relax and not to bear down.

   b. With a needleless syringe, gently push the medication through the tube.

   c. Once the medication has been delivered, remove and dispose of the tube.

8. Monitor the patient's condition and document the medication given, route, time of administration, and patient response.

Administering Parenteral Medications

Parenteral medications are those given through any route other than the GI tract. Parenteral routes used by the AEMT include subcutaneous, intramuscular, IV bolus, IO, sublingual, transcutaneous, and transdermal. Of the parenteral drug routes, IV administration is the most common route used in the prehospital setting and generally is the quickest route for getting medication into the central circulation.

Equipment

A variety of needles and syringes are used for administering parenteral medications. Most syringes come prepackaged in color-coded packs with a needle already attached. The needles and syringes may also be packaged separately. Choose the appropriate size of syringe and appropriate needle length for the desired route. Syringes consist of a plunger, body or barrel, flange, and tip **FIGURE 7-7**. All hypodermic syringes are marked with 10 calibrations per milliliter on one side of the barrel. Each small line represents 0.1 mL. The 3 mL syringe is the most commonly used for injections, but others are available as needed. Needle lengths vary from three eighths to 1 inch for standard injections.

> *Parenteral medications* Drug administration through any route other than through the gastrointestinal tract; includes IV, IO, subcutaneous, intramuscular, sublingual, buccal, transcutaneous, intranasal, and inhalation routes.

Packaging

Parenteral medications are most commonly packaged in ampules, vials, and prefilled syringes. *Ampules* are breakable sterile glass containers designed to carry a single dose of medication **FIGURE 7-8**. *Vials* may contain single or multiple doses **FIGURE 7-9**. Vials have a rubber-stopper top and are made of glass or plastic. Many drugs used in prehospital care are carried in vials. Prefilled syringes are designed for

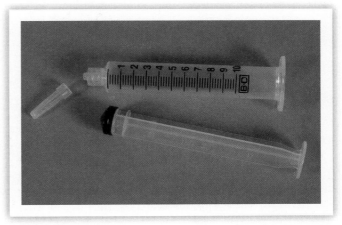

FIGURE 7-7 A syringe consists of a plunger, body or barrel, flange, and tip.

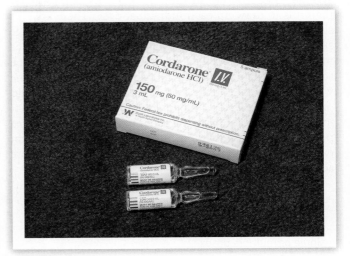

Courtesy of AAOS
FIGURE 7-8 Medication stored in ampules.

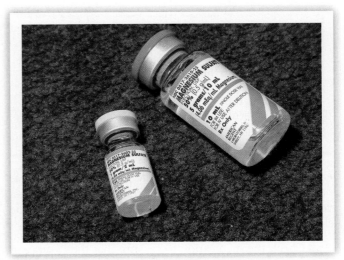

Courtesy of AAOS
FIGURE 7-9 Vials (single-dose and multidose).

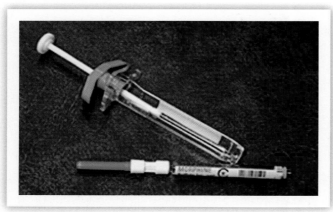

Courtesy of AAOS
FIGURE 7-10 A Tubex syringe.

ease of use. It is much easier and quicker to use a prefilled syringe when you are treating a patient in cardiac arrest than it is to draw up each individual dose. There are also single-dose disposable cartridges that use a reusable syringe such as a Tubex or Abojet **FIGURE 7-10**. Some medications may need to be reconstituted, such as methylprednisolone sodium succinate (Solu-Medrol) and glucagon. These come with two vials, one with a powdered form of the drug and one with sterile water. *Drug reconstitution* involves injecting the sterile water from one vial into a vial containing the powder, making a solution for injection. Glucagon is an example of a medication that must be reconstituted before administration.

> *Ampules* Small glass containers that are sealed and the contents sterilized.
> *Vials* Small glass bottles for medications; may contain single or multiple doses.
> *Drug reconstitution* Injecting sterile water (or saline) from one vial into another vial containing a powdered form of a drug.

Transition Tip

Any time you are using a needle to draw up medication, always hold the syringe against your palm with the needle pointing up and draw the vial down onto the needle using the thumb and forefinger of the palm the syringe is braced against to avoid sticking yourself. This especially applies if you are in a moving ambulance.

Ampules Some medications an AEMT administers, such as naloxone (Narcan), come in the form of an ampule. When you are drawing medication from an ampule, follow the steps in **SKILL DRILL 7-1**:

1 Check the medication to be sure that the expiration date has not passed and that it is the correct drug and concentration.

2 Shake the medication down into the base of the ampule. If some of the drug appears to be stuck in the neck, gently thump or tap the stem (**Step 1**).

3 Using a 4×4-inch gauze pad or an alcohol prep, grip the neck of the ampule and snap it off. Drop the stem in the sharps container (**Step 2**).

4 Insert the needle into the ampule without touching the outer sides of the ampule. Draw the solution into the syringe and dispose of the ampule in the sharps container (**Step 3**).

5 Hold the syringe with the needle pointing up. Gently tap the barrel to loosen air trapped inside and cause it to rise (**Step 4**). Press gently on the plunger to dispel any air bubbles (**Step 5**).

6 If not using a needleless system, recap the needle using the one-handed method to avoid contamination.

Vials Epinephrine and naloxone (Narcan) are two examples of medications that may come in vials. When you are administering a vial of medication, you must first determine how much of the drug you will need and how many doses are in the vial. For a single-dose vial, you will draw up the entire amount in the vial. For multiple-dose vials, you should draw out only the amount needed. Once you remove the cover from a vial, it is no longer sterile. If you need a second dose, the top of the vial should be cleaned with alcohol before withdrawing the medication.

When you are drawing medication from a vial, follow the steps in **SKILL DRILL 7-2**:

1 Check the medication to be sure that the expiration date has not passed, and that it is the correct drug and concentration. Check that it is not discolored (**Step 1**).

2 Remove the sterile cover, or clean the top with alcohol if it was previously opened.

3 Determine the amount of medication that you will need, and draw that amount of air into the syringe (**Step 2**). Allow a little extra room to expel some while removing air bubbles.

4 Invert the vial, and insert the needle through the rubber stopper into the medication. Expel the air in the syringe into the vial and then release the plunger, keeping the tip of the needle within the medication (**Step 3**).

5 Once you have the correct amount of medication in the syringe, withdraw the needle and expel any air in the syringe (**Step 4**).

6 Recap the needle using the one-handed method to avoid contamination (**Step 5**).

Medications that need to be reconstituted come in two separate vials or in a single vial divided into two

SKILL DRILL 7-1

Drawing Medication From an Ampule

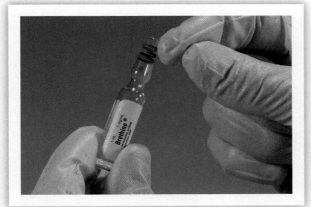

1 Check the medication to be sure that the expiration date has not passed and that it is the correct drug and concentration. Gently thump or tap the stem of the ampule to shake medication down into the base.

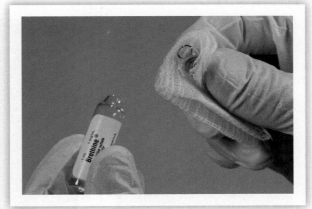

2 Grip the neck of the ampule using a 4×4-inch gauze pad and snap off the neck.

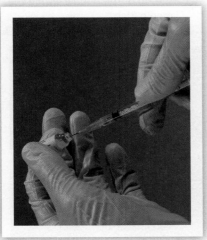

3 Without touching the outer sides of the ampule, insert the needle into the medication in the ampule. Draw the solution in the syringe.

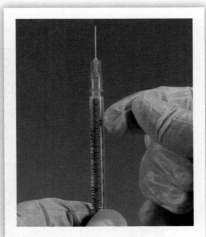

4 Holding the syringe with the needle pointing up, gently tap the barrel to loosen air trapped inside.

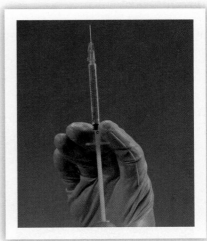

5 Gently press on the plunger to dispel any air bubbles. If not using a needleless system, recap the needle using the one-handed method.

compartments by a rubber stopper. These may also be known as Mix-o-Vials **FIGURE 7-11**. With Mix-o-Vials, you simply squeeze the two vials together, which releases the center stopper and allows the contents to mix. Shake vigorously to mix the contents before drawing out the medication. To mix the contents of two separate vials, draw the fluid out of the first vial in the same manner previously described. Insert the syringe into the top of the second vial and expel all of the fluid into it. Shake vigorously to mix. Once the medication is reconstituted, regardless of the manner, draw up the medication as described for single- and multiple-dose vials.

SKILL DRILL 7-2

Drawing Medication From a Vial

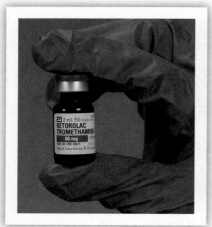

1 Check the medication and its expiration date. Confirm that it is the correct drug and concentration, and that it is not discolored.

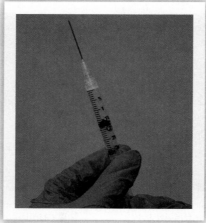

2 Determine the amount of medication needed and draw that amount of air into the syringe.

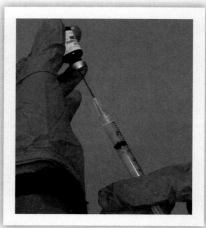

3 Invert the vial and insert the needle through the rubber stopper. Expel the air in the syringe and release the plunger, keeping the tip of the needle within the medication.

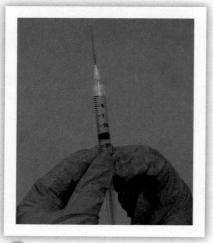

4 Withdraw the needle, and expel any air in the syringe.

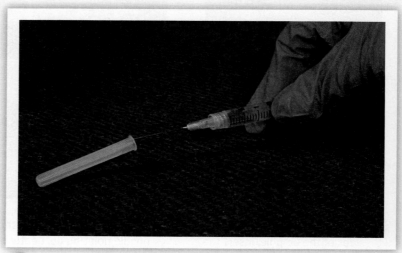

5 Recap the needle using the one-handed method.

Prefilled Syringe Prefilled syringes come in tamper-proof boxes and are separated into the glass drug cartridge and a syringe **FIGURE 7-12**. $D_{50}W$ is an example of a drug that comes as a prefilled syringe. Pop the tops off of the syringe and the drug cartridge, then screw them together. Remove the needle cover and expel air in the manner previously described. Follow the steps for the route the medication is to be given.

Subcutaneous Administration

Subcutaneous injections are given into the loose connective tissue between the dermis and the muscle layer **FIGURE 7-13**. Volumes of a drug administered subcutaneously are usually 1 mL or less. The injection is performed using a 24- to 26-gauge one half- to 1-inch needle. Common sites include the upper part of the arms, anterior part of

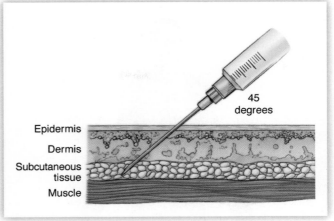

© American Academy of Pediatrics

FIGURE 7-13 A subcutaneous injection is below the dermis and above the muscle.

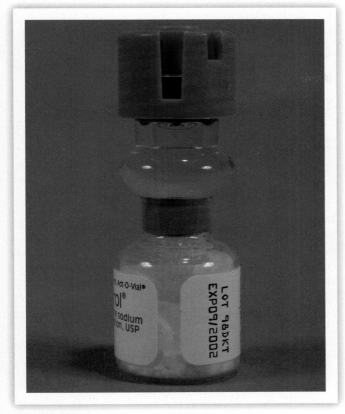

FIGURE 7-11 A Mix-o-Vial.

the thighs, and the abdomen **FIGURE 7-14**. Patients who take insulin injections usually vary the sites because of the multiple number of injections they require (usually daily). An example of an AEMT medication that is administered subcutaneously is epinephrine.

> *Subcutaneous* Into the tissue between the skin and muscle; a medication delivery route.
> *Aseptic technique* A method of cleansing used to prevent contamination of a site when performing an invasive procedure, such as inserting an IV line.

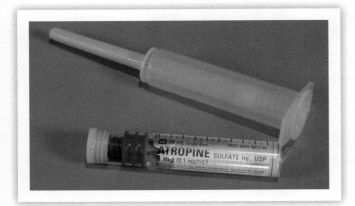

FIGURE 7-12 Prefilled syringes come in two parts, the glass drug cartridge and a syringe.

When you are preparing to administer fluid or medication, you will need to use *aseptic technique*, also called sterile technique. This is a method of cleansing used to prevent site contamination when performing an invasive procedure such as starting an IV line or administering a medication. Aseptic technique may be accomplished through the use of sterilization of equipment, antiseptics, or disinfectants.

Follow the steps in **SKILL DRILL 7-3** to administer a medication via the subcutaneous route:

1. Take standard precautions.

2. Determine the need for the medication based on patient presentation.

3. Obtain a history including any drug allergies and vital signs.

4. Follow standing orders or contact medical control for permission.

5. Check the medication to be sure that it is not cloudy, that the expiration date has not passed, and that it is the correct drug and concentration. Determine the appropriate dose (**Step 1**).

6. Advise the patient of potential discomfort while explaining the procedure.

7. Assemble and check the equipment needed: alcohol preps and a 3-mL syringe with a 24- to 26-gauge needle. Draw up the correct dose of medication (**Step 2**).

8. Cleanse the area for the administration (usually the upper part of the arm or thigh) with an alcohol swab or other disinfectant (**Step 3**).

9. Pinch the skin surrounding the area, advise the patient of a stick, and insert the needle at a 45° angle.

10. Pull back on the plunger to aspirate for blood. The presence of blood in the syringe indicates you may have entered a vein. Remove the needle, and hold pressure over the site. Discard the syringe and needle

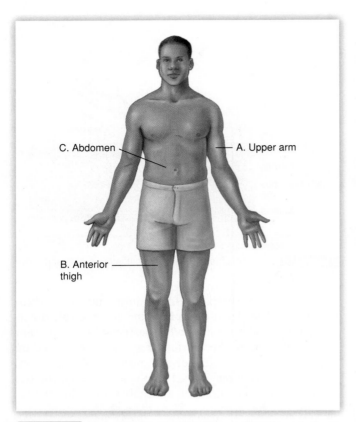

FIGURE 7-14 Common sites for subcutaneous injections. **A.** Upper part of the arm. **B.** Anterior part of the thigh. **C.** Abdomen.

in the sharps container. Prepare a new syringe and needle and select another site.

11 If there is no blood in the syringe, inject the medication and remove the needle. Immediately place it in the sharps container (**Step 4**).

12 To disperse the medication through the tissue, rub the area in a circular motion with your gloved hand.

13 Properly store any unused medication.

14 Monitor the patient's condition and document the medication given, route, administration time, and patient response (**Step 5**).

Intramuscular Administration

Intramuscular (IM) injections are made by penetrating a needle through the dermis and subcutaneous tissue into the muscle layer. This allows administration of a larger volume of medication (up to 5 mL) than the subcutaneous route. There is also the potential for damage to nerves because of the depth of the injection, so it is important to choose the appropriate site. Common anatomic sites for IM injections for adults and children include the following **FIGURE 7-15**:

- **Deltoid muscle**—the muscle of the upper part of the arm that covers the prominence of the shoulder. The site for injection is approximately 1.5 to 2 inches below the acromion process on the lateral side.

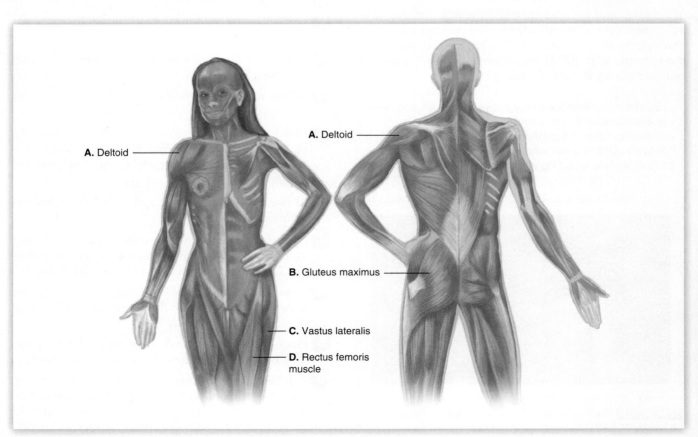

FIGURE 7-15 Common sites for intramuscular injections. **A.** Deltoid muscles. **B.** Gluteal area. **C.** Vastus lateralis muscle. **D.** Rectus femoris muscle.

SKILL DRILL 7-3

Administering Medication Via the Subcutaneous Route

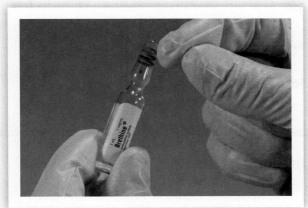

1 Check the medication to be sure that it is the correct one, that it is not discolored, and that the expiration date has not passed.

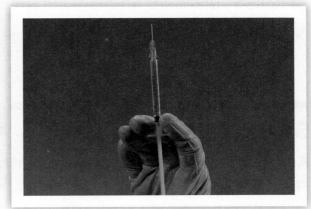

2 Assemble and check the equipment. Draw up the correct dose of medication.

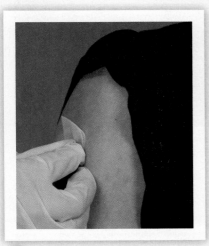

3 Cleanse the injection area using aseptic technique.

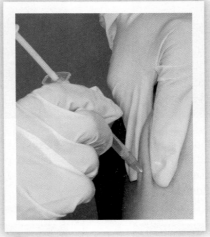

4 Pinch the skin surrounding the area, and insert the needle at a 45° angle. Pull back on the plunger to aspirate for blood. If there is no blood, inject the medication, remove the needle, and hold pressure over the area.

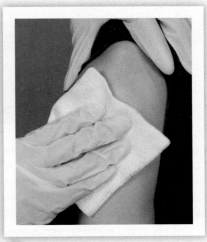

5 To disperse the medication, rub the area in a circular motion. Monitor the patient's condition.

Intramuscular (IM) Injection into a muscle; a medication delivery route.

- **Gluteal area**—the buttocks, specifically the upper lateral aspect of either side
- **Vastus lateralis muscle**—the large muscle on the lateral side of the thigh
- **Rectus femoris muscle**—the large muscle on the anterior side of the thigh

AEMT medications that may be administered intramuscularly include epinephrine and glucagon. Follow the steps in **SKILL DRILL 7-4** to administer an IM injection:

1. Take standard precautions.
2. Determine the need for the medication based on patient presentation.
3. Obtain a history including any drug allergies and vital signs.
4. Follow standing orders or contact medical control for permission.

SKILL DRILL 7-4

Administering Medication Via the Intramuscular Route

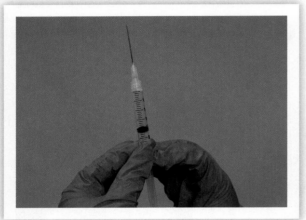

1. Check the medication to be sure that it is the correct one, that it is not discolored, and that the expiration date has not passed. Assemble and check the correct dose of medication.

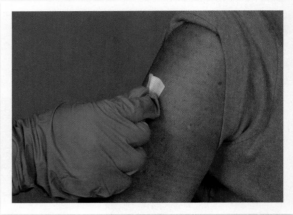

2. Using aseptic technique, cleanse the injection area.

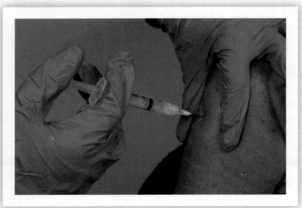

3. Stretch the skin over the area, and insert the needle at a 90° angle. Pull back on the plunger to aspirate for blood. If there is no blood, inject the medication and remove the needle.

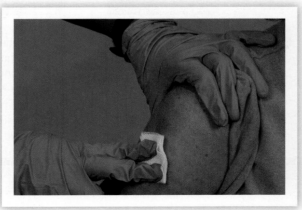

4. To disperse the medication, rub the area in a circular motion. Monitor the patient's condition.

5 Check the medication to be sure it is the correct one, that it is not discolored, and that the expiration date has not passed. Determine the appropriate dose.

6 Advise the patient of potential discomfort while explaining the procedure.

7 Assemble and check equipment needed: alcohol preps and a 3- to 5-mL syringe with a 21-gauge, 1- or 2-inch needle. Draw up the correct dose of medication (**Step 1**).

8 Cleanse the area for the administration (usually the upper part of the arm or the hip) using aseptic technique (**Step 2**).

9 Stretch the skin over the cleansed area, advise the patient of a stick, and insert the needle at a 90° angle.

10 Pull back on the plunger to aspirate for blood. The presence of blood in the syringe indicates you may have entered a blood vessel. Remove the needle and hold pressure over the site. Discard the syringe and needle in the sharps container. Prepare a new syringe and needle, and select another site.

11 If there is no blood in the syringe, inject the medication and remove the needle. Immediately place it in the sharps container (**Step 3**).

12 To disperse the medication through the tissue, rub the area in a circular motion with your gloved hand.

13 Store any unused medication properly.

14 Monitor the patient's condition and document the medication given, route, administration time, and patient response (**Step 4**).

Sublingual Administration

Sublingual and *buccal* medications enter the circulatory system much faster than those that travel through the enteral route. There is a vast network of vessels under the tongue (sublingual) and in the cheek (buccal). In order for a sublingual or buccal medication to work effectively, mucous membranes must be moist to allow the medication to dissolve. Medications given via the sublingual or buccal route may also be taken up in the proximal part of the GI tract without reaching the intestines.

> *Sublingual*　Under the tongue; a medication delivery route.
> *Buccal*　Relating to the cheek or mouth.

Medications given by the sublingual route come in tablet, liquid, and spray forms. Nitroglycerin is a drug that is commonly given via the sublingual route; it comes in tablet and spray forms. To administer a sublingual medication, follow the steps in **SKILL DRILL 7-5**:

1 Take standard precautions.

2 Determine the need for the medication based on patient presentation.

SKILL DRILL 7-5

Administering Medication Via the Sublingual Route

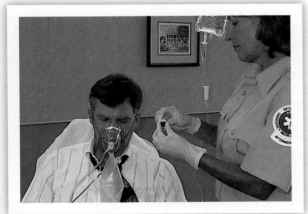

1 Check the medication for drug type and its expiration date. Determine the appropriate dose. Have the patient rinse his or her mouth with a little water if the mucous membranes are dry.

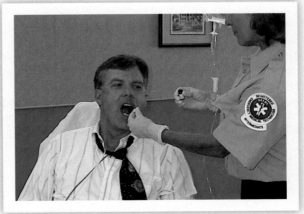

2 Explain the procedure and ask the patient to lift his or her tongue. Place the tablet or spray the dose underneath the tongue or have the patient do so. Advise the patient not to chew or swallow the tablet but to let it dissolve slowly. Monitor the patient and document the medication given, the route, administration time, and the patient's response.

3 Obtain a history including any drug allergies and vital signs.

4 Follow standing orders or contact medical control for permission.

5 Check the medication to make sure that it is the correct one and that its expiration date has not passed. Determine the appropriate dose.

6 Ask the patient to rinse his or her mouth with a little water if the mucous membranes are dry (**Step 1**).

7 Explain the procedure, and ask the patient to lift his or her tongue. Place the tablet or spray the dose under the tongue or ask the patient to do so.

8 Advise the patient not to chew or swallow the tablet, but to let it dissolve slowly.

9 Monitor the patient's condition and document the medication given, route, administration time, and patient response (**Step 2**).

Oral glucose is an example of an AEMT medication administered via the buccal route. The technique for administering oral glucose is shown in the chapter, *Endocrine and Hematologic Emergencies*.

Intranasal Administration

Intranasal (within the nose) medications include nasal spray for congestion or solutions to moisten the nasal mucosa. In recent years, this route of medication administration has become increasingly popular in the prehospital setting. Intranasally administered medications are rapidly absorbed, providing a more rapid onset of action than IM injections. Administration of emergency medications via the intranasal route is performed with a *mucosal atomizer device* `FIGURE 7-16`. The device attaches to a syringe and allows you to spray (atomize) select medications into the nasal mucosa.

> *Intranasal* A delivery route in which a medication is pushed through a specialized atomizer device called a mucosal atomizer device into a nostril.
>
> *Mucosal atomizer device* A device that attaches to the end of a syringe used to spray (atomize) certain medications via the intranasal route.

Because of the molecular structure of drugs, only a few emergency medications can be given intranasally, including naloxone (Narcan). Follow local protocols or consult with medical control about the appropriate doses of these medications and any other medications that may be administered intranasally.

To administer a drug via the intranasal route, follow these steps:

1. Check the medication to ensure that it is the correct one, that it is not cloudy or discolored, and that the expiration date has not passed.

2. Draw up the appropriate dose of medication in the syringe.

3. Attach the mucosal atomizer device to the syringe.

4. Explain the procedure to the patient (or to a relative if the patient is unconscious) and the need for the medication.

5. Spray *half* of the medication dose into each nostril.

6. Dispose of the atomizer device and syringe in the appropriate container.

7. Monitor the patient's condition and document the medication given, route, time of administration, and patient response.

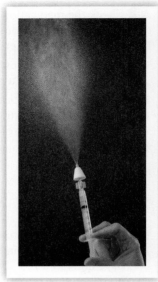

Courtesy of LMA North America

`FIGURE 7-16` Mucosal atomizer device.

Administering by Inhalation

Many medications used in the treatment of respiratory emergencies are administered via the *inhalation* route. This is the fastest method for medication reaching the brain. The most common inhaled medication is oxygen. Bronchodilator (beta-agonist) medications are often administered in the prehospital setting for patients experiencing respiratory distress caused by certain obstructive airway diseases such as asthma, bronchitis, and emphysema. Nitrous oxide, which can be administered by AEMTs for patients in pain, is also delivered via inhalation. Check your drug reference guide or the package insert for indications, contraindications, and precautions before giving any medication. In order for the inhalation route to be effective, the patient must have a patent airway and good tidal volume to be able to pull the medication into the lungs. A disadvantage of inhalers is that it is difficult to regulate the amount of drug the patient receives.

> *Inhalation* The active, muscular part of breathing that draws air into the airway and lungs.

A patient with a history of respiratory problems will usually have a *metered-dose inhaler (MDI)* to use on a regular basis or as needed `FIGURE 7-17`. An MDI is a miniature spray canister used to direct medications through the mouth and into the lungs. For more severe problems, liquid bronchodilators may be aerosolized in a *nebulizer* for inhalation. Small-volume nebulizers (also called updraft or handheld nebulizers) produce a fine spray or mist to deliver inhaled medication, and are the most commonly used method of administration of inhaled medications in the prehospital arena `FIGURE 7-18`. Oxygen or a compressed air source is connected to the nebulizer to produce the aerosolized mist.

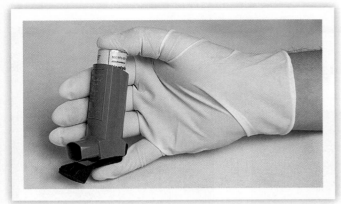

Courtesy of AAOS

FIGURE 7-17 Some medications are inhaled into the lungs with a metered-dose inhaler so that they can be absorbed into the bloodstream more quickly.

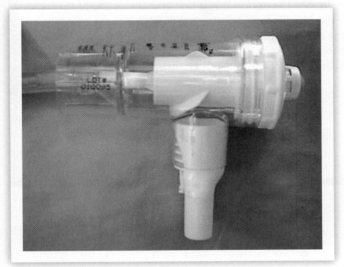

Courtesy of AAOS

FIGURE 7-18 A small-volume nebulizer is used to deliver medications via aerosolized mist.

The mist may be delivered through a mouthpiece held by the patient or by a mask for young children and those who are unable to hold the mouthpiece.

The chapter, *Respiratory Emergencies*, discusses how to help a patient self-administer medication from an inhaler, as well as how to administer medication with a small-volume nebulizer.

> *Metered-dose inhaler (MDI)* A miniature spray canister used to direct medications through the mouth and into the lungs.
> *Nebulizer* A device for producing a fine spray or mist that is used to deliver inhaled medications.

IV Administration

The *intravenous (IV)* route places the drug directly into the circulatory system. This is the fastest route of medication administration for AEMTs to administer because it bypasses most barriers to drug absorption. This also means that there is no room for error. Drugs are administered by direct injection with a needle and syringe into an established peripheral IV line. Many services now use needleless systems to provide protection against needle sticks. In a needleless system, the syringe simply screws into the injection port.

In terms of medication administration, a *bolus* is a single dose given by the IV route. A bolus (in one mass) can be a small or large quantity of a drug. Some medications require an initial bolus and then a continuous IV infusion to maintain a therapeutic level of the drug. Complications may arise from using the IV route including the local and systemic complications discussed earlier in this chapter.

> *Intravenous (IV)* Into a vein; a medication delivery route.
> *Bolus* A term used to describe "in one mass"; in medication administration, a single dose given by the IV route; may be a small or large quantity of a drug.

Follow the steps in **SKILL DRILL 7-6** when administering a medication via the IV bolus route:

1. Take standard precautions.
2. Determine the need for the medication based on patient presentation.
3. Obtain a history including any drug allergies and vital signs.
4. Follow standing orders or contact medical control for permission.
5. Check the medication to be sure that it is the correct one, that it is not cloudy or discolored, and that its expiration date has not passed. Determine the appropriate dose.
6. Explain the procedure to the patient and the need for the medication.
7. Assemble needed equipment and draw up the medication. Expel any air in the syringe. Draw up 20 mL of normal saline to use as a flush for the medication.
8. Cleanse the injection port with alcohol and remove the protective cap from the needleless system (**Step 1**).
9. Attach the syringe to the port and pinch off the IV tubing proximal to the administration port. Failure to shut off the line will result in the medication taking the pathway of least resistance and potentially flowing into the bag instead of the patient.
10. Administer the correct dose of the medication at the appropriate rate. Some medications must be administered very quickly, whereas others must be pushed slowly to prevent adverse effects (**Step 2**).
11. Place the syringe into the sharps container.
12. Unclamp the IV line to flush the medication into the vein. Allow it to run briefly wide open or flush with a 20-mL bolus of normal saline.

SKILL DRILL 7-6

Administering Medication Via the IV Bolus Route

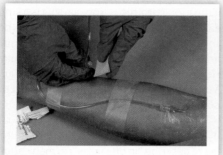

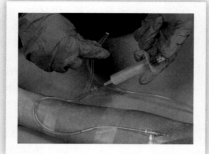

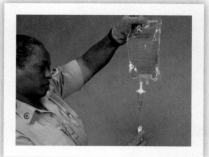

1 Check that the medication is correct, ensure that it is not cloudy or discolored, and check the expiration date. Determine the appropriate dose. Explain the procedure to the patient. Assemble and check the equipment. Cleanse the injection port, or remove the protective cap if using the needleless system.

2 Insert the needle into the port, and pinch off the IV tubing proximal to the administration port. Administer the correct dose at the appropriate rate.

3 Unclamp the IV line to flush the medication into the vein, allowing it to run briefly wide open, or flush with a 20-mL bolus of normal saline. Readjust the IV flow rate to the original setting, and monitor the patient's condition.

13 Readjust the IV flow rate to the original setting.

14 Properly store any unused medication.

15 Monitor the patient's condition and document the medication given, route, time of administration, and patient response (**Step 3**).

Follow these steps to administer a medication through a saline lock, or intermittent site:

1. Take standard precautions.
2. Determine the need for the medication based on patient presentation.
3. Obtain a history including any drug allergies and vital signs.
4. Follow standing orders or contact medical control for permission.
5. Check the medication to be sure it is the correct one, that it is not cloudy or discolored, and that its expiration date has not passed. Determine the appropriate dose.
6. Explain the procedure to the patient and the need for the medication.
7. Assemble needed equipment and draw up the medication. Draw up 20 mL of normal saline to use as a flush for the medication.
8. Cleanse the injection port with alcohol and remove the protective cap from the needleless system.
9. Attach the syringe to the port while holding it carefully.
10. Pull back slightly on the syringe plunger and observe for blood return. If blood appears, slowly inject the medication while watching for infiltration. If resistance is felt, or if the patient complains of any discomfort, discontinue administration immediately. A new site will need to be established.
11. Place the syringe into the sharps container.
12. Clean the port and attach the syringe containing the flush.
13. Flush the saline lock and place the syringe in the sharps container or a biohazard bag.
14. Store any unused medication properly.
15. Monitor the patient's condition and document the medication given, route, time of administration, and patient response.

Intraosseous Administration

Finally, medication may be administered through the IO route. The technique for administering medication via the IO route is discussed in the chapter, *Special Populations*.

PREP KIT

Ready for Review

- Follow a set procedure when you administer any medication. A safe procedure begins with obtaining an order from medical control and making sure you understand the physician's orders.
- A certified AEMT is allowed to administer or help patients self-administer numerous medications: oxygen, oral glucose, glucagon, 50% dextrose, epinephrine, MDI medications, nebulized medications, nitroglycerin, nitrous oxide, naloxone, aspirin, and possibly others based on local protocol.
- Successful IV administration technique takes practice. Take your time when you practice inserting an IV line and gain a solid understanding of what you are doing.
- During IV therapy, it is critical to always keep equipment sterile.

- Possible complications of IV therapy include local reactions and systemic reactions.
- Good math skills, along with an understanding of the metric system, are imperative to providing the correct dose for the patient. Practice your math skills frequently to stay proficient.
- As an AEMT, you should be familiar with the various routes of medication administration. This includes an understanding of the proper use of equipment and proper anatomic locations for administration.
- Enteral administration includes the administration of all drugs that may be given through any portion of the digestive tract. The parenteral route includes any method of drug administration that does not go through the digestive tract.
- When in doubt, always follow local protocols or contact medical control for direction.

Case Study

Your crew is called out for a patient with respiratory distress. After arriving on scene at a local bank, you find a 26-year-old female sitting in the president's office presenting with rapid shallow respirations, audible wheezing, and accessory muscle use. The president tells you she is an employee and has a history of asthma. Her MDI is empty, and she has not been to her physician to get a refill. She encountered a customer wearing a strong perfume that triggered the attack. After a quick assessment you place the patient on oxygen via nonrebreathing mask at 15 L per minute while your partner assembles a nebulizer with 2.5 mg of albuterol. The patient is transported to the local hospital and is breathing much easier upon arrival.

1. What are the six "rights" of medication administration?

2. Documentation is an important part of medication administration. What should be documented after administering a medication?

3. List the steps for preparing a successful IV.

4. What is the purpose of a saline lock?

5. What is the difference between the *enteral* and *parenteral* routes of medication administration?

CHAPTER 8

Airway Management and Oxygenation

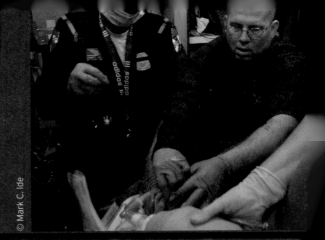

© Mark C. Ide

National EMS Education Standard

Airway Management, Respiration, and Artificial Ventilation

Applies knowledge of upper airway anatomy and physiology to patient assessment and management in order to assure a patent airway, adequate mechanical ventilation, and respiration for patients of all ages.

Anatomy and Physiology

Applies comprehensive knowledge of the anatomy and function of all human systems to the practice of EMS.

Pathophysiology

Applies comprehensive knowledge of the pathophysiology of respiration and perfusion to patient assessment and management.

Pharmacology

Applies fundamental knowledge of the medications that the AEMT may assist with/administer to a patient during an emergency.

Review

Perfusion of all cells in the body with oxygen remains the number one priority in patient care. The most critical patients are those with problems involving their ABCs—airway, breathing, and circulation. If the patient is unable to maintain an open airway, insert an oropharyngeal or nasopharyngeal airway; if he or she is not breathing, insert an airway adjunct and provide positive-pressure ventilations; and if the circulation of the blood is absent, perform CPR. For any patient with secretions or fluid in the airway, suction the oropharynx to prevent aspiration.

Patients often need supplemental oxygen. A nonrebreathing mask can deliver high-flow oxygen to the patient, whereas a nasal cannula provides a lesser amount. Artificial ventilations can be provided using a bag-mask device, a pocket face mask, or a manually triggered ventilation device. There are also certain airway devices that can be inserted blindly and result in better airway management and ventilation.

What's New

Even as a seasoned AEMT, it is important to understand the anatomy and physiology of the respiratory system in detail to fully understand the airway and respiratory conditions a patient may have. In addition, understanding the pathophysiology of ventilation, oxygenation, and respiration will help you better understand the signs and symptoms associated with certain conditions as well as management techniques for caring for a patient presenting with such conditions.

The AEMT has numerous options for providing oxygenation and ventilation to a patient, including the use of continuous positive airway pressure, single-lumen and multilumen airways, and supraglottic devices. To prevent drying of the mucous membranes in the nose, humidification of oxygen may be indicated. It is also important to recognize certain indications for providing nebulized medications to individuals experiencing respiratory distress and to provide prompt treatment and transport for these patients. Medication administration is covered in the chapter, *Respiratory Emergencies*.

Introduction

The single most important steps in caring for any patient are to obtain and maintain a patent airway and to ensure that the patient is breathing adequately. Within a few minutes of being deprived of oxygen, vital organs such as the heart and brain may not function normally. Brain cell death occurs within 4 to 6 minutes after being deprived of oxygen. Basic airway management skills tend to be taken for granted as more advanced skills are learned, yet they are among the most crucial skills any EMS provider learns.

Anatomy of the Respiratory System

The respiratory system consists of all the structures in the body that make up the airway and help us breathe **FIGURE 8-1**. Ventilation is the exchange of air between the lungs and environment.

The upper airway includes the nose, mouth, jaw, oral cavity, and pharynx (throat). The larynx is considered the dividing line between the upper and lower airways. The major functions of the upper airway are to warm, filter, and humidify air brought into the body.

The function of the lower airway is to exchange oxygen and carbon dioxide. Its external boundaries are the fourth cervical vertebra and the xiphoid process, or the narrow cartilaginous lower tip of the sternum. Internally, it spans the glottis to the pulmonary capillary membrane.

In addition to the respiratory and circulatory structures found in the chest cage, an important structure of the nervous system is also found in the thorax—the *phrenic nerve*. Originating from the cervical plexus of nerves in the neck, the phrenic nerve is one of the most important nervous structures in the body. It innervates the diaphragm muscle, allowing it to contract. Contraction of the diaphragm occurs in a downward direction and is necessary for adequate inspiration to occur. When the phrenic nerve stops stimulation of the diaphragm, the diaphragm relaxes and rises upward, causing exhalation to occur.

> *Phrenic nerve* The nerve that innervates the diaphragm; important for adequate breathing.

The respiratory and cardiovascular systems work together to ensure that a constant supply of oxygen and nutrients are delivered to every cell in the body and that carbon dioxide and waste products are removed from every

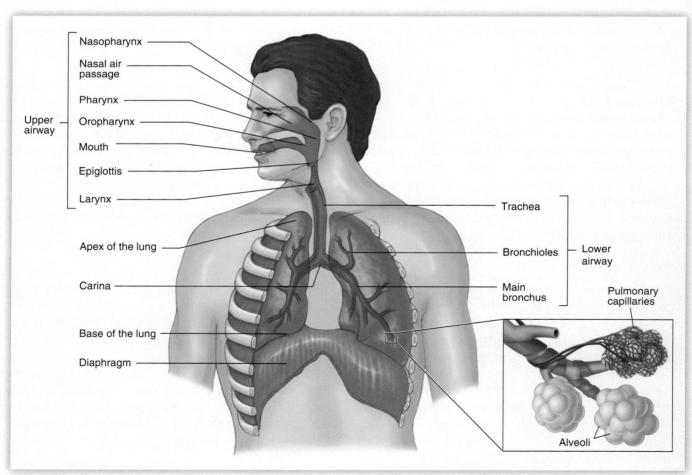

FIGURE 8-1 The upper and lower airways contain the body structures that help us breathe.

cell. When one of these systems is compromised, oxygen delivery is not effective and cellular death could result.

Physiology of the Respiratory System: A Review

While the terms are often used interchangeably, ventilation, oxygenation, and respiration are three distinct processes. If a problem arises in any one of these processes, it can affect other body processes and systems, possibly leading to permanent damage or death TABLE 8-1.

Ventilation

Pulmonary ventilation is the process of moving air into and out of the lungs through inhalation and exhalation. It is necessary for oxygenation and respiration to occur. Adequate, continuous ventilation is essential for life and therefore remains one of the highest priorities in patient care. If the patient has inadequate or absent breathing, immediate action is necessary. Signs of inadequate ventilation include the following:

- Altered mental status
- Inadequate minute volume (shallow or deep respirations)
- Excessive use of accessory muscles
- Fatigue from labored breathing
- Cyanosis
- Inability to speak in complete sentences (one- or two-word dyspnea)

> *Pulmonary ventilation* The process of moving air into and out of the lungs through inhalation and exhalation.

Inhalation

Inhalation is the active part of ventilation or breathing in which a person takes air into the body through the mouth and nose. During this process, the diaphragm and intercostal muscles contract, the thoracic cavity enlarges, and air moves into the trachea and to the lungs via the bronchi, bronchioles, and eventually the alveoli.

Because the lungs have no muscle tissue, they cannot move on their own. Instead, they need the help of other structures to be able to expand and contract during inhalation and exhalation. As such, their ability to function properly depends on the movement of the chest and supporting structures including the thorax, thoracic cavity (chest), diaphragm, intercostal muscles, and accessory muscles of breathing.

> ### Transition Tip
>
> Air can reach the lungs only if it travels through the trachea. As such, maintaining a clear and open airway is essential FIGURE 8-2. This is done by removing obstructing material, tissue, or fluids from the mouth, nose, and throat so that air can enter and leave the lungs freely.

The air pressure outside the body—that is, the atmospheric pressure—is normally higher than the air pressure within the thorax. During inhalation, the thoracic cavity expands, decreasing the air pressure and creating a slight vacuum. This vacuum pulls air in through the trachea, causing the lungs to fill. When the air pressure equalizes, air stops moving and inhalation stops.

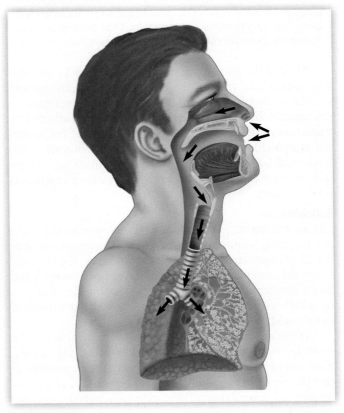

FIGURE 8-2 Air reaches the lungs only if it travels through the trachea. Maintaining the airway means keeping the airway patent so that air can enter and leave the lungs freely.

Table 8-1 Ventilation, Oxygenation, and Respiration	
System	**Function**
Ventilation	The physical act of moving air into and out of the lungs through inhalation and exhalation
Oxygenation	The process of loading oxygen molecules onto hemoglobin molecules in the bloodstream
Respiration	The actual exchange of oxygen and carbon dioxide in the aveoli as well as in the tissues of the body

The entire process of inspiration is focused on delivering oxygen to the alveoli (*alveolar ventilation*). However, not all the air you breathe actually reaches the alveoli. Some air remains in the mouth, nose, trachea, bronchi, and bronchioles; these areas are is called dead space. Alveolar ventilation is determined by subtracting the amount of dead space air from the tidal volume.

> *Alveolar ventilation* The volume of air that reaches the alveoli. It is determined by subtracting the amount of dead space air from the tidal volume.

Tidal volume is the amount of air that moves into or out of the lungs during a single breath. It is measured in milliliters (mL). The average tidal volume for a man is approximately 500 mL; of that amount, 150 mL typically remains in dead space and never reaches the alveoli for gas exchange.

Minute ventilation, or minute volume, is the amount of air that moves through the lungs in 1 minute, minus the dead space. It is calculated as follows:

$$\text{Minute Ventilation} = \text{Tidal Volume} \text{ (minus Dead Space)} \times \text{Respiratory Rate}$$

> *Minute ventilation* The volume of air moved through the lungs in 1 minute minus the dead space air; it is calculated by multiplying the tidal volume (minus the dead space air) and the respiratory rate. Also referred to as minute volume.

Thus, if the patient is breathing at a rate of 12 breaths/min, with a tidal volume of 500 mL per breath, the minute ventilation would be 4,200 mL (4.2 L). It is important to understand, however, that minute ventilation is affected by variations in tidal volume and respiratory rate. For example, if a patient has shallow respirations, the minute ventilation will be decreased. Likewise, the minute ventilation will increase if the patient has deep breathing (increased tidal volume).

Exhalation

Unlike inhalation, exhalation is a passive process that does not normally require muscular effort. During exhalation, the diaphragm and intercostal muscles relax, the thoracic cavity decreases in size, and air in the lungs is compressed into a smaller space. The air pressure within the thorax is then higher than the outside pressure, and the air is pushed out through the trachea.

Vital capacity refers to the amount of air that can be forcibly expelled from the lungs after breathing deeply. Even after forceful exhalation, however, it is impossible to completely empty the lungs of air. The amount of air that remains—known as the *residual volume*—averages approximately 1,200 mL in the average adult male. This residual volume is one of the reasons why CPR can circulate oxygen without providing ventilations.

Regulation of Ventilation

The body's need for oxygen is dynamic, meaning it changes constantly. The respiratory system must be able to accommodate these changes in oxygen demand by altering the rate and depth of ventilation. Such changes are regulated primarily by the cerebrospinal fluid (CSF) pH, which is directly related to the amount of carbon dioxide dissolved in the plasma portion of the blood. The regulation of ventilation involves a complex series of receptors and feedback loops that sense gas concentrations in the body fluids and send messages to the respiratory center in the brain to adjust the rate and depth of ventilation accordingly. Failure to meet the body's needs for oxygen may result in hypoxia, a dangerous condition in which the tissues and cells of the body do not receive enough oxygen. If this process is not corrected quickly, the patient may die.

For most people, the drive to breathe is based on pH changes (related to carbon dioxide levels) in the blood and CSF. However, patients with chronic obstructive pulmonary disease (COPD) have difficulty eliminating carbon dioxide through exhalation; thus they always have higher levels of carbon dioxide and therefore lower pH. This factor may potentially alter their drive for breathing because the respiratory center in the brain gradually accommodates the high levels of carbon dioxide. In patients with COPD, the body uses a backup system to control breathing called *hypoxic drive*, which is based on levels of oxygen dissolved in plasma. This mechanism differs from the primary control of breathing, which uses carbon dioxide as the driving force. Hypoxic drive is typically found in end-stage COPD. Providing high concentrations of oxygen over time will increase the amount of oxygen dissolved in plasma, which could potentially negatively affect the body's drive to breathe.

> *Vital capacity* The amount of air that can be forcibly expelled from the lungs after breathing in as deeply as possible.
> *Residual volume* The air that remains in the lungs after maximal expiration.
> *Hypoxic drive* A condition in which chronically low levels of oxygen in the blood stimulate the respiratory drive; it is seen in patients with chronic lung diseases.

Because increased oxygen levels could eliminate a patient's hypoxic drive, caution should be taken when administering high concentrations of oxygen to patients with COPD. At the same time, it is important to remember that high concentrations of oxygen should never be withheld from any patient who needs it. Patients with severe respiratory or circulatory compromise should receive high concentrations of oxygen regardless of their underlying medical conditions. Just remember that you must be prepared to support ventilations for patients whose drive to breathe is suppressed by high concentrations of oxygen. Such ventilation support may be no more than simply reminding them to breathe regularly.

Oxygenation

Oxygenation is the process of loading oxygen molecules onto hemoglobin molecules in the bloodstream. Although adequate oxygenation is required for internal respiration to take place, it does not *guarantee* that internal respiration is taking place. Oxygenation requires that the air used for ventilation contain an adequate percentage of oxygen. Although it is difficult to oxygenate without ventilation, it is possible to ventilate without oxygenation. This situation occurs when oxygen levels in the air have been depleted, such as in mines and confined spaces. It also takes place in carbon monoxide poisoning, where the excess number of carbon monoxide molecules in the body prevent tissue oxygenation. Ventilation without adequate oxygenation also occurs in climbers who ascend too quickly to an altitude of lower atmospheric pressure. At high altitudes, the percentage of oxygen remains the same, but the atmospheric pressure makes it difficult to adequately bring sufficient amounts of oxygen into the body.

> *Oxygenation* The process of delivering oxygen to the blood by diffusion from the alveoli following inhalation into the lungs.

Transition Tip

Oxygenation can be disrupted through carbon monoxide poisoning. Carbon monoxide has a much greater affinity for hemoglobin than oxygen (200 to 250 times more). As such, carbon monoxide molecules will bind tightly to the hemoglobin in the red blood cells blocking the oxygen molecules, thereby preventing the proper transport of oxygen to tissues and ultimately resulting in tissue death.

Respiration

All living cells perform a specific function and need energy to survive. Cells take energy from nutrients through a series of chemical processes. The name given to these processes as a whole is *metabolism*, or *cellular respiration*. During metabolism, each cell combines nutrients such as sugar with oxygen and produces energy and waste products, primarily water and carbon dioxide. Each cell in the body requires a continuous supply of oxygen and a regular means of disposing of waste (carbon dioxide). The body provides for these requirements through respiration.

Respiration is the process of exchanging oxygen and carbon dioxide. This exchange occurs by diffusion, during which a gas moves from an area of higher concentration to an area of lower concentration. In the body, gases diffuse rapidly across a short distance of only micrometers, and the diffusion occurs rapidly **FIGURE 8-3**.

External Respiration

External respiration, also known as pulmonary respiration, is the process of breathing air into the respiratory system and exchanging oxygen and carbon dioxide between the alveoli and the blood in the pulmonary capillaries **FIGURE 8-4**.

> *Metabolism (cellular respiration)* The biochemical processes that result in production of energy from nutrients within the cells.
> *Respiration* The process of exchanging oxygen and carbon dioxide.
> *External respiration* The exchange of gases between the lungs and the blood cells in the pulmonary capillaries; also called pulmonary respiration.

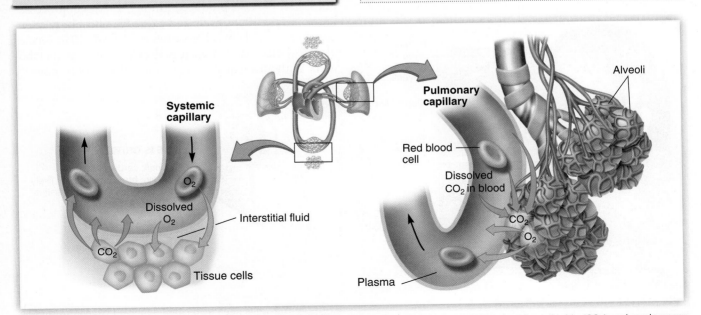

FIGURE 8-3 In the capillaries of the lungs, oxygen (O_2) passes from the blood to the tissue cells, and carbon dioxide (CO_2) and wastes pass from the tissue cells to the blood. Diffusion occurs when molecules move from an area of higher concentration to an area of lower concentration.

Once the oxygen crosses the alveolar membrane, it is bound to hemoglobin, an iron-containing molecule with a great affinity for oxygen molecules. Through their presence in red blood cells, hemoglobin molecules low in oxygen concentration are pumped from the right side of the heart into the capillaries of the pulmonary circulation. The capillaries surround alveoli containing high concentrations of oxygen (from inspired air). The hemoglobin molecules pick up fresh oxygen as it crosses the alveolar membrane and transport it back to the left side of the heart, where it is pumped out to the rest of the body.

Internal Respiration

Internal respiration is the exchange of oxygen and carbon dioxide between the systemic circulatory system and the cells of the body. Via its circulation through the body, blood supplies oxygen and nutrients to various tissues and cells. As the oxygenated blood travels through the arteries and capillaries, the oxygen passes from the blood in the capillaries to tissue cells, while carbon dioxide and cell wastes pass in the opposite direction, from tissue cells through capillaries and into the veins **FIGURE 8-5** .

Every cell in the body needs a constant supply of oxygen to survive. Whereas some tissues are more resilient than others, eventually all cells will die if they are deprived of

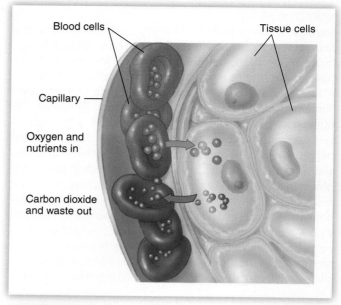

FIGURE 8-5 Internal respiration.

oxygen **FIGURE 8-6** . To deliver adequate amounts of oxygen to the tissues of the body, sufficient levels of external ventilation and perfusion must take place.

> *Internal respiration* The exchange of gases between the blood cells and the tissues.
> *Aerobic metabolism* Metabolism that can proceed only in the presence of oxygen.

In the presence of oxygen, the mitochondria of the cells convert glucose into energy through the process of *aerobic metabolism*. Energy in the form of adenosine triphosphate (ATP) is produced through a series of processes known as the Krebs cycle and oxidative phosphorylation. Together, these chemical processes yield nearly 40 molecules of energy-rich ATP for each molecule of glucose metabolized. Without adequate oxygen, the cells do not completely

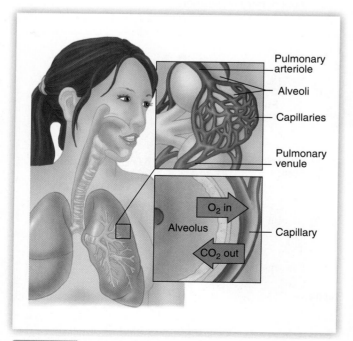

FIGURE 8-4 External respiration.

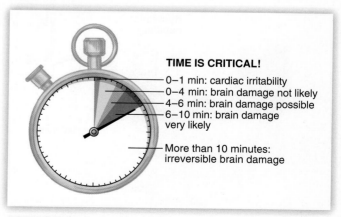

TIME IS CRITICAL!
- 0–1 min: cardiac irritability
- 0–4 min: brain damage not likely
- 4–6 min: brain damage possible
- 6–10 min: brain damage very likely
- More than 10 minutes: irreversible brain damage

FIGURE 8-6 Cells need a constant supply of oxygen to survive. Some cells may be severely or permanently damaged after going 4 to 6 minutes without oxygen.

convert glucose into energy, allowing lactic acid and other toxins to accumulate in the cell. This process, called *anaerobic metabolism*, cannot meet the metabolic demands of the cell. Although another intracellular process, glycolysis, also contributes to ATP production and does not require oxygen, it results in less ATP production and also produces lactic acid waste products and toxins. If this process is not corrected, the cells will eventually die. This phenomenon explains why adequate levels of *perfusion* (circulation of oxygenated blood within an organ or tissue) and external ventilation must be present for aerobic internal respiration to take place. However, while these elements are necessary for internal respiration, they do not guarantee that aerobic internal respiration will take place.

> *Anaerobic metabolism* Metabolism that takes place in the absence of oxygen; its principal product is lactic acid.
> *Perfusion* The circulation of oxygenated blood within an organ or tissue.

When the mitochondria within each cell use oxygen to convert glucose to energy, carbon dioxide—the main waste product—accumulates in the cell. Carbon dioxide is then transported through the circulatory system and back to the lungs for exhalation.

The process of ventilation, oxygenation, and respiration is an important concept for all AEMTs to understand. The overall goal of these mechanisms is to deliver an adequate supply of oxygen to the cells of the body. When one of these processes fails or becomes disrupted, cells die. By recognizing the signs and symptoms of inadequate tissue perfusion and oxygenation, you can immediately intervene and correct a potentially life-threatening condition.

Pathophysiology of Respiration

Multiple conditions inhibit the body's ability to effectively deliver oxygen to the cells. Disruption of pulmonary ventilation, oxygenation, and respiration will cause immediate effects on the body. As an AEMT, you need to recognize these conditions and correct them in a timely manner.

Neural Control

The neural control of breathing originates in the brain and brainstem. Primary control comes from the medulla and pons. The medulla is the primary involuntary respiratory center. The medullary respiratory centers control the rate, depth, and rhythm of breathing in a negative feedback interaction with centers in the pons.

The apneustic center of the pons is the secondary control center if the medulla fails to initiate respiration. The apneustic center influences the respiratory rate by increasing the number of inspirations per minute. This is balanced by the pneumotaxic center, which has an inhibitory influence on inspiration. The respiratory rate results from the interaction between these two centers. In times of increased demand, the pneumotaxic center decreases its influence, thereby increasing the respiratory rate.

Chemical Stimuli

The goal of the respiratory system is to keep the blood's concentrations of oxygen and carbon dioxide and its acid-base balance within very narrow normal ranges. The body has a number of receptors that monitor variables and provide feedback to the respiratory centers to modify the respiratory rate and depth based on the body's needs. These *chemoreceptors* have important effects on respiratory rate and depth.

> *Chemoreceptors* Receptors in the blood vessels, kidneys, brain, and heart that respond to changes in chemical composition of the blood to help maintain homeostasis.

Chemoreceptors that constantly monitor the chemical composition of body fluids are located throughout the body to provide feedback on many metabolic processes. Three sets of chemoreceptors affect respiratory function. The first two, which monitor the carbon dioxide level in the blood and the pH of the CSF, have a much greater effect on ventilatory depth and rate than the third.

The chemoreceptors that measure the carbon dioxide in arterial blood are located in the carotid bodies and the aortic body (located within the aortic arch). These receptors sense minute changes in the carbon dioxide level and send signals to the respiratory center via the glossopharyngeal nerve (9th cranial nerve) in the case of the carotid bodies and the vagus nerve (10th cranial nerve) in the case of the aortic bodies.

Central chemoreceptors, which constantly monitor the pH of the CSF, are located adjacent to the respiratory centers in the medulla. The CSF acidity is an indirect measure of the amount of carbon dioxide in arterial blood because the carbon dioxide in the blood readily diffuses across the blood-brain barrier and combines with water to form carbonic acid (H_2CO_3). The carbonic acid dissociates and the pH drops as the hydrogen ion (H^+) concentration increases. An increase in the CSF acidity triggers the central chemoreceptors to increase the rate and depth of respiration. These central chemoreceptors are very sensitive to small changes in pH and provide for fine tuning of the body's acid-base balance.

While the primary control of ventilation is the pH of the CSF, the amount of oxygen dissolved in the plasma (PaO_2) has a secondary and protective role. The chemoreceptors located in the aortic arch and carotid bodies also respond to decreases in PaO_2 by sending messages to the respiratory control center to increase respiration. Under normal conditions, these chemoreceptors serve as a backup to the primary control of ventilation, which is based on the level of carbon dioxide in the blood and the CSF pH.

When serum carbon dioxide or hydrogen ion levels increase because of medical or traumatic conditions involving the respiratory system, chemoreceptors stimulate the dorsal and ventral respiratory groups in the medulla to increase the respiratory rate, thus removing more carbon dioxide or acid from the body. The *dorsal respiratory group (DRG)* is responsible for initiating inspiration based on the information received from the chemoreceptors. The *ventral respiratory group (VRG)* is primarily responsible for motor control of the inspiratory and expiratory muscles.

Failure to meet the body's needs for oxygen may result in *hypoxia*. Hypoxia is an extremely dangerous condition in which the tissues and cells of the body do not get enough oxygen. If this process is not corrected, patients may die quickly.

Patients with COPD have difficulty eliminating carbon dioxide through exhalation; thus, they always have higher levels of carbon dioxide. This potentially can alter their drive for breathing. The theory is that respiratory centers in the brain gradually accommodate to a high level of carbon dioxide. In patients with COPD in the end stage of their disease, the body uses a backup system to control breathing. This theory of secondary control of breathing, called *hypoxic drive*, stimulates breathing when the arterial oxygen level falls. However, the nerves in the brain, the walls of the aorta, and the carotid arteries that act as oxygen sensors are easily satisfied with a minimal level of oxygen. Therefore, the hypoxic drive is much less sensitive and less powerful than the carbon dioxide sensors in the brainstem. Hypoxic drive is typically found in end-stage COPD and not in the recently diagnosed patient. Providing high concentrations of oxygen over time will increase the amount of oxygen dissolved in plasma. While some people believe this could potentially negatively affect the body's drive to breathe, this principle should never drive you to withhold supplemental oxygen from a patient whose clinical condition otherwise suggests that he needs it.

> *Dorsal respiratory group (DRG)* A portion of the medulla oblongata where the primary respiratory pacemaker is found.
> *Ventral respiratory group (VRG)* A portion of the medulla oblongata that is responsible for modulating breathing during speech.
> *Hypoxia* A dangerous condition in which the body's cells do not have enough oxygen.
> *Hypoxic drive* A backup system to control respirations when the oxygen level falls.

Regardless of the current research, caution should be taken when administering high concentrations of oxygen to patients with obstructive pulmonary disease. However, it is important to remember that a high concentration of oxygen should never be withheld from any patient who needs it. Patients with severe respiratory and/or circulatory compromise should receive high concentrations of oxygen via nonrebreathing mask or bag-mask ventilations regardless of their underlying medical conditions. Be prepared to

assist their ventilations if they become sleepy or develop respiratory depression.

Patients who are breathing inadequately will show varying signs and symptoms of hypoxia. The onset and degree of tissue damage caused by hypoxia often depend on the quality of ventilations. Early signs of hypoxia include restlessness, irritability, apprehension, fast heart rate (tachycardia), and anxiety. Late signs of hypoxia include mental status changes, a weak (thready) pulse, and cyanosis. Responsive patients will report shortness of breath (*dyspnea*) and may not be able to talk in complete sentences. The best time to give patients oxygen is before signs and symptoms of hypoxia appear.

> *Dyspnea* Shortness of breath or difficulty breathing.

Transition Tip

A patient who is breathing inadequately (hypoventilating) requires oxygen regardless of history. Withholding oxygen from a patient with COPD in an attempt to preserve the hypoxic drive could actually kill the patient. If vital organs are not perfused, cells and tissue may die, resulting in irreversible damage. Even after the cause of the problem is addressed, if substantial damage has occurred, the patient may not recover. By ventilating the hypoxic patient, vital organs are perfused. If the hypoxic drive is eliminated, organs are still oxygenated. Once the cause of the original problem is corrected, the patient can be weaned off the ventilator and may return to a normal, productive life.

Ventilation/Perfusion Ratio and Mismatch

The lungs have a functional role of placing ambient air in proximity to circulating blood to permit gas exchange by simple diffusion. To accomplish this action, air and blood flow must be directed to the same place at the same time. In other words, ventilation and perfusion must be matched. A failure to match ventilation and perfusion, or $\dot{V}/\dot{Q}$ mismatch, lies behind several abnormalities in oxygen and carbon dioxide exchange.

> $\dot{V}/\dot{Q}$ *mismatch* A measurement that examines how much gas is being moved effectively and how much blood is gaining access to the alveoli.

In most patients, the normal resting minute ventilation is approximately 6 L/min. About one third of this volume fills dead space; therefore, resting alveolar ventilation is approximately 4 L/min. However, pulmonary artery blood flow is approximately 5 L/min. This yields an overall ratio of ventilation to perfusion of 4/5 L, or 0.8 L. Neither ventilation nor perfusion is distributed equally; both are distributed to dependent regions at rest. However, the increase in gravity-dependent flow is more marked with perfusion (blood) than with ventilation (air). Hence, the ratio of ventilation to perfusion is highest at the apex of the lung and lowest at the base.

When ventilation is compromised but perfusion continues, blood passes over some alveolar membranes without gas exchange taking place; therefore, not all alveoli are enriched with oxygen. This in turn results in a lack of oxygen diffusing across the membrane and into blood circulation. Along the same lines, carbon dioxide is also not able to diffuse across the membrane and is recirculated in the bloodstream. This V/Q mismatch can lead to severe hypoxemia if the problem is not recognized and treated.

Similar problems can occur when perfusion across the alveolar membrane is disrupted. Even though the alveoli are filled with fresh oxygen, disruption in blood flow does not allow for optimal exchange in gases across the membrane. This results in less oxygen absorption in the bloodstream and less carbon dioxide removal. This can also lead to hypoxemia. The patient needs immediate intervention to prevent further damage or death.

Factors Affecting Ventilation

Maintaining a patent airway is critical to the delivery of oxygen to the body tissues. There are many intrinsic and extrinsic factors that cause airway obstructions. Intrinsic conditions such as infections, allergic reactions, and unresponsiveness (possibly leading to airway obstruction by the tongue) can cause significant restrictions on the ability to maintain an open airway. Swelling from infections and allergic reactions can be fatal if not aggressively managed with medications and possibly advanced airway maneuvers. The tongue is the most common airway obstruction in an unresponsive patient. This airway obstruction, while easily corrected, can result in hypoxia and hinder adequate tissue perfusion. Snoring respirations and the position of the head and/or neck are good indicators that the tongue may be obstructing the airway. Prompt correction of this obstruction is necessary for adequate oxygenation.

Some factors affecting pulmonary ventilation are not necessarily directly part of the respiratory system. The central and peripheral nervous systems have key roles in breathing regulation. Interruptions to these systems can have a drastic effect on the ability to breathe efficiently. Medications that depress the central nervous system lower the respiratory rate and tidal volume. This lower rate and volume will decrease the overall minute volume and alveolar ventilation. As a result, the amount of carbon dioxide in the respiratory and circulatory systems is increased, resulting in an overall increase of the carbon dioxide level in the bloodstream, known as *hypercarbia*. Trauma to the head and spinal cord can also interrupt nervous control of ventilation, resulting in decreased respiratory function and even failure. In addition to medications and trauma, conditions such as muscular dystrophy can also affect nervous

control. This disease causes degeneration of muscle fibers, resulting in a gradual weakening of muscles, slowing motor development, and loss of muscle contractility. Curvature of the spine also occurs in patients with muscular dystrophy resulting in decreased thoracic volume, which impairs pulmonary function.

> *Hypercarbia* Increased carbon dioxide level in the bloodstream.

Patients with allergic reactions might have not only a potential airway obstruction from swelling, but also a decrease in pulmonary ventilation from bronchoconstriction. As the bronchioles constrict, air is forced through smaller lumens, resulting in decreased ventilation. This condition is also found in patients with COPD and asthma.

Extrinsic factors affecting pulmonary ventilation can include trauma and foreign body airway obstruction. Trauma to the airway or chest requires immediate evaluation and intervention. Blunt or penetrating trauma and burns can disrupt airflow through the trachea and into the lungs, quickly resulting in oxygenation deficiencies. In addition, trauma to the chest wall can result in structural damage to the thorax, leading to inadequate pulmonary ventilation. Swelling, punctures, and bruising have a tremendous effect on the ability to deliver oxygen to the alveoli and into the bloodstream. Proper airway management and high concentrations of oxygen are crucial to the outcome in these situations.

Factors Affecting Respiration

External elements in the environment can affect the overall process of respiration. For proper respiration to take place at the cellular level, both oxygenation and perfusion need to function efficiently.

External Factors

Adequate respiration requires proper ventilation and oxygenation. Here, external factors such as atmospheric pressure and the partial pressure of oxygen in the ambient air have a key role in the overall process of respiration. At high altitudes, the percentage of oxygen remains the same, but the partial pressure decreases because the total atmospheric pressure decreases. The low partial pressure of oxygen can make it difficult (or impossible) to adequately oxygenate tissue, thus interrupting internal respiration. In addition, closed environments, such as mines and trenches, may have significant decreases in ambient oxygen, resulting in poor oxygenation and respiration.

Carbon monoxide, along with other toxic gases, displaces oxygen in the environment and makes proper oxygenation and respiration difficult. Carbon monoxide, in particular, has a much greater affinity for hemoglobin than does oxygen (200 to 250 times more), thus not allowing for proper transport of oxygen to tissues and causing false pulse oximeter readings.

Internal Factors

Conditions that reduce the surface area for gas exchange also decrease the body's oxygen supply, leading to inadequate tissue perfusion. Medical conditions such as pneumonia, *pulmonary edema*, and COPD may also result in a disturbance of cellular metabolism. These conditions decrease the surface area of the alveoli by damaging the alveoli or by leading to an accumulation of fluid in the lungs.

Nonfunctional alveoli inhibit the diffusion of oxygen and carbon dioxide. As a result, blood entering the lungs from the right side of the heart bypasses the alveoli and returns to the left side of the heart in an unoxygenated state, a condition called *intrapulmonary shunting*.

> *Pulmonary edema* A buildup of fluid in the lungs, usually a result of congestive heart failure.
>
> *Intrapulmonary shunting* Bypassing of oxygen-poor blood past nonfunctional alveoli to the left side of the heart.

Submersion (previously called near drowning) victims and patients with pulmonary edema have fluid in the alveoli. This accumulation of fluid inhibits adequate gas exchange at the alveolar membrane and results in decreased oxygenation and respiration. In addition, exposure to certain environmental conditions like high altitudes, or occupational hazards such as epoxy resins, over time can result in fluid accumulation or other abnormal conditions, resulting in an overall decrease in respiration. These conditions can interrupt the process of aerobic respiration at the cellular level, resulting in anaerobic respiration and an increase in lactic acid accumulation.

Respirations increase or decrease based on the body's need at any given time. As body temperature rises, respirations increase in response to the increased metabolic activity. Certain medications cause the respiratory rate to increase or decrease, depending on their physiologic action. Pain and strong emotions can also increase respirations. Hypoxia, which is a powerful stimulus to breathe, increases respirations in an effort to bring in more oxygen. Conversely, in an effort to eliminate carbon dioxide from the body, respirations increase when there is increased carbon dioxide production. Respirations decrease as metabolism slows, such as during sleep.

Other conditions affecting cells of the body include hypoglycemia (low blood glucose level) and infection. As oxygen and glucose levels decrease, the body is unable to maintain a homeostatic balance with regard to energy production. At this point, the energy production cannot meet the needs of the body, and cellular death is likely if the condition is not quickly corrected. Infection also increases the metabolic needs of the body and disrupts homeostasis. If not corrected, the cells will die as well.

Circulatory Compromise

For respiration to take place, the circulatory system must function efficiently to deliver oxygen to the body tissues.

When this system becomes compromised, the perfusion of oxygen is not enough to meet the oxygen demands of the tissues.

Obstruction of blood flow to individual cells and tissue often occurs in trauma emergencies you may encounter. These conditions include a simple or tension *pneumothorax*, open pneumothorax (sucking chest wound), hemothorax, and hemopneumothorax. All of these conditions limit the ability for gas exchange at the tissue level as a result of their effects on the respiratory and circulatory systems. In addition, conditions such as pulmonary embolism, heart failure, and cardiac tamponade inhibit the ability of the heart to effectively pump oxygenated blood to the tissues.

Blood loss and anemia, a deficiency of red blood cells, result in a decreased ability of blood to carry oxygen. Without sufficient circulating red blood cells, there are not enough hemoglobin molecules for binding to oxygen.

When the body is in a state of shock, oxygen is not being delivered to the cells efficiently. *Hypovolemic shock* is an abnormal decrease in blood volume that causes inadequate oxygen delivery to the body. In contrast, *vasodilatory shock* is not determined by the amount of circulating blood but by the size of the blood vessels. As the diameter of the blood vessels increases, the blood pressure in the circulatory system decreases. As the systemic blood pressure falls, oxygen is not delivered to the tissues in an effective manner. Both forms of shock result in poor tissue perfusion that leads to anaerobic metabolism. Any patient suspected of being in shock should be treated aggressively to prevent further interruptions in tissue perfusion.

> *Pneumothorax* A partial or complete accumulation of air in the pleural space.
>
> *Hypovolemic shock* Shock caused by fluid or blood loss.
>
> *Vasodilatory shock* A type of shock related to relaxation of the blood vessels, allowing blood to pool and impairing circulation.

▮Acid-Base Balance

Disruptions in the acid-base balance in the body caused by hypoventilation and hyperventilation, along with hypoxia, may lead to rapid deterioration and death. The respiratory system and the renal system have roles in maintaining homeostasis in the body. Homeostasis is a tendency toward stability in the body's internal environment and requires a balance between the acids and bases in the body. When there is an excess of acid in the body, the fastest way to get rid of it is through the respiratory system. Excess acid can be expelled as carbon dioxide from the lungs. Conversely, slowing respirations will increase the level of carbon dioxide. The renal system regulates pH by filtering out more hydrogen and retaining bicarbonate when needed, or doing the reverse as necessary. Remember that an acid is any molecule that gives up a hydrogen ion and is often referred to as H^-, and a base is any molecule that can accept a hydrogen ion and is often referred to as OH⁻.

The acidity of a solution is defined by the amount of free hydrogen found in the solution. The *pH* is the measurement of the level of a solution's acidity (from acidic substances) or alkalinity (from base substances). Normal body functions work best within a very narrow range of pH: between 7.35 and 7.45. Cellular function deteriorates and death can occur when the pH drops below 6.9 or rises above 7.8.

> *pH* The measure of acidity or alkalinity of a solution.

Concentrations of H⁺ ions can be increased by adding more H⁺ ions to a solution or by removing OH⁻. To make a solution more acidic, or to decrease its pH, a higher concentration of H⁺ and a lower concentration of OH⁻ are needed. If the solution needs to be more basic, or to increase the pH level, we have two options:

1. Decrease the amount of H⁺.
2. Increase the amount of OH⁻.

Let's say, for example, that strong coffee is acidic and weak coffee is basic. To make the coffee stronger (more acidic), more coffee grounds are added (add H⁺) or less water is used (remove OH⁻). Conversely, to make the coffee weaker (more basic), fewer grounds are used (remove H⁺) or more water is added (add OH⁻).

Ion Shifts

To function properly, acid-base balance, or a balance of charges, must exist on both sides of the cell. If intracellular pH is low, excess H⁺ ions exist in the extracellular fluid (fluid outside the cells) and H⁺ ions move into the cell. This causes the cell to have an overall positive charge. To return its overall charge to neutral, the cell begins to shift cations (ions with a positive charge) into the interstitial fluid. Potassium shifts out into the extracellular fluid until no more potassium can safely be shifted out. This shift has significant consequences and can lead to hyperkalemia, a serious medical emergency.

Calcium ions also shift out of the cell in response to the influx of hydrogen. A high serum calcium level (hypercalcemia) decreases neural transmissions (the speed at which an impulse travels through the nerve cell), whereas a low serum calcium level (hypocalcemia) leads to hypersensitive nerve cells and increased neural transmissions. An increase in extracellular H⁺ ions results in *acidosis*; a decrease in extracellular H⁺ ions results in *alkalosis*.

↓pH Means ↑H⁺ Ion Concentration = Acidosis
↑pH Means ↓H⁺ Ion Concentration = Alkalosis

> *Acidosis* A pathologic condition resulting from the accumulation of acids in the body.
> *Alkalosis* A pathologic condition resulting from the accumulation of bases in the body.

Buffers

A buffer is a compound that can repeatedly neutralize excess acids or bases to prevent the pH from going beyond an acceptable level. For example, circulating proteins can bind with excess acids or bases, thus neutralizing their effects. Bone acts as a buffer by absorbing excess acids and bases and by releasing calcium into the circulation.

Acids can be classified as strong or weak, depending on how completely they *dissociate* in water. It is the ability of weak acids to bond weakly to hydrogen ions that makes them ideal buffers because they can accept or donate hydrogen ions, depending on the needs of the body.

> *Dissociate* To lose a hydrogen atom in the presence of water. Acids are classified as strong or weak, depending on how completely they dissociate in water.

An analogy for understanding a buffer system is to imagine it as a bucket **FIGURE 8-7**. Like a bucket, the buffer system can hold only a certain amount of acid before it reaches the point at which it is saturated (the bucket is full) and overflows. The body responds to shifts in the pH level by absorbing or releasing small amounts of acid into the blood. Problems begin when the amount of acid in circulation is too great and the buffer system becomes overwhelmed.

There are three main components to the buffer system in the body:

- The circulating bicarbonate (HCO_3^-) buffer component
- The respiratory component
- The renal component

The following equation illustrates the balance among these three components:

$$CO_2 + H_2O \leftrightarrow H_2CO_3 \leftrightarrow HCO_3^- + H^+$$

| Respiratory Component | Circulating bicarbonate buffer component | Renal component |

The Circulating Bicarbonate Buffer Component

The circulating bicarbonate buffer component is the bucket that holds and neutralizes excess acid. The circulating bicarbonate buffer system is found in the intracellular and

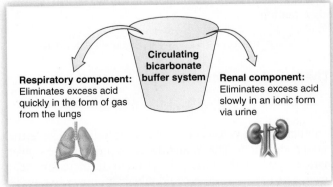

Respiratory component: Eliminates excess acid quickly in the form of gas from the lungs

Circulating bicarbonate buffer system

Renal component: Eliminates excess acid slowly in an ionic form via urine

FIGURE 8-7 Bucket analogy of the body's buffer system.

extracellular fluids and is the fastest-acting segment of the buffer system.

$$H_2CO_3 \leftrightarrow H^+ + HCO_3^-$$

Carbonic acid is a weak acid that can give up an extra H^+ ion to reform as the bicarbonate ion (HCO_3^-). Through metabolic processes, the extra H^+ ion is then converted into compounds that are easily expelled from the body, eliminating the extra acid.

The Respiratory Component

The fastest way the body can get rid of the excess H^+ ions is to create water and carbon dioxide, which can be expelled as gases from the lungs. The following equation illustrates this process, which occurs in the lungs:

$$H_2CO_3 \leftrightarrow CO_2 + H_2O$$

The main reason for breathing is to bring oxygen in for aerobic metabolism and to remove excess carbon dioxide from the blood. Carbon dioxide combines with the circulating water in the blood to create carbonic acid. Chemoreceptors in the brain sense the rising level of carbonic acid and signal the respiratory center to increase respirations and to reduce the available amount of circulating carbon dioxide. Although the respiratory component reacts within minutes, it is much slower to respond than the circulating buffer system. Consider the buffer bucket example again: The respiratory component can be thought of as a large faucet that allows acid to spill out of the buffer bucket, returning the pH to a normal level.

Anything that limits respirations can lead to acid retention and acidosis. Any time a patient is in respiratory distress or is unable to breathe, acidosis quickly develops:

$$\uparrow H^+ \rightarrow \uparrow H_2CO_3 \rightarrow \uparrow CO_2 \rightarrow \text{Tachypnea}$$

A patient can develop acidosis as a result of respiratory difficulty. The following equation demonstrates this:

$$\downarrow \text{Respirations} \rightarrow \uparrow CO_2 \rightarrow \uparrow H_2CO_3 \rightarrow \text{Acidosis}$$

Alkalosis can also develop if the respiratory rate is too high (or the volume too much), as shown in the following equation:

$$\uparrow \text{Respiration} \rightarrow \downarrow CO_2 \rightarrow \downarrow H_2CO_3 \rightarrow \text{Alkalosis}$$

The Renal Component

$$H_2CO_3 \leftrightarrow H^+ + HCO_3^-$$

Another smaller faucet connected to the buffer bucket is the renal component. The smaller faucet represents the slower nature by which the kidneys respond to the increasing acid level. The renal response could take from hours to days to restore the body's pH to normal. Kidneys account for every molecule, ion, and electrolyte found in the circulation; they maintain homeostasis by retaining certain products and filtering out others.

As with the respiratory system, the renal system can control the increasing acid level in the blood by excreting the acid. The kidneys excrete acid in an ionic form, unlike the respiratory system, which excretes acid as a gas.

If the patient experiences decreased urine output, excess acid cannot be removed from the blood and acidosis can develop.

$$\downarrow \text{Output} \rightarrow \uparrow H^+ \rightarrow \text{Acidosis}$$

If urine output becomes excessive, alkalosis can develop.

$$\uparrow \text{Output} \rightarrow \downarrow H^+ \rightarrow \text{Alkalosis}$$

Pathophysiology of Acid-Base Balance

There are four main clinical presentations of acid-base disorders:

- Respiratory acidosis
- Respiratory alkalosis
- Metabolic acidosis
- Metabolic alkalosis

Fluctuations in pH caused by the available bicarbonate level result in metabolic acidosis or alkalosis, whereas fluctuations in pH because of respiratory disorders result in respiratory acidosis or alkalosis.

Acid-base disorders not immediately correctable by the body's buffering systems initiate compensatory mechanisms to help return levels to normal. For example, metabolic acidosis may create respiratory alkalosis as a compensatory response. Often, patient management involves treating more than one form of acid-base imbalance.

Respiratory Acidosis

Recall the following equation from earlier in this section, which demonstrates how decreased respirations can result in acidosis:

$$\downarrow \text{Respirations} \rightarrow \uparrow CO_2 \rightarrow \uparrow H_2CO_3 \rightarrow \text{Acidosis}$$

Respiratory acidosis is always related to hypoventilation of some type. Because the acidosis is a result of insufficient breathing, the compensatory mechanism is the slower-reacting renal system. Some causes for respiratory acidosis include the following:

- Airway obstruction
- Cardiac arrest
- Overdose of a central nervous system depressant drug
- Drowning (submersion)
- Respiratory arrest
- Pulmonary edema
- Closed head injury
- Chest trauma
- Carbon monoxide poisoning

> *Respiratory acidosis* A pathologic condition characterized by a blood pH of less than 7.35, caused by accumulation of acids in the body from a respiratory cause.

Hypoventilation that develops from any of the conditions listed is considered a serious, life-threatening condition. The acidosis that results is quick, overwhelming, and potentially fatal, making it impossible for the slower-reacting renal system to compensate in time for the pH shift. The increasing acidosis causes potassium ions to shift into the extracellular fluid, leading to a potentially fatal cardiac *dysrhythmia*. Calcium also shifts into extracellular spaces, resulting in hypercalcemia. This creates lethargy and a decreasing level of consciousness (LOC) as well as a generalized slowing of the nervous system. This may be evidenced by a delayed pupillary response or a weakened or delayed response to painful stimuli.

Signs and symptoms of respiratory acidosis include the following:

- Systemic or *cerebral vasodilation* or both
- Headaches
- Red, flushed skin
- *Central nervous system (CNS) depression*
- *Bradypnea* (slow respiratory rate)
- Nausea and vomiting
- Hypercalcemia

> *Dysrhythmia* An irregular or abnormal heart rhythm.
> *Cerebral vasodilation* Relaxation of cerebral blood vessels that can lead to pooling of blood and inadequate circulation.
> *Central nervous system (CNS) depression* The slowing of the nervous system function of the brain because of delays in nerve cell transmission. Several factors can influence CNS depression including nerve cell permeability, hypoxia, drugs, and injury.
> *Bradypnea* A slow respiratory rate.

COPD creates respiratory acidosis over time as gradual destruction of lung tissue inhibits the exchange of oxygen and carbon dioxide. With COPD, the normal stimulus for this exchange is absent. Increasing carbon dioxide retention leads to an increasing level of carbonic acid, eventually making chemoreceptors unaware of the presence of metabolic acids. The hypoxic drive is then the only remaining stimulus for respiration. The hypoxic drive stimulates breathing based on the circulating oxygen level in the blood.

The slow onset makes this form of respiratory acidosis in patients with COPD survivable. In these cases, the renal system slowly mitigates the acidosis, preventing the life-threatening cardiac arrhythmias that may result from acute acidosis.

Respiratory Alkalosis

Recall the following equation from earlier in this section, which demonstrates how increased respirations can result in alkalosis:

$$\uparrow \text{Respirations} \rightarrow \downarrow_{CO_2} \rightarrow \downarrow H_2CO_3 \rightarrow \text{Alkalosis}$$

Respiratory alkalosis is always the result of *hyperventilation*. The carbon dioxide level drops in the blood, forcing a reduction of circulating carbonic acid. The renal system then begins retaining H^+ ions to rebalance the depleted acid level. As this is happening, H^+ ions begin to shift from the extracellular to the intracellular fluid compartment. Calcium shifts into the intracellular compartment to rebalance the depleted hydrogen level. Hypocalcemia leads to muscle contractions; the classic sign of carpopedal spasms accompanies hyperventilation.

Treatment for the classic hyperventilation syndrome focuses on restoring the normal respiratory rate to increase the carbon dioxide level. However, increasing the carbon dioxide level can aggravate other more serious medical conditions that cause hyperventilation. Therefore, you must carefully evaluate the patient to determine the underlying cause of the hyperventilation before you attempt to correct it.

Some causes for hyperventilation and respiratory alkalosis include the following:

- Drug overdoses, especially aspirin
- Fever
- Overzealous bag-mask ventilations

Some signs and symptoms of respiratory alkalosis include the following:

- Decreased LOC
- Light-headedness
- Carpopedal spasms
- Tingling lips and face
- Chest tightness
- Confusion
- Vertigo
- Blurred vision
- Hypocalcemia
- Nausea and vomiting

> *Respiratory alkalosis* A pathologic condition characterized by a blood pH of greater than 7.45 and resulting from the accumulation of bases in the body from a respiratory cause.
> *Hyperventilation* Rapid or deep breathing.
> *Metabolic acidosis* A pathologic condition characterized by a blood pH of less than 7.35; caused by accumulation of acids in the body from a metabolic cause.

Metabolic Acidosis

The following equation demonstrates how an increased carbonic acid level can result in *metabolic acidosis*:

$$\uparrow H_2CO_3 \rightarrow \uparrow H^+ + HCO_3^- \rightarrow \text{Acidosis}$$

Any acidosis that is not related to the respiratory system is considered metabolic. Increased respiration (tachypnea) is the compensatory mechanism for this condition as the respiratory system attempts to restore acid-base balance by eliminating carbon dioxide. Patient presentations for metabolic acidosis are similar to those for respiratory acidosis.

As with any acidosis, the extracellular hydrogen level increases and the extracellular buffers attempt to neutralize the excess acid. Ion shifts occur, hydrogen leaks into the cell, and potassium shifts into the extracellular spaces, raising the serum potassium level, which can lead to potentially life-threatening cardiac arrhythmias. Along with the potassium ion shift, calcium also shifts into extracellular spaces. The resulting hypercalcemia obstructs impulses to muscle and nerve cells, and the patient becomes lethargic with a decreased LOC.

Causes for metabolic acidosis include the following:

- *Lactic acidosis* created by anaerobic cellular respiration caused by *hypoperfusion* of tissues and organs, as seen with shock and cardiac arrest.
- Ketoacidosis results when cells are forced to switch to metabolizing fatty acids for energy because they are unable to utilize glucose due to insulin insufficiency or desensitization of the cells to insulin. The by-products of fat metabolism are *ketones*, which are extremely acidic.
- Aspirin (acetylsalicylic acid) overdose (10 to 30 g for adults). Acetylsalicylic acid directly stimulates the respiratory centers of the brain, creating tachypnea and leading to respiratory alkalosis. Compensatory mechanisms involve the renal system, resulting in metabolic acidosis.
- Alcohol ingestion. Ingestion of ethyl alcohol can lead to *alcoholic ketoacidosis*. Methanol (wood alcohol) and ethylene glycol can produce fatal forms of acidosis, often with amounts as small as 30 mL.
- Gastrointestinal losses. Diarrhea, for example, removes bases from the lower intestinal tract.

Lactic acidosis The metabolic acidotic state resulting from the accumulation of lactic acid during anaerobic cellular metabolism.
Hypoperfusion A condition that develops when the circulatory system is not able to deliver sufficient blood and oxygen to body organs, resulting in organ failure and eventual death if untreated.
Ketones The by-products of fat metabolism when fatty acids are used, rather than glucose, by body cells. An excess can lead to ketoacidosis.
Alcoholic ketoacidosis The metabolic acidotic state that manifests from the poor nutritional habits associated with chronic alcohol abuse. The liver and the body experience inadequate fuel reserves of glycogen and thus have to switch to fatty acid metabolism.

Signs and symptoms of metabolic acidosis include the following:

- Vasodilation
- CNS depression
- Headaches
- Hot, red, flushed skin
- Hypercalcemia

- Tachypnea
- Nausea and vomiting
- Arrhythmias

Metabolic Alkalosis

The following equation demonstrates how decreased hydrogen ions can result in alkalosis:

$$\downarrow H^+ \rightarrow \downarrow H_2CO_3 \rightarrow \text{Alkalosis}$$

Metabolic alkalosis results any time there is excessive loss of acid from excessive urination or from a decreased acid level in the stomach. Several factors related to upper gastrointestinal losses can lead to metabolic alkalosis:

- Excessive vomiting
- Excessive water intake
- Nasogastric suctioning
- Excessive intake of base
- Eating disorders

Metabolic alkalosis A pathologic condition characterized by a blood pH of greater than 7.45, and resulting from the accumulation of bases in the body from a metabolic cause.

Causes for metabolic alkalosis include the following:

- Upper gastrointestinal losses of acid resulting from illness or anorexia. When the patient expels a great deal of acid from the stomach, a complex metabolic pathway can lead to metabolic alkalosis.
- Drinking large amounts of water during heavy exertion. The water not only dilutes the stomach acid, it also stimulates the digestive system to prepare for incoming food from the stomach. This stimulation causes a dump of very basic digestive enzymes into the lower gastrointestinal tract, adding to the acid-base imbalance. As with respiratory alkalosis, there is a shift of calcium out of the cell—hypercalcemia—causing overstimulation of the nervous system and leading to muscle cramping. This cramping is analogous to carpopedal spasms except it occurs in the abdominal area and is referred to as heat cramps.
- Excessive intake of basic substances such as antacids **FIGURE 8-8**. This is important to remember when dealing with cardiac patients because one of their main complaints tends to be feelings of nausea or indigestion. Often, the patient has self-medicated for hours or days with over-the-counter antacids, which can result in metabolic alkalosis. Another cause of excessive base intake is the excessive administration of sodium bicarbonate during resuscitation. Introducing excessive amounts of sodium bicarbonate intravenously can seriously alter the pH level.

The compensatory mechanism for metabolic alkalosis is the respiratory system. To correct the reduced hydrogen

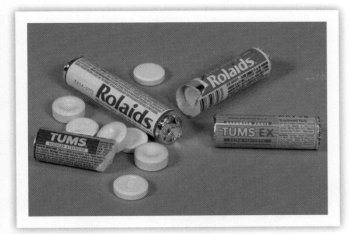

FIGURE 8-8 Excessive intake of basic substances such as antacids can result in metabolic alkalosis.

level, bradypnea develops to retain carbon dioxide and drive up the levels of circulating acids.

Signs and symptoms of metabolic alkalosis include the following:

- Confusion
- Muscle tremors and cramps
- Bradypnea
- Hypotension

Patient Assessment: Airway Evaluation

Recognizing Adequate Breathing

Think of a normal breathing pattern as a bellows system. Breathing should appear easy, not labored. As with a bellows used to move air to start a fire, breathing should be a smooth flow of air into and out of the lungs. A patient with adequate breathing should be able to speak in full sentences and in a normal voice. Generally, if you can see or hear a patient breathe, there is a problem.

> **Transition Tip**
>
> Recognition of a very rapid rate, a very slow rate, any unusual respiratory pattern, or poor tidal volume should immediately lead to consideration of bag-mask ventilations if the patient will tolerate it.

Normal respirations in an adult are characterized by a rate of between 12 and 20 breaths/min with adequate depth (tidal volume, a regular pattern of inhalation and exhalation, and clear and equal lung sounds on both sides of the chest [bilateral]). Irregular respiratory patterns are clinically significant until proven otherwise. Breathing at rest should be effortless; changes may be subtle in rate or regularity. Patients often compensate for respiratory distress with preferential positioning, such as an upright sniffing position (tripoding)

or a semi-Fowler (semisitting) position. A patient experiencing breathing difficulty will avoid a supine position because this position increases respiratory distress.

Recognizing Inadequate Breathing

An adult who is awake, alert, and able to talk to you in complete sentences has no immediate airway or breathing problems. However, you should always have supplemental oxygen and ventilation equipment close at hand to assist with breathing if necessary. An adult who is breathing normally will have respirations of 12 to 20 breaths/min **TABLE 8-2** with a regular pattern of breathing and adequate depth (tidal volume). An adult patient who is breathing fewer than 12 breaths/min or more than 20 breaths/min should be evaluated for other signs of inadequate breathing, such as reduced tidal volume (shallow breathing), an irregular pattern of breathing, altered mentation, or abnormal airway sounds.

Respiratory distress may be the result of upper and/or lower airway obstruction, inadequate ventilation, impairment of the respiratory muscles, or impairment of the nervous system. Any difficulty in respiratory rate, regularity, or effort is defined as dyspnea. Dyspnea may be the result of or result in *hypoxemia*, a deficiency of oxygen in the arterial blood. If left untreated, hypoxemia will progress to hypoxia (lack of oxygen to the body's cells and tissues). Untreated hypoxia will lead to anoxia and death of the body's cells and tissues.

> *Hypoxemia* A deficiency of oxygen in arterial blood.

Recognition and treatment of dyspnea are crucial to patient survival. Careful assessment and management of a patient with dyspnea are essential. The brain can survive only a few minutes of anoxia. After 4 to 6 minutes without oxygen, brain cells may be severely and permanently damaged and may even die. Dead brain cells can never be replaced. Management of the patient will be ineffective if the airway is not patent and the patient is not breathing adequately.

Evaluation of the patient in respiratory distress includes observation, palpation, and auscultation. Visual techniques should be used at first sight of the patient, literally from the door as you are entering the room. The following questions

Table 8-2 Normal Respiratory Rate Ranges	
Adults	12 to 20 breaths/min
Children	15 to 30 breaths/min
Infants	25 to 50 breaths/min
These ranges are per the NHTSA 2009 *EMT National EMS Education Standards*. Ranges presented in other courses may vary.	

should be answered when you are assessing a patient for signs of respiratory distress:

- How is the patient positioned? Is he or she in a tripod position (elbows out)?
- Is the patient *orthopneic*? (Does the patient have positional dyspnea?)
- Is there adequate rise and fall of the chest?
- Is the patient gasping?
- What is the color of the skin?
- Is there any flaring of the nares?
- Are the lips pursed?
- Do verbal or painful stimuli affect the respiratory rate?
- Do you note any retractions (skin pulling in around the ribs during inspiration):
  - Intercostal?
  - At the suprasternal notch?
  - At the supraclavicular fossa?
  - Subcostal?
- Is the patient using accessory muscles to breathe?

A patient with inadequate breathing may appear to be working hard to breathe. This type of breathing pattern is called *labored breathing*. It requires effort and, especially among children, may involve the use of accessory muscles. Accessory muscles include the neck muscles (sternocleidomastoid), the chest pectoralis major muscles, and the abdominal muscles **FIGURE 8-9** .

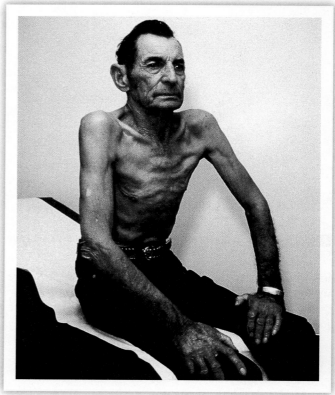

Courtesy of AAOS

FIGURE 8-9 The accessory muscles of breathing are used when a patient is having difficulty breathing, but not during normal breathing. The accessory muscles include the sternocleidomastoid, pectoralis major, and abdominal muscles.

Orthopnea Severe dyspnea experienced when lying down and relieved by sitting up.
Labored breathing Breathing that requires visibly increased effort; characterized by grunting, stridor, and use of accessory muscles.

These muscles are not used during normal breathing. More information about recognizing labored breathing and respiratory distress in children is found in later chapters. Signs of inadequate breathing in adults are as follows:

- Respiratory rate of fewer than 12 breaths/min or more than 20 breaths/min in the presence of shortness of breath (dyspnea)
- Irregular rhythm, such as a patient taking a series of deep breaths followed by periods of apnea
- Diminished, absent, or noisy auscultated breath sounds
- Abdominal breathing
- Reduced flow of expired air at the nose and mouth
- Unequal or inadequate chest expansion, resulting in reduced tidal volume
- Increased effort of breathing—use of accessory muscles
- Shallow depth (reduced tidal volume)
- Skin that is pale, cyanotic (blue), cool, or moist (clammy)

- Skin pulling in around the ribs or above the clavicles during inspiration (*retractions*)
- Staccato speech patterns (one- to two-word dyspnea)

When you are assessing a patient with a potential airway compromise, pay particular attention to the external environment and take that into consideration when examining your patient. Do not forget personal safety if the environment is unsafe. Conditions such as high altitude and enclosed spaces alter the partial pressure of oxygen in the environment, thus making the process of oxygenation difficult for the patient. In addition, poisonous gases such as carbon monoxide displace oxygen in the environment and alter the overall metabolism of the patient. It is important to recognize these potential situations and take them into consideration when deciding on appropriate treatment for the patient.

Next, auscultate breathing with and without a stethoscope. Is air movement noted at the mouth and nose? Can clear, equal, and *bilateral* breath sounds be heard over all lung fields?

Retractions Movements in which the skin pulls in around the ribs during inspiration.
Bilateral A body part or condition that appears on both sides of the midline.

Finally, feel for air movement at the mouth and nose. Observe the chest for symmetry, *paradoxical motion*, and retractions. Paradoxical motion is the inward movement of the chest during inhalation and outward movement during exhalation, which is the opposite of normal chest wall movement during breathing and occurs on the side of injury (flail segment).

> *Paradoxical motion* The motion of the chest wall section that is detached in a flail chest; the motion is exactly the opposite of normal motion during breathing (that is, in during inhalation, out during exhalation).

Evaluate for pulsus paradoxus, a condition in which the systolic blood pressure drops more than 10 mm Hg with inspiration. A change in pulse quality, or even the disappearance of a pulse, may also be detected. Pulsus paradoxus is generally seen in patients with decompensating COPD or severe pericardial tamponade. It may also indicate an increase in intrathoracic pressure.

A history of the present illness is a vital part of your assessment. Determine the evolution of this particular event:

- Was its onset sudden or gradual?
- Is there any known cause or trigger of the event?
- Are there any alleviating or exacerbating factors?
- Are there any other associated symptoms, such as a productive cough (if yes, what does the sputum look like?), chest pain, or fever?
- What interventions have been attempted before EMS arrival?
- What medications does the patient take, and is he or she compliant with the prescribed regimens?
- What is the duration?
- Is this a constant (chronic) or recurrent (episodic) problem?
- Has the patient been evaluated or admitted to the hospital for this condition in the past?
- Has the patient ever been intubated for this problem? If so, how does today's episode compare to that experience? This is one of the most important questions to ask; a condition serious enough to warrant intubation needs urgent attention to prevent a repeated occurrence.

Note protective reflexes of the airway, including coughing, sneezing, and gagging. A cough is a forceful, spastic exhalation that aids in clearing the bronchi and bronchioles. Sneezing clears the nasopharynx and is often caused by an irritant such as dust. The gag reflex is a spastic pharyngeal and esophageal reflex caused by a stimulus of the posterior pharynx to prevent foreign objects from entering the trachea.

Sighing and hiccuping are other modified forms of respiration. Sighing is an involuntary deep breath that increases opening of the alveoli, preventing atelectasis. The average person normally sighs about once per minute. Hiccuping is the intermittent spastic closure of the glottis and is caused by spasm of the diaphragm. Persistent hiccuping may be clinically significant.

Respiratory pattern changes indicate serious injury or illness. **TABLE 8-3** shows various respiratory patterns and causes. Irregular respiratory breathing patterns may be related to a specific condition. For example, Cheyne-Stokes respirations are often seen in patients with stroke and patients with serious head injuries **FIGURE 8-10**. Cheyne-Stokes respirations are an irregular respiratory pattern in which the patient breathes with an increasing rate and depth of respirations that is followed by a period of *apnea*, or lack of spontaneous breathing, followed again by a pattern of increasing rate and depth of respiration.

> *Apnea* Absence of breathing; periods of not breathing.
> *Ketoacidosis* An acidotic state created by the production of ketones via fat metabolism.

Serious head injuries may also cause changes in the normal respiratory rate and pattern of breathing. The result may be irregular, ineffective respirations that may or may not

Table 8-3
Respiratory Pattern Changes

Pattern	Characteristics
Cheyne-Stokes respirations	Rhythmic, gradually increasing rate and tidal volume followed by gradual decrease; associated with brain stem injury
Kussmaul respirations	Deep, gasping respirations; common in diabetic coma and *ketoacidosis*
Biot respirations	Irregular pattern, rate, and volume with intermittent periods of apnea (absence of breathing); results from increased intracranial pressure
Central neurogenic hyperventilation	Deep, rapid respirations similar to Kussmaul; also results from increased intracranial pressure
Agonal gasps	Slow, shallow, irregular, or occasional gasping breaths; results from brain anoxia. Agonal gasps may be seen when the heart has stopped but the brain continues to send signals to the muscles of respiration. This is not considered a form of respiration.

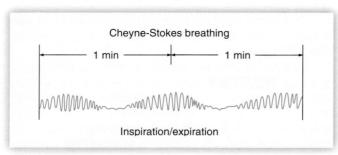

FIGURE 8-10 Cheyne-Stokes breathing shows irregular respirations followed by a period of apnea.

have an identifiable pattern (*ataxic respirations*). Patients experiencing a metabolic or toxic disorder may display other irregular respiratory patterns such as Kussmaul respirations. Kussmaul respirations are characterized as deep, gasping respirations commonly seen in patients with metabolic acidosis.

You should be aware that a patient may appear to take a breath after his or her heart has stopped. These occasional gasps are called *agonal gasps* and for all intents and purposes the patient is not breathing; you must ventilate him or her. They occur when the respiratory center in the brain continues to send signals to the respiratory muscles. These respirations do not provide adequate oxygen because they are infrequent, gasping respiratory efforts.

> *Ataxic respirations* Irregular, ineffective respirations that may or may not have an identifiable pattern.
> *Agonal gasps* Occasional, slow gasps that are ineffective attempts at breathing, occurring after the heart has stopped; sometimes seen in dying patients.

In patients with agonal gasps, you will need to provide artificial ventilations and, most likely, chest compressions.

Whereas rapid breathing is a compensatory mechanism to help patients in respiratory distress, some patients are so ill that their body is not able to compensate for their respiratory distress. The patients may look like they are compensating; however, no clinical improvement will be noticeable. You need to be vigilant when monitoring patients in respiratory distress because their condition may decline rapidly.

Patients with inadequate breathing have inadequate minute volume and need to be treated immediately. This condition is most easily recognized in patients who are unable to speak in complete sentences when at rest or who have a fast or slow respiratory rate, either of which may result in a reduction in tidal volume. Emergency medical care includes airway management, supplemental oxygen, and ventilatory support.

Assessment of Respiration

Respiration is the actual exchange of oxygen and carbon dioxide at the tissue level. Even though a patient may be ventilating appropriately, the process of respiration may be compromised. Therefore, you must assess for signs of adequate and inadequate respiration in your patients. These signs and symptoms will guide you in the overall assessment of patients.

As stated earlier, there are external factors that may disrupt the process of respiration. Areas involving poor oxygenation, such as enclosed spaces, do not provide an adequate oxygen level and as a result hinder respiration. You should be aware of the patient's environment and assess the quality of ambient air when approaching the patient. High altitudes and poisonous gases should always be considered when assessing respiration. These factors can dramatically affect respiration and alter metabolism in your patient. Some EMS services carry hand-held carbon monoxide detectors to aid in the process of assessing ambient air. However, if you believe the quality of the ambient air is not safe, remove yourself and the patient (if possible) from the scene immediately and contact the appropriate resource. If there is more than one patient with similar symptoms, consider the presence of toxic gases. Remove yourself, your partner, and any patients immediately. For example, carbon monoxide may be present in a residence with improperly vented heating systems and may be poisoning the occupants. If more than one family member reports a headache, nausea, vomiting, chest pain, and fatigue, consider an environmental hazard, food, or water, as a culprit first rather than multiple concurrent cases of the flu.

A patient's LOC and skin color are excellent indicators of respiration. During normal respiration, oxygen and carbon dioxide diffuse in and out of tissues and allow aerobic metabolism to take place. When you are assessing the brain and skin tissues, it will be apparent if the patient has adequate oxygen reaching these areas. A patient presenting with an altered LOC may not have adequate oxygen reaching the brain. This lack of oxygen can cause rapid changes in the patient's mental status. Therefore, when treating patients with an altered mental status, always consider the possibility that the patients may not be getting adequate oxygen to the brain and that you need to consider the possible underlying causes. However, remember to determine a baseline mental status on the patient. Some patients naturally have an abnormal mental status because of a previous medical condition. Ask family members what the patient's normal mental status is.

Just as an altered LOC is indicative of inadequate respiration, the same is true for patients with poor skin color. As oxygen fails to reach the skin from a lack of perfusion or poor oxygenation, the color of the skin changes to reflect the inadequate oxygen. Pale skin and mucous membranes, or pallor, are typically associated with poor perfusion caused by illness or shock. As this condition worsens, cyanosis becomes noticeable first peripherally in the fingertips and then centrally in the mucous membranes and around the lips. Eventually, if the poor perfusion or oxygenation is not corrected, anaerobic metabolism will take place. This could cause the skin to become marked with blotches of different colors, commonly referred to as mottling.

Whereas assessment of a patient's baseline mental status and color of the skin and mucous membranes provides good indicators of respiration, you should also consider proper oxygenation when assessing patients. Oxygenation is the process of loading oxygen molecules onto hemoglobin molecules in the bloodstream. Several methods can be used to assess proper oxygenation, including assessing skin color, mental status, and *pulse oximetry*.

Oxygen saturation (Spo₂) is the measure of the percentage of hemoglobin molecules that are bound in arterial blood. Because hemoglobin delivers 97% of the oxygen delivered to the body's tissues, oxygen saturation is an excellent indication of the amount of oxygen available to the end organs.

> **Pulse oximetry** An assessment tool that measures oxygen saturation of hemoglobin in the capillary beds.
> **Oxygen saturation (Spo₂)** The measure of the percentage of hemoglobin binding sites attached to oxygen in arterial blood.

The pulse oximeter is a standard device used in the assessment of patients in emergency situations **FIGURE 8-11**. The pulse oximeter provides a rapid, reliable, noninvasive, real-time indication of respiratory efficiency. Although its results must not be used without conducting an overall clinical assessment of the patient, careful use of the pulse oximeter provides valuable information about a patient's oxygenation status. This device can be used to assess the adequacy of oxygenation during positive-pressure ventilation and assess the overall impact of interventions on your patient. However, it is important to remember that cold environments or carbon monoxide can render pulse oximetry readings inaccurate.

A pulse oximeter measures the percentage of hemoglobin saturation. Under normal conditions, the Spo₂ should be 98% to 100% while breathing room air. Although no definitive threshold for normal values exists, an Spo₂ of less than 96% in a nonsmoker may indicate hypoxemia. An Spo₂ of 90% generally requires treatment unless the patient has a chronic condition causing a perpetually low oxygen

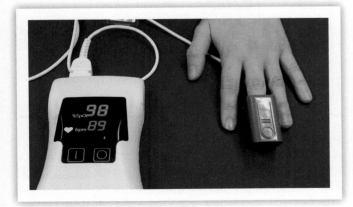

FIGURE 8-11 A pulse oximeter.

saturation. Pulse oximeters are highly reliable in Spo₂ readings of more than 85%; while readings of less than 85% are less reliable, they certainly indicate profound hypoxemia.

Pulse oximetry is considered a routine vital sign and can be used as part of any patient assessment. Whereas there are no true contraindications to using pulse oximetry, you must be aware of the limitations associated with this device. To function properly, the pulse oximeter must find a pulsation in the selected tissue. The most commonly used site is a finger.

> **Transition Tip**
>
> Remember that a pulse oximeter can detect only the saturation of hemoglobin. It cannot identify the gas that is saturating the hemoglobin. For example, a patient in an area rich with carbon monoxide may have a normal Spo₂ measurement. Carbon monoxide, which has an affinity for hemoglobin that is 200 to 250 times greater than that of oxygen for hemoglobin, has similar characteristics to arterial blood. Therefore, the dual wavelengths of infrared light used by the pulse oximeter may not be able to distinguish between carbon monoxide and oxygen, producing a falsely high reading. It is essential to pay close attention to the scene size-up and to treat the patient instead of the diagnostic equipment. The pulse oximeter is designed to detect gross abnormalities, not subtle changes.

In patients with significant vasoconstriction or very low perfusion states (including cardiac arrest), there may not be enough peripheral perfusion to be detected by the sensor. In these cases, move the sensor to a more central location (bridge of the nose or earlobe). Always consult the manufacturer's guidelines for proper placement and troubleshooting of these devices. An inaccurate pulse oximetry reading may be caused by the following:

- Hypovolemia
- Anemia
- Severe peripheral vasoconstriction (chronic hypoxia, smoking, hypothermia)
- Dark or metallic nail polish
- Dirty fingers
- Carbon monoxide poisoning

Carbon monoxide has an affinity for hemoglobin that is 200 to 250 times greater than that of oxygen. When carbon monoxide is present in the inspired gas, it displaces oxygen from the hemoglobin. Because pulse oximetry measures hemoglobin saturation, it is unable to distinguish between oxygen saturation and carbon monoxide saturation. Therefore, in cases of carbon monoxide poisoning, the Spo₂ can be normal in the context of profound hypoxia.

The pulse oximeter is a valuable adjunct to aid in decision making, but it is not a replacement for a complete assessment. Because of many factors, the pulse oximeter may give falsely high or low readings. When you are conducting a complete patient assessment, consider using pulse oximetry readings as one additional measure while obtaining all of the other comprehensive information you need. Assess the patient for signs and symptoms of adequate oxygenation. If a patient has signs such as cyanosis or pale or clammy skin, or symptoms such as shortness of breath and a normal SpO_2 reading, treat the patient's condition, not the diagnostic device.

Supplemental Oxygen

In hypoxia, not enough oxygen is getting to the tissues and cells of the body. Thus all patients who are hypoxic should receive supplemental oxygen. Some tissues and organs such as the heart, central nervous system, lungs, kidneys, and liver require a constant supply of oxygen to function normally. Supplemental oxygen should be administered to any patient with potential hypoxia, regardless of his or her appearance.

An ongoing debate has focused on how much supplemental oxygen a patient requires. In some EMS systems, immediate high-flow oxygen is given to any trauma patient. Other systems require a full assessment prior to making a determination of the patient's oxygen needs. Make sure to know your local protocols regarding oxygen administration.

> ### Transition Tip
>
> Never withhold oxygen from any patient who might benefit from it, especially if you must assist ventilations. When you are ventilating any patient in cardiac or respiratory arrest, always use high-concentration supplemental oxygen.

Oxygen Cylinders

Oxygen has traditionally been stored in seamless steel or aluminum cylinders of various sizes **FIGURE 8-12**. As an AEMT, you should be familiar with the various sizes of cylinders, safety considerations, and operating procedures when providing supplemental oxygen using an oxygen cylinder.

Liquid Oxygen

Liquid oxygen is oxygen that has been cooled to a liquid state. When warmed, it converts to a gaseous state. Liquid oxygen is becoming more commonly used as an alternative to compressed gas oxygen. Liquid oxygen containers tend to be more expensive than compressed oxygen tanks; however, the containers hold a large volume of oxygen and do not need to be filled as often. Liquid oxygen units also weigh less than aluminum or steel tanks. For these reasons, many people who receive long-term oxygen therapy use liquid oxygen units. Unfortunately, liquid oxygen tanks generally need to be kept upright and have special requirements for filling, large-volume storage, and cylinder transfer.

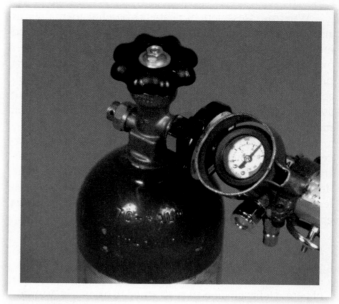

FIGURE 8-12 Oxygen tanks are made of steel or aluminum and come in various sizes.

Oxygen-Delivery Equipment

Traditionally, the oxygen-delivery equipment used in the field has been limited to nonrebreathing masks, bag-mask devices, and nasal cannulas. Today, however, other devices are available to the AEMT, including the partial rebreathing face mask, Venturi mask, and tracheostomy mask. The use of humidification is also new to the AEMT.

Nonrebreathing Masks

The nonrebreathing mask is the preferred way of giving oxygen in the prehospital setting to patients who are breathing adequately but are suspected of having or showing signs of hypoxia **FIGURE 8-13**. With a good mask-to-face seal, this device is capable of providing as much as 90% inspired oxygen at a flow rate of 10 to 15 L/min.

> ### Transition Tip
>
> Ensure that the reservoir bag of the nonrebreathing mask is full before you place the mask on the patient. If oxygen therapy is discontinued, remove the mask from the patient's face. Leaving the mask in place while oxygen is not flowing allows the patient to rebreathe exhaled carbon dioxide.

Nasal Cannulas

A nasal cannula delivers oxygen through two small, tube-like prongs that fit into the patient's nostrils **FIGURE 8-14**. This device can provide 24% to 44% inspired oxygen at a flow rate of 1 to 6 L/min. For the comfort of your patient, flow rates greater than 6 L/min are not recommended with the nasal cannula.

> ### Transition Tip
>
> The nasal cannula delivers dry oxygen directly into the nostrils, which, over prolonged periods, can cause dryness or irritate the mucous membrane lining of the nose. For this reason, you should consider the use of humidification during prolonged transport times.

A nasal cannula is used for patients who simply cannot tolerate a nonrebreathing or partial rebreathing mask and for patients who are not critical but may benefit from supplemental oxygen administered in lower concentrations. It is also useful when transporting a noncritical patient who is on home oxygen via a nasal cannula.

Partial Rebreathing Masks

The partial rebreathing mask is similar to a nonrebreathing mask except that it lacks a one-way valve between the mask and the reservoir **FIGURE 8-15**. Consequently, patients rebreathe a small amount of their exhaled air. This arrangement has some benefit when you want to increase the patient's partial pressure of carbon dioxide, making this device the ideal mask for patients who may develop hyperventilation syndrome. The oxygen enriches the air mixture and delivers a gas mixture consisting of approximately 80% to 90% oxygen and 2% to 3% carbon dioxide. You can easily convert a nonrebreathing mask to a partial rebreathing mask by removing the one-way valve between the mask and the reservoir bag.

Venturi Masks

A Venturi mask has a number of attachments that enable you to vary the percentage of oxygen delivered to the patient while a constant flow is maintained from the regulator **FIGURE 8-16**. This delivery is accomplished by exploiting

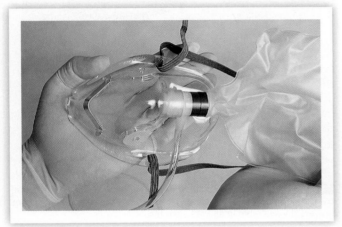

Courtesy of AAOS

FIGURE 8-13 The nonrebreathing mask contains flapper valve ports at the cheek areas of the mask to prevent the patient from rebreathing exhaled gases.

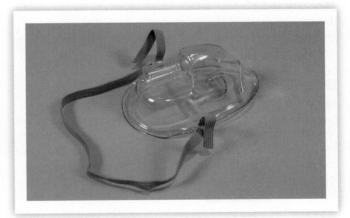

FIGURE 8-15 A partial rebreathing mask.

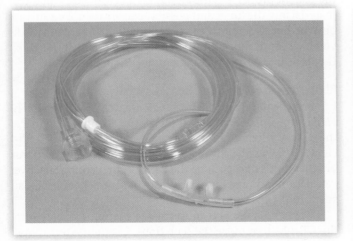

FIGURE 8-14 The nasal cannula delivers oxygen directly through the nostrils.

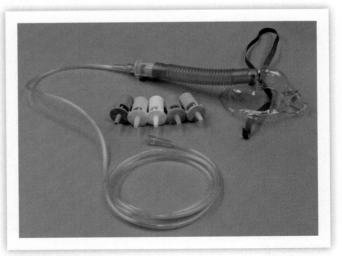

FIGURE 8-16 The Venturi mask.

the Venturi principle, which causes air to be drawn into the flow of oxygen as it passes a hole in the line. The Venturi mask is a medium-flow device that delivers 24% to 40% oxygen, depending on the manufacturer's settings.

The main advantage of the Venturi mask is its fine adjustment capabilities, which has benefits in the long-term management of physiologically stable patients. When it is necessary to adjust the oxygen concentration in an emergency, the health care provider typically changes either the flow rate or the delivery device.

Tracheostomy Masks

Patients with tracheostomies do not breathe through their mouth and nose. As such, a face mask or nasal cannula cannot be used to provide supplemental oxygen to these individuals in the usual fashion. Tracheostomy masks are specially designed to cover the tracheostomy hole; they have a strap that goes around the neck. These masks are usually available in intensive care units, where many patients have tracheostomies, but may not be available in an emergency setting. If you do not have a tracheostomy mask, you can improvise by placing a face mask over the stoma. Even though the mask is shaped to fit the face, you can usually get an adequate fit over the patient's neck by adjusting the strap **FIGURE 8-17**.

Humidification

Although dry oxygen is not considered harmful for short-term use, when longer transport times are expected, the use of humidified oxygen may be beneficial to the patient to prevent drying of the nasal mucosa. An oxygen humidifier consists of a small bottle of water through which the oxygen leaving the cylinder becomes moisturized before it reaches the patient **FIGURE 8-18**. Because the humidifier must be kept in an upright position, however, it is practical only for the fixed oxygen unit in the ambulance.

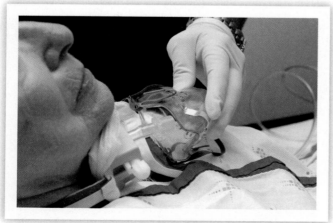

Courtesy of AAOS
FIGURE 8-17 If a tracheostomy mask is not available, use a face mask instead.

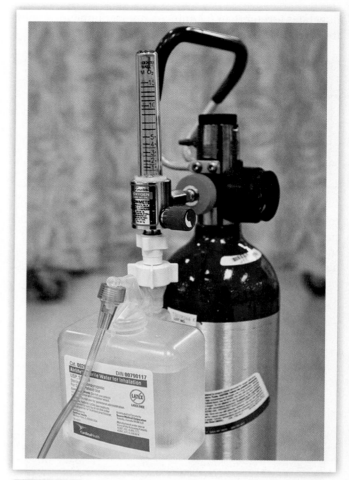

FIGURE 8-18 Giving humidified oxygen may be preferred with long transport times. However, this type of oxygen delivery system is not universally available in all EMS systems.

Suctioning

You must keep the airway clear so that you can ventilate the patient properly. If the airway is not clear, you will force material into the lungs and possibly cause a complete airway obstruction. Therefore, suctioning is your first priority. If you have any doubt about the situation, remember this rule: If you hear gurgling, the patient needs suctioning.

Tracheobronchial Suctioning

Endotracheal (ET) intubation is a paramedic skill in which an ET tube is passed through the glottis opening to manage the airway when other less invasive methods are not sufficient. Following ET intubation, thick pulmonary secretions or other fluids may occlude the ET tube, preventing effective ventilation. You may at times assist with tracheobronchial suctioning of an intubated patient.

In such cases, you must pass a suction catheter into the ET tube to remove the secretions. Use sterile technique if possible; do not reinsert a catheter that is not sterile. Preoxygenation is essential before suctioning. Prelubricate a soft-tip catheter and hyperoxygenate the patient for 30 seconds to 1 minute. It may be necessary to inject 3 to 5 mL of sterile water down the ET tube to loosen secretions. Gently insert the catheter until resistance is felt. Apply suction as the catheter is extracted, taking care not to exceed 15 seconds in an adult patient. Continue to ventilate and oxygenate the patient.

Assisted and Artificial Ventilation

A patient who is not breathing needs artificial ventilation with 100% supplemental oxygen. Assisted and artificial ventilation are probably the most important skills in EMS—at any level. Too often emphasis is placed on advanced airway techniques, making the basic airway maneuvers seem ineffective. This perception could not be further from the truth: basic airway and ventilation techniques are extremely effective when administered appropriately. Mastery of these techniques at the AEMT level is imperative.

Patients who are breathing inadequately (too rapidly or too slowly with reduced tidal volume) are typically unable to speak in complete sentences without becoming winded. These patients, in addition to those with an irregular breathing pattern, may require artificial ventilation to help them maintain adequate minute volume.

> ### Transition Tip
>
> Shallow breathing can be just as dangerous as very slow breathing. Fast, shallow breathing moves air primarily in the larger airway passages (dead air space) and does not allow for adequate exchange of air and carbon dioxide in the alveoli. Patients with inadequate breathing require assisted ventilations with some form of positive-pressure ventilation. Remember to follow standard precautions when managing the patient's airway.

Assisting Ventilation in Respiratory Distress/Failure

A patient exhibiting signs of severe respiratory distress or respiratory failure requires immediate intervention. Two treatment options are available in these situations: assisted ventilation via a bag-mask device and continuous positive airway pressure (CPAP).

The purpose of assisted ventilations is to improve the overall oxygenation and ventilatory status of the patient. Patients who require assisted ventilation are no longer able to maintain adequate oxygen levels for the body and need intervention to prevent further hypoxia. Indicators of inadequate ventilation include altered mental status and inadequate minute volume. In addition, excessive accessory muscle use and fatigue from labored breathing are signs of potential respiratory failure. TABLE 8-4 lists the recommended ventilation rates for apneic patients with a pulse.

Table 8-4
Ventilation Rates for an Apneic Patient With a Pulse

Adult	1 breath every 5 seconds
Child	1 breath every 3 seconds
Infant	1 breath every 3 seconds

Follow these steps to assist a patient with ventilations using a bag-mask device:

1. Explain the procedure to the patient.
2. Place the mask over the patient's nose and mouth.
3. Squeeze the bag each time the patient breathes, maintaining the same rate as the patient.
4. After the initial 5 to 10 breaths, slowly adjust the rate and deliver an appropriate tidal volume.
5. Adjust the rate and tidal volume to maintain an adequate minute volume.

Artificial Ventilation

Patients who are in respiratory arrest need immediate intervention. Without it, they will die. Devices for providing artificial ventilation include the pocket face mask for performing mouth-to-mask ventilations, the bag-mask device, and the manually triggered ventilation device.

Normal Ventilation Versus Positive-Pressure Ventilation

Although artificial ventilations are necessary to sustain life, they are not the same as normal breaths. As discussed earlier, the act of air moving in and out the lungs is based on pressure changes within the thoracic cavity. During normal ventilation, the diaphragm contracts and negative pressure is generated in the chest cavity. In response, air is essentially sucked into the chest from the trachea in an attempt to equalize the pressure in the chest with the atmospheric pressure. In contrast, positive-pressure ventilation generated by a device such as a bag-mask device forces air into the chest cavity from the external environment rather than based on pressure changes. This difference between normal ventilation and positive-pressure ventilation can create some challenges for the AEMT TABLE 8-5.

The physical act of the chest wall expanding and retracting during breathing serves to aid the circulatory system in returning blood back to the heart. During normal ventilation, the chest wall movement works similar to a pump. The pressure changes in the thoracic cavity help draw venous return back to the heart.

When positive-pressure ventilation is initiated, however, more air is needed to achieve the same oxygenation and ventilatory effects that occur during normal breathing. This increase in airway wall pressure pushes the walls of the chest cavity out of their normal anatomic shape. As a result, the

Table 8-5
Normal Ventilation Versus Positive-Pressure Ventilation

	Normal Ventilation	**Positive-Pressure Ventilation**
Air movement	Air is sucked into the lungs as a result of the negative intrathoracic pressure created when the diaphragm contracts.	Air is forced into the lungs through a means of mechanical ventilation.
Blood movement	Normal breathing allows blood to naturally be pulled back to the heart.	Intrathoracic pressure is increased, not allowing blood to be adequately pulled back to the heart. This causes a reduction in the amount of blood pumped by the heart.
Airway wall pressure	Not affected during normal breathing.	More volume is required to have the same effects as normal breathing. As a result, the walls are pushed out of their normal anatomic shape.
Esophageal opening pressure	Not affected during normal breathing.	Air is forced into the stomach, causing gastric distention that could result in vomiting and aspiration.
Overventilation	Overventilation is not typical of normal breathing.	Forcing the volume and rate results in increased intrathoracic pressure, gastric distention, and decrease in cardiac output (hypotension).

overall intrathoracic pressure within the chest cavity increases. This increased pressure in turn causes a decrease in blood flow, resulting in poor venous return to the heart and a reduction in the amount of blood pumped out of the heart. *Cardiac output (CO)* is a function of stroke volume and heart rate:

$$\text{Cardiac Output (CO)} = \text{Stroke Volume} \times \text{Heart Rate}$$

Cardiac output (CO) The amount of blood ejected by the left ventricle in 1 minute.
Stroke volume The volume of blood pumped forward with each ventricular contraction.

Stroke volume is the amount of blood ejected by the ventricle in one cardiac cycle or one beat. The heart rate is assessed by taking the pulse for 1 minute. The CO is the amount of blood ejected by the left ventricle in 1 minute.

Transition Tip

To prevent a drop in cardiac output, it is imperative that the AEMT regulate the rate and volume of artificial ventilations.

Another difference between normal ventilation and positive-pressure ventilation relates to the control of airflow. When a person breathes normally, air enters the trachea but generally not the esophagus. In contrast, the force generated from positive-pressure ventilation allows air to enter both the trachea and the esophagus. Ventilations that are too forceful can lead to gastric distention (excessive air in the stomach).

Transition Tip

Mouth-to-mouth, mouth-to-mask, and bag-mask ventilations are all skills that you should have mastered by now.

Manually Triggered Ventilation Devices

Another method of providing artificial ventilation is with a manually triggered ventilation device **FIGURE 8-19**. Such devices—also known as flow-restricted, oxygen-powered ventilation devices or demand valves—have been widely available for use in EMS systems for decades, although they have not been widely used.

The major advantage associated with this device is that it allows a single rescuer to use both hands to maintain a mask-to-face seal while providing positive-pressure ventilation. It

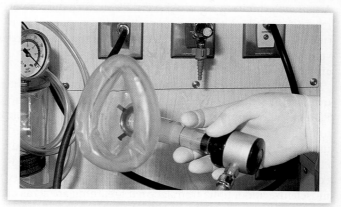

Courtesy of AAOS

FIGURE 8-19 A manually triggered ventilation device can provide as much as 100% oxygen.

also reduces the rescuer fatigue associated with using a bag-mask device on extended transports. Nevertheless, recent findings suggest that manually triggered ventilation devices are associated with difficulty in maintaining adequate ventilation without assistance and should not be used routinely because of the high incidence of gastric distention and possible damage to structures within the chest cavity. Another disadvantage is that a special unit and additional training are required when using the manually triggered ventilation device on infants and children.

Transition Tip

The manually triggered ventilation device should not be used on patients with chronic obstructive pulmonary disease or with suspected cervical spine or chest injuries. This device is typically used only on adult patients. Additional training is necessary prior to using the device on pediatric patients.

SKILL DRILL 8-1 illustrates the sequence for ventilating an apneic patient using the manually triggered ventilation device:

1. Choose the proper mask size to seat the mask from the bridge of the nose to the chin (**Step 1**).

2. Position the mask on the patient's face by the most appropriate method. (**Step 2**).

3. Open the patient's airway and hold the mask in place with one hand, maintaining an adequate mask-to-face seal (**Step 3**).

4. Press the ventilation button until you see visible chest rise (**Step 4**).

5. Allow the patient to exhale passively (**Step 5**).

Transition Tip

The Sellick maneuver, or cricoid pressure, has been used to inhibit the flow of air into the stomach (thereby reducing gastric distention) and to reduce the chance of aspiration by helping block the regurgitation of gastric contents from the esophagus. It has also been used to improve visualization of the vocal cords or positioning of the lighted stylet during intubation. In this maneuver, an AEMT applies cricoid pressure on the patient by placing the thumb and index finger on either side of the cricoid cartilage (located at the inferior border of the larynx) and pressing down.

According to several studies cited in the 2010 American Heart Association Guidelines, cricoid pressure may actually impede ventilation and not completely prevent aspiration. For this reason, the procedure is generally not recommended. Be sure to follow your local protocol regarding the use of the Sellick maneuver.

SKILL DRILL 8-2 shows the steps for administering supplemental oxygen to a spontaneously breathing patient with the manually triggered ventilation device:

1. Prepare your equipment by attaching the appropriately sized mask to the manually triggered ventilation device and ensuring that it is connected to an oxygen source (**Step 1**).

2. Whenever possible, have the patient hold the mask to his or her own face to maintain a good seal (**Step 2**).

3. When the patient inhales, the negative pressure created will trigger the valve within the manually triggered ventilation device and deliver 100% oxygen (**Step 3**).

Automatic Transport Ventilator/Resuscitator

The automatic transport ventilator (ATV) is essentially a manually triggered ventilation device attached to a control box that allows the user to set the ventilation variables **FIGURE 8-20**. Although an ATV lacks the sophisticated control of a hospital ventilator, it frees the AEMT to perform other tasks such as maintaining a mask seal or ensuring continued patency of the airway. You can even perform non–airway-related tasks if the patient has an advanced airway in place and is being ventilated with the ATV. However, even though an ATV is helpful to an AEMT, a bag-mask device and mask should always be prepared and ready for use should a malfunction occur with the ATV.

Like the manually triggered ventilation device, the ATV is generally oxygen powered, although some models may require an external power source. This device generally

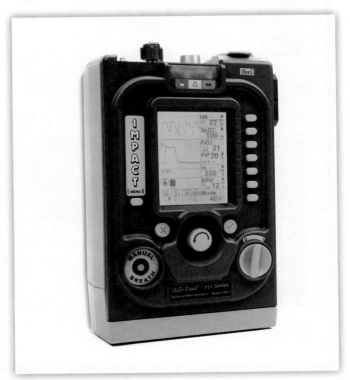

Courtesy of Impact Instrumentation, Inc.

FIGURE 8-20 Automatic transport ventilator (ATV).

SKILL DRILL 8-1

Manually Triggered Ventilation Device for Apneic Patients

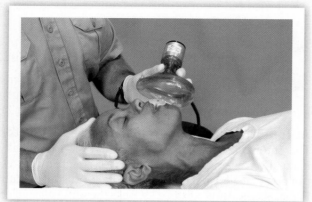

1 Choose the proper mask size to seat the mask from the bridge of the nose to the chin.

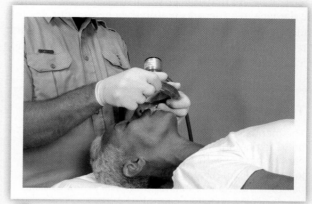

2 Position the mask on the patient's face by the most appropriate method.

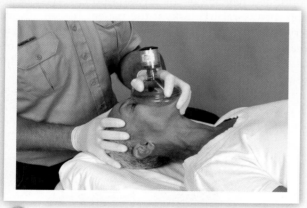

3 Open the patient's airway and hold the mask with one hand.

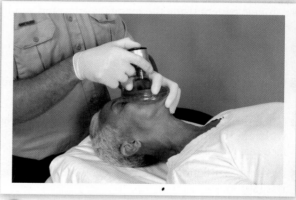

4 Press the ventilation button until you see visible chest rise.

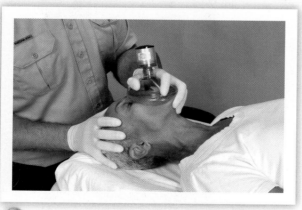

5 Allow the patient to exhale passively.

SKILL DRILL 8-2

Manually Triggered Ventilation for Conscious, Spontaneously Breathing Patients

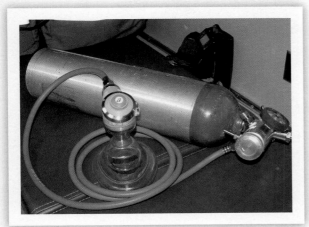

Courtesy of AAOS

 Prepare your equipment.

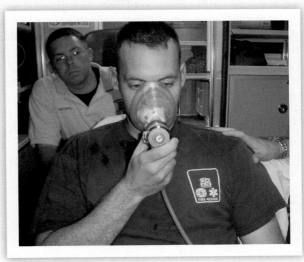

Courtesy of AAOS

 Whenever possible, have the patient hold the mask to his or her own face to maintain a good seal.

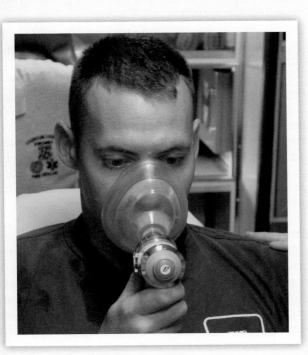

Courtesy of AAOS

3 When the patient inhales, the negative pressure created will trigger the valve within the manually triggered ventilation device and deliver 100% oxygen.

consumes 5 L/min of oxygen; by comparison, a bag-mask device requires 15 to 25 L/min of oxygen. In addition, just like the manually triggered ventilation device, the ATV includes a pressure relief valve, which can lead to hypoventilation in patients with poor lung compliance, increased airway resistance, or airway obstruction. Compliance is the ability of the alveoli to expand when air is drawn in during inhalation; poor lung compliance is the inability of the alveoli to fully expand during inhalation.

Although use of an ATV potentially frees the AEMT to perform other tasks, constant reassessment of the patient is necessary. Barotrauma is a common complication associated with manually triggered ventilation devices and the ATV. In addition, the AEMT needs to assess for full chest recoil when using an ATV. This step is not only essential with patients in respiratory arrest, but also with patients in cardiac arrest receiving chest compressions.

Continuous Positive Airway Pressure

Continuous positive airway pressure (CPAP) is a noninvasive means of providing ventilatory support for patients experiencing respiratory distress. Many people with obstructive sleep apnea wear a CPAP unit at night to maintain their airway while they sleep. During the past several years, the use of CPAP in the prehospital environment has proven to be an excellent adjunct in the treatment of respiratory distress associated with obstructive pulmonary disease and acute pulmonary edema **FIGURE 8-21**. Typically, many of the patients would be managed with advanced airway devices such as ET intubation. Research has shown that there is a significant increase in morbidity and mortality when patients with these conditions receive intubation for their condition in the field; early intervention with CPAP is an alternative means for providing ventilatory assistance and can prevent the need for ET intubation, thereby improving the patient's chance of survival. CPAP offers an alternative means for providing ventilatory assistance to patients and helps to decrease overall morbidity and mortality. Because of the simplicity of the device and its great benefit to patients, CPAP is becoming widely used by AEMTs.

> *Continuous positive airway pressure (CPAP)* A method of ventilation used primarily in the treatment of critically ill patients with respiratory distress; can prevent the need for endotracheal intubation.

CPAP increases pressure in the lungs, opens collapsed alveoli, pushes more oxygen across the alveolar membrane, and forces interstitial fluid back into the pulmonary circulation. Studies of this treatment have shown positive results in patients with obstructive pulmonary diseases and patients with acute pulmonary edema. The therapy is typically delivered through a face mask that is held to the head with a

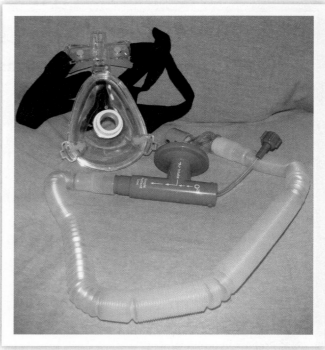

Courtesy of Rhonda Beck

FIGURE 8-21 A CPAP unit can be used as an adjunct in treating respiratory distress associated with obstructive pulmonary disease and acute pulmonary edema.

strapping system. A good seal with minimal leakage between the face and mask is essential.

The face mask is fitted with a pressure-relief valve that determines the amount of pressure delivered to the patient (such as 5 cm of water). The result is similar to hanging your head out the window while driving on the highway. This results in a high inspiratory flow and the need to push a pressure valve open with exhalation. While this may appear to require a great deal of effort on the part of a patient already in distress, many patients make a dramatic turnaround when CPAP is applied.

Indications for CPAP

CPAP is indicated for patients experiencing respiratory distress in which their own compensatory mechanisms are not enough to keep up with their oxygen demand. Whereas the condition of most patients improves after the application of CPAP, it is important to remember that CPAP is merely treating the symptoms and not necessarily the underlying pathology.

The following are some general guidelines for CPAP candidates:

- Patient alert and able to follow commands
- Obvious signs in patient of moderate to severe respiratory distress (such as accessory muscle use or tripod position) from an underlying pathology such as pulmonary edema or obstructive pulmonary disease (such as COPD)

- Rapid breathing (more than 26 breaths/min) such that it affects overall minute volume
- Pulse oximetry reading less than 90%

Whereas these guidelines should be considered when assessing the need for CPAP, it is important that you follow your local guidelines and protocols.

Contraindications to CPAP

CPAP has proven to be immensely beneficial to patients experiencing respiratory distress from acute pulmonary edema or obstructive pulmonary disease; however, there are times when CPAP is not appropriate.

The following are general contraindications for CPAP use:

- Respiratory arrest
- Signs and symptoms of a pneumothorax or chest trauma
- Tracheostomy
- Active gastrointestinal bleeding or vomiting
- Patient unable to follow verbal commands
- Inability to properly fit the CPAP system mask and strap

In addition to these contraindications, AEMTs should always reassess the patient for signs of deterioration and/or respiratory failure. CPAP is an excellent tool to assist with ventilation; however, not all patients will have an improvement in condition with this device. Once signs of respiratory failure become apparent or the patient is no longer able to follow commands, CPAP should be removed and positive-pressure ventilation with a bag-mask device attached to high-flow oxygen should be initiated.

Application

Several varieties of CPAP units are available to EMS services; however, most follow the same general guidelines for use and set-up. CPAP units are generally composed of a generator, a mask, a circuit that contains corrugated tubing, a bacteria filter, and a one-way valve. During the expiratory phase, the patient exhales against a resistance called *positive end-expiratory pressure (PEEP)*. Within the CPAP generator is a valve that determines the amount of PEEP; however, some CPAP models have PEEP valves that connect separately. Depending on the device, the PEEP is controlled by the AEMT manually adjusting it using a manometer or predetermined by a fixed setting on the PEEP valve. A PEEP of 5.0 to 10.0 cm water is generally an acceptable therapeutic range for a patient using CPAP. Always consult the operations manual of a particular CPAP device for proper assembly instructions.

> *Positive end-expiratory pressure (PEEP)* Mechanical maintenance of pressure in the airway at the end of expiration to increase the volume of gas remaining in the lungs.

Because most CPAP units are powered by oxygen, it is important to have a full cylinder of oxygen when using CPAP. Some CPAP units use a continuous flow of oxygen while others use oxygen on more of a demand basis. Continuously monitor the amount of available oxygen in your cylinder. Some CPAP units will empty a D cylinder in as little as 5 to 10 minutes. Therefore, proper planning for oxygen consumption is necessary when considering applying CPAP. In addition, some of the newer CPAP devices allow the provider to adjust the fraction of inspired oxygen (FIO_2). Most CPAP devices are set to deliver a fixed FIO_2 of 30% to 35%; however, some can deliver as high as 80%.

It is important that you reassess the patient for signs of deterioration. Continually reassess patients for sudden drops in blood pressure, changes in pulse rate and quality, changes in respiratory rate and quality, the work of breathing, and changes in LOC. If the patient is no longer able to follow verbal commands and/or goes into respiratory failure/arrest, you must act quickly to remove CPAP and begin positive-pressure ventilation using a bag-mask device attached to high-flow oxygen.

Complications

The application and administration of CPAP is a relatively easy process. However, some patients may find CPAP claustrophobic and will resist the application. As patients become more hypoxic, the application of a mask to their face is sometimes perceived as suffocation, rather than helping them breathe. In any event, it is important to explain the application to patients and coach them through the process. Do not force the mask on patients. This will create a higher level of anxiety and increase their oxygen demand. Coach patients through the application of CPAP, allowing them to adjust to the situation. Coaching patients is not always an easy task; it takes practice and a willingness to work closely with your patient during a difficult time.

Because of the high volume of pressure generated by CPAP, there is the possibility of causing a pneumothorax. Whereas some literature suggests this is not likely, AEMTs should be aware of this risk and continually assess their patients for signs and symptoms of a pneumothorax.

In addition to a pneumothorax, high pressure in the chest can lower a patient's blood pressure. As the intrathoracic pressure increases, venous blood returning to the heart meets resistance from the increased pressure in the chest. This can result in a sudden drop in blood pressure. While this is not common with lower levels of CPAP, continuous monitoring of blood pressure is necessary.

▋Multilumen Airways

Certain airway devices can be inserted blindly and result in better airway management and ventilation. Two such devices are the *pharyngeotracheal lumen airway (PtL)* and the *Combitube* FIGURE 8-22 . The PtL is the predecessor of the Combitube and now rarely used.

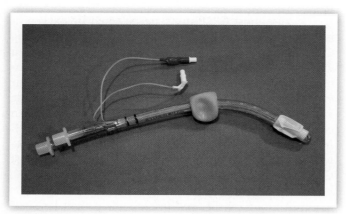

FIGURE 8-22 A Combitube.

> *Pharyngeotracheal lumen airway (PtL)* A dual-lumen airway device that is inserted blindly into the mouth. The patient can be ventilated whether the tube is placed in the esophagus or into the trachea.
>
> *Combitube* A dual-lumen airway device that is inserted blindly; permits ventilation of the patient whether the tube is placed in the esophagus or the trachea.

The PtL and the Combitube have a long tube that is blindly inserted into the airway. In contrast with esophageal airways, the tube can be used for ventilation whether it is inserted into the esophagus or trachea. It can function as an ET tube (if inserted into the trachea). These *multilumen airways* contain two lumens, which function appropriately based on tube position and ventilating through the correct lumen. Each lumen has a 15/22-mm ventilation adapter. The proper port for ventilation depends on where the tube is located. They also contain an oropharyngeal balloon, which eliminates the need for a mask seal.

> *Multilumen airways* Airway devices with a single long tube that can be used for esophageal obturation or endotracheal tube ventilation, depending on where it comes to rest following blind positioning.

Advantages and Disadvantages of Multilumen Airways

Multilumen airways have many advantages and have been engineered to decrease some of the disadvantages. The major advantage is that insertion is technically easier than ET intubation and requires less experience and technical skill. In effect, the airway cannot be improperly placed, because effective ventilation is possible if the tube goes into either the trachea or the esophagus. Because the procedure is performed with the patient in the neutral position, cervical spine movement is kept to a minimum. No mask seal is required to ventilate with either device.

Multilumen airways also provide some patency to the airway. If the tube is placed in the trachea, it allows the airway to be maintained and no upper airway positioning is required. If the tube is placed into the esophagus

(as most commonly occurs), the pharyngeal balloon creates an airtight seal in the oropharynx, making the tongue position less of a factor in the maintenance of a patent airway. A jaw-thrust maneuver should easily alleviate any ventilatory difficulty that occurs if the epiglottis partially obstructs the airway.

When using a multilumen airway, you must pay strict attention to the assessment of ventilation because ventilation in the wrong port results in no pulmonary ventilation. Multilumen airways are usually considered temporary airways. Although in some cases they have been used for prolonged ventilation, these devices are generally replaced as soon as possible.

Indications for Multilumen Airways

Multilumen airways are indicated for the airway management of deeply unresponsive, apneic patients with no gag reflex in whom ET intubation is not possible or has failed.

Contraindiations for Multilumen Airways

Neither of the multilumen airways can be used in pediatric patients younger than 16 years, and they should be used only for patients between 5 and 7 feet tall. (A smaller version of the Combitube, called the Combitube SA [small adult], can be used for adults more than 4 feet tall.) Because most of the time the tube is inserted into the esophagus, the Combitube should not be used in patients with a known pathologic condition of the esophagus, who have ingested a caustic substance, or who have very severe alcoholism with liver dysfunction.

Complications of Multilumen Airways

Research with multilumen airways is still somewhat limited. Use of a multilumen airway does not necessarily prevent the occurrence of *laryngospasm*, vomiting, and possible hypoventilation. Trauma may also result from improper insertion technique.

> *Laryngospasm* A severe constriction of the larynx and vocal cords.

Ventilation may be difficult if the pharyngeal balloon pushes the epiglottis over the glottic opening. In such cases, ventilation should become easier if the device is withdrawn 2 to 4 cm.

Insertion Techniques

The Combitube consists of a single tube with two lumens, two balloons, and two ventilation attachments. One of the lumens is open at its distal end and the other is closed. The closed lumen has side holes distal to the pharyngeal balloon. The proximal balloon is designed to be inflated with 100 to 140 mL of air and provide a pharyngeal seal. The distal balloon is inflated with 15 mL of air and makes an airtight seal with the walls of the trachea in case of tracheal placement or leads to esophageal obturation in case of esophageal placement **FIGURE 8-23**.

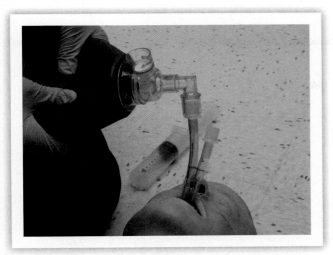

FIGURE 8-23 Ventilation with a Combitube in place.

pharynx. The Combitube is inserted until the incisors are between the two black lines printed on the tube. Be gentle, and stop advancing the tube if you meet resistance.

- **Inflate the cuffs.** The Combitube has two independent inflation valves that must be inflated sequentially. The first inflation valve goes to the pharyngeal balloon and is inflated with 100 mL of air (this is printed on the pilot balloon). The second inflation valve inflates the distal balloon and is filled with 15 mL of air.

Remember that when inserting a multilumen airway, confirmation of ventilation is very important. If you used the wrong port, the patient would receive no pulmonary ventilation.

The steps for insertion of a Combitube are described in **SKILL DRILL 8-3**:

1 Take standard precautions (gloves and face shield) (**Step 1**).

2 Preoxygenate the patient whenever possible with a bag-mask device and 100% oxygen (**Step 2**).

3 Gather your equipment (**Step 3**).

4 Place the patient's head in the neutral position (**Step 4**).

5 Open the patient's mouth with the tongue–jaw lift maneuver, and insert the Combitube in the midline of the patient's mouth. Insert the tube until the incisors or alveolar ridge lie between the two reference marks (**Step 5**).

6 Inflate the pharyngeal cuff with 100 mL of air (**Step 6**).

Before inserting a multilumen airway, check and prepare all equipment. Check both cuffs to ensure that they hold air. The patient should be preoxygenated before insertion. Ventilation should not be interrupted for longer than 30 seconds to accomplish airway placement. For insertion, the patient's head should be placed in the neutral position.

- **Forwardly displace the jaw.** With the patient's head in the neutral position, insert the thumb of your gloved nondominant hand into the patient's mouth and lift the jaw. This action lifts the hyoid bone and pulls the base of the tongue off the posterior pharyngeal wall.
- **Insert the device.** Following the curvature of the tube, insert the device blindly into the posterior

SKILL DRILL 8-3

Insertion of the Combitube

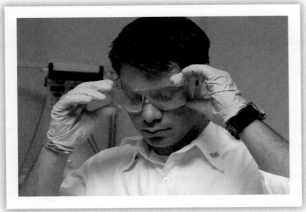

1 Take standard precautions (gloves and face shield).

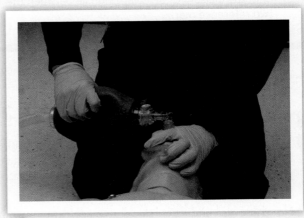

2 Preoxygenate the patient whenever possible with a bag-mask device and 100% oxygen.

(continues)

SKILL DRILL 8-3

Insertion of the Combitube (*continued*)

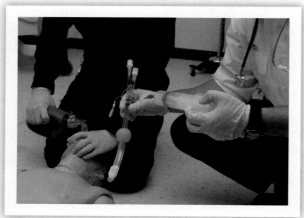

3 Gather your equipment.

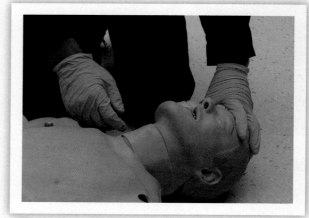

4 Place the patient's head in the neutral position.

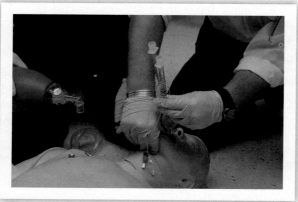

5 Open the patient's mouth with the tongue–jaw lift maneuver, and insert the Combitube in the midline of the patient's mouth. Insert the tube until the incisors or alveolar ridge lie between the two reference marks.

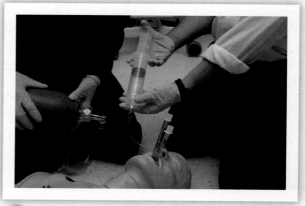

6 Inflate the pharyngeal cuff with 100 mL of air.

7 Inflate the distal cuff with 10 to 15 mL of air (**Step 7**).

8 Ventilate the patient through the longest tube (pharyngeal) first. Chest rise indicates esophageal placement of the distal tip (continue to ventilate) (**Step 8**).

9 No chest rise indicates tracheal placement (switch ports and ventilate) (**Step 9**). Confirm placement by listening for breath sounds over the lungs and for gastric sounds over the abdomen.

Following inflation of the balloons, begin to ventilate the patient. With the Combitube, ventilate the longer (blue) tube. Confirm the patient's chest rise and the presence of breath sounds. If there are no breath sounds and the chest does not rise and fall with ventilation, switch immediately to the other inflation port. Be sure to continuously monitor ventilation. Both multilumen airways are generally secure in the airway owing to the large pharyngeal balloons. However, it is still important to secure the device in place once ventilations are confirmed.

SKILL DRILL 8-3

Insertion of the Combitube (*continued*)

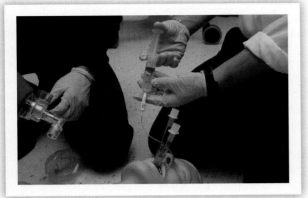

7 Inflate the distal cuff with 10 to 15 mL of air.

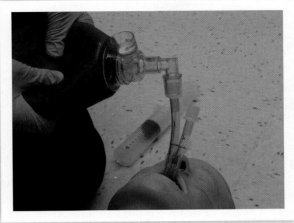

8 Ventilate the patient through the longest tube (pharyngeal) first. Chest rise indicates esophageal placement of the distal tip (continue to ventilate).

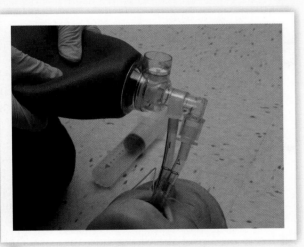

9 No chest rise indicates tracheal placement (switch ports and ventilate). Confirm placement by listening for breath sounds over the lungs and for gastric sounds over the abdomen.

King LT Airway

The *King LT airway* is a latex-free, single-use, single-lumen airway that is blindly inserted into the esophagus FIGURE 8-24. It consists of a curved tube with ventilation ports located between two inflatable cuffs. Both cuffs are inflated using a single valve/pilot balloon. When the airway is properly placed in the esophagus, the distal cuff seals the esophagus and the proximal cuff seals the oropharynx FIGURE 8-25. Openings located between these two cuffs

provide ventilation of the lungs once positioning is confirmed. Studies show that the King LT is easier and quicker to insert than the Combitube and that it can be used successfully as a rescue airway device.

> *King LT airway* A single-lumen airway that is blindly inserted into the esophagus; when properly placed in the esophagus, one cuff seals the esophagus and the other seals the oropharynx.

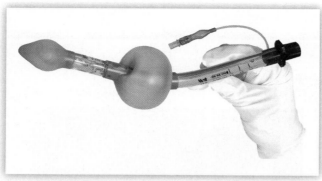

Courtesy of King Systems

FIGURE 8-24 The King LT is a single-lumen airway that is blindly inserted into the esophagus.

Indications for the King LT Airway

The King LT airway should be considered as a possible alternative to bag-mask ventilation in the place of a Combitube or when a rescue device is required for a failed intubation attempt. The King LT airway is intended for airway management in patients who are taller than 4 feet. It has the same disadvantages, complications, and special considerations as the Combitube.

Contraindications for the King LT Airway

The King LT airway does not protect the airway from the effects of vomiting and aspiration. High airway pressures may cause air to leak into the stomach or out of the mouth. The King LT airway should not be used in patients with an intact gag reflex, patients with known esophageal disease, or patients who have ingested caustic substances. As with

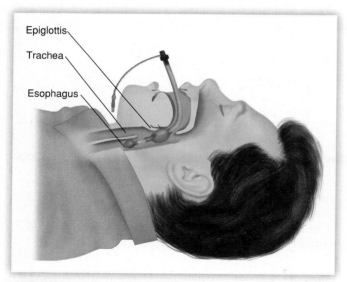

FIGURE 8-25 Placement of the King LT airway. When properly placed, the distal cuff seals the esophagus and the proximal cuff seals the oropharynx.

other advanced airway devices, confirm proper placement by observing chest rise, auscultating the epigastrium and lungs, and using a secondary confirmation device.

Complications of the King LT Airway

As with multilumen devices, it is reasonable to assume that laryngospasm, vomiting, and possible hypoventilation may occur. Trauma may also result from improper insertion technique. Ventilation may be difficult if the pharyngeal balloon pushes the epiglottis over the glottic opening. While gently bagging the patient to assess ventilation, withdraw the device until ventilation is easy and free flowing.

Insertion Technique

The King LT airway comes in many sizes; the patient's size and weight determine the size that should be used. **SKILL DRILL 8-4** shows the steps for inserting a King LT Airway:

1. Take standard precautions (gloves and face shield at a minimum) (**Step 1**).

2. Preoxygenate the patient with a bag-mask device and 100% oxygen (**Step 2**).

3. Gather your equipment (**Step 3**).

4. Choose the proper size King LT airway for the patient. Test the bulbs for proper inflation. Ensure that all air is removed from bulbs before insertion. Lubricate the tip of the device with a water-based lubricant for easy insertion and minimal airway damage.

5. Place the patient's head in a neutral position unless contraindicated (use a jaw-thrust maneuver if trauma is suspected). In your dominant hand, hold the King LT at the connector. With your other hand, hold the patient's mouth open while positioning the head (**Step 4**).

6. Insert the tip of the device into the corner of the mouth and continue to advance it behind the base of the tongue while rotating the device. When rotation is complete, the blue line on the device should face the patient's chin.

7. Continue to gently advance the device until the base of the connector is aligned with the patient's teeth or gums. Do not use excessive force.

8. Inflate the cuffs to the recommended amount of air or to just seal the device (**Step 5**).

9. Attach the tube to the bag-mask device and confirm tube placement. Add additional air to the cuffs to maximize airway seal, if needed.

10. Once placement is confirmed, secure the tube and begin ventilating the patient (**Step 6**).

SKILL DRILL 8-4

Insertion of a King LT Airway

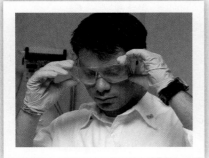

1 Take standard precautions (gloves and face shield at a minimum).

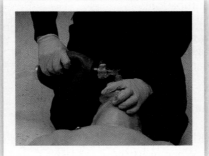

2 Preoxygenate the patient with a bag-mask device and 100% oxygen.

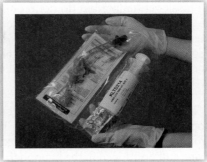

3 Gather your equipment.

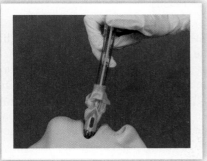

4 Place the patient's head in a neutral position unless contraindicated. Open the patient's mouth and insert the King LT airway in the corner of the mouth.

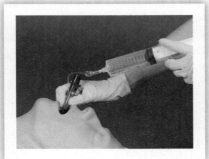

5 Advance the tip behind the base of the tongue while rotating the tube back to midline so the blue line on the device faces the patient's chin. Gently advance the device until the base of the connector is aligned with the teeth or gums. Do not use excessive force. Inflate the cuffs to the recommended amount of air or to just seal the device.

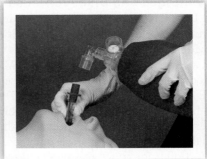

6 Attach the tube to the bag-mask device, and confirm tube placement. Once placement is confirmed, secure the tube and begin ventilating the patient.

Supraglottic Devices

The Laryngeal Mask Airway

The *laryngeal mask airway (LMA)* **FIGURE 8-26** was originally developed for use in the operating room. It provides a viable option for cases that require more airway support than mask ventilation but do not require intubation.

> *Laryngeal mask airway (LMA)* An airway device that is inserted into the mouth blindly and comes to rest at the glottic opening. A flexible cuff is inflated, creating an almost airtight seal.

The LMA is designed to provide a conduit from the glottic opening to the ventilation device. This is achieved by surrounding the opening of the larynx with an inflatable silicone cuff positioned in the hypopharynx. When properly inserted, the opening of the LMA is positioned right at the glottic opening. The inflatable cuff conforms to the contours of the airway and makes a relatively airtight seal **FIGURE 8-27**.

Advantages and Disadvantages of the LMA

The LMA has many advantages compared with ventilating the unprotected airway with a mask. It has been shown to provide better oxygenation than mask ventilation with an oral airway, and ventilation with an LMA does not require the continual maintenance of a mask seal. Compared with an ET tube, LMA insertion is easier. There is significantly less risk of soft-tissue, vocal cord, tracheal wall, and dental trauma than with ET intubation and other forms of intubation that rely on blocking the esophagus. The LMA provides protection from upper airway secretions, and the tip of the LMA wedged into the proximal esophagus most likely provides some obturation.

The main disadvantage of the LMA, especially in emergencies, is that it does not provide the same level of protection against aspiration as does an ET tube or tube that completely occludes the esophagus. In fact, the LMA actually increases the risk of aspiration if the patient regurgitates

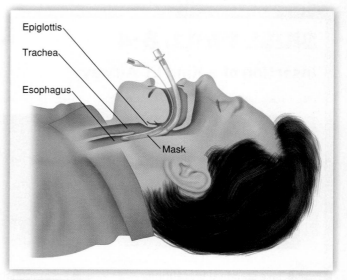

FIGURE 8-27 When properly positioned, the opening of the laryngeal mask airway is at the glottic opening, the tip is at the entrance of the esophagus, the lateral portion is in the pyriform fossae, and the upper border is at the base of the tongue.

because the patient's stomach contents would most likely be directed into the trachea.

During prolonged LMA ventilation, some air may be insufflated into the stomach because the seal made in the airway is not airtight. Because of the risk of aspiration, it is unlikely that the LMA will ever replace ET intubation in prehospital emergency care. The LMA should not be considered a primary airway for emergency patients, but it may have a role. For a patient who cannot be intubated, the LMA should be considered superior to mask ventilation.

Indications for the LMA

The LMA should be considered as one possible alternative to mask ventilation only when the patient cannot be intubated.

Contraindications for the LMA

The LMA is less effective in obese patients and should not be used in patients with morbid obesity. Patients who are pregnant or have a hiatal hernia are at an increased risk for regurgitation and must be evaluated carefully if LMA use is considered. The LMA is ineffective for the ventilation of patients requiring high pulmonary pressures.

Complications of Using the LMA

The biggest complications involve regurgitation and subsequent aspiration. Technically the LMA should be used only in fasting patients. Unfortunately, this would eliminate all emergency patients. You must weigh the risk of aspiration against the risk of hypoventilation with mask ventilation in the context of a given clinical scenario.

You should observe the patient for clinical indications of adequate ventilation (chest rise, breath sounds) during LMA ventilation. Hypoventilation of patients who require high ventilatory pressures can also occur. A few cases of upper airway swelling have been reported.

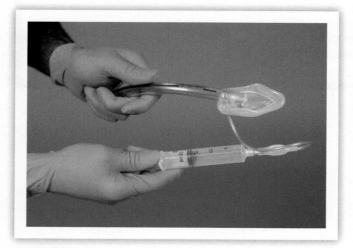

FIGURE 8-26 The laryngeal mask airway.

Equipment for the LMA

The LMA comes in seven sizes and is sized based on the patient's weight. The device consists of a tube and a mask or inflatable cuff. The cuff provides a collar designed to position the opening of the tube at the glottic opening when inflated. Two vertical bars are present at the opening of the tube to prevent occlusion. The proximal end of the tube is fitted with a standard 15/22-mm adapter. The cuff has a one-way valve assembly and should be inflated with a predetermined volume of air (based on the size of the airway).

Insertion Technique

Before insertion, check and prepare all equipment. The steps for using an LMA are summarized in **SKILL DRILL 8-5**:

1. Take standard precautions. Check the cuff of the LMA by inflating it with 50% more air than required for the size of airway to be used. Then deflate the cuff completely (**Step 1**). The cuff should be completely deflated so that no folds appear near the tip. Deflation is best accomplished by pressing the device, cuff down, on a flat surface **FIGURE 8-28**.

2. Lubricate the base of the device with water-soluble lubricant (**Step 2**).

3. Preoxygenate the patient before insertion. Ventilation should not be interrupted for more than 30 seconds to accomplish airway placement. Place the patient in the sniffing position (**Step 3**).

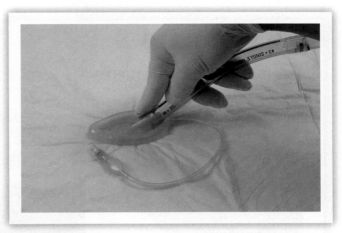

FIGURE 8-28 Press the laryngeal mask airway against a flat surface to remove all wrinkles from the cuff.

4. Insert the LMA along the roof of the mouth. The key to proper insertion is to slide the convex surface of the airway along the roof of the mouth. Use your finger to push the airway against the hard palate (**Step 4**). Once it slides past the tongue, the LMA will move easily into position.

5. Inflate the cuff with the amount of air indicated for the size of airway being used (**Step 5**). If the LMA is properly positioned, it will move out of the airway slightly

SKILL DRILL 8-5

LMA Insertion

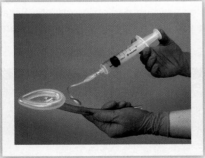

1. Take standard precautions. Check the cuff of the LMA by inflating it with 50% more air than required for the size of airway to be used. Then deflate the cuff completely.

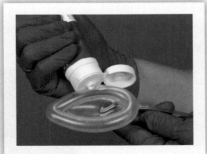

2. Lubricate the base of the device.

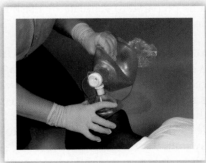

3. Preoxygenate the patient before insertion. Ventilation should not be interrupted for more than 30 seconds to accomplish airway placement. Place the patient in the sniffing position.

(continues)

SKILL DRILL 8-5

LMA Insertion (*continued*)

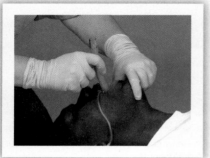 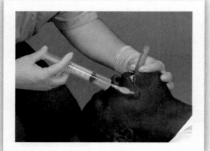 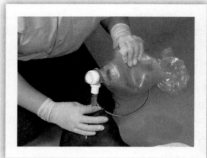

4 Insert the LMA along the roof of the mouth. Use your finger to push the airway against the hard palate.

5 Inflate the cuff with the amount of air indicated for the airway being used.

6 Begin to ventilate the patient. Confirm chest rise and the presence of breath sounds. Continuously and carefully monitor the patient.

(1 to 2 cm) as it moves into position. This is a good indication that the LMA is in the correct position.

6 Begin to ventilate the patient. Confirm chest rise and the presence of breath sounds. Continuously and carefully monitor the patient (**Step 6**).

Continuously and carefully monitor for regurgitation in the tube. The LMA can be easily dislodged because it was not designed for patients who are being transported. Carefully attend to the airway during any patient movement, and be prepared to ventilate by mask if the LMA becomes dislodged.

The Cobra Perilaryngeal Airway

The *Cobra perilaryngeal airway (CobraPLA)* was first introduced as a device to ventilate patients with difficult airways. It is so named because of the cobra shape of the distal part of the airway **FIGURE 8-29**. This shape allows the device to slide easily along the hard palate and to hold the soft tissue away from the laryngeal inlet (hence, "perilaryngeal") once in place. It is a supraglottic device with a tube for ventilation and a circumferential cuff that sits in the hypopharnyx at the base of the tongue proximal to the distal end, which is the ventilation outlet. It also has a 15-mm standard adapter and the distal widened end that holds soft tissue apart and allows for ventilation of the trachea. The distal tip is proximal to the esophagus and seals the hypopharnyx. When the cuff is inflated, it raises the tongue and creates an airway seal, allowing for ventilation. Because the insertion technique is very simple, personnel with little or no experience often are successful.

> *Cobra perilaryngeal airway (CobraPLA)* A supraglottic airway device with a shape that allows the device to slide easily along the hard palate and to hold the soft tissue away from the laryngeal inlet.

The CobraPLA is available in eight sizes. Proper size is determined by the one that comfortably fits through the patient's mouth.

Indications for the CobraPLA

The CobraPLA is used in a similar manner to other supraglottic airways and can be used on pediatric patients. Because the device does not provide protection against aspiration,

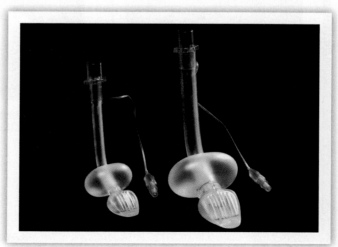

Courtesy of Pulmodyne, Inc.

FIGURE 8-29 The Cobra perilaryngeal airway.

it is recommended for use only in patients who are not at risk of vomiting.

Contraindications to the CobraPLA

Contraindications include risk for aspiration and massive trauma to the oral cavity.

Complications of the CobraPLA

If the patient has an intact gag reflex, laryngospasm may occur. If the CobraPLA is not inserted far enough, inflation of the cuff may cause the tongue to protrude from the mouth, disrupting an adequate seal. Using the proper size is vital because the patient cannot be ventilated if the device is too small and passes into the laryngeal inlet. However, in such an instance it can be removed and another size inserted with minimal trauma to the oropharynx.

Insertion Technique

SKILL DRILL 8-6 shows the steps for inserting a CobraPLA:

1. Take standard precautions (gloves and face shield).
2. Preoxygenate the patient whenever possible with a bag-mask device and 100% oxygen.
3. Gather, inspect, and prepare your equipment.
4. Fully deflate the cuff of the CobraPLA and fold back against the breathing tube.
5. Apply a water-soluble lubricant liberally to the front and back of the CobraPLA head and to the cuff.
6. Place the patient's head and neck in the sniffing position.

SKILL DRILL 8-6

Insertion of a Cobra Perilaryngeal Airway (CobraPLA)

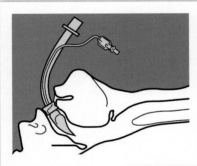

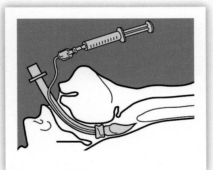

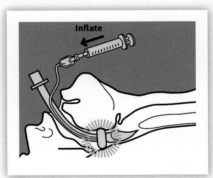

1. Take standard precautions. Preoxygenate the patient. Gather, inspect, and prepare your equipment. Fully deflate the cuff of the CobraPLA and fold back against the breathing tube. Apply a water-soluble lubricant liberally to the front and back of the CobraPLA head and to the cuff. Place the patient's head and neck in the sniffing position. Open the patient's mouth with a scissor maneuver with your nondominant hand, gently pulling the mandible upward. Direct the distal end of the CobraPLA straight back between the tongue and hard palate while lifting the jaw.

2. Continue advancing the CobraPLA until modest resistance is encountered.

3. Inflate the cuff with only enough air to achieve a good seal. Never overinflate the cuff. Ventilate the patient to confirm correct placement and to measure the pressure at which an audible leak occurs. Confirm placement by observing for chest rise and auscultating over the neck, chest, and epigastric region.

7 Open the patient's mouth with a scissor maneuver with your nondominant hand, gently pulling the mandible upward. Do not direct the CobraPLA tip against the hard palate; instead, direct the distal end straight back between the tongue and hard palate with your dominant hand while lifting the jaw with your nondominant hand (**Step 1**).

8 Continue advancing the CobraPLA until modest resistance is encountered as the device tip reaches the glottis (**Step 2**).

9 Inflate the cuff with only enough air to achieve a good seal (**Step 3**). Never overinflate the cuff. Inflate with less than the maximum volume recommended until there is no leak obtained with positive-pressure ventilation.

10 Ventilate the patient to confirm correct placement and to measure the pressure at which an audible leak occurs. Confirm placement by observing for chest rise and auscultating over the neck, chest, and epigastric region.

11 Secure the tube in place.

PREP KIT

Ready for Review

- To fully understand the respiratory conditions a patient may have, the AEMT must understand the anatomy and physiology of the respiratory system in more detail.
- Understanding the pathophysiology of ventilation, oxygenation, and respiration will also help the AEMT better understand the signs and symptoms associated with certain conditions as well as management techniques for caring for a patient presenting with such conditions.
- The respiratory system and the renal system have roles in maintaining a balance between acids and bases in the body. The respiratory system works to quickly remove excess acid as carbon dioxide from the lungs. Conversely, slowing the respirations will increase carbon dioxide. The renal system regulates pH by filtering out more hydrogen and retaining bicarbonate when needed, or by doing the reverse.
- Imbalances in pH can lead to serious medical emergencies. An increase in extracellular H^+ ions results in acidosis; a decrease in extracellular H^+ ions results in alkalosis.
- Factors that may affect pulmonary ventilation include airway obstruction; swelling from infection or allergic reaction; bronchoconstriction; medications that may depress the CNS, leading to a lower respiratory rate and tidal volume; trauma; and muscular dystrophy.
- External factors that may affect respiration include the atmospheric pressure and the partial pressure of oxygen in the ambient air. Internal factors include pneumonia, pulmonary edema, and COPD/emphysema.
- Adequate breathing for an adult is equivalent to a rate of 12 to 20 breaths/min and includes a regular pattern of inhalation and exhalation, adequate depth, bilaterally clear and equal lung sounds, and regular and equal chest rise and fall.
- Inadequate breathing for an adult is defined as fewer than 12 breaths/min or more than 20 breaths/min and includes shallow depth (reduced tidal volume), an irregular pattern of inhalation and exhalation, and breath sounds that are diminished, absent, or noisy.
- Patients with inadequate breathing must be treated immediately. Emergency medical care includes airway management, supplemental oxygen, and ventilatory support.

- Oxygen-delivery devices include nonrebreathing masks, nasal cannulas, partial rebreathing masks, Venturi masks, tracheostomy masks, and humidified oxygen.
- Artificial ventilation devices include the pocket face mask for performing mouth-to-mask ventilations, the bag-mask device, the manually triggered ventilation device, and the automatic transport ventilator.
- The use of cricoid pressure (Sellick maneuver) during artificial ventilation is no longer recommended.
- Suctioning is a priority after opening the patient's airway. AEMTs may also need to perform tracheobronchial suctioning in patients who have been intubated by paramedics.
- CPAP is a noninvasive method of providing ventilator support for patients in respiratory distress or suffering from sleep apnea.
- It is imperative that you are familiar with indications, contraindications, advantages, disadvantages, and special considerations when choosing the appropriate device. This is especially important when you are treating pediatric patients. Regardless of the method, aggressive airway management is essential to a positive patient outcome.
- Advanced devices that can be used by AEMTs to provide definitive airway management to patients unable to maintain their own airway include esophageal airways and multilumen airways.
- Multilumen airways have two tubes and can be inserted blindly. The Combitube is an example of such a device. The multilumen airway can be used to ventilate via the esophagus or the trachea, based on placement.
- The King LT is a single-lumen airway that is blindly inserted into the esophagus. When it is placed into the esophagus, the distal cuff seals the esophagus while the proximal cuff seals the oropharynx. Openings located between these two cuffs provide ventilation of the lungs.
- The LMA is designed to provide a conduit from the glottis opening to the ventilation device. When inserted, the opening of the LMA is positioned right at the glottis opening. The inflatable cuff conforms to the contours of the airway and makes a relatively airtight seal.
- The CobraPLA is designed to slide easily along the hard palate and to hold the soft tissue away from the laryngeal inlet once in place. The distal tip is proximal to the esophagus and seals the hypopharynx.

Case Study

You arrive at the scene of a 56-year-old woman having trouble breathing. As you approach the patient, you immediately see she is in respiratory distress. Her husband tells you that she has emphysema and is on several medications to help control her illness. He informs you that the patient has been struggling with increasing trouble breathing for the past 2 days and now is at a point where she can no longer breathe without significant difficulty. The patient is alert, oriented, and able to follow commands, but is only able to speak in one- or two-word phrases. She is in a tripod position and her skin appears pale. As your partner places the patient on oxygen and obtains vital signs, you listen to the lung sounds. You hear diminished sounds in all fields with slight inspiratory and expiratory wheezes in the apices of the lungs. Her vital signs are as follows: pulse rate, 108 beats/min; respirations, 32 breaths/min; blood pressure, 152/96 mm Hg; and a pulse oximetry reading of 87%.

1. Is this patient a candidate for CPAP? Explain your answer.

2. Some CPAP units will empty a D oxygen cylinder in as little as:
A. 5 to 10 minutes.
B. 10 to 15 minutes.
C. 15 to 20 minutes.
D. 20 to 25 minutes.

3. Compare and contrast the differences between oxygenation, respiration, and ventilation.

4. Explain how the Venturi mask works and how this can benefit patients.

5. What are the conditions that may give you an inaccurate pulse oximetry reading?

CHAPTER 9

Shock and BLS Resuscitation

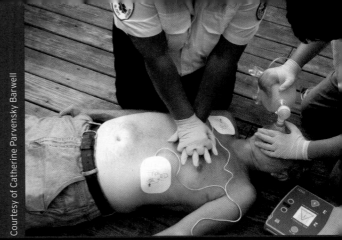

Courtesy of Catherine Parvensky Barwell

National EMS Education Standard

Anatomy and Physiology

Applies fundamental knowledge of the anatomy and function of all human systems to the practice of EMS.

Pathophysiology

Applies comprehensive knowledge of the pathophysiology of respiration and perfusion to patient assessment and management.

Medicine

Applies fundamental knowledge to provide basic and selected advanced emergency care and transportation based on assessment findings for an acutely ill patient.

Shock and Resuscitation

Applies fundamental knowledge to provide basic and selected advanced emergency care and transportation based on assessment findings for a patient in shock, respiratory failure or arrest, cardiac failure or arrest, and post resuscitation management.

Review

Perfusion is the circulation of oxygen-rich blood to cells, tissue, and organs. Shock, also known as hypoperfusion, occurs when the circulation of blood in the body becomes inadequate, and the oxygen and nutrient needs of the cells cannot be met. In the early stages of shock, the body will undergo a series of changes in its various functions in an attempt to maintain homeostasis (a balance of all systems of the body). A drop in blood pressure is a late sign of shock and occurs when the body is no longer able to compensate for blood loss.

Cardiovascular pulmonary resuscitation (CPR) is used to establish artificial ventilation and circulation in a patient who is not breathing and has no pulse, so as to supply vital organs with oxygen. The goal of CPR is to restore spontaneous breathing and circulation; however, advanced procedures such as medications and defibrillation are often necessary to achieve this outcome. Ideally, only seconds should pass between the time when you recognize that a patient needs BLS and the time when you start treatment, because more brain cells will die every second that the brain is deprived of oxygen. Permanent brain damage is possible if the brain goes without oxygen for 4 to 6 minutes. After 6 minutes without oxygen, brain damage is likely.

What's New

The term "shock" has been reintroduced as the term meaning hypoperfusion syndrome. It describes a state of collapse and failure of the cardiovascular system. This abnormal state of inadequate circulation of oxygen and nutrients to the cells of the body first causes organs and then organ systems to fail. If not treated promptly, shock can be fatal. It can occur due to several medical or traumatic events, including heart attack or severe allergic reaction (now referred to as anaphylactic shock or anaphylaxis).

The standards for CPR and Emergency Cardiac Care changed in October 2010. In addition to other important changes, the process of assessment for CPR, which once focused on ABCs, has changed to CAB (chest compressions, airway open, breaths), with emphasis placed on early chest compressions for victims of cardiac arrest.

Introduction

Shock has a number of meanings. In this chapter, *shock* (hypoperfusion) describes a state of collapse and failure of the cardiovascular system. When the circulation of blood in the body becomes inadequate, the oxygen and nutrient needs of the cells cannot be met. In the early stages of shock, the body will attempt to maintain *homeostasis*; however, as shock progresses, blood circulation slows and eventually ceases. This abnormal state of inadequate oxygen and nutrient delivery to the cells of the body causes organs and then organ systems to fail. If not treated promptly, shock can be fatal.

Shock can occur because of several medical or traumatic events such as a heart attack, severe allergic reaction, an automobile crash, or a gunshot wound. As an AEMT, you will respond to these different types of emergencies to provide care and transportation for these patients. Therefore, you must be constantly alert to the signs and symptoms of shock. Maintain a high index of suspicion. The goal is to recognize shock in its early stages and provide appropriate treatment.

Physiology of Perfusion

Perfusion is the circulation of blood within an organ or tissue in adequate amounts to meet the cells' current needs for oxygen, nutrients, and waste removal. Perfusion requires having a working cardiovascular system. It also requires adequate gas exchange in the lungs, adequate nutrients in the form of glucose in the blood, and adequate waste removal, primarily through the lungs.

> **Shock** A condition in which the circulatory system fails to provide sufficient circulation to enable every body part to perform its function; also called hypoperfusion.
>
> **Homeostasis** A tendency to constancy or stability in the body's internal environment.
>
> **Perfusion** The circulation of oxygenated blood within an organ or tissue in adequate amounts to meet the cells' current needs.

The body is perfused via the circulatory system. The circulatory system is a complex arrangement of connected tubes, including the arteries, arterioles, capillaries, venules, and veins. There are two circuits in the body: the systemic circulation in the body and the pulmonary circulation in the lungs. The systemic circulation, the circuit in the body, carries oxygen-rich blood from the left ventricle through the body and back to the right atrium. In the systemic circulation, as blood passes through the tissues and organs, it gives up oxygen and nutrients and absorbs cellular wastes and carbon dioxide. Carbon dioxide is one of the primary waste products of cellular work (metabolism) in the body and is removed from the body by the lungs. This is the reason why one of your primary concerns for your patient should be ensuring adequate ventilation and oxygenation.

> ## Transition Tip
>
> The following elements are collectively known as the *Fick principle*, which states that the movement and use of oxygen in the body are dependent on:
> 1. Adequate concentration of inspired oxygen (FIO_2; fraction of inspired oxygen)
> 2. Appropriate movement of oxygen across the alveolar–capillary membrane into the arterial bloodstream
> 3. Adequate number of red blood cells to carry the oxygen
> 4. Proper tissue perfusion
> 5. Efficient off-loading of oxygen at the tissue level

> *Fick principle* States that the movement and use of oxygen in the body are dependent on adequate concentration of inspired oxygen (FIO_2; fraction of inspired oxygen), appropriate movement of oxygen across the alveolar–capillary membrane into the arterial bloodstream, adequate number of red blood cells to carry the oxygen, proper tissue perfusion, and efficient off-loading of oxygen at the tissue level.

Respiration and Oxygenation

Each time you take a breath, the alveoli (microscopic, thin-walled air sacs within the lungs) receive a supply of oxygen-rich air. The oxygen then dissolves in the blood plasma and attaches to the blood's hemoglobin. In order to accomplish the exchange of gases, the blood passes adjacent to the alveolar wall via a fine network of pulmonary capillaries that are in close contact with the alveoli. Oxygenated blood is then circulated to the cells and organs to allow them to receive proper nutrients necessary to sustain life.

Oxygen and carbon dioxide pass rapidly across thin tissue layers both in the lungs and in the cells throughout the body through diffusion. Diffusion is a passive process in which molecules move from an area with a higher concentration of a particular substance to an area of lower concentration. There are more oxygen molecules in the alveoli than in the blood. Therefore, the oxygen molecules move from the alveoli into the blood. Because there are more carbon dioxide molecules in the blood than in the inhaled air, carbon dioxide moves from the blood into the alveoli.

Just like oxygen, carbon dioxide is dissolved in the plasma and attaches to the blood's hemoglobin. The body takes the carbon dioxide, combines it with water, and creates carbonic acid. Carbonic acid concentrations become very high just as the blood is moving toward the lungs. Once it reaches the lungs, the carbonic acid breaks down and the carbon dioxide is exhaled. All of this action takes place to maintain the delicate balance between the gases and maintain the pH of the body.

Regulation of Blood Flow

Blood flow through the capillary beds is regulated by the capillary sphincters, circular muscular walls that constrict and dilate, acting as a gate to increase or decrease flow. These *sphincters* are under the control of the *autonomic nervous system (ANS)*, which regulates involuntary functions such as sweating and digestion. Capillary sphincters also respond to other stimuli such as heat, cold, the need for oxygen, and the need for waste removal. Under normal circumstances, not all cells have the same needs at the same time. For example, the stomach and intestines have a high need for blood flow during and shortly after eating, when digestion is at its peak. Between meals, blood flow is lessened, and blood is diverted to other areas. The brain, by contrast, needs a constant and consistent supply of blood to function.

Regulation of blood flow is determined by cellular need and is accomplished by vessel constriction or dilation, which is accomplished through sphincter constriction or dilation. Maintenance of blood flow, or perfusion, is accomplished by the heart, blood vessels, and blood working together.

Cardiac Output

Cardiac output (CO) is the volume of blood that the heart can pump per minute, and it is dependent on several factors. First, the heart must have adequate strength, which is largely determined by the ability of the heart muscle to contract. This ability to contract is referred to as *myocardial contractility*. Second, the heart must receive adequate blood to pump. As the volume of blood coming to the heart increases, the precontraction pressure in the heart builds up. This precontraction pressure is known as *preload*. As preload increases, the volume of blood within the ventricles increases, which causes the heart muscle to stretch. When the muscle is stretched, myocardial contractility improves, leading to greater force of contraction and increased cardiac output. Lastly, the resistance to flow in the peripheral circulation must be appropriate. The force or resistance against which the heart pumps is known as *afterload*.

Sphincters Circular muscles that encircle and, by contracting, constrict a duct, tube, or opening. Examples are found within the rectum, bladder, and blood vessels.
Autonomic nervous system (ANS) The part of the nervous system that regulates functions that are not controlled consciously, such as digestion and sweating.
Cardiac output (CO) The amount of blood pumped through the circulatory system in 1 minute.
Myocardial contractility The ability of the heart muscle to contract.
Preload The amount of blood returned to the heart to be pumped out; directly affects myocardial contractility.
Afterload The pressure in the aorta against which the left ventricle must pump blood.

Blood pressure, the pressure that is generated by the contractions of the heart and the dilation and constriction of the blood vessels, is usually carefully controlled by the body so that there is always sufficient circulation to the various tissues and organs. It is a rough measure of perfusion. Because the heart cannot pump out what is not in its holding chambers, blood pressure varies directly with cardiac output, *systemic vascular resistance (SVR)*, and blood volume. (Systemic vascular resistance is the resistance to blood flow within all of the blood vessels except the pulmonary vessels.) Remember that blood pressure is the pressure of blood within the vessels at any one time. The systolic pressure is the peak arterial pressure, or pressure generated every time the heart contracts; the diastolic pressure is the pressure maintained within the arteries while the heart rests between heartbeats.

Perfusion depends on cardiac output, SVR, and transport of oxygen.

$$CO = HR \times SV$$

Cardiac Output = Heart Rate × Stroke Volume

$$BP = CO \times SVR$$

Blood Pressure = Cardiac Output × Systemic Vascular Resistance

Mean arterial pressure (MAP) is generally considered to be the patient's blood pressure. However, MAP is ultimately the blood pressure required to sustain organ perfusion and is roughly 60 mm Hg in the average person. If the MAP falls significantly below 60 mm Hg for an appreciable amount of time, the result will be ischemia of the organ(s) from lack of perfusion.

MAP is determined with this formula:

$$MAP = (CO \times SVR) + CVP$$

Systemic vascular resistance (SVR) The resistance that blood must overcome to be able to move within the blood vessels; related to the amount of dilation or constriction in the blood vessel.
Mean arterial pressure (MAP) The average pressure against the arterial wall during a cardiac cycle; generally considered to be the same as blood pressure.

However, the central venous pressure (CVP) is negligible and is usually left out of the equation.

■ Pathophysiology

Shock can result from inadequate cardiac output, decreased SVR, or the inability of red blood cells to deliver oxygen to tissues. If there is a disturbance in the transportation of oxygen and removal of carbon dioxide, dangerous waste products will build up, leading to cellular death and eventually death of the entire organ. If the shock state persists, it will ultimately lead to death of the entire organism (body). As mentioned, shock, or hypoperfusion, is a state of collapse and failure of the cardiovascular system that leads to inadequate circulation. To protect vital organs, the body attempts to compensate by shunting (directing) blood flow from organs that are more tolerant of low flow (such as the skin and intestines) to vital organs that cannot tolerate hypoperfusion (such as the heart, brain, and lungs). If the cause of shock is not promptly addressed, the patient will soon die.

The cardiovascular system consists of three parts: a pump (the heart), a set of pipes (the blood vessels or arteries that act as the container), and the contents of the container (the fluid or blood) **FIGURE 9-1**. These three parts can be referred to as the "perfusion triangle" **FIGURE 9-2**.

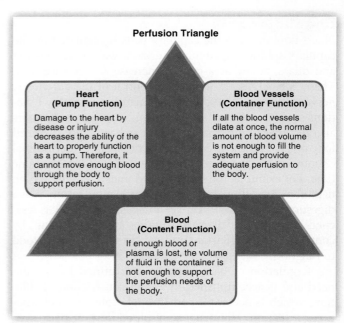

Perfusion Triangle

Heart (Pump Function)
Damage to the heart by disease or injury decreases the ability of the heart to properly function as a pump. Therefore, it cannot move enough blood through the body to support perfusion.

Blood Vessels (Container Function)
If all the blood vessels dilate at once, the normal amount of blood volume is not enough to fill the system and provide adequate perfusion to the body.

Blood (Content Function)
If enough blood or plasma is lost, the volume of fluid in the container is not enough to support the perfusion needs of the body.

FIGURE 9-2 The heart, the blood vessels, and the blood represent the three legs of the perfusion triangle.

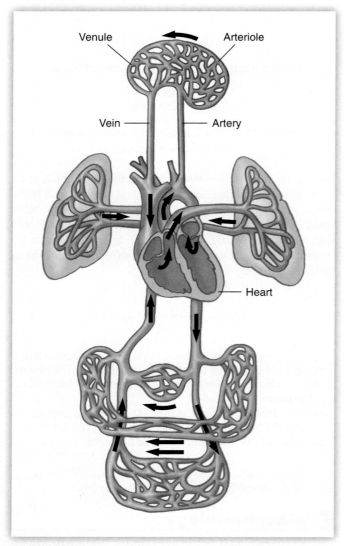

FIGURE 9-1 The cardiovascular system consists of three parts: the pump (heart), the container (vessels), and the contents (blood). The blood carries oxygen and nutrients through the vessels to the capillary beds, where they are exchanged for waste products.

When a patient is in shock, one or more of the three parts is not working properly.

Blood is the vehicle for carrying oxygen and nutrients through the vessels to the capillary beds to tissue cells, where these supplies are exchanged for waste products created during metabolism. For this process to happen, the vessels (container) must be intact. Blood contains red blood cells, white blood cells, platelets, and plasma (the liquid portion of the blood). Red blood cells, specifically hemoglobin, are responsible for the transportation of oxygen to the cells and for transporting carbon dioxide (a waste product of cellular metabolism) away from the cells to the lungs where it is exhaled and removed from the body. White blood cells help the body to fight infection. Platelets are responsible for forming blood clots.

Blood clots are an important response from the body to control blood loss. In the body, a blood clot forms depending on one of the following principles: retention of blood because of blockage in blood circulation (blood stasis), changes in the vessel wall (such as a wound), and the blood's ability to clot (as the result of a disease process or medication). When injury occurs to tissues in the body, platelets begin to aggregate at the site of injury; this causes the red blood cells to become sticky and clump together. As the red blood cells begin to clump, another substance in the body called fibrinogen reinforces the red blood cells. This is the final step in the formation of a blood clot. However, clots are unstable and prone to rupture because blood is continually moving as a result of the blood pressure.

The body's neural and hormonal mechanisms, including the autonomic nervous system and hormones, are triggered when the body senses that the pressure in the system is falling and there is an increased need for perfusion of vital organs. The sympathetic side of the autonomic nervous system, which is responsible for the fight-or-flight response, will assume more control of the body's functions during a state of shock. The parasympathetic nervous system is a division of the autonomic nervous system that controls involuntary functions by sending signals to the cardiac, smooth, and glandular muscles. The autonomic nervous system causes the release of hormones such as epinephrine and norepinephrine. These hormones cause changes in certain body functions such as an increase in the heart rate and in the strength of cardiac contractions and vasoconstriction in nonessential areas, primarily in the skin, muscles, and gastrointestinal tract (peripheral vasoconstriction). Together, these actions are designed to maintain pressure in the system and, as a result, sustain perfusion of the vital organs (ie, brain, heart, lungs, kidneys, and liver).

Eventually, there is also a shifting of body fluids to help maintain pressure within the system. However, the response of the autonomic nervous system and hormones comes within seconds. It is this response that causes all the signs and symptoms of shock in a patient.

Compensation for Decreased Perfusion

This section takes a more in-depth look at the body's neural and hormonal mechanisms for regulating blood pressure. As mentioned, maintenance of blood pressure is one of the most important homeostatic mechanisms to regulate cardiovascular dynamics. When any event results in decreased perfusion, the body must respond immediately in an attempt to preserve the vital organs. *Baroreceptors* located in the aortic arch and carotid sinuses (as well as in most of the large arteries of the neck and thorax) sense the decreased pressure and activate the vasomotor center in the medulla oblongata, which oversees changes in the diameter of blood vessels, to begin constriction of the vessels and, therefore, increase blood pressure.

> *Baroreceptors* Receptors in the blood vessels, kidneys, brain, and heart that respond to changes in pressure in the heart or main arteries to help maintain blood pressure.

Normally, stimulation occurs when the systolic pressure is between 60 and 80 mm Hg and even lower in children. A decrease in systolic pressure to less than 80 mm Hg stimulates the vasomotor center to increase arterial pressure by constricting vessels. As the arterial pressure drops, the walls of the arteries are not stretched as much, thereby decreasing baroreceptor stimulation. Normally, baroreceptor stimulation prevents the vasoconstrictor center of the medulla from constricting the vessels, leading to vasodilation in the peripheral circulatory system and a decrease in heart rate and contractility. This causes a decrease in arterial pressure. With dropping pressure, the baroreceptors are not stimulated to allow for vasodilation, so the vessels constrict to raise the blood pressure. The sympathetic

nervous system is also stimulated at this time as the body recognizes a potential catastrophic event.

Short-term control of blood pressure is mediated by the nervous system and bloodborne chemicals to counteract fluctuations in blood pressure by altering SVR. *Chemoreceptors* located in the carotid and aortic bodies are stimulated by decreases in PaO_2 and increases in $PaCO_2$ and are more important in regulating respiration than blood pressure. However, they also contribute to controlling blood pressure on a smaller scale. When the pH of the blood drops sharply as the carbon dioxide level rises, impulses are sent to the cardio-acceleratory center to increase cardiac output and to the vasomotor center to stimulate vasoconstriction. Long-term control of blood pressure is also regulated by the slower-acting renal system, which helps regulate blood volume and acid–base balance.

> *Chemoreceptors* Receptors in the blood vessels, kidneys, brain, and heart that respond to changes in chemical composition of the blood to help maintain homeostasis.

As perfusion decreases, the sympathetic nervous system is stimulated, initiating the fight-or-flight response. The adrenal medulla secretes two catecholamines, epinephrine and norepinephrine. The alpha-1 response to the release of epinephrine includes vasoconstriction, increased peripheral vascular resistance, and an increased afterload from the arteriolar constriction. Alpha-2 effects ensure a regulated release of alpha-1. Beta responses from the release of epinephrine primarily effect the heart and lungs. Increases in heart rate, contractility, conductivity, and automaticity occur in tandem with bronchodilation. Effects of norepinephrine are primarily alpha-1 and alpha-2 and are centered on vasoconstriction and increasing peripheral vascular resistance. **TABLE 9-1** lists the alpha and beta effects of epinephrine and norepinephrine.

Failure of compensatory mechanisms to preserve perfusion leads to decreases in preload and cardiac output. Myocardial blood supply and oxygenation decrease, reducing myocardial perfusion. As cardiac output further decreases, coronary artery perfusion also decreases, leading to myocardial ischemia.

Transition Tip

Starling's Law of the Heart states that the length of the muscle fibers constituting the heart's muscular wall is the primary determinant of the force of the heartbeat. In other words, an increase in diastolic filling increases the force of the contraction, whereas a decrease in diastolic filling decreases the force of the contraction. Decreased perfusion in shock is usually associated with a decrease in cardiac contraction, which may be the result of loss of fluid, increased container size, or a damaged pump.

Table 9-1 Effects of Epinephrine and Norepinephrine	
Epinephrine	
Alpha-1	Vasoconstriction
	Increase in peripheral vascular resistance
	Increased afterload from arteriolar constriction
Alpha-2	Regulated release of alpha-1
Beta-1	Positive *chronotropic effects* (increase in the heart's rate of contraction)
	Positive *inotropic effects* (increase in the contractility of the heart muscle)
	Positive *dromotropic effects* (increase in the heart's velocity of conduction)
Beta-2	Bronchodilation
	Gastrointestinal smooth muscle dilation
Norepinephrine	
Alpha-1 and alpha-2	Vasoconstriction
	Increase in peripheral vascular resistance
	Increased afterload from arteriolar constriction

Capillary and Cellular Changes

Recall that capillary sphincters regulate blood flow through the capillary beds. Regulation of blood flow is determined by cellular need and is accomplished by vessel constriction or dilation, together with sphincter constriction or dilation. Cellular ischemia occurs as perfusion decreases. There is minimal blood flow through the capillaries, causing the cells to go from *aerobic metabolism* to *anaerobic metabolism*, which can quickly lead to metabolic acidosis. With less circulation in the capillaries, the blood stagnates there. The precapillary sphincter relaxes in response to the buildup of lactic acid, vasomotor center failure, and increased amounts of carbon dioxide. The postcapillary sphincters remain constricted, causing the capillaries to engorge with fluid.

Chronotropic effects Affecting the heart's rate of contraction.

Inotropic effects Affecting the contractility of the heart muscle.

Dromotropic effects Affecting the heart's velocity of conduction.

Aerobic metabolism Metabolism that can proceed only in the presence of oxygen.

Anaerobic metabolism The metabolism that takes place in the absence of oxygen; the principal product is lactic acid.

Ischemia stimulates carbon dioxide production by the tissues. The higher the body's metabolic rate, the higher the carbon dioxide level in hypoperfused states. The excess carbon dioxide combines with intracellular water to produce carbonic acid. Increased tissue acids will, in turn, react with other buffers to form more intracellular acidic substances.

As anaerobic metabolism continues, increasing lactic acid production causes the pH of the blood to significantly fall. Because arteries deprived of oxygenated blood cannot remain constricted, more vasodilation occurs. There is an aggregation, or accumulation, of red blood cells and formation of microemboli (small clots). Because the capillary walls are stretched, they lose their ability to retain large molecules, allowing leaking into the surrounding interstitial spaces. Hydrostatic pressure forces plasma into the interstitial spaces, further increasing the distance from the capillaries to the cells, and, as a result, oxygen transport decreases, increasing cellular hypoxia. Capillary hydrostatic pressure tends to force fluids through capillary walls whereas interstitial fluid hydrostatic pressure pushes fluid back into the cells.

Oncotic pressure pulls fluids from the surrounding tissue into the capillaries as a result of a difference in the concentration of solutes in the fluid inside the capillaries. Fluid leaves the capillaries as a result of hydrostatic pressure, while albumin and other large proteins remain inside, resulting in a greater concentration of solutes inside the capillaries. The oncotic pressure rises, pulling more water into the capillaries in order to balance the solute concentration. If capillary hydrostatic pressure is greater, fluid will leave the capillaries. If capillary oncotic pressure is greater, fluid will be pulled into the capillaries.

The continuing buildup of lactic acid and carbon dioxide acts as a potent vasodilator, leading to relaxation of the postcapillary sphincters. The accumulated hydrogen, potassium, carbon dioxide, and thrombosed (clotted) red blood cells wash out into the venous circulation, increasing the metabolic acidosis. The result is an even further drop in cardiac output.

Multiple-Organ Dysfunction Syndrome

Multiple-organ dysfunction syndrome (MODS) is a progressive condition characterized by combined failure of several organs, such as the lungs, liver, and kidney, along with some clotting mechanisms, which occurs after severe illness or injury. It is a major cause of death following septic, traumatic, and burn injuries.

Multiple-organ dysfunction syndrome (MODS) A progressive condition usually characterized by combined failure of several organs, such as the lungs, liver, and kidney, along with some clotting mechanisms, which occurs after severe illness or injury.

The net outcome of overactivity in these systems is maldistribution of systemic and organ blood flow. Often tissues attempt to compensate by accelerating their metabolism.

The result is an oxygen supply–demand imbalance that leads to tissue hypoxia, tissue hypoperfusion, exhaustion of the cells' fuel supply (adenosine triphosphate), metabolic failure, lysosome breakdown, anaerobic metabolism, acidosis, and impaired cellular function. As MODS progresses, various organs begin to malfunction as a result of the cell and tissue hypoxia.

MODS typically develops within hours to days following resuscitation. Over a 14- to 21-day period, renal and liver failure can develop, along with collapse of the gastrointestinal and immune systems. If the patient does not respond to treatment of the underlying condition, cardiovascular collapse and death typically occur within days to weeks of the initial injury.

Signs and symptoms of MODS include hypotension, insufficient tissue perfusion, uncontrollable bleeding, and multisystem organ failure caused mainly by hypoxia, tissue acidosis, and severe local alterations of metabolism. Patients can have a low-grade fever from the inflammatory response and are tachycardic and dyspneic. They may prove difficult to oxygenate because of the presence of adult respiratory distress syndrome.

Causes of Shock

Shock can result from many conditions, including bleeding, respiratory failure, acute allergic reactions, and overwhelming infection. In all cases, however, the damage occurs because of insufficient perfusion of organs and tissues. As soon as perfusion stops or becomes impaired, tissues start to die, affecting all local body processes. If the conditions causing shock are not promptly arrested and reversed, death soon follows.

You should have a high index of suspicion for shock in many emergency medical situations. For example, you would expect hemorrhagic shock to accompany massive external or internal bleeding. You should also expect shock if a patient has any one of the following conditions:

- Multiple severe fractures
- Abdominal or chest injury
- Spinal injury
- A severe infection
- A major heart attack
- Anaphylaxis

Transition Tip

Shock is a complex physiologic process that gives subtle signs to its presence before it becomes severe. These early signs relate very closely to the events that lead to more severe shock, so it is important for you to know the underlying processes thoroughly. If you understand what causes shock, you will be able to recognize it in many patients before it becomes out of control.

Understanding the basic physiologic causes of shock will better prepare you to treat it. There are three basic causes of shock FIGURE 9-3.

Types of Shock

Shock may be the result of a variety of causes, but hypovolemia from blood or fluid loss is a common culprit. TABLE 9-2 explains the differences between the types of shock and how to differentiate them from hypovolemic shock. Specific types of shock are discussed next.

Cardiogenic Shock

Cardiogenic shock is caused by inadequate function of the heart, or pump failure. Circulation of blood throughout the vascular system requires the constant pumping action of a normal and vigorous heart muscle. Many diseases or injury can cause destruction or inflammation of this muscle. Within certain limits, the heart can adapt to these problems. If too much muscular damage occurs, however, as sometimes happens after a massive heart attack, the heart no longer functions well. A major effect is the backup of blood into the lungs. The resulting buildup of fluid within the pulmonary tissue is called pulmonary edema. *Edema* is the presence of abnormally large amounts of fluid between cells in body tissues, causing swelling of the affected area

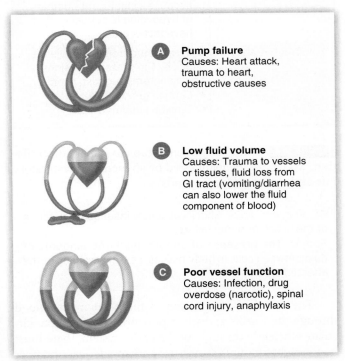

A **Pump failure**
Causes: Heart attack, trauma to heart, obstructive causes

B **Low fluid volume**
Causes: Trauma to vessels or tissues, fluid loss from GI tract (vomiting/diarrhea can also lower the fluid component of blood)

C **Poor vessel function**
Causes: Infection, drug overdose (narcotic), spinal cord injury, anaphylaxis

FIGURE 9-3 There are three basic causes of shock and impaired tissue perfusion. **A.** Pump failure occurs when the heart is damaged by disease, injury, or obstructive causes. The heart may not generate enough energy to move the blood through the system. **B.** Low fluid volume, often a result of bleeding, leads to inadequate perfusion. **C.** Poor vessel function—if blood vessels dilate excessively, the blood within them, even though it is of normal volume, is inadequate to fill the system and provide efficient perfusion.

Table 9-2 Differentiating Types of Shock	
Type	**How to Differentiate**
Cardiogenic shock	Differentiated from hypovolemic shock by the presence of one or more of the following: ■ Chief complaint: chest pain, dyspnea, tachycardia ■ Heart rate: bradycardia or excessive tachycardia ■ Signs of congestive heart failure: jugular vein distention, rales ■ Arrhythmias
Distributive shock	Differentiated from hypovolemic shock by the presence of one or more of the following: ■ Mechanism that suggests vasodilation: spinal cord injury, drug overdose, sepsis, anaphylaxis ■ Warm, flushed skin, especially in dependent areas ■ Lack of tachycardic response: This is not reliable, however, because a significant number of hypovolemic patients never have tachycardia.
Obstructive shock	Differentiated from hypovolemic shock by the presence of signs and symptoms suggestive of: ■ Cardiac tamponade ■ Tension pneumothorax

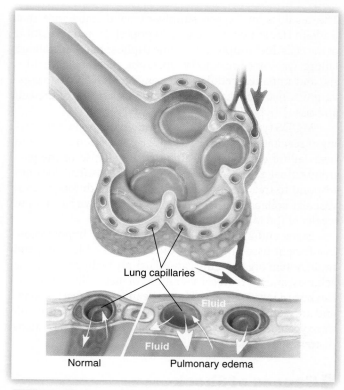

FIGURE 9-4 Pulmonary edema develops as a result of fluid buildup within the pulmonary tissue. The edema causes swelling and leads to impaired ventilation.

FIGURE 9-4. Pulmonary edema leads to impaired ventilation, which may be manifested by an increased respiratory rate and abnormal lung sounds.

> **Cardiogenic shock** Shock caused by inadequate function of the heart, or pump failure.
> **Edema** The presence of abnormally large amounts of fluid between cells in body tissues; causing swelling of the affected area.

The muscular contraction of the heart moves blood through the vessels at distinct pressures. For blood to circulate efficiently throughout the entire system, there must be the right amount of pressure and an adequate number of heartbeats. For this reason, the heart has its own electrical system that initiates and regulates its beating. Disease or injury can damage or destroy this system, causing irregular and uncoordinated beats, beats that are too slow (fewer than 60 beats/min), or beats that are too fast (more than 100 beats/min).

Cardiogenic shock develops when the heart cannot maintain sufficient output (cardiac output) to meet the demands of the body. In general, as afterload increases, cardiac output decreases. Increased afterload may also cause the heart to overwork while trying to maintain adequate cardiac output. High afterload is often the reason that heart failure develops in patients with hypertension. Cardiogenic shock may result from low cardiac output caused by high afterload, low preload, poor contractility, or any combination of the three.

Obstructive Shock

Obstructive shock results when conditions that cause mechanical obstruction of the cardiac muscle also impact pump function. Two of the most common examples of obstructive shock are cardiac tamponade and tension pneumothorax, described next.

> **Obstructive shock** Shock that occurs when there is a block to blood flow in the heart or great vessels, causing an insufficient blood supply to the body's tissues.
> **Cardiac tamponade** Compression of the heart caused by a buildup of blood or other fluid in the pericardial sac.

Cardiac tamponade, or pericardial tamponade, occurs when blood leaks into the tough fibrous membrane known as the pericardium, causing an accumulation of blood within the pericardial sac. It is caused by blunt or penetrating trauma and can progress rapidly. This accumulation leads to compression of the heart. Because the pericardium has a limited ability to stretch, each contraction of the heart allows more blood accumulation between the heart and the sac. The accumulated blood prevents the heart from opening up to allow complete refilling. Continued pressure within the pericardial sac obstructs the flow of blood into the heart, resulting in decreased outflow from the heart. Signs and symptoms of cardiac tamponade are referred to as Beck's triad, and include the presence of jugular vein distention, muffled heart sounds, and a narrowing *pulse pressure* (the difference between the systolic and diastolic pressures).

Another obstructive condition occurs with a *tension pneumothorax*. A tension pneumothorax is caused by damage to the lung tissue. This damage allows air normally held within the lung to escape into the chest cavity. If a pneumothorax is allowed to continue untreated, a sufficient amount of air can accumulate within the chest cavity to cause pressure on the structures in the mediastinum. The primary organs in this area are the heart and great vessels (aorta and vena cava). When the trapped air begins to shift the chest organs toward the uninjured side, a pneumothorax becomes known as a tension pneumothorax, which is a very serious and life-threatening condition. As pressure from one side of the chest begins to push the mediastinum toward the other side, the vena cava loses its ability to stay fully expanded. This mechanical compression of the vessel leads to reduced return of blood to the heart. The patient becomes anxious and short of breath. The heart and respiratory rates increase and become shallower. Blood pressure drops. You may notice difficulty when attempting to ventilate the patient with a bag-mask device. The affected side will have decreased or absent lung sounds and the patient will become cyanotic. Tracheal deviation may be a late sign of tension pneumothorax.

Distributive Shock

Distributive shock results when there is widespread dilation of the small arterioles, small venules, or both. As a result, the circulating blood volume pools in the expanded vascular beds and tissue perfusion decreases. The four most common types of distributive shock are septic shock, neurogenic shock, anaphylactic shock, and psychogenic shock.

Septic Shock

Septic shock occurs as a result of severe infections, usually bacterial, in which toxins (poisons) are generated by the bacteria or by infected body tissues. In this condition, the toxins damage the vessel walls, causing increased cellular permeability. The vessel walls leak and are unable to contract well. Widespread dilation of vessels, in combination with plasma loss through the injured vessel walls, results in shock.

Septic shock is a complex problem. First, there is an insufficient volume of fluid in the container because much of the plasma has leaked out of the vascular system (hypovolemia). Second, the fluid that has leaked out often collects in the respiratory system, interfering with ventilation. Third, the vasodilation leads to a larger-than-normal vascular bed to contain the smaller-than-normal volume of intravascular fluid.

Septic shock is almost always a complication of a very serious illness, injury, or surgery.

> *Pulse pressure* The difference between the systolic and diastolic pressures.
> *Tension pneumothorax* An accumulation of air or gas in the pleural space that causes collapse of one lung and compression of the mediastinum with potentially fatal results.
> *Distributive shock* A condition that occurs when there is widespread dilation of the small arterioles, small venules, or both.
> *Septic shock* Shock caused by severe infection, usually a bacterial infection.
> *Neurogenic shock* Circulatory failure caused by paralysis of the nerves that control the size of the blood vessels, leading to widespread dilation; seen in patients with spinal cord injuries.

Neurogenic Shock

Damage to the spinal cord, particularly at the upper cervical levels, may cause significant injury to the part of the nervous system that controls the size and muscular tone of the blood vessels. *Neurogenic shock* is usually the result. Although not as common, there are medical causes as well. These include brain conditions, tumors, pressure on the spinal cord, and spina bifida. In neurogenic shock, the muscles in the walls of the blood vessels are cut off from the sympathetic nervous system and nerve impulses that cause them to contract. This prevents the natural catecholamine release that is seen with other types of shock, resulting in the classic symptoms. As a result of the lack of sympathetic innervation, all vessels below the level of the spinal injury dilate widely, increasing the size and capacity of the vascular system **FIGURE 9-5** and causing blood to pool. The available 6 L of blood in the body can no longer fill the enlarged vascular system.

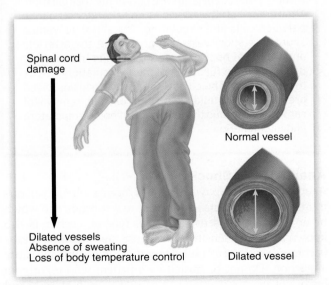

FIGURE 9-5 Damage to the spinal cord can result in nerves no longer being able to make the vessels contract. Instead, vessels dilate widely. The blood in the body can no longer fill the enlarged vessels; inadequate perfusion results.

Spinal cord damage

Dilated vessels
Absence of sweating
Loss of body temperature control

Normal vessel

Dilated vessel

Even though no blood or fluid has been lost, perfusion of organs and tissues becomes inadequate, and shock occurs. In this condition, a radical change in the size of the vascular system has caused shock. Characteristic signs of this type of shock are the absence of sweating below the level of injury, normal warm skin, and the lack of a tachycardia response.

Transition Tip

With neurogenic shock, many other functions under the control of the same part of the nervous system are also lost. The most important of them, in an acute injury setting, is the ability to control body temperature. Body temperature in a patient with neurogenic shock can rapidly fall to match that of the environment. In many situations, significant hypothermia occurs, severely complicating the situation. *Hypothermia* is a condition in which the internal body temperature falls below 95°F (35°C), usually after prolonged exposure to cool or freezing temperatures. Maintenance of body temperature is always an important element of treatment for a patient in shock.

Hypothermia A condition in which the internal body temperature falls below 95°F (35°C), usually as a result of prolonged exposure to cool or freezing temperatures.

Transition Tip

Microcirculation is a term used to describe the small vessels in the vasculature that are embedded within organs and responsible for the distribution of blood within tissues. Capillaries are part of microcirculation. They branch off the arterioles and allow for exchange between cells and circulation. The arteriole–venule shunts are short vessels that connect the arteriole and venule at opposite sides, bypassing the capillary beds. The main functions of microcirculation include the regulation of blood flow and tissue perfusion, blood pressure, tissue fluid, delivery of oxygen, removal of carbon dioxide, and the regulation of body temperature and inflammation.

Anaphylactic Shock

Anaphylaxis, or *anaphylactic shock*, occurs when a person's immune system reacts abnormally to a substance to which he or she has been sensitized. This type of reaction is also known as a hypersensitivity response. *Sensitization* means becoming sensitive to a substance that did not initially cause a reaction. Do not be misled by a patient who reports no history of allergic reaction to a substance on first or second exposure. Each subsequent exposure after sensitization tends to produce a more severe reaction.

Anaphylaxis An extreme, possibly life-threatening systemic allergic reaction that may include shock and respiratory failure. Also known as a hypersensitivity reaction.
Anaphylactic shock Severe shock caused by an allergic reaction.
Sensitization Developing a sensitivity to a substance that initially caused no allergic reaction.

Instances that cause severe allergic reactions commonly fall into the following four categories of exposure:

- Injections (tetanus antitoxin, penicillin)
- Stings (honeybee, wasp, yellow jacket, hornet)
- Ingestion (shellfish, nuts, fruit, medication)
- Inhalation (dust, pollen)

Anaphylactic reactions can develop within minutes or even seconds after contact with the substance to which the patient is allergic. The signs of such allergic reactions are very distinct and not seen with other forms of shock. **TABLE 9-3** lists the signs of anaphylactic shock in the order in which they typically occur. Note that cyanosis (bluish color of the skin) is a late sign of anaphylactic shock.

In anaphylactic shock, there is no loss of blood, no mechanical vascular damage, and only a slight possibility of direct cardiac muscular injury. Instead, there is widespread vascular dilation, increased permeability, and bronchoconstriction. The combination of poor oxygenation and poor perfusion in anaphylactic shock may easily prove fatal.

Psychogenic Shock

A patient in *psychogenic shock* has had a sudden reaction of the nervous system that produces a temporary, generalized vascular dilation, resulting in fainting, or syncope (vasovagal syncope). Blood pools in the dilated vessels, reducing the blood supply to the brain; as a result, the brain ceases to function normally, and the patient faints. Whereas there are many causes of syncope, it is important to realize that some are of a serious nature but others are not. Causes of syncope that are potentially life threatening result from events such as an irregular heartbeat or a brain *aneurysm*. Other non–life-threatening events that cause syncope may be the receipt of bad news or experiencing fear or unpleasant sights (such as the sight of blood).

Hypovolemic Shock

Hypovolemic shock is the result of an inadequate amount of fluid or volume in the system. There are hemorrhagic and nonhemorrhagic causes of hypovolemic shock. Injuries may result in hemorrhagic shock, while vomiting and diarrhea may result in nonhemorrhagic hypovolemic shock.

Psychogenic shock Shock caused by a sudden, temporary reduction in blood supply to the brain that causes fainting (syncope).
Aneurysm A swelling or enlargement of a part of an artery, resulting from weakening of the arterial wall.
Hypovolemic shock Shock caused by fluid or blood loss.

**Table 9-3
Signs of Anaphylactic Shock**

System	Sign
Skin	■ Flushing, itching, or burning, especially over the face and upper part of the chest ■ Urticaria (hives), which may spread over large areas of the body ■ Edema, especially of the face, tongue, and lips ■ Pallor ■ Cyanosis (a bluish cast to the skin resulting from poor oxygenation of circulating blood) about the lips
Circulatory System	■ Dilation of peripheral blood vessels ■ Increased vessel permeability ■ A drop in blood pressure ■ A weak, barely palpable pulse ■ Dizziness ■ Fainting and coma
Respiratory System	■ Sneezing or itching in the nasal passages ■ Tightness in the chest, with a persistent dry cough ■ Wheezing and dyspnea (difficulty breathing) ■ Secretions of fluid and mucus into the bronchial passages, alveoli, and lung tissue, causing coughing ■ Constrictions of the bronchi; difficulty drawing air into the lungs ■ Forced expiration, requiring exertion and accompanied by wheezing ■ Cessation of breathing

Hypovolemic shock also occurs with severe thermal burns. In this case, it is intravascular plasma (the colorless part of the blood) that is lost, leaking from the circulatory system into the burned tissues that lie adjacent to the injury. Likewise, crushing injuries may result in the loss of blood and plasma from damaged vessels into injured tissues.

Dehydration, the loss of water or fluid from body tissues, can cause or aggravate shock. Fluid loss may be a result of severe vomiting and/or diarrhea. Patients who are very young or elderly are particularly susceptible to fluid loss and therefore at risk for developing shock through dehydration. People who exercise in hot weather and are not accustomed to it may experience dehydration if they do not drink enough fluids. In these circumstances, the common factor is an insufficient volume of blood within the vascular system to provide adequate circulation to the organs of the body. **TABLE 9-4** lists signs and symptoms of hypovolemic shock.

Transition Tip

You should consider any patient exhibiting signs and symptoms of shock without obvious external injury to have probable internal bleeding, usually in the abdominal cavity.

Respiratory Insufficiency

A patient with a severe chest injury, such as flail chest or obstruction of the airway, may be unable to breathe in an adequate amount of oxygen. This affects the ventilation process of respiration; enough oxygen cannot be inspired to meet the metabolic demand.

An insufficient concentration of oxygen in the blood can produce shock as rapidly as vascular causes, even if the volume of blood, the volume of the vessels, and the action of the heart are all normal. Without oxygen, the organs in the body cannot survive, and their cells promptly start to deteriorate.

Certain types of poisoning may affect the ability of cells to metabolize or carry oxygen. Carbon monoxide has a 200 to 250 times greater affinity for hemoglobin than oxygen. If a patient is in an environment where carbon monoxide is inhaled, it will bind to the hemoglobin, forming

**Table 9-4
Signs and Symptoms of Hypovolemic Shock**

■ Rapid, weak pulse
■ Thirst
■ Low blood pressure (late sign)
■ Mental status change
■ Cool, clammy, pale skin

carboxyhemoglobin rather than allowing oxygen to bind. This results in a hypoxic state if not corrected. Cyanide impairs the ability of cells to metabolize oxygen within the cell, and cellular asphyxia may occur.

Anemia occurs when there is an abnormally low number of red blood cells. Red blood cells contain hemoglobin, an iron-containing pigment. Hemoglobin transports oxygen from the lungs to the tissues. Each hemoglobin molecule is able to carry four molecules of oxygen. Anemia may be the result of either chronic or acute bleeding, a deficiency in certain vitamins or minerals, or an underlying disease process. If anemia is present, tissues may be hypoxic because the blood may not be able to carry adequate oxygen, even though the hemoglobin is fully saturated. In this situation, a pulse oximeter may indicate that there is adequate saturation, even though the tissues are hypoxic. This type of hypoxia is known as hypoxemic hypoxia.

Patient Assessment of Shock

Scene Size-up

Ensure that the scene is safe and follow standard precautions. If this is a trauma scene or bleeding is suspected, put on gloves and eye protection, at a minimum. Put several pairs of gloves in your pocket for easy access in case your gloves tear or there are multiple patients with bleeding.

Transition Tip

When you are caring for a bleeding patient, be sure to take necessary precautions to protect yourself from splashing or splattering. Wear appropriate protective equipment including gloves, gown, mask, and eye protection. This is especially essential when arterial bleeding is present. Also remember that frequent, thorough handwashing between patients and after every call is a simple yet important protective measure.

Observe the scene and patient for clues to determine the nature of the illness or the mechanism of injury (MOI). Remember that the more traumatic injuries a patient has sustained, the less likely the patient will be able to compensate.

Primary Assessment

Form a general impression of the patient. How does the patient look? A patient with suspected shock should undergo a rapid scan to determine level of consciousness, identify and manage life threats, and determine priority of the patient and transport. Perform cervical spine stabilization when necessary. Always carry out a thorough, careful primary assessment of the ABCs. In some situations, significant bleeding may require management before applying oxygen for a person with adequate breathing. Significant bleeding, internal or external, is an immediate life threat. Obvious external bleeding must be controlled quickly and treatment of shock begun as quickly as possible.

Administer high-flow oxygen to assist in perfusion of damaged tissues. If the patient has signs of hypoperfusion, treat aggressively and provide rapid transport to the hospital. Request paramedic backup as necessary to assist with more aggressive shock management. Do not delay transport to apply a splint or perform any other non-lifesaving treatment; complete these types of treatments during transport.

An increased respiratory rate is often an early sign of impending shock. With a stethoscope, listen for wheezes or other abnormal breath sounds. Administer high-flow oxygen, or, if needed, assist respirations with a bag-mask device at a normal rate. Hyperventilation is contraindicated. Maintain the SpO_2 at greater than 90%.

Check for the presence of a distal pulse. If you cannot obtain a distal pulse, assess for a central pulse. Make a rapid determination if the pulse is fast, slow, weak, strong, or altogether absent. A rapid pulse suggests compensated shock. In shock or compensated shock, the skin may be cool, clammy, or ashen. If the patient has no pulse and is not breathing, immediately begin CPR.

Look for signs of internal hemorrhage and consider the potential for loss in the area of suspected hemorrhage. For example, a patient may lose up to 1 L of blood in the tissues of the thigh in a closed femur fracture. Maintain a high index of suspicion for occult injuries, especially when the patient is exhibiting signs of shock with no obvious cause.

Trauma patients with shock or a suspicious MOI generally should be transported to a trauma center. Gain IV access and provide all treatments en route. Provide psychological support en route. Even unresponsive patients can sometimes hear and understand. Remember to speak calmly and reassuringly to the patient throughout assessment, care, and transport.

Transition Tip

You should provide rapid transport and avoid any unnecessary scene delays. Gain IV access and administer fluid en route.

History Taking

After the life threats have been managed during the primary assessment, determine the chief complaint. You should obtain a medical history and be alert for injury-specific signs and symptoms as well as any pertinent negatives such as loss of sensation.

Obtain a SAMPLE history from the patient. Note that patients taking beta blockers or calcium channel blockers are less able to compensate because their vessels do not vasoconstrict as well. Also, blood thinners can make bleeding injuries considerably worse.

Secondary Assessment

The secondary assessment begins by repeating the primary assessment followed by a focused assessment. In some instances, such as a critically injured patient or short transport time, you may not have time to conduct a secondary assessment.

If significant trauma has likely affected multiple systems, start with a full-body scan to be sure that you have identified all injuries. Assess the patient's vital signs, including heart rate, rhythm, and quality; respiratory rate, rhythm, and quality; skin color, temperature, and condition; and blood pressure. Listen for air movement at the patient's mouth and nose. Then listen to breath sounds with a stethoscope. Breath sounds should be clear and equal bilaterally, anteriorly, and posteriorly. Finally, assess asymmetrical chest wall movement. Assess the neurologic system to gather baseline data on your patient. This examination should include:

- Level of consciousness—use AVPU
- Pupil size and reactivity
- Motor response
- Sensory response

Assess the musculoskeletal system by conducting a detailed full-body scan. Look for DCAP-BTLS. Assess the chest, abdomen, and extremities for hidden bleeding and injuries. Log roll the patient and assess the posterior torso for injuries as well. Once the back has been assessed, the patient can be log rolled back down onto a backboard, followed by complete spinal immobilization. Log-rolling and securing the patient to a backboard or other full-body immobilization device should take into consideration injuries found during the primary assessment.

Assess all anatomic regions looking for the following signs/symptoms:

- Be alert for raccoon eyes, Battle's sign, and/or drainage of blood or fluid from the ears or nose.
- Check the neck for jugular vein distention and tracheal deviation. Be alert for patients with a stoma or tracheostomy.
- Check the chest for symmetry and crepitus. Listen to breath sounds and heart tones.
- Check the abdomen, feeling all four quadrants for tenderness or rigidity. If the abdomen is tender, expect internal bleeding.
- Check the pelvis for stability.
- Check the extremities and record pulse, motor, and sensory function.

If your patient is a trauma patient with a significant MOI or multiple injuries, or is one who gives you a poor general impression, or if you found problems in the primary assessment, perform a rapid full-body scan. If your patient has a medical problem but is not responsive or problems were noted in the primary assessment, perform a rapid full-body scan. These scans should be performed quickly but thoroughly to ensure that you do not miss any significant or life-threatening problems or delay needed care. In addition to hands-on assessment, you should use monitoring devices to quantify the patient's oxygenation and circulatory status.

> **Transition Tip**
>
> Just as they make for thorough written reporting, taking and recording frequent vital signs—and observing perfusion indicators such as skin condition and mental status—will give you a window into the progression of shock in your patient. Use your documentation to remind you to suspect shock early and treat it aggressively.

Reassessment

Assess the patient to determine whether the interventions you performed are having any effect on the patient. Accurately record the patient's vital signs every 5 minutes if the patient's condition is unstable and every 15 minutes if the patient's condition is stable.

You must determine what interventions are needed for your patient at this point based on the findings of your assessment. Your focus should be on supporting the cardiovascular system. Treating for shock early and aggressively will help to prevent inadequate perfusion from harming your patient. Provide oxygen and put the patient in the position dictated by local protocol for shock patients. Provide warmth, gain IV access, and administer fluid as needed. Determine, based on the signs and symptoms found in your assessment, whether your patient is in compensated or decompensated shock. Document these findings after you have treated the patient for shock. Specific interventions are discussed in the next section on emergency medical care.

> **Transition Tip**
>
> In older patients, dizziness, syncope, or weakness may be the first sign of nontraumatic internal hemorrhage or cardiac dysrhythmia.

Emergency Medical Care for Shock

You must begin immediate treatment for shock as soon as you realize that the condition may exist. Follow the steps in **SKILL DRILL 9-1**:

1 As with any type of patient care, you should begin by following standard precautions and by making sure the patient has an open airway. Maintain manual in-line stabilization if necessary, and check breathing and pulse. Comfort, calm, and reassure the patient, while maintaining the patient in the supine position. Never allow patients to eat or drink anything prior to being evaluated by a physician. Patients who have had a severe heart attack or who have lung disease may find it easier to breathe in a sitting or semisitting position (**Step 1**).

2 Next, control all obvious external bleeding. Place dry, sterile dressings over the bleeding sites and secure with bandages. If direct pressure is not rapidly successful in the control of bleeding from an extremity, apply a tourniquet proximal to the bleeding site according to local protocol (**Step 2**).

3 Splint the patient on a backboard. Do not delay transport by applying individual splints in the field. If possible, splint individual extremity fractures during transport. This minimizes pain, bleeding, and discomfort, all of which can aggravate shock. It also prevents the broken bone ends from further damaging adjacent soft tissue. In general, splinting will make it easier to move the patient. Handle the patient gently and no more than is necessary (**Step 3**).

4 Remember that inadequate ventilation may be the primary cause of shock or a major factor in its development. Always provide oxygen, assist with ventilations, and use airway control adjuncts as needed, and continue to monitor the patient's breathing. To prevent the loss of body heat, place blankets under and over the patient. Be careful not to overload the patient with covers or attempt to warm the body too much; it is best for the patient to maintain a normal body temperature. Do not use external heat sources, such as hot water bottles or heating pads. They may harm a patient in shock by causing vasodilation and decreasing blood pressure even more (**Step 4**).

5 Once you have positioned the patient on a backboard or a stretcher, consider placing the patient in the Trendelenburg position. This technique is easily accomplished by raising the foot of the backboard or stretcher about 6 to 12 inches. If the patient is not on a backboard and no lower extremity fractures are suspected, place the patient in the shock position. This is accomplished by elevating the patient's legs 6 to 12 inches by propping them up on several blankets or other stable objects. These positions may help to return blood from the extremities back to the core of the body where it is needed most. Raising the lower extremities any higher may aggravate a patient's breathing because the abdominal organs push against the diaphragm. Take care not to use the Trendelenburg position or shock position for patients who have associated chest injury or intra-abdominal injury; this may be aggravated by causing the abdominal contents to push against the diaphragm and further impair breathing.

6 Transport the patient and treat additional injuries en route. Gain IV access en route, preferably using two large-bore catheters, and administer fluid, as described in the next section.

Do not give the patient anything by mouth, no matter how urgently you are asked. To relieve the intense thirst that often accompanies shock, give the patient a moistened piece of gauze to chew or suck. Never give a patient in shock an alcoholic drink or other depressant. A stimulant, such as coffee, also has no value in treating shock.

Accurately record the patient's vital signs approximately every 5 minutes throughout treatment and transport. It is essential to transport trauma patients to the emergency department as rapidly as possible for definitive treatment. The Golden Hour refers to the first 60 minutes after injury, which is thought to be a critically important period for the early resuscitation and treatment of severely injured trauma patients. This concept underscores the importance of rapid evaluation, stabilization, and transport. The goal of EMS is to limit on-scene time (time on-scene until transport to hospital is started) to 10 minutes or less (the platinum ten). Remember to speak calmly and reassuringly to a conscious patient throughout assessment, care, and transport.

SKILL DRILL 9-1

Treating Shock

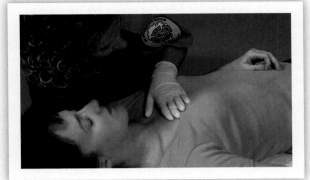

1 Keep the patient supine, open the airway, and check breathing and pulse.

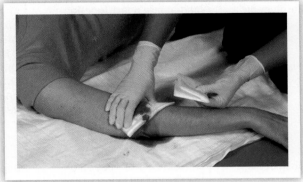

2 Control obvious external bleeding. Apply a tourniquet, if necessary, to achieve rapid control of severe blood loss from extremities.

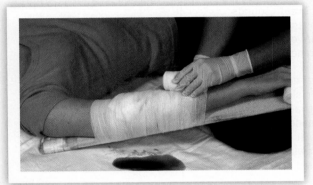

3 Splint the patient on a backboard. Splint any broken bones or injuries during transport.

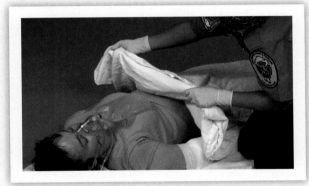

4 Administer high-flow oxygen if you have not already done so, and place blankets under and over the patient.

TABLE 9-5 lists the general supportive measures for the major types of shock. Not every measure is used for every type of shock.

Transition Tip

The skin's structure includes tension lines, which make the skin become taut with movement. If the skin is cut in a direction perpendicular to a tension line (such as over a knee), it will be more difficult to control bleeding in that area because the tension lines will tend to pull the cut open. Splinting injuries helps address this situation and helps to control bleeding.

Fluid Administration

As mentioned previously, starting an IV and administering fluids is part of treating a patient who is in shock. Hypovolemic shock should be treated with IV volume expanders to replace what has been lost or to "fill the container" in relative hypovolemia. For cardiogenic shock, cautious use of volume expanders may increase preload and, subsequently, cardiac output.

Establish IV access with two large-bore catheters (14 or 16 gauge) and administer IV volume expanders (warmed if possible) to replace blood loss. Isotonic crystalloids, such as normal saline or lactated Ringer's, should be used (synthetic solutions may also be used). The goal of volume replacement is to maintain perfusion without increasing

Table 9-5
Types of Shock

Type of Shock	Examples of Potential Causes	Signs and Symptoms	Treatment
Cardiogenic	Inadequate heart function Disease of muscle tissue Impaired electrical system Disease or injury	Chest pain Irregular pulse Weak pulse Low blood pressure Cyanosis (lips, under nails) Cool, clammy skin Anxiety Rales Pulmonary edema	Place patient in a position of comfort with legs dependent (hanging downward) if signs of pulmonary edema. Administer oxygen Assist ventilations Transport promptly Gain IV access en route to the hospital; administer fluid at a keep vein open (KVO) rate
Obstructive	Mechanical obstruction of the cardiac muscle causing a decrease in cardiac output 1. Tension pneumothorax 2. Cardiac tamponade	Dependent on cause: ■ Dyspnea ■ Rapid, weak pulse ■ Rapid, shallow breaths ■ Decreased lung compliance ■ Unilateral, decreased, or absent breath sounds ■ Decreased blood pressure ■ Jugular vein distention ■ Subcutaneous emphysema ■ Cyanosis ■ Tracheal deviation toward affected side (late sign) ■ Beck's triad (cardiac tamponade): 　• Jugular vein distention 　• Narrowing pulse pressure 　• Muffled heart tones	Dependent on cause: ■ Paramedic assist and rapid transport ■ Gain IV access en route as a medication route; administer fluid at a KVO rate
Septic	Severe bacterial infection	Warm skin Tachycardia Low blood pressure	Transport promptly Administer oxygen en route Provide full ventilatory support Consider elevating legs Keep patient warm Gain IV access en route; administer fluid boluses to maintain radial pulses
Neurogenic	Damaged cervical or thoracic spinal cord, which causes widespread blood vessel dilation	Bradycardia (slow pulse) or normal pulse Low blood pressure Signs of neck or thoracic spinal injury	Secure airway. Spinal stabilization Assist ventilations. Administer high-flow oxygen. Preserve body heat Transport promptly Gain IV access en route; administer warmed IV fluids to maintain radial pulses

**Table 9-5
Types of Shock** (*continued*)

Type of Shock	Examples of Potential Causes	Signs and Symptoms	Treatment
Anaphylactic	Extreme life-threatening allergic reaction	Can develop within seconds Mild itching or rash Burning skin Vascular dilation Generalized edema Coma Rapid death	Manage the airway Assist ventilations Administer high-flow oxygen Determine cause Assist with administration of epinephrine Gain IV access en route as a medication route; administer fluid at a KVO rate Transport promptly
Psychogenic (fainting)	Temporary, generalized vascular dilation Anxiety, bad news, sight of injury or blood, prospect of medical treatment, severe pain, illness, tiredness	Rapid pulse Normal or low blood pressure	Determine duration of unresponsiveness Record initial vital signs and mental status Suspect head injury if patient is confused or slow to respond Transport promptly
Hypovolemic	Loss of blood or fluid	Rapid, weak pulse Low blood pressure Change in mental status Cyanosis (lips, under nails) Cool, clammy skin Increased respiratory rate	Secure airway Assist ventilations Administer high-flow oxygen Control external bleeding Consider elevating legs Keep warm Transport promptly Gain IV access en route; provide fluid resuscitation en route
Respiratory insufficiency	Severe chest injury, airway obstruction	Rapid, weak pulse Low blood pressure Change in mental status Cyanosis (lips, under nails) Cool, clammy skin Increased respiratory rate	Secure airway Clear air passages Assist ventilations Administer high-flow oxygen Transport promptly Gain IV access en route; administer fluid at a KVO rate

internal or uncontrollable external hemorrhage. For this reason, most protocols advise administration of IV fluid in boluses of 20 mL/kg up to 30 mL/kg in 250- to 500-mL increments until there is a return of radial pulses. The presence of radial pulses equates to a systolic blood pressure of 80 to 90 mm Hg, which, in most people, is sufficient to perfuse the brain and other vital organs. Raising blood pressure further may result in worsening internal hemorrhage. Monitor the patient's response to IV therapy carefully and document any changes. Never delay transport to start an IV. It is perfectly acceptable and in fact far preferable to wait until transport has begun prior to initiating an attempt to establish IV access.

If vital signs return to within normal limits or reach the desired status, slow IV fluid administration to a KVO rate and reassess frequently, adjusting the flow as needed. If the patient's response to initial treatment is one of no improvement or slow deterioration, there may be ongoing uncontrolled blood loss. Maintain the patient's blood pressure around 90 mm Hg systolic depending on local protocol.

Call early for paramedic intervention to administer vasopressors if needed, but don't delay transport to definitive care. The vasodilation that accompanies distributive shock creates relative hypovolemia. Regardless of the cause, the problem is still a lack of fluid for the size of the container. Treatment involves the administration of volume expanders and positive cardiac inotropic drugs. Volume expanders are also indicated for obstructive shock and neurogenic shock.

> ### Transition Tip
>
> Using larger-diameter and shorter-length catheters results in greater fluid flow. Choose a large-bore catheter (14 to 16 gauge) no longer than 1 to 1½ inches. For maximum volume infusion, use a blood set or macrodrip set (10 to 15 drops/min) without a saline lock that restricts flow.

Special Considerations in Fluid Resuscitation

In instances where increasing blood pressure may be detrimental to the patient, such as cardiogenic shock or massive internal bleeding, it may be preferable to maintain a level of hypotension. Aggressive fluid therapy increases the workload on the heart, worsening cardiogenic shock and increasing internal bleeding by breaking up forming clots or increasing the pressure in the vessels.

> ### Transition Tip
>
> An unstable pelvis is the primary indication for use of the pneumatic antishock garments (PASG). The PASG serves as an air splint and is inflated only until firm. Conditions of decreased SVR not corrected by other means, such as increasing fluid volume in cases of neurogenic shock, may also benefit from use of the PASG. Pulmonary edema and uncontrolled bleeding above the level of the PASG are contraindications to PASG use. PASG use is highly controversial and has never been demonstrated to increase survival; always follow local protocols.

Temperature control is vital to maintaining perfusion in children and infants. If fluid replacement is required and IV access cannot be obtained, consider using intraosseous infusion. Use a Broselow tape or other reference to remember normal vital signs by age. Infuse a 20 mL/kg bolus of a warmed isotonic crystalloid solution, considering a second infusion if there is no response to the first. While administering fluids, it is imperative to remember that a patient who has lost blood needs replacement of red blood cells. Carefully monitor patient status and treat conservatively in instances of uncontrolled hemorrhage. Use a continuous infusion to maintain adequate perfusion levels of critical organs en route to the hospital. A third infusion of 20 mL/kg may be considered in patients with controlled hemorrhage.

Geriatric patients can present a challenge when providing IV therapy in instances of shock. Patients who have chronic hypertension may require a higher blood pressure to achieve the same level of end organ perfusion than those who maintain a normal blood pressure. The geriatric patient may be in shock and his or her systolic blood pressure may be above 100 mm Hg. Even modest amounts of blood loss can be detrimental and lead to shock in these patients because of a reduced circulating blood volume. Geriatric patients may also be less able to tolerate excessive fluids that may cause harmful electrolyte alterations. Anemia may be yet another complication because aggressive fluid resuscitation may further reduce the relative concentrations of red blood cells. For these patients, rapid transport is essential.

When you are treating obstetric patients, it is imperative to remember that there are two patients involved, the pregnant woman and the fetus. Because shock states lead to shunting of blood away from the fetus, the only way to maintain fetal perfusion is to aggressively treat the woman. Remember to place the patient in a left lateral recumbent position, or tilt the backboard if the patient is immobilized, to increase perfusion. Provide fluid resuscitation to maintain radial pulses of the mother. The closer the maternal blood pressure is to normal, the better the perfusion of the fetus.

> ### Transition Tip
>
> Treating a pediatric or geriatric patient in shock is no different than treating any other shock patient:
> 1. Provide in-line spinal stabilization if indicated. If spinal immobilization is not indicated, maintain the patient in a position of comfort.
> 2. Suction as necessary and provide high-flow oxygen via a nonrebreathing mask.
> 3. Control bleeding.
> 4. Maintain body temperature.
> 5. Provide rapid transportation.

■ BLS Resuscitation

Introduction

The principles of BLS were introduced in 1960. Since then, the specific techniques have been reviewed and revised every 4 to 5 years. The updated guidelines are published in the *Journal of the American Medical Association* (*JAMA*). The most recent revision occurred as a result of the 2010 Conference on Cardiopulmonary Resuscitation and Emergency Cardiovascular Care. The following information highlights the changes made between the 2005 guidelines and the new 2010 guidelines. For a general review of BLS resuscitation and topics not covered in this chapter, refer to a 2010 CPR manual.

Pathophysiology of Cardiac Arrest

By definition, cardiac arrest is the cessation of systemic blood flow because of the absent or ineffective contraction of the ventricles of the heart. As discussed earlier in this chapter, there are many reasons why the heart may suddenly fail to work effectively. In some cases, cardiac arrest is caused by untreated respiratory failure, which may be constrictive, obstructive, or destructive in nature. It can also result from a traumatic injury, either directly to the heart or to another body system, ultimately leading to the inadequate tissue perfusion.

Shock, regardless of its cause, if left untreated, can ultimately result in cardiac arrest. As such, any of the conditions described in this chapter can cause cardiac arrest. Once the heart stops contracting, systemic blood flow ceases and oxygen is no longer delivered to body tissues. The result is irreversible damage and, without immediate and definitive treatment of the underlying condition, death.

In the pediatric patient, research has shown that the leading cause of cardiac arrest is respiratory arrest. If not immediately recognized and managed, acute respiratory failure, regardless of the cause, will result in cardiovascular changes and ultimately cardiac arrest in infants and children.

Different organs respond differently to the lack of oxygen caused by cardiac arrest. The brain is the first organ to suffer permanent damage from a lack of blood flow. Research has shown that brain damage begins 4 to 6 minutes after circulation stops and that the damage becomes irreversible, resulting in brain death, within 8 to 10 minutes. While it may be possible to revive the heart after 10 minutes, brain function will likely be impaired, and neurologic functioning, including the ability to breathe on one's own, may be compromised.

The heart is the second organ to suffer permanent damage as a result of the lack of blood flow. Other body systems, such as the gastrointestinal, renal, integumentary, and musculoskeletal systems, are better able to manage decreased perfusion for a longer period of time, and they rarely suffer permanent damage in patients who are successfully resuscitated.

CPR seeks to "buy time" when perfusion fails. CPR entails providing artificial respirations to supply the blood with oxygen and manual chest compressions to squeeze the heart, thereby simulating a contraction in an effort to circulate the oxygenated blood to the brain and other vital organs and sustain life until definitive treatment is available.

Patient Assessment of Cardiac Arrest

Within 15 seconds of the onset of cardiac arrest, the patient will lose consciousness. Agonal gasps can continue for a minute or so. You may also note incontinence or the loss of bowel or bladder control immediately after the onset of arrest. Most often, by the time you arrive at the scene of a cardiac arrest, you will find the patient unresponsive, pulseless, and apneic, with skin that is cool and cyanotic.

Although immediate intervention is certainly the priority in caring for a patient in cardiac arrest, obtaining information at the scene may provide clues about the cause of the arrest, which could ultimately assist in resuscitation efforts. For example, if it is known that the patient has an allergy to bees and was stung by a bee just prior to cardiac arrest, administration of epinephrine may be necessary to relieve swelling of the airway. If the patient is known to have been choking prior to losing consciousness, focus on relieving the airway obstruction would be the priority over use of the automated external defibrillator (AED).

The priority at the scene of a cardiac arrest is always immediate and definitive treatment. If adequate resources are available, however, assign a team member to ask bystanders or family members about relevant past medical history or events leading to the arrest:

- Was the arrest witnessed?
- When did the arrest occur?
- How long after the arrest was CPR initiated?
- What was the patient doing prior to the arrest?
- What is the patient's past medical history?

Elements of BLS

While the elements of CPR have not changed, the manner in which they are provided has been modified in the most recent guidelines.

As you are aware, BLS is noninvasive, emergency lifesaving care that is used to treat medical conditions including airway obstruction, respiratory arrest, and cardiac arrest. Traditionally, the process of assessment for CPR focused on the ABCs—airway (obstruction), breathing (respiratory arrest), and circulation (cardiac arrest or severe bleeding). The same sequence—establish unresponsiveness; open the airway; look, listen, and feel for breathing; provide two breaths; check for a pulse, and if there is no pulse, begin CPR—was imprinted on the minds of AEMTs for many years. With the 2010 guidelines, however, this approach has changed to CAB, with the emphasis now being placed on early compressions when cardiac arrest is suspected.

■ Key Changes to CPR

This section highlights the key changes of the 2010 CPR guidelines.

CAB Instead of ABC

On the basis of a wealth of research findings, it was decided that the key to a successful outcome in patients with cardiac arrest is the speed at which chest compressions are initiated. Notably, a delay or interruption in chest compressions is associated with reduced survival rates. With that point in mind, the sequence was changed. As per the new guidelines, after establishing unresponsiveness and the lack of "normal" breathing (ie, agonal gasps or absent breathing), the AEMT should spend no more than 10 seconds determining pulselessness and immediately begin CPR by delivering 30 chest compressions at a rate of at least 100 compressions/min.

Elimination of "Look, Listen, and Feel" for Breathing

Again, in an attempt to decrease the delay to provision of the first chest compression, the steps of opening the airway and taking 5 to 10 seconds to check for breathing have been eliminated. Instead, the AEMT should briefly check for breathing when checking responsiveness to detect signs of cardiac arrest.

Opening the patient's airway and delivering two breaths now *follows* the delivery of 30 chest compressions.

Pulse Check

The new guidelines call for the provision of chest compressions when the AEMT is unsure whether the patient has a pulse. Under the new guidelines, the AEMT should perform a pulse check for no more than 10 seconds. If a pulse is not clearly recognizable within that time frame, begin chest compressions.

Rate of Chest Compressions

The 2005 standards called for a rate of compression of 80 to 100/min. More recently, research has shown that delivery of more compressions during resuscitation efforts is associated with increased survival rates, and especially with survival with good neurologic function. As a result, the guideline was changed and now calls for delivery of chest compressions at a rate of at least 100/min.

Depth of Chest Compressions

Physiologically, the process of chest compressions creates blood flow by increasing intrathoracic pressure and directly compressing the heart, which circulates blood throughout the body. Research has shown that adequate compression depth was often not achieved during CPR and that deeper compressions may be more effective for circulating oxygen to vital organs. The guideline now calls for compressions to a depth of at least 2 inches in adults and one third of the chest depth in infants and children.

Automated External Defibrillation Use

Prior to the 2010 changes, use of an AED was contraindicated in infants. Research suggests, however, that even high-energy defibrillation may be successfully performed in infants and children with no significant adverse effects. Thus the new standard states that AED use is appropriate for infants as well, although use of an AED with a pediatric dose-attenuator is preferred. Because cardiac arrest in a newborn is most likely asphyxial in nature, however, resuscitation of a newborn should continue to focus on ventilation and compressions. This point is discussed in more detail in the *Special Populations* chapter.

The following guidelines should be used for AED use:

- Adults: Use a standard adult AED unit.
- Children (ages 1 to 8): Use an AED with pediatric dose-attenuation if available. If no pediatric dose-attenuator system is available, use a standard adult AED.
- Infants (ages 1 month to 1 year): A manual defibrillator should be used if available; however, its application is a paramedic-level skill. If ALS personnel are not immediately available, use a pediatric dose-attenuator system. If neither is available, use a standard adult AED.
- Newborns (birth to 1 month of age): Focus attention on CPR with emphasis on ventilation.

In all patients, you should begin CPR by starting with chest compressions and attach the AED as soon as it is available. CPR should be resumed immediately after delivering a shock, beginning with chest compressions. **FIGURE 9-6** provides the AED algorithm.

Although for ease of teaching there has been no change in AED pad placement techniques, any of four pad positions are now acceptable, with anterior-lateral placement designated as the default. The other options, based on individual patient characteristics, are anterior-posterior, anterior-left infrascapular, and anterior-right infrascapular placement.

Ventilations With Advanced Airways

Once the ALS provider inserts an advanced airway, ventilations should be administered every 6 to 8 seconds (8 to 10 breaths/min), taking approximately 1 second to deliver each breath. Breaths are asynchronous with chest compressions, so there should be no pause in chest compressions once an advanced airway is in place. Ensure that the chest rises with each ventilation, as advanced airways may become displaced during CPR.

Compression-to-Ventilation Ratio

There is no change in the compression-to-ventilation ratio. Once an advanced airway is placed, however, ventilations are delivered asynchronously, so there is no longer a pause in compressions. The ratios are as follows:

- Adult: 30:2 (one or two rescuers)
- Child or infant: 30:2 (one rescuer) and 15:2 (two rescuers)

Additional Changes

Additional changes to the CPR guidelines include the following:

- **Cricoid Pressure:** Although the use of cricoid pressure can reduce the risk of aspiration from regurgitation during bag-mask ventilations, research has shown that it may also impede ventilation. In addition, cricoid pressure has been shown to delay or prevent placement of advanced airways; even when it is used, some aspiration may occur. For all these reasons, the routine use of cricoid pressure in patients with cardiac arrest is no longer recommended.
- **Lay Rescuer CPR Instructions:** The new guidelines emphasize "hands-only CPR" for the lay rescuer. Research has shown that bystander CPR substantially improves the survival rates for patients in cardiac arrest. Furthermore, there does not appear to be any substantial difference in survival rates between patients who receive hands-only CPR and those who receive traditional CPR with rescue breaths. Given that it is easier to teach hands-only CPR, dispatchers are encouraged to provide instructions emphasizing compressions only for victims who are unresponsive, with no breathing or no "normal" breathing, unless it is suspected that the victim suffered cardiac arrest due to asphyxia, such as a drowning or suffocation. A pulse check is not taught to, or performed by, lay rescuers.

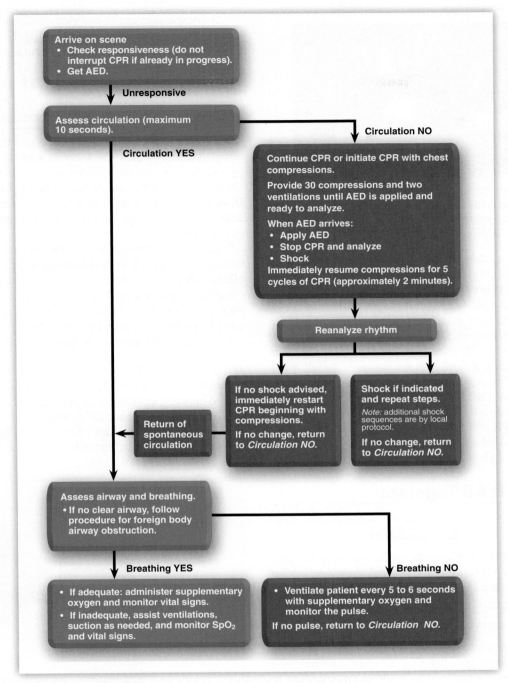

Arrive on scene
- Check responsiveness (do not interrupt CPR if already in progress).
- Get AED.

Unresponsive

Assess circulation (maximum 10 seconds).

Circulation YES

Circulation NO

Continue CPR or initiate CPR with chest compressions.

Provide 30 compressions and two ventilations until AED is applied and ready to analyze.

When AED arrives:
- Apply AED
- Stop CPR and analyze
- Shock

Immediately resume compressions for 5 cycles of CPR (approximately 2 minutes).

Reanalyze rhythm

If no shock advised, immediately restart CPR beginning with compressions.

If no change, return to *Circulation NO*.

Shock if indicated and repeat steps.

Note: additional shock sequences are by local protocol.

If no change, return to *Circulation NO*.

Return of spontaneous circulation

Assess airway and breathing.
- If no clear airway, follow procedure for foreign body airway obstruction.

Breathing YES
- If adequate: administer supplementary oxygen and monitor vital signs.
- If inadequate, assist ventilations, suction as needed, and monitor SpO_2 and vital signs.

Breathing NO
- Ventilate patient every 5 to 6 seconds with supplementary oxygen and monitor the pulse.

If no pulse, return to *Circulation NO*.

FIGURE 9-6 Automated external defibrillator algorithm for an adult victim of cardiac arrest.

Transition Tip

Because lay rescuers do not provide ventilations, it is important to take over CPR, with the inclusion of ventilations, immediately upon your arrival.

- **Activation of EMS:** Although AEMTs are most likely to be responding to a cardiac arrest because

of activation of the emergency response system, it is also important to understand the new guidelines that health care providers are required to follow upon finding a victim in cardiac arrest. Upon simultaneously establishing unresponsiveness and lack of "normal" breathing (ie, agonal gasps or absent breathing), the rescuer should activate the emergency response system and obtain an AED or send someone else to obtain this device. A pulse check is then performed

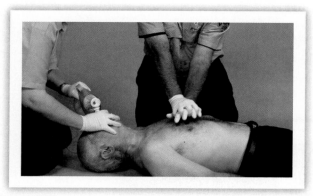

FIGURE 9-7 If multiple rescuers are present at the scene, divide and perform tasks simultaneously.

and, if no pulse is found within 10 seconds, CPR should begin, starting with chest compressions.

- **Emphasis on Team Resuscitation:** Although CPR was traditionally taught as a specific sequence of tasks, the new standards call for more of a team approach to resuscitation, reflecting the reality that multiple health care providers usually arrive at the scene of a cardiac arrest together **FIGURE 9-7**. Although rescuers need to know all the tasks of CPR, they should be able to divide and perform such tasks simultaneously. For example, one rescuer should begin CPR while another obtains a history, another retrieves and applies the AED unit, and yet another assembles a bag-mask device and begins ventilations.

Putting It All Together

The new CPR sequence for an adult, based on the 2010 guidelines, is as follows **SKILL DRILL 9-2**:

1. Establish unresponsiveness while assessing for lack of "normal" breathing (ie, agonal gasps or absent breathing) (**Step 1**). Call for help.

2. Position the patient properly and check for a carotid pulse for no more than 10 seconds (**Step 2**).

3. If there is no pulse, begin CPR until an AED becomes available. Begin by delivering 30 chest compressions hard and fast at a rate of at least 100 per minute (**Step 3**).

4. Open the patient's airway using the appropriate technique and deliver two breaths (1 second each) (**Step 4**). Observe for chest rise.

5. Continue the process of 30 compressions and two breaths until an AED becomes available or ALS support arrives and an advanced airway is in place.

6. Research has shown that the effectiveness of compressions is dramatically reduced after 2 minutes because of rescuer fatigue. Whenever possible, the rescuer providing compressions should be switched every 2 minutes to allow time for rest.

A comparison of the key elements of adult, child, and infant CPR is provided in **TABLE 9-6**. Neonatal resuscitation is discussed in the *Special Populations* chapter. For complete understanding of the 2010 CPR standards, it is suggested that you participate in a CPR renewal course.

Devices to Assist Circulation

The effectiveness of CPR depends on the amount of blood circulated throughout the body as a result of chest compressions. Even under ideal conditions, however, manual chest compressions cannot equate normal cardiac output. In addition, factors such as rescuer fatigue or inaccurate depth or rate of compressions can further impede the resuscitation process.

Several mechanical devices are now available to assist emergency responders in delivering improved circulatory efforts when providing CPR. Although improved patient outcomes have not yet been documented with their use, these devices may be considered as an adjunct to CPR when used by properly trained personnel for patients in cardiac arrest in the prehospital or in-hospital setting.

Impedance Threshold Device

An *impedance threshold device (ITD)* is a valve device that is placed between an endotracheal tube and bag-mask device. It is designed to limit the air entering the lungs during the recoil phase between chest compressions **FIGURE 9-8**. Its use results in negative intrathoracic pressure that draws

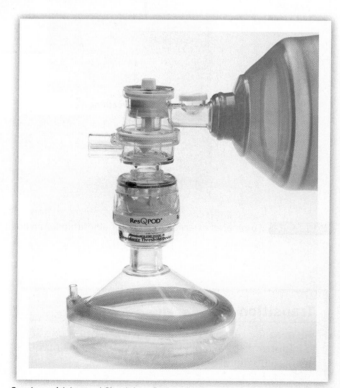

Courtesy of Advanced Circulatory Systems, Inc.
FIGURE 9-8 An impedance threshold device.

SKILL DRILL 9-2
CPR Sequence for an Adult

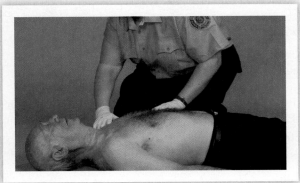

1 Establish unresponsiveness while assessing for lack of "normal" breathing (ie, agonal gasps or absent breathing).

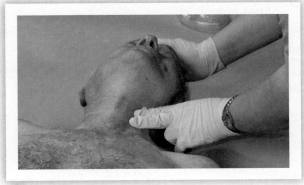

2 Position the patient properly and check for a carotid pulse for no more than 10 seconds.

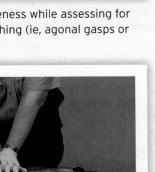

3 If there is no pulse, begin CPR until an AED becomes available. Begin by delivering 30 chest compressions hard and fast at a rate of at least 100 per minute.

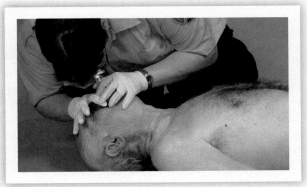

4 Open the patient's airway using the appropriate technique and deliver two breaths (1 second each).

more blood toward the heart, ultimately resulting in improved cardiac filling and circulation during each chest compression.

With a patient who is not intubated, studies suggest that the ITD could be used in conjunction with a face mask; however, a tight seal is essential to achieve the desired effect. Although increased survival rates have not been definitively documented, the use of ITDs may improve the effectiveness of CPR when used by trained rescuers.

Mechanical Piston Device

A *mechanical piston device* depresses the sternum via a compressed gas-powered plunger mounted on a backboard **FIGURE 9-9**. The patient is positioned supine on the backboard, with the piston placed on top of the patient and

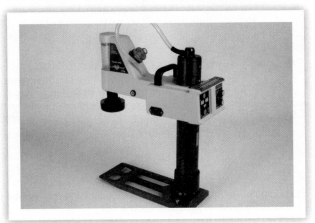

Courtesy of Michigan Instruments, Inc.
FIGURE 9-9 A mechanical piston device.

Table 9-6
Key Elements of CPR for Adults, Children, and Infants, 2010 Standards

Procedure	Adults	Children (1 to 8 Years)	Infants (Younger Than 1 Year[a])
Circulation			
Recognition	Unresponsive with no breathing, or only agonal (gasping) respirations		
Pulse check	Carotid artery		Brachial artery
Compression location	In the center of the chest, in between the nipples		Just below the nipple line
Compression area	Heel of both hands	Heel of one or both hands	Two fingers or two-thumb encircling-hands technique
Compression depth	At least 2 inches	At least one-third of chest depth Approximately 2 inches	At least one-third of chest depth Approximately 1½ inches
Compression rate	At least 100/min		
Chest wall recoil	Allow full chest recoil in between compressions Rotate professional rescuers delivering compressions every 2 minutes		
Interruptions	Limit interruptions in delivery of chest compressions to less than 10 seconds		
Ratio of compressions to ventilations (until an advanced airway is inserted)	30:2 (one or two rescuers)	30:2 (one rescuer); 15:2 (two professional rescuers)	
Airway			
	Head tilt–chin lift maneuver; jaw-thrust maneuver if spinal injury is suspected		
Breathing			
Untrained rescuer	Compressions only		
Ventilations without advanced airway	2 breaths with a duration of 1 second each, with enough volume to produce chest rise[b]		
Ventilations with advanced airway	1 breath every 6–8 seconds (8–10/min) Asynchronous with chest compressions Duration of 1 second each, with enough volume to produce chest rise		
Rescue breaths	1 breath every 5 seconds (12 breaths/min)	1 breath every 3 seconds (20 breaths/min)	1 breath every 3 seconds (20 breaths/min)
Defibrillation			
Device	Adult AED	Use pediatric dose-attenuator unit if available; if not available, use adult unit	Use manual defibrillator if available; if not, use unit with pediatric dose-attenuator; if neither is available, use adult unit
Procedure	Attach AED as soon as it is available. If two rescuers are available, one should immediately begin CPR while the second retrieves and applies the AED. Minimize CPR interruptions. Resume CPR immediately after shock, beginning with chest compressions.		
Airway Obstruction			
Foreign body obstruction	Conscious: abdominal thrusts Unconscious: CPR[c]	Conscious: abdominal thrusts	Conscious: back slaps and chest thrusts

[a]Excluding newborns, in whom arrest is usually the result of asphyxiation and requires the rescue ventilations.
[b]Pause compressions to deliver ventilations.
[c]Look in the mouth for objects before delivering breaths on a patient with a known or suspected airway obstruction.

the plunger centered over the patient's thorax in the same manner as with manual chest compressions. The device is then secured to the backboard.

> *Impedance threshold device (ITD)* A valve device that is placed between an endotracheal tube and a bag-mask device to limit the amount of air entering the lungs during the recoil phase between chest compressions.
> *Mechanical piston device* A device that depresses the sternum via a compressed gas-powered plunger mounted on a backboard.

The mechanical piston device allows rescuers to configure the depth and rate of compressions, resulting in uniform delivery. As a consequence, it frees the rescuer to complete other tasks and eliminates rescuer fatigue that might otherwise result from continuous delivery of manual chest compressions.

Load-Distributing Band CPR or Vest CPR

The *load-distributing band (LDB)* is a circumferential chest compression device that consists of a constricting band and backboard **FIGURE 9-10**. This device is either electrically or pneumatically driven to compress the heart by putting inward pressure on the thorax.

> *Load-distributing band (LDB)* A circumferential chest compression device that consists of a constricting band and backboard; it is either electrically or pneumatically driven to compress the heart by putting inward pressure on the thorax.

As with the mechanical piston device, use of the LDB frees the rescuer to complete other tasks. The LDB is lighter than the mechanical piston device and is easier to apply. The end result is improved hemodyamics in the patient when the device is used by properly trained emergency responders, although studies have demonstrated no improvement in short-term survival and worse neurologic outcome when the device is used. Further studies are needed to determine the utility of the LDB.

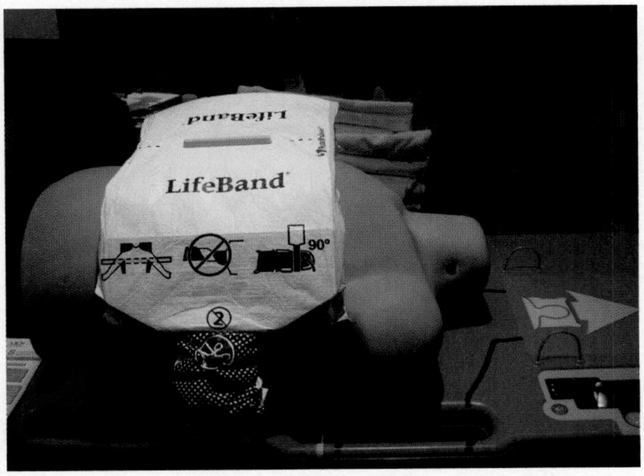

Improved CPR Performance

Several new devices are available to assist health care professionals not only learn CPR, but also improve effectiveness when performing CPR **FIGURE 9-11**. Such devices can be used during training or while performing CPR on a patient. The device alerts the rescuer to the effectiveness of compressions in terms of depth and rate. Apps **FIGURE 9-12** are also offered that provide the same function and may be held in the rescuer's hand during compressions.

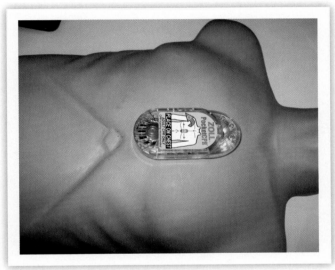

Courtesy of Catherine Parvensky Barwell
FIGURE 9-11 The Pocket CPR.

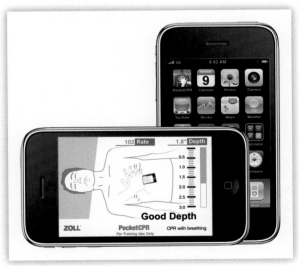

Courtesy of Bio-Detek, Inc.
FIGURE 9-12 A CPR app.

Courtesy of Catherine Parvensky Barwell
FIGURE 9-10 A load-distributing band.

Ready for Review

- There are several types of shock: cardiogenic, obstructive, septic, neurogenic, anaphylactic, psychogenic, and hypovolemic.
- Signs of compensated shock include anxiety or agitation; tachycardia; pale, cool, moist skin; increased respiratory rate; nausea and vomiting; and increased thirst. If there is any question about the patient's condition, treat for shock.
- Signs of decompensated shock include labored or irregular respirations, ashen gray or cyanotic skin color, weak or absent distal pulses, dilated pupils, and profound hypotension.

- Hypotension is a late sign of shock, usually signifying an advanced state.
- Anticipate shock in patients who have the following conditions:
  - Severe infection
  - Significant blunt force or penetrating trauma
  - Massive external bleeding or index of suspicion for major internal bleeding
  - Spinal injury
  - Chest or abdominal injury
  - Major heart attack
  - Anaphylaxis

- Treat a pediatric or geriatric patient in shock the same as any other patient in shock.
- Treat all patients suspected to be in shock, regardless of the cause, in this order:
  - Open and maintain the airway.
  - Provide high-flow oxygen and, as needed, assisted ventilations.
  - Call for ALS assistance, if available.
  - Control all obvious external bleeding.
  - Consider placing the patient in the shock position or, if on a backboard or stretcher, in the Trendelenburg position.
  - Use blankets to maintain normal body temperature.
  - Provide prompt transport to an appropriate hospital.
- The sequence of CPR has changed from ABC to CAB (circulation, airway, breathing) when cardiac arrest is suspected.

- Upon arrival at a scene where a patient is suspected to have experienced sudden cardiac death, immediately and simultaneously assess for unresponsiveness and breathlessness. If no "normal" breathing is noted (ie, only agonal gasps), assess the patient's pulse for no more than 10 seconds. If no clear pulse is noted within 10 seconds, begin CPR with 30 chest compressions (at a rate of at least 100 per minute), followed by opening the airway and delivering two breaths.
- An AED should be applied to any nontrauma cardiac arrest patient older than 1 month of age as soon as this device becomes available.
- For infants aged 1 month to 1 year, a manual defibrillator is preferred. If not available, a pediatric unit should be used. For a child between 1 and 8 years of age, use pediatric-sized pads and a dose-attenuating system (energy reducer). If these items are not available, an adult AED can be used.

Case Study

You respond to a motor vehicle crash involving two vehicles at an intersection known for frequent traffic incidents. When you arrive on scene, you are directed by the EMS officer to a vehicle on the side of the road that appears to have rolled several times. Fire fighters and emergency medical responders are currently extricating the patient. They inform you the patient is a 29-year-old male who is alert but confused. He complains of right leg pain and abdominal pain. Once the patient is extricated, he is fully immobilized on a long backboard with a cervical collar and head immobilization device in place. He is currently receiving high-flow oxygen. When you ask him about the incident, the patient tells you he does not remember anything. You perform a rapid head-to-toe scan to look for any obvious injuries. A firm abdomen with pain in the left upper quadrant and an obvious deformity to the right thigh are noted in your exam. The vital signs are as follows: pulse, 120 beats/min; respirations, 26 breaths/min; blood pressure, 96/60 mm Hg; and cool, pale, clammy skin. You immediately provide rapid transport to the local trauma center where the patient is found to have a lacerated spleen and a fractured right femur.

1. What are the signs and symptoms of hypovolemic shock?

2. Explain the basic pathophysiology behind shock.

3. Along with hypovolemic shock, neurogenic shock can also be seen in trauma patients. Explain the pathophysiology of neurogenic shock.

4. If this patient would go into cardiac arrest while in your care, it would be considered "witnessed" and an AED could be used right away. However, if this was an unwitnessed arrest, it is recommended that 2 minutes of CPR be performed before application of an AED. Explain the rationale behind this.

5. What is the basic pathophysiology of cardiac arrest?

CHAPTER 10

Respiratory Emergencies

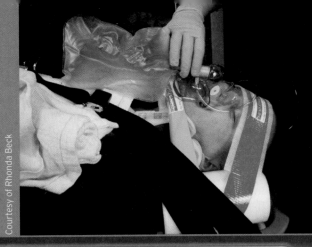

Courtesy of Rhonda Beck

National EMS Education Standard

Anatomy and Physiology

Applies complex knowledge of the anatomy and function of all human systems to the practice of EMS.

Pathophysiology

Applies complex knowledge of the pathophysiology of respiration and perfusion to patient assessment and management.

Pharmacology

Applies complex knowledge of the medications that an AEMT may assist/administer to a patient during a respiratory emergency.

Medicine

Applies complex knowledge to provide advanced emergency care and transportation based on assessment findings for an acutely ill patient.

Review

In your EMT-I class, you learned about the basic anatomy and physiology of the respiratory system and how to assess patients with respiratory problems. You also learned about causes of dyspnea and when it is appropriate to administer oxygen, the available modes of oxygen administration, and when to assist a patient with his or her prescribed inhaler.

What's New

The *National EMS Education Standards* include more in-depth evaluation of a patient with respiratory problems. It also includes more complex depth of the anatomy and physiology of the respiratory system so that you can better understand the pathophysiology of conditions that may lead to respiratory emergencies. In addition, specific respiratory conditions including asthma, obstructive/restrictive disease, and pneumonia are included in the new standards.

The immediate administration of high-flow oxygen (15 L/min) via nonrebreathing mask has been a standard form of treatment for most serious traumatic injuries and medical conditions. However, there have been studies that show detrimental effects of prolonged hyperoxygenation. As such, some states have modified their protocols to call for oxygen delivery titrated to a pulse oximetry reading greater than or equal to 94%. Make certain to refer to your local protocols regarding administration of oxygen.

Introduction

Dyspnea, or difficulty breathing, is a complaint that you will encounter often. It is a symptom of many different conditions, from the common cold and asthma to heart failure and pulmonary embolism. Several different problems occurring at the same time may contribute to a patient's dyspnea, including some that are serious or life threatening. You may or may not be able to determine the cause of dyspnea in a particular patient. Regardless, you may still be able to save a life.

Dyspnea Shortness of breath or difficulty breathing.

Anatomy and Physiology

The respiratory system consists of all the structures of the body that contribute to the breathing process. The upper airway includes all anatomic airway structures above the level of the vocal cords. These include the nose, mouth, jaw, oral cavity, pharynx, and larynx. Air enters the upper airway primarily through the nares (nostrils) of the nose, whose hairs filter the air we breathe **FIGURE 10-1**. The upper airway ends at the larynx, where it is protected by the epiglottis. This leaf-shaped valve diverts food and fluid into the esophagus and air into the trachea. Air then moves through the trachea and to the lower airway. The larynx (voicebox) and glottis (opening at the top of the trachea) are typically considered the dividing line between the upper airway and the sterile lower airway.

When air reaches the lower airway, it travels through the trachea, to the bronchi (larger airways), then on to the bronchioles (smaller airways), and finally into the alveoli **FIGURE 10-2**. Cilia in the bronchi and bronchioles help move particulate matter up and out of the airway.

Gas transfer is probably most efficient in the alveoli, but a significant amount of gas is also exchanged across the respiratory bronchioles. These terminal bronchioles are very thin and have little structure. This is helpful for gas exchange, but it also means that these bronchioles lack cilia, a mucus blanket, smooth muscle, or rigid structures. Once foreign material gets into the terminal bronchioles

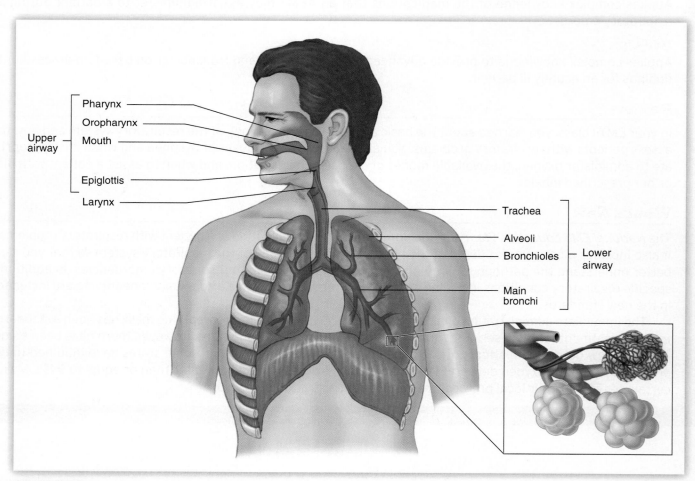

FIGURE 10-1 The upper airway includes the nasopharynx, nasal air passages, pharynx, oropharynx, mouth, and epiglottis. The larynx is considered the dividing line between the upper and lower airways. The lower airway includes the trachea, alveoli, bronchioles, and main bronchi.

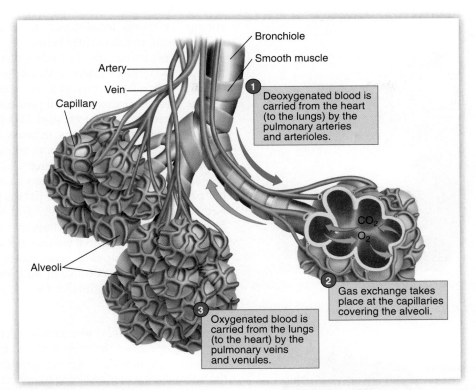

Bronchiole

Smooth muscle

Artery

Vein

Capillary

1 Deoxygenated blood is carried from the heart (to the lungs) by the pulmonary arteries and arterioles.

CO_2
O_2

Alveoli

2 Gas exchange takes place at the capillaries covering the alveoli.

3 Oxygenated blood is carried from the lungs (to the heart) by the pulmonary veins and venules.

FIGURE 10-2 An enlarged view of a single alveolus (air sac) showing where the exchange of oxygen and carbon dioxide between air in the sac and blood in the pulmonary capillaries takes place.

and alveoli, it typically never comes out. Emphysema may affect this area of the lungs, damaging or destroying the few structural components that are present. When that happens, the terminal branches of the tracheobronchial tree become so weak that they collapse during exhalation and trap air in the alveoli.

Respiration

The principal function of the lungs is *respiration*, which is the exchange of oxygen and carbon dioxide. The two processes that occur during respiration are inspiration, the act of breathing in or inhaling, and expiration, the act of breathing out or exhaling.

Respiration The exchange of gases that occurs at both the pulmonary level and the cellular level. At the pulmonary level, oxygen in the alveoli is exchanged for carbon dioxide in the bloodstream, and the opposite occurs at the cellular level, when oxygen in the bloodstream is exchanged for carbon dioxide in the cells.

Ventilation is the process of moving air into and out of the lungs. During respiration, oxygen is provided to the blood, and carbon dioxide is removed from it. This exchange of gases takes place rapidly in normal lungs at the level of the alveoli. Oxygen and carbon dioxide must

be able to pass freely between the alveoli and the capillaries. Oxygen entering the alveoli from inhalation passes through tiny passages in the alveolar wall into the capillaries, which carry the oxygen to the heart. This is known as pulmonary respiration. The heart, in turn, pumps oxygenated blood throughout the body. Carbon dioxide produced by the body's cells **FIGURE 10-3A** returns to the lungs in the blood that circulates through and around the alveolar air spaces. The exchange of gases that moves oxygen into the cells and carbon dioxide into the capillaries is known as cellular respiration. The carbon dioxide diffuses back into the alveoli and travels back up the bronchial tree and out the upper airways during exhalation **FIGURE 10-3B**. Again, carbon dioxide is exchanged for oxygen, which travels in exactly the opposite direction (during inhalation).

Ventilation The movement of air into and out of the lungs, spontaneously by the patient or with assistance.

Inspiration

The stimulus to breathe comes from the respiratory center located in the medulla. The involuntary control of breathing originates in the brain stem, specifically in the pons and medulla. The impulses for automatic breathing descend through the spinal cord and can be overridden (to a point)

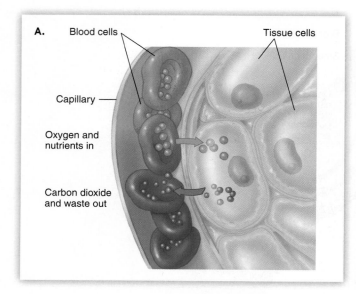

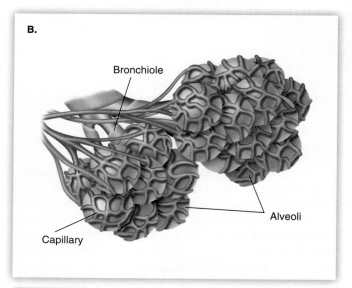

FIGURE 10-3 The exchange of oxygen and carbon dioxide during respiration. **A.** Oxygen passes from the blood through capillaries to tissue cells. Carbon dioxide passes from tissue cells through capillaries to the blood. **B.** In the lungs, oxygen is picked up by the blood and carbon dioxide is given off.

enlarge the thorax in all directions, causing intrapulmonary pressure to fall slightly below atmospheric pressure. The air pressure outside the body, called the atmospheric pressure, is normally equal to the air pressure within the thorax. As the diaphragm and intercostal muscles contract and the thoracic cage expands, air pressure within the thorax decreases, creating a slight vacuum. This pulls air in through the trachea and fills the lungs, inflating the alveoli. When the air pressure outside the thorax equals the air pressure inside the thorax, air stops moving. Gases such as oxygen and carbon dioxide will move from an area of higher partial pressure to an area of lower partial pressure until the partial pressures are equal. Oxygen and carbon dioxide diffuse across the alveolar membrane in opposite directions. Normal inspiratory reserve volume, the amount of air that can be inhaled in addition to normal tidal volume (about 500 mL), is about 3,000 mL in a typical adult male and 2,300 mL in a typical adult female.

Expiration

As the chest expands, mechanical receptors, known as stretch receptors, in the chest wall and bronchioles send a signal to the apneustic center via the vagus nerve to inhibit the inspiratory center and expiration occurs. This feedback loop, a combination of mechanical and neural control, is known as the *Hering-Breuer reflex* and terminates inhalation to prevent overexpansion of the lungs. The diaphragm and intercostal muscles relax, which increases intrapulmonary pressure. The natural elasticity, or recoil, of the lungs and chest wall results in exhalation. Normal expiratory reserve volume, the amount of air that can be exhaled following normal exhalation, is about 1,200 mL.

> *Hering-Breuer reflex* A protective mechanism that terminates inhalation, thus preventing overexpansion of the lungs.

TABLE 10-1 lists the characteristics of adequate breathing, and **TABLE 10-2** lists characteristics of inadequate breathing.

by voluntary control. The motor nerves of respiration are the phrenic nerves, which innervate the diaphragm, and the intercostal nerves, which innervate the intercostal muscles (muscles between the ribs).

The diaphragm is the primary muscle of respiration and separates the thoracic cavity from the abdominal cavity. During inspiration, the diaphragm and intercostal muscles contract. When the diaphragm contracts, it flattens and descends, increasing the vertical dimension of the thoracic cage. When the intercostal muscles contract, they raise the ribs up and out. The combined actions of these structures

Table 10-1
Signs of Adequate Breathing

- A normal rate (between 12 and 20 breaths/min)
- A regular pattern of inhalation and exhalation
- Good audible breath sounds on both sides of the chest
- Regular and equal (symmetric) chest rise and fall on both sides of the chest
- Adequate depth (tidal volume)
- Pink, warm, dry skin

Table 10-2
Signs and Symptoms of Inadequate Breathing

- A rate of breathing that is slower than 12 breaths/min or faster than 20 breaths/min in an adult
- Two- to three-word dyspnea (inability to speak more than a few words between breaths)
- Reduced flow of expired air at the nose and mouth
- Muscle retractions above the clavicles, between the ribs, and below the rib cage, especially in children
- Accessory muscle use
- Excessive coughing
- Diminished, noisy, or absent breath sounds
- Abnormal breath sounds (wheezing, rales, rhonchi, stridor, gurgling, or snoring)
- Unequal (asymmetric) chest wall movement, which results in reduced tidal and minute volume
- Pale or cyanotic skin or conjunctivae
- Cool, damp (clammy) skin
- Shallow respirations (reduced tidal volume)
- Irregular respirations, such as a patient taking a series of deep breaths followed by periods of apnea
- Pursed lips
- Nasal flaring
- Altered mental status
- Anxiousness or restlessness
- Tripod position
- Barrel-shaped chest

▌Pathophysiology

For the body to receive the required nutrients and oxygen and to dispose of waste products, adequate ventilation, *diffusion*, and *perfusion* must occur. There are multiple complications that interfere with ample ventilation. These can be separated into four areas:

1. Upper airway obstruction may be from a foreign body obstruction, trauma, or an inflammation such as tonsillitis or epiglottitis.
2. Lower airway obstruction may be caused by trauma. Obstructive lung disease and other complications, such as mucus accumulation, smooth-muscle spasm, and airway edema, can also create narrowing and blockage of the lower airways.
3. Chest wall impairment is another cause of impaired ventilation. Trauma, hemothorax, pneumothorax, empyema (pleural effusion), pleural inflammation, and neuromuscular diseases such as multiple sclerosis or muscular dystrophy prevent adequate chest wall excursion.
4. Problems in neurologic control can impair ventilation. These include brain stem malfunction from CNS depressant drugs, stroke or other medical neurologic condition, or trauma. Trauma and neuromuscular diseases can also cause phrenic or spinal nerve dysfunction, preventing normal neurologic control.

By rapidly assessing the patient and providing the necessary interventions, problems associated with oxygenation and ventilation can be minimized or avoided altogether.

> *Diffusion* The movement of solutes (molecules) from an area of higher concentration to an area of lower concentration.
> *Perfusion* The circulation of oxygenated blood to target tissues and organs in order to meet cellular demands.

Regardless of the reason for breathing difficulty, the critical issue is that you must be able to immediately recognize the signs and symptoms of inadequate breathing and know what to do.

Carbon Dioxide Retention and Hypoxic Drive

The level of carbon dioxide in arterial blood can rise for a number of reasons. Various types of lung disease may impair the exhalation process. The body may also produce too much carbon dioxide, either temporarily or chronically, depending on the disease or abnormality.

If, over a period of years, arterial carbon dioxide levels rise slowly to an underlying disease process and remain there (as in late COPD), the respiratory center in the brain, which senses carbon dioxide levels and controls breathing, may work less efficiently. This is called chronic *carbon dioxide retention*. If the condition is severe, a secondary drive called the *hypoxic drive* stimulates the respiratory center. In these patients, low blood oxygen levels cause the respiratory center to respond and stimulate respiration. If the arterial level of oxygen then is raised, as happens when the patient is given additional oxygen, there is no longer any stimulus to breathe; both the high carbon dioxide and low oxygen drives are lost. Patients with chronic lung diseases frequently have a chronically high level of blood carbon dioxide. Therefore, giving supplemental oxygen to these patients may actually depress, or completely stop, their respirations. However, as will be discussed later in this chapter, you should never withhold oxygen from a patient who needs it. Instead, these patients need to be reminded to breathe, and respirations may need to be assisted to compensate if a loss of respiratory drive develops.

> *Carbon dioxide retention* A condition characterized by a chronically high level of carbon dioxide in blood as the result of a respiratory disease.
> *Hypoxic drive* A backup system to control respirations when the oxygen level falls.

Causes of Dyspnea

Dyspnea is shortness of breath or difficulty breathing. Many different medical problems may cause dyspnea. Be aware that if the problem is severe and the brain is deprived of oxygen, the patient may not be conscious and alert enough to complain of shortness of breath. More commonly, altered mental status is a sign of *hypoxia* of the brain.

> *Hypoxia* A dangerous condition in which the body's cells do not have enough oxygen.

Patients with the following medical conditions often experience breathing difficulty, or hypoxia:

- Acute pulmonary edema
- Obstruction of the airway
- COPD
- Asthma or allergic reaction
- Rib fractures
- Spontaneous pneumothorax
- Upper or lower airway infection
- Pleural effusion
- Epiglottitis
- Pertussis
- Cystic fibrosis
- Pulmonary thromboembolism
- Hyperventilation syndrome
- Prolonged seizures
- Use of CNS depressant drugs (such as narcotics, barbiturates, or benzodiazepines)
- Neuromuscular disease (such as multiple sclerosis or muscular dystrophy)
- Environmental or industrial exposure to toxic gases

As you treat patients with disorders of the lungs, be aware that one or more of the following situations may exist:

- Gas exchange between the alveoli and pulmonary circulation is obstructed by fluid in the lung, infection, or collapsed alveoli (*atelectasis*).
- The alveoli are damaged and cannot transport gases properly across their own walls.
- The air passages are obstructed by muscle spasm, mucus, or weakened floppy airway walls.
- Blood flow to the lungs is obstructed by blood clots.
- The pleural space is filled with air or excess fluid, so the lungs cannot properly expand.

> *Atelectasis* Collapse of the alveoli; prevents the use of that portion of the lung for ventilation and oxygenation.

All of these conditions prevent the proper exchange of oxygen and carbon dioxide. In addition, the pulmonary blood vessels themselves may have abnormalities that interfere with blood flow and thus with the transfer of gases.

Besides shortness of breath, a patient with dyspnea may also report the sensation of chest tightness and air hunger. Air hunger is when a person reports the feeling of "not getting enough air" and has a strong need to breathe. Chest tightness is described as an uncomfortable feeling in the chest; it is commonly reported by patients with asthma.

Dyspnea is also a common complaint in patients with cardiopulmonary diseases. In some cases, it may be caused by physical exertion that has been made difficult because the patient's heart is damaged. Congestive heart failure is a troublesome cause of breathlessness because the heart is not pumping efficiently, and therefore the body does not have adequate oxygen. Another condition commonly associated with congestive heart failure is pulmonary edema, in which the alveoli are filled with fluid.

Severe pain itself can cause a patient to experience rapid, shallow breathing without the presence of a primary pulmonary problem. In some patients, breathing deeply causes pain because it causes expansion of the chest wall.

When you assess your patient for complaints of dyspnea, ask about chest pain; conversely, when you are evaluating your patient for chest pain, ask about dyspnea. Never withhold oxygen from any patient exhibiting signs of distress. If a patient with COPD stops breathing spontaneously (rare) because of increased levels of oxygen, it is a simple matter to coach breathing or to ventilate the patient and continue oxygenating organs and tissues. Withholding oxygen may result in an insufficient amount of inspired oxygen, and as a result of the decreased rate, depth, or other obstructive problem, vital organ damage may occur.

Upper and Lower Airway Infection

Infectious diseases causing dyspnea may affect all parts of the airway. Some cause mild discomfort. Others obstruct the airway to the point that patients require total respiratory support. In general, the problem is always some form of obstruction, either to the flow of air in the major passages (colds, diphtheria, epiglottitis, and croup) or to the exchange of gases between the alveoli and the capillaries (pneumonia).

Acute Pulmonary Edema

Pulmonary edema is an accumulation of fluid in the lungs and has various causes. The fluid accumulation causes a decrease in gas exchange and results in severe dyspnea. Severe myocardial damage caused by an acute problem (such as acute myocardial infarction) or a chronic problem (such as cardiomyopathy) results in reduced contractile force of the myocardium. In these cases, the left side of the heart cannot remove blood from the lungs as fast as the right side delivers it. As a result, fluid eventually backs up into the alveoli and in the lung tissue between the alveoli and the pulmonary capillaries. By physically separating the alveoli from the pulmonary capillary vessels, the edema interferes with the exchange of carbon dioxide and oxygen **FIGURE 10-4**. There is not enough room left in the lung for slow, deep breaths.

> *Pulmonary edema* A buildup of fluid in the lungs, often as a result of congestive heart failure.

Pulmonary edema can develop quickly, especially following a major cardiovascular insult. The patient usually experiences dyspnea with rapid, shallow respirations. In

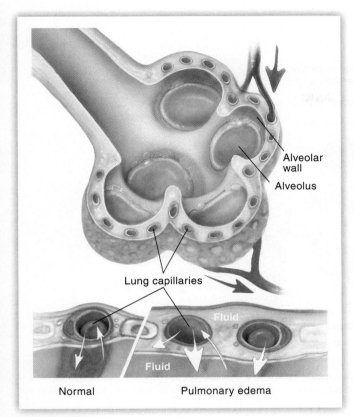

Alveolar wall

Alveolus

Lung capillaries

Fluid

Fluid

Normal   Pulmonary edema

FIGURE 10-4 In pulmonary edema, fluid fills the alveoli and separates the capillaries from the alveolar wall, interfering with the exchange of oxygen and carbon dioxide.

the most severe instances, you will see frothy pink sputum at the nose and mouth.

Not all patients with pulmonary edema have heart disease. Poisonings from smoke or toxic chemical fumes or other pulmonary irritants can produce pulmonary edema, as can traumatic injuries of the chest and exposure to high altitudes. In these cases, fluid collects in the alveoli and lung tissue in response to damage of the tissues of the lung or the bronchi.

Regardless of the initial cause, the resulting assessment findings are similar. Patients with pulmonary edema that is cardiogenic in origin may present with signs and symptoms of a cardiac emergency. Patients with noncardiogenic pulmonary edema tend to have a history of associated factors such as a hypoxic episode, shock, chest trauma, recent acute inhalation of toxic gases or particles, or recent ascent to a high altitude without acclimatizing. In both cases, patients may also present with dyspnea, *orthopnea* (severe dyspnea experienced when lying down or in a position that is not upright, and relieved by sitting or standing up), fatigue, reduced exercise capacity, and pulmonary rales.

> *Orthopnea* Severe dyspnea experienced when lying down and relieved by sitting up.

Chronic Obstructive Pulmonary Disease

Chronic obstructive pulmonary disease (COPD) is a common lung condition. It is the end of a slow process, which over several years results in disruption of the airways, the alveoli, and the pulmonary blood vessels. The process most often results from cigarette smoking. COPD may result from chronic bronchitis or emphysema. Obstruction occurs in the bronchioles. The cilia are unable to remove excess mucus, creating a buildup. The bronchioles dilate naturally on inspiration, enabling air to enter the alveoli despite the presence of obstruction. The bronchioles naturally constrict on expiration, and air becomes trapped distal to the obstruction on exhalation.

> *Chronic obstructive pulmonary disease (COPD)* A progressive and irreversible disease of the airway that causes destructive changes in the alveoli and bronchioles in the lungs, resulting in decreased inspiratory and expiratory capacity.

Tobacco smoke itself is a bronchial irritant and can create *chronic bronchitis*, an ongoing irritation of the trachea and bronchi. Chronic bronchitis results from overgrowth of the airway mucous glands and excess secretion of mucus, which blocks the airway. Patients have a chronic productive cough. The clinical definition of chronic bronchitis is a productive cough for at least 3 months per year for 2 or more consecutive years.

> *Chronic bronchitis* Irritation and inflammation of the major lung passageways from either infectious disease or irritants such as smoke.

Pneumonia develops easily when the passages are persistently obstructed. Ultimately, repeated episodes of irritation and pneumonia cause scarring in the lungs and some dilation of the obstructed alveoli, leading to COPD **FIGURE 10-5**.

Another type of COPD is *emphysema*. Emphysema is a degenerative condition characterized by destruction of the alveolar walls related to a deficiency of pulmonary surfactant. Surfactant is a substance that lines and lubricates the alveolar walls, allowing them to easily expand and recoil. Once the amount of surfactant is reduced, elasticity is diminished and the walls of the alveoli eventually fall apart, leaving large "holes" in the lung that resemble a large air pocket or cavity.

> *Emphysema* A disease of the lungs in which there is extreme dilation and eventual destruction of pulmonary alveoli with poor exchange of oxygen and carbon dioxide; it is one form of chronic obstructive pulmonary disease.

Emphysema is an irreversible condition. It also makes the alveoli prone to collapsing (atelectasis). Chronically low oxygen levels associated with emphysema stimulate

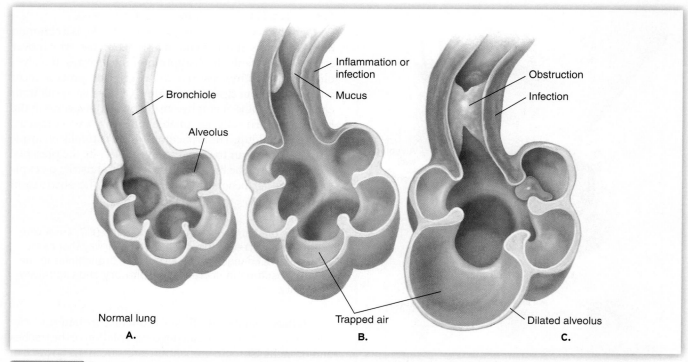

FIGURE 10-5 Repeated episodes of irritation and inflammation in the alveoli result in the obstruction, scarring, and some dilation of the alveolar sac characteristic of COPD. **A.** Normal alveolus. **B.** Infection produces mucus and swelling. **C.** A mucus plug creates an obstruction and further dilation of the alveolus.

the production of red blood cells, sometimes in excessive quantity (polycythemia). As a result, the patient's skin tends to remain pink.

Most patients with COPD have elements of both chronic bronchitis and emphysema. They have a history of recurring lung problems and are almost always long-term cigarette smokers. Some patients will have more elements of one condition than the other; few patients will have only emphysema or bronchitis. Therefore, most patients with COPD will consistently produce sputum, have a chronic cough, and have difficulty expelling air from their lungs, with long expiratory phases and wheezing.

The patient in an acute COPD episode will complain of shortness of breath with gradually increasing symptoms over a period of days. The patient often exhales through pursed lips. Patients with COPD may complain of tightness in the chest and constant fatigue. Because air has been gradually and continuously trapped in their lungs in increasing amounts, their chests often have a barrel-like appearance **FIGURE 10-6** . If you listen to the chest with a stethoscope, you will hear abnormal breath sounds.

Asthma

Asthma is an acute spasm of the smaller air passages called bronchioles that is associated with excessive mucus production and spasm of the bronchiolar muscles **FIGURE 10-7** . It is a common but serious disease. Asthma is a reversible

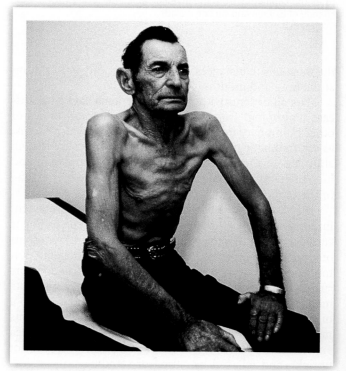

Courtesy of AAOS

FIGURE 10-6 Typically, a patient with COPD has a barrel-shaped chest and uses accessory muscles and pursed lips for breathing. Notice also that the patient is sitting in the tripod position.

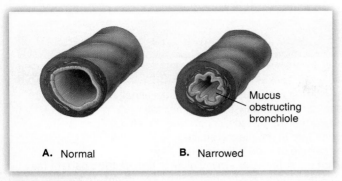

A. Normal   **B.** Narrowed

Mucus
obstructing
bronchiole

FIGURE 10-7 Asthma is an acute spasm of the bronchioles. **A.** Cross-section of a normal bronchiole. **B.** The bronchiole in spasm; a mucus plug has formed and partially obstructed the bronchiole.

obstruction that is caused by a combination of smooth-muscle spasm (bronchospasm), mucus production, and edema. *Status asthmaticus* is a severe, prolonged asthmatic attack that cannot be broken with conventional treatment. It is a dire medical emergency.

Asthma A disease of the lungs in which muscle spasm in the small air passageways and the production of large amounts of mucus result in airway obstruction.
Status asthmaticus A prolonged exacerbation of asthma that does not respond to conventional therapy.

Asthma produces a characteristic wheezing sound as patients attempt to exhale through partially obstructed air passages. These same air passages open more easily during inspiration. In early or more mild cases, when patients inhale, breathing appears relatively normal; the wheezing is heard only when they exhale. This wheezing may become so loud that you can hear it without a stethoscope, which is known as "audible wheezing." In severe cases, wheezing occurs during both inspiration and expiration and is diffuse, or heard throughout the lungs, not just over one particular lobe. In other cases, the airways are so blocked that no air movement is heard (a silent chest). In the worst cases, the actual work of exhaling is very tiring, and cyanosis, respiratory arrest, or both may develop.

Asthma affects people of all ages and is usually the result of an allergic reaction to an inhaled, ingested, or injected substance. It may also be induced by exercise, severe emotional stress, or an upper respiratory infection.

Most patients with asthma are familiar with their symptoms and know when an attack is imminent. Typically, they will have appropriate medication with them or at home. You should listen carefully to what these patients tell you; they often know exactly what they need.

Environmental/Industrial Exposure

Many potentially toxic substances can be inhaled, often at industrial sites. Such substances include pesticides, cleaning solutions, chemicals, chlorine, and other gases. Carbon monoxide is another toxic, odorless, highly poisonous gas that is produced in industrial settings by vehicles, gasoline-powered tools, and heaters.

The type of damage from the substance depends in large part on the water solubility of the toxic gas. Highly water-soluble gases such as ammonia will react with the moist mucous membranes of the upper airway and cause swelling and irritation. If the substance gets in the patient's eyes, they will also burn and feel inflamed and irritated. Less water-soluble gases such as phosgene and nitrogen dioxide may get deep into the lower airway, where they may cause pulmonary edema up to 24 hours later.

Cystic Fibrosis

Cystic fibrosis (CF) is a genetic disorder of the endocrine system that primarily targets the respiratory and digestive systems. The disease is usually fatal, with most children not living past their teens; however, because of advances in treatment, the life expectancy for patients with CF becomes better each year. With aggressive management and careful monitoring, patients occasionally live into their 30s.

Cystic fibrosis (CF) A genetic disorder of the endocrine system that makes it difficult for chloride to move through cells; primarily targets the respiratory and digestive systems.

CF is caused by a defective gene, which makes it difficult for chloride to move through cells. This causes unusually high sodium loss and abnormally thick mucus secretions. The secretions in the lungs cause breathing difficulties and provide an ideal growth environment for bacteria, leaving the patient highly susceptible to infection. Ultimately, the lung damage from the condition represents the primary cause of death in affected persons.

In CF, the child's symptoms range from sinus congestion to wheezing and asthma-like complaints. The child may develop a chronic cough that produces thick, heavy, discolored mucus. He or she may also present with tachypnea, shortness of breath, barrel chest, clubbed fingers, and cyanosis. The thick mucus may also collect in the intestines. The child often has dyspnea; this occasionally results in the need to call EMS. Treat the child with suction and oxygen using age-appropriate adjuncts. Keep a keen eye out for respiratory insufficiency, signs of a respiratory infection, and intestinal blockage.

CF often causes death in childhood because of chronic pneumonia secondary to the very thick, pathologic mucus in the airway. Adults with CF are predisposed to other medical conditions, including arthritis, osteoporosis, diabetes, and liver problems.

TABLE 10-3 shows infectious diseases associated with some degree of dyspnea.

Table 10-3
Infectious Diseases Associated With Dyspnea

Disease	Characteristics
Bronchitis	■ An acute or chronic inflammation of the lung that may damage lung tissue, usually associated with cough and production of sputum and, depending on its cause, sometimes fever. ■ Fluid also accumulates in the surrounding normal lung tissue, separating the alveoli from their capillaries. (Sometimes fluid can also accumulate in the pleural space.) ■ The lung's ability to exchange oxygen and carbon dioxide is impaired. ■ The breathing pattern in bronchitis does not indicate major airway obstruction, but the patient may experience tachypnea, or an increase in the breathing rate in an attempt to compensate for the reduced amount of normal lung tissue and for the buildup of fluid.
Common cold	■ A viral infection usually associated with swollen nasal mucous membranes and the production of fluid from the sinuses and nose. ■ Dyspnea is not severe; patients complain of "stuffiness" or difficulty breathing through the nose.
Croup	■ Inflammation and swelling of the whole airway (pharynx, larynx, and trachea) typically seen in children between ages 6 months and 3 years **FIGURE 10-8**. ■ The common signs of croup are stridor and a seal-bark cough, which signal a significant narrowing of the air passage of the larynx that may progress to significant obstruction. ■ Croup often responds well to the administration of humidified oxygen. ■ Croup is rarely seen in adults because the airways are larger.
Diphtheria	■ Although well controlled during the past decade, it is still highly contagious and serious when it occurs. ■ The disease causes the formation of a diphtheritic membrane lining the pharynx that is composed of debris, inflammatory cells, and mucus. This membrane can rapidly and severely obstruct the passage of air into the larynx.
Epiglottitis	■ Inflammation of the epiglottis caused by a bacterial infection that can produce severe swelling of the flap over the larynx; severe, rapidly progressive infection of the epiglottis and surrounding tissue that may be fatal because of sudden respiratory obstruction. ■ In preschool and school-aged children (ages 4 to 7 years) especially, the epiglottis can swell to two or three times its normal size. ■ The airway may become almost completely obstructed, sometimes quite suddenly **FIGURE 10-9**. ■ Stridor (harsh, high-pitched, continued, rough, barking inspiratory sounds) may be heard late in the development of airway obstruction. ■ Acute epiglottitis in the adult is characterized by a severe sore throat. ■ Less common in children than it was 20 years ago because of a vaccine that can help to prevent most cases.
Influenza type A	■ A virus that has crossed the animal/human barrier and has infected humans. ■ Flu that has the potential to spread at a pandemic level.
Meningococcal meningitis	■ An inflammation of the meningeal coverings of the brain and spinal cord that can be highly contagious. ■ The bacteria can be spread through the exchange of respiratory and throat secretions from coughing and sneezing. ■ The effects are lethal in some cases. Patients who survive can be left with brain damage, hearing loss, or learning disabilities. ■ Patients may present with flulike symptoms, but unique to meningitis are high fever, severe headache, photophobia (light sensitivity), and a stiff neck in adults. Patients sometimes have an altered level of consciousness and can have red blotches on the skin. ■ Use respiratory protection and report any potential cases.
Methicillin-resistant Staphylococcus aureus (MRSA)	■ A bacterium that can cause infections in different parts of the body. ■ Transmitted by different routes, including the respiratory route; can enter the body through nonintact skin or respiratory droplets when patients cough. ■ Difficult to treat because it is resistant to many commonly used antibiotics. ■ Most common in people with weakened immune systems, including those in hospitals and nursing homes.

Table 10-3
Infectious Diseases Associated With Dyspnea (*continued*)

Disease	Characteristics
Pertussis (whooping cough)	■ An airborne bacterial infection that affects mostly children younger than 6 years. ■ Patient will be feverish and exhibit a "whoop" sound on inspiration after a coughing attack. ■ Highly contagious through droplet infection. ■ Coughing spells can last for more than a minute; child may turn red or purple. ■ Does not cause the typical whooping illness in adults; causes severe upper respiratory infection that could lead to pneumonia in older persons.
Pneumonia	■ An acute bacterial or viral infection of the lungs that damages lung tissue, usually associated with fever, cough, and production of sputum. ■ Fluid also accumulates in the surrounding normal lung tissue, separating the alveoli from their capillaries. (Sometimes fluid can also accumulate in the pleural space.) ■ The lungs' ability to exchange oxygen and carbon dioxide is impaired. ■ The breathing pattern does not indicate major airway obstruction, but the patient may experience tachypnea, an increase in the breathing rate, which is an attempt to compensate for the reduced amount of normal lung tissue and for the buildup of fluid.
Respiratory syncytial virus (RSV)	■ A major cause of illness in young children. ■ Causes an infection of the lungs and breathing passages. ■ Can lead to other serious illnesses that affect the lungs or heart, such as bronchiolitis and pneumonia. ■ Highly contagious and spread through droplets. ■ Survives on surfaces, including hands and clothing. ■ Look for signs of dehydration. ■ Humidified oxygen is helpful if available.
Severe acute respiratory syndrome (SARS)	■ A serious, potentially life-threatening viral infection caused by a recently discovered family of viruses. ■ Usually starts with flulike symptoms, which may progress to pneumonia, respiratory failure, and, in some cases, death. ■ Thought to be transmitted primarily by close person-to-person contact.
Tuberculosis	■ A disease that can lay dormant in a person's lungs for decades, then reactivate. ■ Dangerous because many tuberculosis strains are resistant to many antibiotics. ■ Spread by cough; droplet nuclei can remain intact for decades. ■ Use a high-efficiency particulate air (HEPA) respirator to reduce risk of transmission and infection.

Common cold A viral infection usually associated with swollen nasal mucous membranes and the production of fluid from the sinuses.

Croup An infectious disease of the upper respiratory system that may cause partial airway obstruction and is characterized by a barking cough; usually seen in children; also called laryngotracheobronchitis.

Diphtheria An infectious disease in which a membrane lining the pharynx is formed that can severely obstruct passage of air into the larynx.

Influenza type A A virus that has crossed the animal/human barrier and has infected humans, recently reaching a pandemic level with the H1N1 strain.

Meningococcal meningitis An inflammation of the meningeal coverings of the brain and spinal cord; can be highly contagious.

Methicillin-resistant Staphylococcus aureus (MRSA) A bacterium that causes infections in different parts of the body and is often resistant to commonly used antibiotics. It can be found on the skin, in surgical wounds, and in the bloodstream, lungs, and urinary tract.

Severe acute respiratory syndrome (SARS) A potentially life-threatening viral infection that usually starts with flulike symptoms.

Tuberculosis A chronic bacterial disease caused by *Myobacterium tuberculosis* that usually affects the lungs but also can affect other organs such as the brain or kidneys.

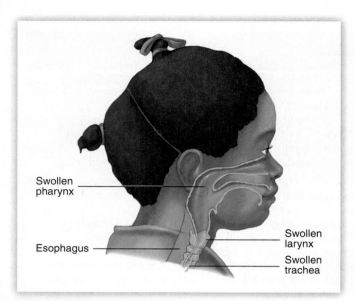

FIGURE 10-8 Croup swells the lining of the larynx, which is the narrowest point in the child's airway.

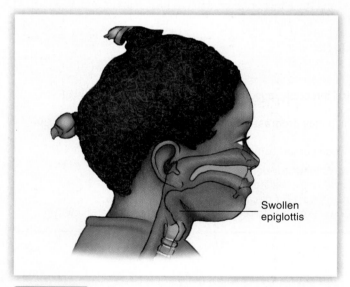

FIGURE 10-9 Epiglottitis is caused by a bacterial infection resulting in severe swelling of the epiglottis.

Age-Related Conditions

Bronchiolitis

Bronchiolitis is an inflammation of the small airways (bronchioles) in the lower respiratory tract caused by viral infection. The most common source of this disease is respiratory syncytial virus, although a new virus, *Metapneumovirus,* has also been found to cause this illness. These viruses occur with highest frequency during the late fall and winter months, and they primarily affect infants and children younger than 2 years. Severity ranges from mild to moderate respiratory distress with hypoxia and respiratory failure.

> *Bronchiolitis* Inflammation of the bronchioles that usually occurs in children younger than 2 years and is often caused by the respiratory syncytial virus.

The signs and symptoms of bronchiolitis can be difficult to distinguish from those of asthma, but note the child's age. Asthma is rare in children younger than 1 year; an infant with a first-time wheezing episode occurring in late fall or winter likely has bronchiolitis. Mild to moderate retractions, tachypnea, diffuse wheezing, diffuse crackles, and mild hypoxia are characteristic findings. As with asthma, a sleepy or obtunded patient or one with severe retractions, diminished breath sounds, or moderate to severe hypoxia (oxygen saturation <90%) is in danger of respiratory failure and requires immediate transport.

Respiratory Syncytial Virus

As mentioned, *respiratory syncytial virus (RSV)* is a major cause of illness in young children, creating an infection in the lungs and breathing passages. The more serious infections found in premature infants and children with depressed immune systems can lead to other serious illnesses that affect the lungs or heart. An RSV infection can cause respiratory illnesses like bronchiolitis and pneumonia.

> *Respiratory syncytial virus (RSV)* A virus that causes an infection of the lungs and breathing passages; can lead to other serious illnesses that affect the lungs or heart such as bronchiolitis and pneumonia; highly contagious and spread through droplets.

RSV is highly contagious and spread through droplets when the patient coughs or sneezes. The virus can also survive on surfaces, including hands and clothing. The infection tends to spread rapidly through schools and in child care centers.

RSV can also cause severe upper respiratory infections and typical asthma symptoms in adults and geriatric patients.

Croup

Croup is caused by inflammation and swelling of the pharynx, larynx, and trachea. This disease is often secondary to an acute viral infection of the upper respiratory tract and is typically seen in children between ages 6 months and 3 years. It is easily passed between children.

The disease starts with a cold, cough, and a low-grade fever that develop over 2 days. The hallmark signs of croup are stridor and a seal-bark cough, which is a signal of significant narrowing of the air passage of the trachea that may progress to significant obstruction. Peak seasonal outbreaks of this disease occur in the late fall and during the winter.

Croup is rarely seen in adults because their breathing passages are larger and are able to accommodate the inflammation and mucus production without producing symptoms. The airways of adults are wider, and the supporting tissue is firmer than in children.

Croup often responds well to the administration of humidified oxygen.

Epiglottitis

Epiglottitis is a serious inflammation of the epiglottis, usually caused by a bacterial infection that produces severe swelling of the flap over the larynx. Although it may be seen at any age, it is much more predominant in children. In preschool and school-aged children especially, the epiglottis can swell to two to three times its normal size. The airway is at risk of becoming completely obstructed. Patients with epiglottitis will look very sick. Epiglottitis usually has a sudden onset in an otherwise healthy child; children with this infection look ill, complain of a very sore throat, and have a high fever. They will usually be in the tripod position and drooling. Patients will also have stridor, high-pitched inspiratory sounds indicating partial airway obstruction.

> *Epiglottitis* An acute bacterial infection that results in rapid swelling of the epiglottis and surrounding tissues, and that may cause upper airway obstruction; also called acute supraglottic laryngitis.

Occasionally the constellation of symptoms of epiglottitis can also appear in an adult or a geriatric patient, especially if the patient has other issues such as diabetes, which may affect his or her ability to fight off disease. In adults, epiglottitis, or supraglottitis, can be caused by different bacterial or viral organisms. Acute epiglottitis in an adult or geriatric patient can be potentially life threatening and not recognized because it more commonly occurs in pediatric patients. Deterioration can occur quickly in adults with acute epiglottitis. You should be very concerned if your patient is an adult presenting with stridor or any other sign of anatomic airway obstruction.

Pneumonia

Pneumonia is a ventilation disorder caused by an infection of the lung parenchyma, which is the tissue of the lung itself. It is the fifth leading cause of death in the United States and is not a single disease, but a group of specific infections. Very young children are at risk for pneumonia because of their immature immune systems. Elderly people are also at risk because of age-related weakening of the immune system.

> *Pneumonia* An inflammation/infection of the lung from a bacterial, viral, or fungal cause.

Pneumonia presents as a localized infection in the lungs that may cause atelectasis, or alveolar collapse. If not treated promptly, the infection may become systemic, leading to sepsis and septic shock. Typical findings with pneumonia include an acute onset of fever and chills, productive cough with purulent (thick) sputum, pleuritic chest pain, and excessive mucus causing pulmonary consolidation that may be detected by auscultation in the form of rales or rhonchi.

Pertussis

Pertussis (whooping cough) is an airborne bacterial infection that mostly affects children younger than 6 years. It is highly contagious and is passed through droplet infection.

> *Pertussis (whooping cough)* An airborne bacterial infection that causes fever and a "whoop" sound on inspiration after a coughing attack; affects mostly children younger than 6 years; highly contagious through droplet infection.

A patient with pertussis will be feverish and exhibit a "whoop" sound on inspiration after a coughing attack. Symptoms are generally similar to those of colds, but coughing spells may last for more than a minute, in which the child may turn red or purple. This may frighten the parents into calling 9-1-1.

Airway Obstruction

Always consider upper airway obstruction from a foreign body first when a young child becomes short of breath. This is especially true of crawling babies, who might have swallowed and choked on a small object. Inflammation of the tonsils may also partially occlude the airway, creating an obstruction. Dysfunction of a tracheostomy may also create an upper airway obstruction, especially if it is plugged with mucus or other secretions.

The obstruction may be in the lower airway, below the vocal cords. Trauma to the trachea may result in a crushing injury, fractured larynx, or edema that obstructs the lower airway. Obstruction may also be in the form of obstructive lung disease, mucus accumulation, or smooth muscle spasm. Edema also may be present when a patient has been exposed to toxic chemicals or superheated air, as in a structural fire.

Congestive Heart Failure

After a heart attack or other illness, the heart muscle may be so injured that it cannot circulate blood properly. The heart is not able to maintain cardiac output that meets the needs of the body; thus the heart is failing as a pump.

In these cases, the left side of the heart cannot remove blood from the lungs as fast as the right side delivers it. As a result, fluid builds up within the alveoli and in the lung tissue between the alveoli and the pulmonary capillaries. This results in pulmonary edema.

Patient risk factors for congestive heart failure include hypertension and a history of coronary artery disease and/or atrial fibrillation, a condition in which the atria no longer contract, but instead quiver.

In most cases, patients have a long-standing history of chronic congestive heart failure that can be kept under control with medication. However, an acute onset may occur if the patient stops taking the medication, eats food that is too salty, or has a stressful illness, a new heart attack, or an abnormal heart rhythm.

Signs and symptoms of congestive heart failure include the patient reporting difficulty breathing with exertion because the heart cannot keep up with the body's need for oxygen. Patients may also report a sudden attack of respiratory distress that wakes them at night when they are in a reclining position. This is caused by fluid accumulation in the lungs. Patients also complain of coughing, feeling suffocated, cold sweats, and tachycardia.

Wet Lungs Versus Dry Lungs and "Cardiac Asthma"

Confusion sometimes exists between the concepts *wet lungs* in pulmonary edema, caused most often by congestive heart failure, and *dry lungs* in COPD. **TABLE 10-4** compares the differences between COPD and congestive heart failure.

Suppose you are called to assist an 80-year-old man who has had shortness of breath for 45 minutes. Physical examination reveals that his pulse and respirations are elevated, and you can see that he has pedal edema and jugular vein distention. His lung sound check reveals wheezing. He has a history of hypertension, congestive heart failure, and myocardial infarction; however, he has no history of smoking.

Are patients with congestive heart failure supposed to have rales rather than wheezing? Lung sounds are very helpful but can also be confusing. In a case in which the alveoli are so full of fluid, bubbles (the condition that gives the sound of rales) cannot form. The bronchi also become constricted, which produces wheezing. This patient is experiencing "cardiac asthma," which is all the more confusing because the patient has no history of asthma.

Patients with COPD wheeze because of bronchial constriction and present with shortness of breath. Their breathing becomes progressively worse over time, and they have the most trouble breathing on exertion. Patients with COPD have chronic coughing and thick sputum. They do not have jugular vein distention or dependent edema and are usually long-term smokers with a thin, barrel chest appearance. Their medications would include home oxygen, bronchodilators, and corticosteroids.

You should suspect congestive heart failure in this patient because of the patient's elevated blood pressure, pedal edema, and history of congestive heart failure. Unlike a typical patient with COPD, he has no history of smoking and takes diuretics and medications to reduce preload.

Patients with COPD have a slower onset of symptoms because their disease is worsened by infection and other stressors. Patients with congestive heart failure experience a fluid overload in the lung, which develops quickly from a failing pump.

As you try to discern between COPD and congestive heart failure, do not assume that *all* COPD patients have wheezing and *all* congestive heart failure patients have rales; keep an open mind so that you do not miss other important differences. The best advice is to treat the patient, not the lung sounds. In some cases, a patient with COPD may have air passages that are so constricted that you do not hear anything.

Table 10-4
Differences Between Chronic Obstructive Pulmonary Disease (COPD) and Congestive Heart Failure

COPD	Congestive Heart Failure
A disease of the lung characterized by shortness of breath and wheezing	A disease of the heart characterized by shortness of breath, edema, and weakness
Home oxygen, bronchodilators, and corticosteroids used for treatment	Diuretics prescribed to help promote cardiac function and to reduce fluid loads on the heart
Breathing progressively worse over time	Sudden onset of shortness of breath
Usually in long-term smokers	Patient may or may not smoke
Shortness of breath mostly on exertion	Shortness of breath all the time
Chronic coughing	Coughing
Sputum may be thick	Sputum may be pink and frothy
No jugular vein distention or dependent edema	Jugular vein distention and dependent edema
Patient usually thin with a barrel chest	May have distended abdomen

Transition Tip

Normal aging processes alter the respiratory system and the ability to exchange oxygen and carbon dioxide. The geriatric patient is at an increased risk of pneumonia or a worsening of asthma or COPD if the airways have lost muscle mass or tone. Secretions might not be expelled from the airways, allowing pneumonia to develop. Provide adequate ventilation and oxygenation according to the patient's needs. Geriatric patients may need ventilatory support for conditions that, in younger adults, are easily accommodated by the respiratory system.

Geriatric patients may also have a decreased ability to generate heat during a fever. Even a low-grade fever in a geriatric patient may have a serious underlying cause. Fever may also result in confusion or an altered mental status.

Patient Assessment of Respiratory Conditions

Assessment of patients in respiratory distress should be conducted as a calm and systematic process. Patients in respiratory distress are usually quite anxious, and they may be some of the most ill and challenging patients you will encounter.

> **Transition Tip**
>
> Scene safety is crucial in a toxic environment, but you will not always be told that you are entering a toxic environment. Stay alert for clues. If you enter a house for a patient who is not feeling well and you notice others with the same symptoms, suspect a toxic emergency. Remain alert for clues throughout the call; clues may not always be apparent when you first arrive.

Scene Size-up

Your first thought as an AEMT should always be the consideration of standard precautions and use of personal protective equipment (PPE). PPE is vital any time there is a potential for exposure to blood, body fluids, or respiratory secretions. The patient may have a respiratory infection that could be passed to you through sputum and air droplets. The minimum PPE when treating patients with respiratory distress and a productive cough or sputum production should be examination gloves, eye protection, and a HEPA respirator.

Pulmonary complaints may be associated with exposure to a wide variety of toxins, including carbon monoxide, toxic products of combustion, or environments that have deficient ambient oxygen (such as silos and enclosed storage spaces). It is critical to ensure a safe environment for all EMS personnel before making patient contact. If necessary, personnel with specialized training and equipment should remove the patient from a hazardous environment.

Once you have determined that the scene is safe, determine how many patients there are and whether you need additional or specialized resources. Frequently, in situations where there are multiple people with dyspnea, you should consider the possibility of an airborne hazardous material release.

Primary Assessment

As you approach and begin interacting, form a general impression of the patient. A variety of pulmonary conditions pose a high risk for death. Treat any immediate life threats. Signs of life-threatening respiratory distress in adults, listed from most ominous to least severe, include the following:

- Altered mental status
- Severe cyanosis
- Absent or abnormal breath sounds

- Audible stridor
- One- to two-word dyspnea
- Coughing
- Tachycardia of more than 130 beats/min
- Abdominal breathing
- Change in respiratory rate or rhythm
- Pallor and diaphoresis
- The presence of retractions and/or the use of the accessory muscles
- Tripod positioning

> **Transition Tip**
>
> In children, foreign bodies such as pencil erasers, candy, and beans frequently obstruct a nostril. These items often sit in the nose for a day or two before the child presents with pain and a foul-smelling nasal discharge. Do not try to remove the obstruction yourself.

Note whether the patient is responsive. Note the position of the patient's body. The more distress a dyspneic patient is in, the more the patient will want to sit up. Patients in severe respiratory distress may be in the tripod position. Does the patient appear calm? Is he or she anxious or restless? Does the patient appear listless and tired? How severe is his or her breathing complaint?

This initial impression will help you decide whether the patient's condition is stable or unstable. A stable condition generally will not deteriorate during treatment and transport, for example, a patient who has had pneumonia for 3 days and is being transported to the hospital to receive IV antibiotics. Conversely, an unstable condition may deteriorate during treatment and transport, for example, a patient who has been stung by a bee and is experiencing increasing difficulty in breathing.

Determine the patient's level of consciousness using the AVPU scale. If the patient is alert or responding to verbal stimuli, you know that the brain is still receiving oxygen. Now is a good time to ask the patient about his or her chief complaint. If the patient is responsive only to painful stimuli or unresponsive, the brain may not be oxygenating well and the potential for an airway or breathing problem is more likely. If there is no gag or cough reflex, you need to immediately assess the patient's airway status.

Is the airway open and clear? Is the patient breathing? If not, you must take action. Assess the airway and give two ventilations.

As you ventilate, you need to ask another series of questions, as follows:

1. Is air going into the lungs? Look for clues in the rise and fall of the chest, the respirations, and the heart rate.

2. When you squeeze the bag-mask device, does the chest wall expand?

3. When you release the bag, does the chest fall?

If the answer to any of these questions is "no," something is wrong. Try to reposition the patient and insert an airway adjunct to keep the tongue from blocking the airway. Reposition the head. Reassess your hand position and face mask seal.

Next, assess the rate at which you are assisting the patient's ventilation. You need to give breaths at roughly the same rate as the patient would if he or she were breathing spontaneously (12 to 20 breaths/min). Rescuers often get excited and ventilate the patient too rapidly. Breathing for the patient too rapidly can cause harm. With rapid squeezing of the bag, higher pressures force the air rapidly into the lungs. Higher pressures can fill the stomach, as well as the lungs, with air. If the air and fluid in the stomach are regurgitated from the esophagus, vomitus may enter the lungs, which can cause airway obstruction or aspiration pneumonia—pneumonia that develops as a result of aspirating a caustic substance (such as vomitus) into the lungs. Have suction readily available. Adults should be given one breath every 5 to 6 seconds. Infants and children need a smaller breath every 3 to 5 seconds. Use the appropriately sized bag-mask device for each age group.

If the patient is breathing, you need to decide whether the breathing is adequate. Is he or she able to speak? Does the patient present with one- to two-word dyspnea, or is he or she able to speak freely? Rapid, rambling speech is a sign of anxiety and fear. What is the respiratory effort like? Hard work may indicate an obstruction. Do you note any retractions or the use of accessory muscles? What is the patient's skin color? Is the patient diaphoretic? Is central or peripheral cyanosis present? If the breathing rate and tidal volume are adequate, apply 100% supplemental oxygen with a nonrebreathing mask and continue your assessment.

Determine whether your patient's breath sounds are normal (*vesicular breath sounds* represent air moving in and out of the alveoli, and *bronchial breath sounds* represent air moving through the bronchi) or decreased, absent, or abnormal (*adventitious breath sounds*). With your stethoscope, check lung sounds on the right and left sides of the chest, and compare each apex (top) of the lung with the opposite apex and each base (bottom) of the lung with the opposite base **FIGURE 10-10**. When you are listening on the patient's back, place the stethoscope head between and below the scapulae, not over them, or you will not have an accurate assessment.

> *Vesicular breath sounds* Normal breath sounds made by air moving in and out of the alveoli; heard over a normal lung.
>
> *Bronchial breath sounds* Normal breath sounds made by air moving through the bronchi.
>
> *Adventitious breath sounds* Abnormal breath sounds such as wheezes, rhonchi, rales, stridor, and pleural friction rubs.

Make sure that you listen for a full respiratory cycle so you can detect the adventitious sounds that may be heard at the end of the inspiratory or expiratory phase. When you are assessing the patient for fluid collection, pay special attention to the lower lung fields. Start from the bottom up and determine at which level you start hearing clear breath sounds.

You want to hear clear flow of air in both lungs. Not hearing the flow of air is considered an absent lung sound. The lack of air movement in the lung is a significant finding. Listen carefully and do not confuse absent lung sounds with clear lung sounds. **TABLE 10-5** provides examples of lung sounds, the diseases that may be associated with them, and important signs and symptoms.

Assess the pulse rate, quality, and rhythm. If the patient has a pulse, continue to support respirations. If the pulse rate is too fast (more than 100 beats/min) or too slow (fewer

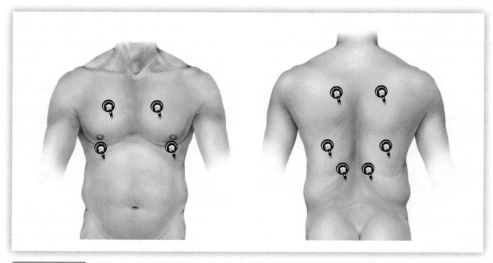

FIGURE 10-10 Stethoscope placement for auscultation of breath sounds.

Table 10-5
Signs, Symptoms, and Adventitious Lung Sounds Associated With Specific Respiratory Diseases

Lung Sounds	Disease	Signs and Symptoms
Wheezes	• Asthma • Chronic obstructive pulmonary disease • Congestive heart failure/pulmonary edema • Pneumonia • Bronchitis • Anaphylaxis	Dyspnea Productive or nonproductive cough Dependent edema, pink frothy sputum Fever, pleuritic chest pain Clear or white sputum Hives and stridor, nonproductive cough
Rhonchi	• Chronic obstructive pulmonary disease • Pneumonia • Bronchitis	Productive cough Fever, pleuritic chest pain Clear or white sputum
Rales (crackles)	• Congestive heart failure/pulmonary edema • Pneumonia	Dependent edema, pink frothy sputum Fever, pleuritic chest pain
Stridor	• Croup • Epiglottitis	Fever, barking cough Fever, sore throat, drooling
Decreased or absent breath sounds	• Asthma • Chronic obstructive pulmonary disease • Pneumonia • Hemothorax: shock, respiratory distress • Pneumothorax: fever, pleuritic chest pain • Atelectasis: fever, decreased oxygen saturation	Nonproductive cough, dyspnea Productive cough Fever, pleuritic chest pain Blood in chest Air in chest Collapsed lung

than 60 beats/min), the patient may not be getting enough oxygen. An increased pulse rate is the body's way of responding to respiratory distress and can be an indicator of shock.

Tachycardia is also a normal response to pain, fear, excitement, and exertion.

A rate of less than 60 beats/min is described as bradycardia. A slow pulse rate could mean problems with the cardiac conduction system, a medication reaction, organophosphate poisoning, or decompensation. If the pulse rate is normal, the patient is most likely receiving enough oxygen to support life. If the pulse rate is too fast or too slow, the patient may not be getting enough oxygen. Check the radial pulse in an adult. If no radial pulse is felt, palpate the carotid pulse. In a child 1 year old or younger, palpate a brachial pulse.

Determine the quality of the pulse. You must also determine whether the rhythm is regular or irregular. When the interval between each ventricular contraction of the heart is short, the pulse is rapid. When the interval is longer, the pulse is slower. No matter what the rate, the interval between each contraction should be the same, and the pulse that results should occur at a constant, regular rhythm. Irregular beats could indicate a cardiac problem.

Assessing a patient's circulation includes an evaluation for the presence of shock and bleeding. Respiratory distress

Transition Tip

Not everyone should be ventilated the same way. If you are ventilating a patient who has severe obstructive disease, such as those with either decompensated asthma or COPD, remember that these patients have difficulty exhaling. If each breath is not allowed to come back out before the delivery of the next, then pressure in the thorax will continually go up. This phenomenon, which is called auto-PEEP (positive end-expiratory pressure), can eventually cause pneumothorax or cardiac arrest. If the pressure in the chest exceeds the pressure of blood returning to the heart, thus limiting venous return, cardiac arrest may occur.

Such patients should be ventilated as little as 4 to 6 breaths/min to avoid "bagging them to death." This is difficult to do when your partner, bystanders, the BLS crew, and your own epinephrine release are all telling you to hyperventilate the patient, but it is an absolute necessity if you hope to avoid the dire consequences of raising the thoracic pressure more with each breath. Seek guidance from your medical director and follow local protocols when you encounter patients with severe COPD or asthma who are in cardiac arrest or near arrest. However, also remember that the standard ventilation rate for adults is 10 to 12 breaths/min.

in a patient could be caused by an insufficient number of red blood cells to transport the oxygen. Assess capillary refill in infants and children. Normal capillary refill is less than 2 seconds; abnormal capillary refill is greater than 2 seconds. Capillary refill is not considered a reliable assessment tool in the adult patient.

Assess the patient's perfusion by evaluating skin color, temperature, and condition. The patient's skin color is assessed by looking at the nail beds, lips, and eyes. In a white person, normal skin is pink. Abnormal skin conditions are pale, cyanotic or blue-gray, flushed or red, and jaundiced or yellow.

Assess the patient's skin temperature by feeling the skin. Normal is warm. Abnormal skin temperatures are hot, cool, cold, and clammy. Assess the patient's skin condition. Normal is dry; abnormal is moist or wet.

If the patient's condition is unstable and there is a possible life threat, address the life threat and proceed with rapid transport. Patients with the following signs or symptoms require rapid transport:

- Problems with the ABCs
- Poor initial general impression
- Unresponsiveness
- Potential hypoperfusion or shock
- Chest pain associated with a low blood pressure
- Severe pain anywhere
- Excessive bleeding

History Taking

After you form your general impression and have completed the primary assessment, ask the patient to describe the problem to determine the chief complaint. Is there any dyspnea or chest pain? Begin by asking an open-ended question: "What can you tell me about your breathing?" Use the OPQRST mnemonic: when the problem began (Onset), what makes the breathing difficulty worse or better (Provocation or Palliation), how the breathing feels (Quality), and whether the discomfort, if present, moves (Radiation). How much of a problem is the patient having (Severity)? On a scale of 1 to 10, with 10 being the worst pain the patient has ever had, how bad is it? Is the problem continuous or intermittent (Time)? If it is intermittent, how long does it last? Does the patient have a cough? Is it productive or nonproductive? If it is productive, what color is the sputum? Is there any hemoptysis? Wheezing? Fever? Chills? Any increased sputum production? Has there been any exposure to smoke or is there a smoking history?

Find out what the patient has already done for the breathing problem. Does the patient use a prescribed inhaler? If so, when was it used last? How many doses have been taken? Does the patient use more than one inhaler? When was the last time the patient saw a physician for this problem? Does the patient take any type of corticosteroid or steroid medication on a regular basis? Find out whether the patient has any allergies or history of medication reactions.

What are the patient's vital signs? What is the pulse rate? Tachycardia is a sign of hypoxemia or might be a result of sympathomimetic medications taken for respiratory difficulty. Bradycardia in a patient experiencing dyspnea is an ominous sign of severe hypoxemia and imminent cardiac arrest. What is the patient's blood pressure? Hypertension may be associated with the use of sympathomimetic medication.

What is the patient's respiratory status? The respiratory rate is not an accurate indicator of respiratory status unless it is very slow. However, respiratory trends are essential for evaluating chronically ill patients. A slowing respiratory rate in the face of an unimproved condition suggests physical exhaustion and impending respiratory failure. The patient's respiratory pattern should be noted as follows:

- Eupnea (normal breathing pattern)
- Tachypnea (rapid respiratory rate)
- Cheyne-Stokes respirations (a rhythmic breathing pattern characterized by periods of rapid and slow respirations alternating with periods of apnea; commonly seen in patients with head injury)
- Central neurogenic hyperventilation (deep, rapid respirations commonly seen in patients with head injury)
- Kussmaul respirations (deep, rapid respirations accompanied by an acetone or fruity odor on the patient's breath; seen in patients with diabetic ketoacidosis)
- Ataxic (Biot) respirations (rapid, irregular respirations with periods of apnea)
- Apneustic respirations (impaired respirations with sustained inspiratory effort)
- Apnea (cessation of breathing)

Transition Tip

The presence of corticosteroids or other steroids in the patient's daily medication regimen strongly suggests severe, chronic disease.

Different respiratory complaints offer different clues and different challenges. Patients with chronic conditions may have long periods in which they are able to live relatively normal lives but then sometimes experience acute worsening of their conditions. That is when you are called, and it is important for you to be able to determine your patient's baseline status, or his or her normal condition, and what is different this time that made the patient call you. For example, patients with COPD (emphysema and chronic bronchitis) do not cope well with pulmonary infections because the existing airway damage makes them unable to cough up the mucus or sputum produced by the infection. The chronic lower airway obstruction makes it difficult for the patient to breathe deeply enough to clear the lungs.

Gradually, the arterial oxygen level falls, and the carbon dioxide level rises. If a new infection of the lung occurs in a patient with COPD, the arterial oxygen level may fall rapidly. In a few patients, the carbon dioxide level may become high enough to cause sleepiness. In these cases, patients require respiratory support and careful administration of oxygen.

Patients with COPD usually have a long history of dyspnea with a sudden increase in shortness of breath. There is rarely a history of chest pain. More often, they will remember having had a recent "chest cold" with fever and either an inability to cough up mucus or a sudden increase in sputum. If the patient is able to cough up sputum, it will be thick and is often green or yellow. The blood pressure of patients with COPD is normal; however, the pulse is rapid and occasionally irregular. Pay particular attention to the respirations. They may be rapid, or they may be very slow.

Patients with asthma may have different "triggers," meaning different causes of acute attacks. These include allergens, cold, exercise, stress, infection, and noncompliance with medication prescriptions. It is important to try to determine what may have triggered the attack so that it can be treated appropriately. For example, an asthma attack that occurred while your patient was jogging in the cold will probably not respond to antihistamines, whereas one brought on by a reaction to pollen might.

Patients with congestive heart failure often walk a fine line between compensating for their diminished cardiac capacity and decompensating. Many take several medications, most often including diuretics ("water pills") and blood pressure medications. Your history taking should include obtaining a list of all their medications and paying special attention to the events leading up to the present problem.

With patients in respiratory distress, the SAMPLE history can be obtained from the family or bystanders if they are present. Limit the number of questions to pertinent ones—a patient who is in respiratory distress does not need to be using any additional air to answer questions.

Be sure to ask the following questions about a patient in respiratory distress:

- What is the patient's general state of health?
- Has the patient had any childhood or adult diseases?
- Have there been any surgeries or recent hospitalizations?
- Are there any psychiatric or mental health illnesses?
- Have there been any traumatic injuries?

If time allows, also ask about the patient's immunization history.

Because chronically ill patients live with their condition every day, when they call EMS, something has changed for the worse. Ask about previous episodes, medication allergies, and current medications. The patient's subjective description of the problem is an accurate indicator of the acuity of this episode if the disease is chronic. Any history

of intubation is an accurate indicator of severe pulmonary disease and suggests that intubation by paramedics may be required again.

Pay close attention to the medications the patient is currently taking. Are there any pulmonary medications, and if so, are they inhaled, oral, or parenteral? The patient probably has prescribed medications to use that are delivered by an inhaler. Consult medical control. Remember to report the name of the medication, when the patient last took a puff, how many puffs were used at that time, and what the label states regarding dosage. If medical control permits, you may administer a bronchodilator via nebulizer, which is discussed later.

If the patient does not have a prescribed inhaler, continue with the history taking and secondary assessment. Despite use of the inhaler, the patient's condition may continue to worsen. You need to reassess breathing frequently and be prepared to assist ventilations in severe cases.

Secondary Assessment

As always, you should only proceed to history taking and the secondary assessment once all life threats have been identified and treated during the primary assessment. If you are busy treating airway or breathing problems, you may not have the opportunity to proceed to a physical examination prior to arriving at the emergency department. Never compromise the assessment and treatment of airway and breathing problems to conduct a physical examination.

Sometimes it is not possible to quickly and definitively determine what is causing your patient's respiratory distress. Keep an open mind, gather as complete a history as possible, and perform a physical examination.

Additional pieces to the assessment and treatment puzzle may be revealed during the physical examination. As you perform your physical examination, look for signs of increased work of breathing. Are the patient's lips pursed? Do you see any accessory muscle use in the neck?

When you are examining the chest, are there any obvious signs of trauma? Any retractions? Is the chest symmetric? A barrel chest indicates the presence of longstanding COPD. Next, listen to the breath sounds. Are they normal or abnormal? Do you hear stridor, wheezing, rhonchi, or rales? Examine the extremities for skin color, condition, and temperature. Numbness, tingling, and carpopedal spasm may be associated with hypocapnia, resulting from periods of rapid, deep respiration.

Conduct an in-depth assessment when a patient complains of shortness of breath. In addition to the signs of air hunger present in all patients with respiratory distress, such as tripod positioning, rapid breathing, and use of accessory muscles, restriction of the small lower airways in patients with asthma often causes wheezing. Patients may have a prolonged expiratory phase of breathing as they attempt to exhale trapped air from the lungs. In severe cases, you may actually not hear wheezing because of insufficient air flow. As your patient tires from the effort of breathing and oxygen levels drop, the respiratory and heart rates may actually drop, and your patient may seem to relax or go to sleep. These signs indicate impending respiratory arrest, and you must act immediately.

When patients with congestive heart failure decompensate, they will often experience pulmonary edema as fluid backs up in their circulatory system and into the lungs. High blood pressure and low cardiac output often trigger this "flash" (sudden) pulmonary edema. These patients are among the most sick, frightened, and worrisome patients you will encounter. They are literally drowning in their own fluid. In addition to the classic signs of respiratory distress, they may have pink, frothy sputum coming from the mouth. They will have adventitious lung sounds, most often wet (rales, rhonchi, crackles) but sometimes dry sounding (wheezes). Their legs and feet may be swollen (pedal edema) from the backup of fluid.

When the blood contains inadequate oxygen, the body will attempt to divert blood from the extremities to the core to help keep the vital organs, including the brain, functioning. This action by the body will result in pale skin and delayed capillary refill in the hands and feet. Capillary refill that takes longer than 2 seconds is considered delayed. Feel for the skin temperature and look for color changes in the extremities and in the core of the body. Cyanosis is a late sign and can be seen first in the lips and mucous membranes. Cyanosis is an ominous sign that requires immediate, aggressive intervention.

In addition to determining the presence and quality of the pulse and respirations, and assessing the skin and lung sounds, obtain a baseline blood pressure reading.

Pulse oximetry is an effective diagnostic tool for evaluating or confirming the adequacy of oxygen saturation. However, pulse oximetry readings may be inaccurate in the presence of conditions that abnormally bind hemoglobin, such as carbon monoxide poisoning or any condition that causes a decrease in perfusion. Using a peak flow meter provides a baseline assessment of expiratory airflow for patients with obstructive lung disease. Many patients with chronic asthma may already use a peak flow meter at home. Encourage these patients to take their records and medications with them to the hospital for evaluation of the progression of their illness.

Reassessment

Once the assessment and treatment have been completed, repeat the primary assessment, monitor the patient's breathing, and reassess circulation.

Determine whether the patient's condition has changed in any way, and confirm the adequacy of interventions and patient status. Is the current treatment improving the patient's condition? Are there any new problems?

If the changes you find are improvements, simply continue the treatments; however, if your patient's condition

deteriorates, prepare to modify treatments. Be prepared to assist ventilations with a bag-mask device. Monitor the skin color and temperature. Reassess and record vital signs at least every 5 minutes for a patient in unstable condition and/or after the patient uses an inhaler. If the patient's condition is stable and no life threat exists, vital signs should be obtained at least every 15 minutes.

Interventions may be based on standing orders, or you should contact the hospital and ask for specific directions. Remember, interventions for immediate life threats should have been completed during the primary assessment and should not require contacting the hospital first. Interventions for respiratory problems may include the following:

- Providing oxygen via a nonrebreathing mask at 15 L min
- Providing positive-pressure ventilations using a bag-mask device, pocket mask, or a flow-restricted, oxygen-powered ventilation device
- Using airway management techniques such as an oropharyngeal airway, a nasopharyngeal airway, suctioning, or airway positioning
- Positioning the patient in a high Fowler's position or a position of choice to facilitate breathing
- Assisting with respiratory medications found in a patient-prescribed metered-dose inhaler or a small-volume nebulizer

Some of these interventions were performed in the primary assessment to address life threats. Others are used to support breathing problems until definitive care can be provided at the hospital. Some of your interventions may even correct the problem.

Contact medical control with any change in level of consciousness or difficulty breathing. Depending on local protocol, contact medical control prior to assisting with any prescribed medications. Be sure to document any changes (and at what time) and any orders given by medical control.

▮ Emergency Medical Care

When you are taking the initial vital signs of a person with dyspnea, pay particular attention to respirations. Always speak with assurance and assume a concerned, professional approach to reassure the patient, who no doubt will be very frightened.

If the patient complains of breathing difficulty, administer high-flow supplemental oxygen. If breathing difficulty is severe, put a nonrebreathing face mask on the patient and supply oxygen at a rate of 12 to 15 L/min (enough to keep the reservoir bag inflated). Reevaluate the patient's response to treatment frequently, at least every 5 minutes, until you reach the emergency department.

As stated previously, there is some concern about suppression of the hypoxic drive to breathe in some patients with COPD. Be prepared to intervene by coaching breathing or assisting ventilations in the event that respiratory drive is suppressed by supplemental oxygen, but don't withhold oxygen. In stable patients who have longstanding COPD and probable carbon dioxide retention, administration of low-flow oxygen (2 L/min) is a good place to start, with adjustments to 3 L/min, then 4 L/min, and so on, until symptoms have improved (for example, the patient has less dyspnea or an improved mental status). When in doubt, err on the side of more oxygen and monitor the patient closely.

Never withhold oxygen from a patient who needs it for fear of depressing or stopping breathing, even in patients with COPD. Slowing of respirations after oxygen administration does not necessarily mean that the patient's condition is improving; it may be deteriorating. If respirations slow and perfusion diminishes after oxygen administration, simply coach breathing or assist breathing with a bag-mask device.

If the patient has altered mental status, open the airway using manual maneuvers. Suction any secretions or blood from the airway. Insert an oropharyngeal or nasopharyngeal adjunct as needed to maintain airway patency. If the patient's tidal volume is inadequate (for example, shallow breathing), provide positive-pressure ventilation with a bag-mask device attached to 100% oxygen.

Consider insertion of an advanced airway in unresponsive patients. Call for paramedic backup if needed.

Gain IV access and consider a 20 mL/kg bolus of normal saline if the patient is not hypertensive and no rales are present when the lungs are auscultated. For patients with COPD or asthma, the fluid can help to thin secretions. A patient with pneumonia or other conditions may also be dehydrated.

> ### Transition Tip
>
> If humidified oxygen is not available, use a nebulizer with a mask and add normal saline to humidify the oxygen and help thin secretions. This is especially helpful with patients who have COPD, epiglottitis, and croup.

Metered-Dose Inhalers and Small-Volume Nebulizers

A patient may have a prescribed *metered-dose inhaler (MDI)* or small-volume nebulizer. An MDI is a miniature spray canister used to direct medication through the mouth and into the lungs. If the patient has not done so, he or she should be advised to use the MDI. For more severe problems, liquid bronchodilators may be aerosolized in a nebulizer for inhalation. A *small-volume nebulizer* contains a mouthpiece through which the patient inhales a mist of aerosolized medicine. When breathed in correctly, the medicine goes deep into the patient's lungs, allowing it to start to work quickly. Oxygen or a compressed air source is connected to the nebulizer to produce the aerosolized mist.

> *Metered-dose inhaler (MDI)* A miniature spray canister used to direct medications through the mouth and into the lungs.
>
> *Small-volume nebulizer* A respiratory device that holds liquid medicine that is turned into a fine mist. The patient inhales the medication into the airways and lungs as a treatment for conditions like asthma.

Some of the medications most commonly used for shortness of breath are called inhaled beta-agonists, which, through stimulation of selective beta-2 receptors in the lungs, dilate the bronchioles. Typical trade names are Proventil, Ventolin, Alupent, Metaprel, and Brethine. The generic name for Proventil and Ventolin is albuterol; for Alupent and Metaprel, it is metaproterenol; and for Brethine, it is terbutaline. The action of most of these medications is to relax the smooth muscles within the bronchioles in the lungs, leading to enlargement (dilation) of the airways and easier passage of air.

TABLE 10-6 lists medications used for acute and chronic symptoms. Those used for acute symptoms are designed to give the patient rapid relief from symptoms if the condition is reversible. Medications used for chronic symptoms are administered for preventive measures or as maintenance doses. The medications for chronic use will provide little relief of acute symptoms. Common side effects of inhalers used for acute shortness of breath include increased pulse rate, nervousness, and muscle tremors.

Indications and Contraindications

If a patient with shortness of breath has a prescribed MDI, read the label carefully to make sure that the medication has been prescribed to the patient and that it is not expired. The patient should take repeated doses of the medication if the maximum dose has not been exceeded and he or she is still experiencing shortness of breath. Contraindications for the use of an MDI include the following:

- The patient is unable to help coordinate inhalation with depression of the trigger on an MDI or is too confused to effectively administer medication through a small-volume nebulizer. These devices will be only minimally effective when patients are in respiratory failure and have only minimal air movement.
- The MDI or small-volume nebulizer is not prescribed for this patient.
- The medication is expired.
- The patient had already met the maximum prescribed dose before your arrival (typically two to four puffs).
- There are other contraindications specific to the medication.

Table 10-6
Respiratory Inhalation Medications

Medication		Indications			Usage: Acute vs Chronic	
Generic Drug Name	**Trade Names**	**Asthma**	**Bronchitis**	**Chronic Obstructive Pulmonary Disease**	**Acute**	**Chronic**
Albuterol	Proventil, Ventolin, Volmax	Yes	Yes	Yes	Yes	No
Beclomethasone dipropionate	Beclovent	Yes	No	No	No	Yes
Cromolyn sodium	Intal	Yes	No	No	No	Yes
Fluticasone propionate	Flovent	Yes	No	No	No	Yes
Fluticasone propionate, salmeterol xinafoate	Advair Diskus	Yes	No	No	No	Yes
Ipratropium bromide	Atrovent	Yes	Yes	Yes	Yes	No
Metaproterenol sulfate	Alupent	Yes	Yes	Yes	Yes	No
Montelukast sodium	Singulair	Yes	No	No	No	Yes
Salmeterol xinafoate	Serevent	Yes	Yes	Yes	No	Yes

Transition Tip

Positioning the patient in an upright position to loosen mucus and relieve buildup can be very effective in treating a patient with a respiratory emergency.

Medication from an inhaler is delivered through the respiratory tract to the lung. The dose is one puff for an MDI and continuation of the small-volume nebulizer until all the medication has been administered or the patient no longer feels the need for the medication.

Administration of a Metered-Dose Inhaler

To help a patient self-administer medication from an inhaler, follow the steps in **SKILL DRILL 10-1**.

1. Follow standard precautions.

2. Obtain an order from medical control or follow local protocol.

3. Check that you have the right medication, right patient, right dose, right route, and that the medication is not expired.

4. Make sure that the patient is alert enough to use the inhaler.

5. Check to see whether the patient has already taken any doses.

6. Make sure the inhaler is at room temperature or warmer (**Step 1**).

7. Shake the inhaler vigorously several times.

8. Stop administering supplemental oxygen and remove any mask from the patient's face.

9. Ask the patient to exhale deeply and, before inhaling, to put his or her lips around the opening of the inhaler (**Step 2**).

10. If the patient has a spacer, attach it to allow more effective use of the medication **FIGURE 10-11**.

11. Have the patient depress the hand-held inhaler as he or she begins to inhale deeply.

12. Instruct the patient to hold his or her breath for as long as he or she comfortably can to help the lungs absorb the medication (**Step 3**).

SKILL DRILL 10-1

Assisting a Patient With a Metered-Dose Inhaler

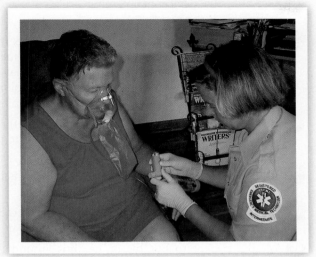

Courtesy of Rhonda Beck

1 Check to make sure you have the correct medication for the correct patient. Check the expiration date. Ensure the inhaler is at room temperature or warmer.

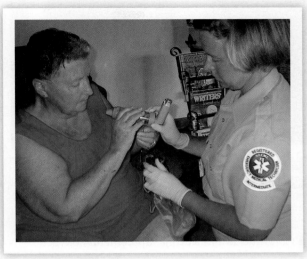

Courtesy of Rhonda Beck

2 Remove any mask. Hand the inhaler to the patient. Instruct about breathing and lip seal. Use a spacer if the patient has one.

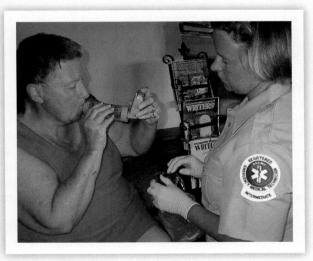

Courtesy of Rhonda Beck

3 Instruct the patient to press the inhaler and inhale one puff. Instruct about breath holding.

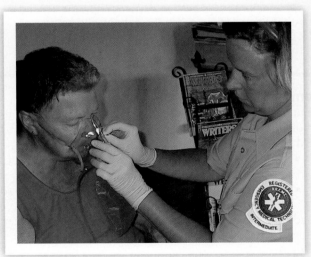

Courtesy of Rhonda Beck

4 Reapply oxygen. After a few breaths, have the patient repeat the dose if medical control or local protocol allows.

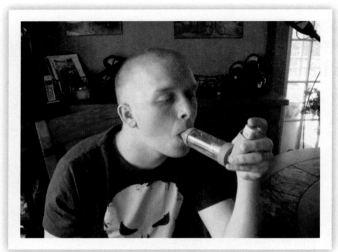

Courtesy of Rhonda Beck

FIGURE 10-11 Using a spacer can increase the benefit of an inhaled medication.

13 Continue administering supplemental oxygen.

14 Allow the patient to breathe a few times, then give the second dose per direction from medical control or according to local protocol (**Step 4**).

Transition Tip

While one AEMT is getting oxygen ready, the second AEMT should try to coach the patient with asthma or COPD to use pursed-lip breathing. This further opens the bronchioles to help air to escape.

Administration of a Small-Volume Nebulizer

Albuterol is one of the most commonly administered bronchodilators given via nebulizer and can be administered by AEMTs. Dosages are as follows:

- **Adult:** Administer 2.5 mg diluted with 2.5 mL of normal saline.
- **Pediatric:** Administer 0.01 to 0.03 mL (0.05 to 0.15 mg/kg) diluted with 2 mL of normal saline.

To administer medication from a small-volume nebulizer, follow the steps in **SKILL DRILL 10-2**.

1 Follow standard precautions.

2 Obtain an order from medical control or follow local protocol.

3 Check that you have the right medication, right patient, right dose, and right route and that the medication is not expired. Ensure there are no issues with contamination, discoloration, or clarity of the medication (**Step 1**).

4 Make sure that the patient is alert enough to use the device.

5 Check to see whether the patient has already taken any treatments.

6 Assemble the device maintaining an aseptic technique.

7 Open the medication container on the nebulizer and insert the medication (generally, the whole volume of the medication). In some cases, sterile saline may be added (about 3 mL) to achieve the optimum volume of fluid for the nebulized application (**Step 2**).

8 Attach the medication container to the nebulizer, mouthpiece, and tubing. Attach oxygen tubing to the oxygen tank.

9 Adjust oxygen flow to 6 L/min to establish a misting effect (**Step 3**).

10 Stop administering supplemental oxygen and remove nonrebreathing mask from the patient's face.

11 Ask the patient to put his or her lips around the mouthpiece of the device, inhale the mist, and hold it for 3 to 5 seconds before exhaling (**Step 4**).

12 When the mist dissipates and the medication has been used or the patient is no longer experiencing shortness of breath, discontinue use of the device.

13 Place the nonrebreathing mask back on the patient.

14 Reassess vital signs, and document your actions and the patient's response.

15 Consult with medical control and/or follow local policy if repeated doses are necessary.

Reassessment

You must carefully monitor patients with shortness of breath. About 5 minutes after the patient uses an inhaler, repeat the vital signs and the focused assessment. Ask the patient whether the treatment made any difference. Look at the patient's chest to see whether the patient is still using accessory muscles to breathe. Listen to the patient's speech pattern. Be prepared to assist ventilations with a bag-mask device if the patient's condition deteriorates.

After helping the patient with the inhaler treatment or administering a bronchodilator via nebulizer, transport the patient to the closest, most appropriate emergency department. While en route, continue to assess the patient's breathing.

Provide reassurance and continue to give supplemental oxygen. In cases of severe distress, do not delay transport. Using MDIs as well as administering nebulized treatments may be done en route.

SKILL DRILL 10-2

Administering Medication With a Small-Volume Nebulizer

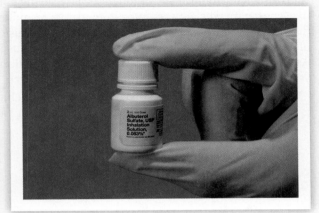

1 Check to make sure you have the correct medication for the correct patient. Check the expiration date. Confirm you have the correct patient.

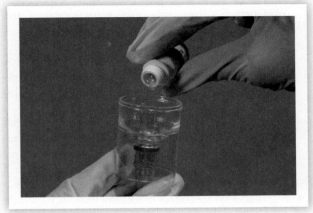

2 Insert the medication into the container on the nebulizer. In some cases, sterile saline may be added (about 3 mL) to achieve the optimum volume of fluid for the nebulized application.

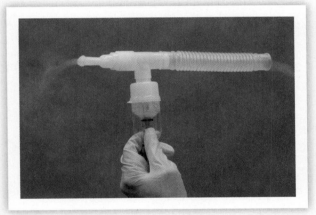

3 Attach the medication container to the nebulizer, mouthpiece, and tubing. Attach oxygen tubing to the oxygen tank. Set the flow meter at 6 L/min.

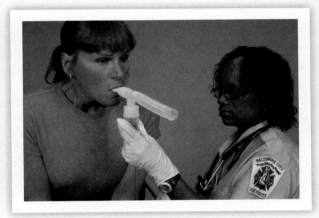

4 Instruct the patient on how to breathe.

PREP KIT

Ready for Review

- Dyspnea is a common complaint that may be caused by numerous medical problems, including infections of the upper or lower airways, acute pulmonary edema, COPD, spontaneous pneumothorax, asthma or allergic reactions, pleural effusions, mechanical obstruction of the airway, pulmonary embolism, and hyperventilation.
- Lung disorders interfere in one way or another with the exchange of oxygen and carbon dioxide that takes place during respiration through problems with ventilation, diffusion, perfusion, or a combination of these.
- Pulmonary complaints may be associated with exposure to a wide variety of toxins. Suspect toxic inhalation if more than one patient has dyspnea, and immediately remove yourself from the scene until it is safe.
- Signs and symptoms of breathing difficulty include unusual breath sounds (wheezing, stridor, rales, and rhonchi), nasal flaring, pursed-lip breathing, cyanosis, inability to talk, use of accessory muscles to breathe, and sitting in the tripod position.
- Assessment of patients in respiratory distress should be conducted as a calm, systematic process. The patients are usually quite anxious.
- In treating dyspnea, it is important to reassure the patient and provide supplemental oxygen. Remember to maintain the patient in a position that is comfortable for breathing, usually sitting upright.
- Interventions for respiratory problems may include the following:
  - Oxygen administration via a nonrebreathing mask, nasal cannula, or Venturi mask, or positive-pressure ventilations using a bag-mask device, pocket mask, or a manually triggered ventilation device (flow-restricted, oxygen powered ventilation device)
  - Airway management techniques such as use of an oropharyngeal airway, a nasopharyngeal airway, suctioning, or airway positioning
  - Placing the patient in a high Fowler's position or a position of comfort to facilitate breathing
  - Assistance with respiratory medications found in a prescribed MDI or small-volume nebulizer (consult medical control to assist with appropriate use of the inhaler or injector)
- Remember that a patient who is breathing rapidly may not be getting a sufficient amount of oxygen as a result of respiratory distress from a variety of problems. In every case, prompt recognition of the problem, giving oxygen or providing ventilatory support, and prompt transport are essential.

Case Study

As you are nearing the end of what feels like a very long shift, you and your partner are dispatched to a local residence for a person with "trouble breathing." When you arrive on scene, you find a 62-year-old woman sitting slightly forward on a living room chair; although she is receiving home oxygen therapy, she appears to be in moderate respiratory distress. The patient is able to tell you that she has a history of COPD and that her distress today is worse than usual. As your partner obtains the patient's vital signs, he informs you that her pulse oximetry reading is 88% on oxygen.

1. COPD includes emphysema and chronic bronchitis. How are these two conditions differenct from each other?

2. Patients with COPD are prone to developing a spontaneous pneumothorax. What are some of the signs that would suggest your patient might be experiencing a spontaneous pneumothorax?

3. Explain why "cardiac asthma" can be confused with conditions like COPD.

4. Explain the pathophysiology behind cystic fibrosis.

5. Which of the following medications is used to treat chronic asthma, bronchitis, and COPD?
   A. Albuterol
   B. Salmeterol
   C. Alupent
   D. Fluticasone

CHAPTER 11

Cardiovascular Emergencies

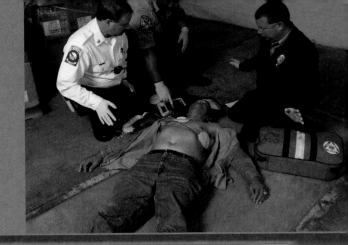

National EMS Education Standards

Anatomy and Physiology
Applies fundamental knowledge of the anatomy and function of all human systems to the practice of EMS.

Pathophysiology
Applies fundamental knowledge of the pathophysiology of respiration and perfusion to patient assessment and management.

Pharmacology
Applies fundamental knowledge of the medications that the AEMT may assist/administer to a patient during an emergency.

Medicine
Applies fundamental knowledge to provide advanced emergency care and transportation based on assessment findings for an acutely ill patient.

Review

The most common calls for EMS systems involve chest pain and difficulty breathing. Patients with a history of chest pain may take nitroglycerin. As an EMT-I, you should already know how to assist a patient in taking nitroglycerin. Because one of the effects of nitroglycerin is vasodilation of coronary arteries leading to a drop in blood pressure, it is essential that the patient's systolic blood pressure be a minimum of 90 mm Hg. In addition, if the patient takes an erectile dysfunction medication such as Viagra, Levitra, or Cialis within 24 to 48 hours of taking nitroglycerin, a significant fall in blood pressure may lead to sudden cardiac death.

In general, emergency care for a patient experiencing cardiovascular symptoms involves administering high-flow oxygen, placing the patient in a position of comfort, requesting paramedic assistance, and ensuring rapid transport to the hospital. Continual monitoring of the patient and emergency intervention in the event of sudden death are essential.

What's New

For AEMTs, it is important to enhance knowledge of the anatomy and physiology of the cardiovascular system to better understand the pathophysiology of the diseases that may be encountered. This chapter discusses the relationship between chest pain and ischemic heart disease. It also covers specific cardiovascular conditions including acute myocardial infarction (classic heart attack) and its complications—sudden death, cardiogenic shock, and congestive heart failure (CHF). Finally, the administration of aspirin and nitroglycerin to a patient experiencing a possible heart attack is discussed. Current AHA guidelines for cardiopulmonary resuscitation (CPR) and automated external defibrillator (AED) are also included.

Introduction

The American Heart Association (AHA) reports that cardiovascular disease claimed 831,272 lives in the United States in 2006. This is 34.3% of all deaths, or approximately 1 of every 2.8 deaths. Heart disease has been the leading killer of Americans since 1900. It is estimated that 81,100,000 people in the United States have one or more forms of cardiovascular disease.

Anatomy and Physiology

The cardiovascular system consists of the heart (the pump), the blood vessels (the container), and the blood (the fluid). All components must interact effectively to maintain life.

Structures of the Heart

The *heart* is a muscular, cone-shaped organ whose function is to pump blood throughout the body. The heart is located behind the sternum and is about the size of the closed fist of the person it belongs to **FIGURE 11-1**. Roughly two thirds of the heart lies in the left part of the *mediastinum*, the area between the lungs that also contains the great vessels (that is, the aorta and vena cavae) and other structures.

> *Heart* A muscular organ that pumps blood throughout the body.
> *Mediastinum* The space between the lungs that contains the heart, great vessels, trachea, mainstem bronchi, vagus nerve, and part of the esophagus.

The heart muscle is referred to as the myocardium. The pericardium, also called the pericardial sac, is a thick fibrous membrane that surrounds the heart **FIGURE 11-2**. The pericardium anchors the heart within the mediastinum and prevents overdistention of the heart. The inner membrane of the pericardium is the serous pericardium. This inner membrane contains two layers: the visceral layer and the parietal layer. The visceral layer of the pericardium lies closely against the heart and is also called the epicardium. The second layer of the pericardium, the parietal layer, is separated from the visceral layer by a small amount of pericardial fluid that reduces friction within the pericardial sac.

The human heart consists of four chambers: two atria and two ventricles. The upper chambers are the atria, and the lower chambers are the ventricles. Each side of the heart contains one atrium and one ventricle. A membrane, the interatrial septum, separates the two atria; a thicker wall, the interventricular septum, separates the right and left ventricles. Each *atrium* receives blood that is returned to the heart from other parts of the body; each *ventricle* pumps blood out of the heart **FIGURE 11-3**.

> *Atrium* One of two (right and left) upper chambers of the heart.
> *Ventricle* One of two lower chambers of the heart.

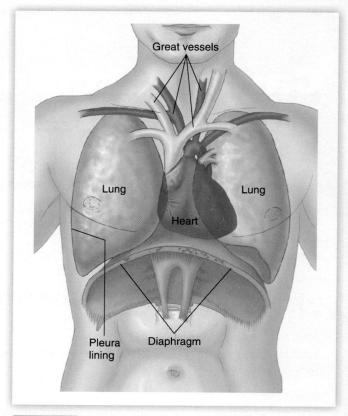

FIGURE 11-1 The anterior aspect of the thorax shows the relative position of the heart beneath the surface.

Blood enters the right atrium via the superior and inferior venae cavae and the coronary sinus, which is the end of the great cardiac vein, and collects blood returning from the walls of the heart. Blood from four pulmonary veins enters the left atrium.

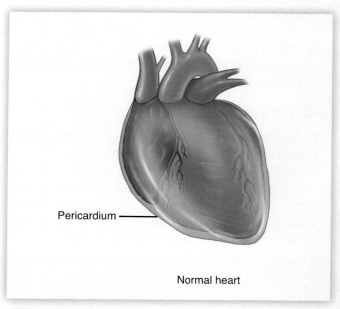

FIGURE 11-2 The pericardial sac surrounds the heart.

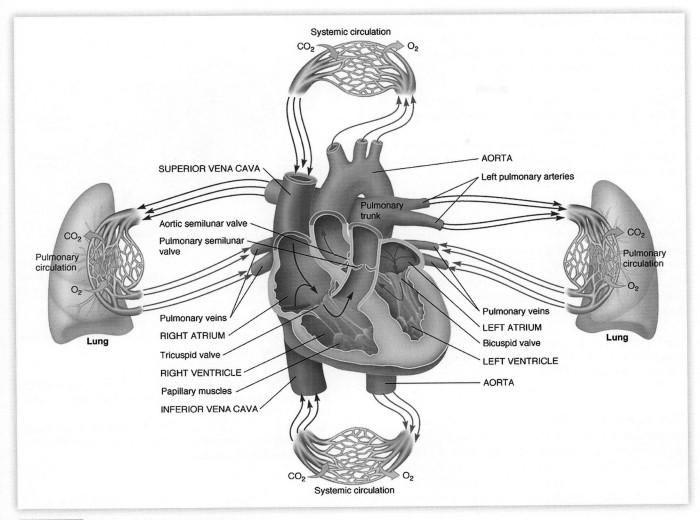

FIGURE 11-3 Blood flows through the heart.

Valves of the Heart

Blood passing from the atria to the ventricles flows through one of two *atrioventricular valves*. The tricuspid valve separates the right atrium from the right ventricle, while the mitral valve, a bicuspid valve, separates the left atrium from the left ventricle. The valves consist of flaps called cusps. Papillary muscles attach to the ventricles and send small muscular strands called chordae tendineae to the cusps. When the papillary muscle contracts, these strands tighten, preventing regurgitation of blood through the valves from the ventricles to the atria.

> *Atrioventricular valves* The two valves through which blood flows from the atria to the ventricles.

Two semilunar valves, the aortic valve and the pulmonic valve, divide the heart from the aorta and the pulmonary artery. The *pulmonic valve* regulates blood flow from the right ventricle to the pulmonary artery. The *aortic valve* regulates blood flow from the left ventricle to the aorta.

The semilunar valves are not attached to papillary muscles. When these valves close, they prevent backflow from the aorta and pulmonary artery into the left and right ventricles, respectively.

> *Pulmonic valve* The semilunar valve that regulates blood flow between the lungs to the left atrium of the heart.
> *Aortic valve* The one-way semilunar valve that regulars blood flow from the left ventricle to the aorta.

Blood Flow Within the Heart

Two large veins, the *superior vena cava* and the *inferior vena cava*, return deoxygenated blood from the body to the right atrium. Blood from the upper part of the body returns to the heart through the superior vena cava, and blood from the lower part of the body returns through the inferior vena cava. The inferior vena cava is the larger of the two veins. From the right atrium, blood passes through the tricuspid valve into the right ventricle. Blood is then pumped by the right ventricle through the pulmonic valve into the pulmonary artery and to the lungs. In the lungs, blood is oxygenated and at the same time carbon dioxide and other waste products are removed.

> *Superior vena cava* One of the two largest veins in the body; carries blood from the upper extremities, head, neck, and chest into the heart.
>
> *Inferior vena cava* One of the two largest veins in the body; carries blood from the lower extremities and the pelvic and the abdominal organs to the heart.

Freshly oxygenated blood is returned to the left atrium through the pulmonary veins. Blood then flows through the mitral valve into the left ventricle, which pumps the oxygenated blood through the aortic valve, into the *aorta*, the body's largest artery, and then to the entire body. The left ventricle is the strongest and largest of the four cardiac chambers because it is responsible for pumping blood through blood vessels throughout the body.

> *Aorta* The main artery that receives blood from the left ventricle and delivers it to all the other arteries that carry blood to the tissues of the body.

The Electrical Conduction System

The mechanical pumping action of the heart can occur only in response to an electrical stimulus. This impulse causes the heart to beat via a set of complex chemical changes within the myocardial cells. The brain partially controls the heart's rate and strength of contraction via the autonomic nervous system. Contractions of myocardial tissue, however, are initiated within the heart itself, in a group of complex electrical tissues that are part of a conduction system. The cardiac conduction system consists of six parts: the sinoatrial (SA) node, the atrioventricular (AV) node, the bundle of His, the right and left bundle branches, and the Purkinje fibers **FIGURE 11-4**.

The *sinoatrial (SA) node* is located high in the right atrium and is the normal site of origin of the electrical impulse. It is the heart's natural pacemaker and has an intrinsic rate of 60 to 100 beats/min. If the SA node is not functioning properly, the AV node may take over as the heart's pacemaker. The intrinsic rate of the AV node is 40 to 60 beats/min. Rhythms originating below the AV node have an intrinsic rate of 20 to 40 beats/min. Impulses originating in the SA node travel through the right and left atria, resulting in atrial contraction. The impulse then travels to the *atrioventricular (AV) node*, located in the right atrium adjacent to the septum, where it transiently slows. Electrical stimulation of the heart muscle then continues toward the bundle of His, which is a continuation of the AV node. From here, it proceeds rapidly to the right and left bundle branches, stimulating the interventricular septum. The impulse then spreads out via the Purkinje fibers to the left,

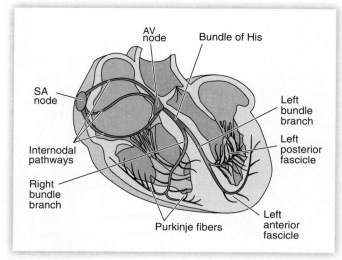

FIGURE 11-4 The electrical conduction system of the heart initiates an electrical impulse throughout the heart. The impulse travels through the six parts of the cardiac conduction system.

then the right ventricular myocardium, resulting in ventricular contraction, or systole.

> *Sinoatrial (SA) node* The normal site of the origin of electrical impulses; located high in the right atrium, it is the heart's natural pacemaker.
>
> *Atrioventricular (AV) node* The site located in the right atrium adjacent to the septum that is responsible for transiently slowing electrical conduction.

Electrical Properties of Cardiac Cells

The ability of cells to respond to electrical impulses is referred to as the property of excitability. The ability of the cells to conduct electrical impulses is referred to as the property of conductivity.

Cardiac muscle cells have a special characteristic called *automaticity* that is not found in any other type of muscle cells. Automaticity allows a cardiac muscle cell to contract spontaneously without a stimulus from a nerve source. Normal impulses in the heart start at the SA node. As long as impulses come from the SA node, the other myocardial cells will contract when the impulse reaches them. If no impulse arrives, however, the other myocardial cells are capable of creating their own impulses and stimulating a contraction of the heart, although at a generally slower rate.

> *Automaticity* The ability of cardiac cells to generate an impulse to contract even when there is no external nervous stimulus.

Regulation of Heart Function

The stimulus, which originates in the SA node, is controlled by impulses from the brain, which arrive by way of the autonomic nervous system (ANS). The autonomic nervous system is the part of the brain that controls the functions of the body that do not require conscious thought, such as the heartbeat, respirations, dilation and constriction of blood vessels, and digestion of food. The heart's chronotropic state (control of the rate of contraction), dromotropic state (control of electrical conduction), and inotropic state (control of the strength of contraction) are controlled by the autonomic nervous system, the hormones of the endocrine system, and the heart tissue.

The autonomic nervous system has two parts, the **sympathetic nervous system** and the **parasympathetic nervous system**. The sympathetic nervous system is also known as the "fight-or-flight" system and makes adjustments to the body to allow for physical activity. The sympathetic nervous system speeds up the heart rate, increases respiratory rate and depth, dilates blood vessels in the muscles, and constricts blood vessels in the digestive system. The parasympathetic nervous system directly opposes the sympathetic nervous system. The parasympathetic nervous system slows the heart and respiratory rates, constricts blood vessels in the muscles, and dilates blood vessels in the digestive system. Normally these two systems balance each other, but in times of stress, the sympathetic nervous system gains primary control, whereas in times of relaxation, the parasympathetic system takes control.

> **Sympathetic nervous system** Subdivision of the autonomic nervous system that governs the body's fight-or-flight reactions by inducing smooth muscle contraction or relaxation of the blood vessels and bronchioles.
> **Parasympathetic nervous system** A subdivision of the autonomic nervous system, involved in control of involuntary, vegetative functions, mediated largely by the vagus nerve through the chemical acetylcholine.

Receptors in the blood vessels, kidneys, brain, and heart constantly monitor body functions to help maintain homeostasis. **Baroreceptors** respond to changes in pressure, usually within the heart or the main arteries. **Chemoreceptors** sense changes in the chemical composition of the blood. If abnormalities are sensed, nerve signals are transmitted to the appropriate target organs, and hormones or neurotransmitters are released to correct the situation. Once conditions normalize, the receptors stop firing and the signals cease.

> **Baroreceptors** Receptors in the blood vessels, kidneys, brain, and heart that respond to changes in pressure in the heart or main arteries to help maintain homeostasis.
> **Chemoreceptors** Receptors in the blood vessels, kidneys, brain, and heart that respond to changes in chemical composition of the blood to help maintain homeostasis.

The Cardiac Cycle

The process that creates the pumping of the heart is known as the cardiac cycle. This cycle begins with myocardial contraction and concludes at the beginning of the next contraction. The heart's contraction results in pressure changes within the cardiac chambers, resulting in the movement of blood from areas of high pressure to areas of low pressure.

Systole is a term that refers to the contraction of the ventricular mass and the pumping of blood into the systemic circulation. During systole, a pressure is created within the arteries that can be recorded; this pressure is known as the systolic blood pressure. A normal systolic blood pressure in an adult is between 110 and 140 mm Hg. A pressure also exists in the vessels during **diastole**, the relaxation phase of the heart cycle; it is called the diastolic blood pressure. A normal diastolic blood pressure in an adult is between 70 and 90 mm Hg.

> **Systole** The contraction, or period of contraction, of the heart, especially that of the ventricles.
> **Diastole** The relaxation phase of the heart, when the ventricles are filling with blood.

Blood pressure is noted as a fraction and the systolic reading is placed above the diastolic reading (for example, a systolic reading of 130 and a diastolic reading of 70 would be noted as 130/70 mm Hg). The unit of measure mm Hg refers to millimeters of mercury and describes the height, in millimeters, to which the blood pressure elevates a column of liquid mercury in a glass tube. Although many blood pressure measurement devices now use dials, blood pressure is still described in millimeters of mercury.

Preload is the amount of blood returned to the heart to be pumped out, and it directly affects the afterload. The pressure in the aorta or the peripheral vascular resistance, against which the left ventricle must pump blood, is called the afterload. The greater the afterload, the harder it is for the ventricle to eject blood into the aorta, reducing the stroke volume (SV), or the amount of blood ejected per contraction. To a large degree, afterload is governed by arterial blood pressure. Afterload is greater with vasoconstriction and less with vasodilation.

Cardiac output (CO) is the amount of blood pumped through the circulatory system in 1 minute. Cardiac output is expressed in liters per minute (L/min). The cardiac output equals the heart rate multiplied by the stroke volume:

$$\text{Cardiac Output} = \text{Stroke Volume} \times \text{Heart Rate}$$

Factors that influence the heart rate, the stroke volume, or both will affect cardiac output and thus **perfusion** to the body's tissues. The presence of pulses is a good indicator of blood pressure. Weak or absent peripheral pulses indicate decreased perfusion. Weak central pulses indicate significant hypotension and decompensated shock.

Increased venous return to the heart stretches the ventricles to some extent, resulting in increased cardiac **contractility**. This relationship is called **Starling's law** of the heart.

> *Cardiac output (CO)* The amount of blood pumped through the circulatory system in 1 minute.
> *Perfusion* The circulation of oxygenated blood within an organ or tissue in adequate amounts to meet the cells' current needs.
> *Contractility* The strength of heart muscle contraction.
> *Starling's law* A principle that states that if a muscle is stretched slightly before stimulation to contract, the muscle will contract harder; describes how increased venous return to the heart stretches the ventricles and allows for increased cardiac contractility.

The heart has several ways of increasing stroke volume. According to Starling's law, the more cardiac muscle is stretched, the greater the force with which it contracts. If for any reason an increased volume of blood is returned from the systemic veins to the right side of the heart or from the pulmonary veins to the left side of the heart, the muscle surrounding the cardiac chambers will have to stretch to accommodate the larger volume. The more the cardiac muscle stretches, the greater will be the force of its contraction, the more completely it will empty, and therefore the greater the stroke volume. The amount of blood returning to the right atrium may vary somewhat from minute to minute, but the normal heart continues to pump out the same percentage of blood returned to the left ventricle. This is called the *ejection fraction*. This system allows the heart to function at the same capacity regardless of changes in the body's position or what the person is doing, whether sitting, moving, sneezing, or any other activity.

> *Ejection fraction* The portion of the blood ejected from the left ventricle during systole.

Transition Tip

Three components are required to have adequate tissue perfusion: pump (heart), container (vessels), and fluid (blood).

Blood and Its Components

Plasma and Formed Elements (Cells)

Blood is the substance that is pumped by the heart through the arteries, veins, and capillaries. Blood consists of plasma and formed elements or cells that are suspended in the plasma. These cells include *red blood cells (RBCs)*, *white blood cells (WBCs)*, and platelets. The purpose of blood is to carry oxygen and nutrients to the tissues and carry cell waste products away from the tissues. In addition, the formed elements are the mainstay of numerous other body functions such as fighting infection and controlling bleeding. Average human adult male bodies contain approximately

70 mL/kg, or about 5 L, of blood, whereas average female bodies contain approximately 65 mL/kg.

Plasma is a watery, straw-colored fluid that accounts for more than half of the total blood volume. Plasma is made up of 92% water and 8% dissolved substances such as chemicals, minerals, and nutrients. Water enters the plasma from the digestive tract, from fluids between cells, and as a by-product of metabolism.

> *Red blood cells (RBCs)* Cells that contain hemoglobin and carry oxygen to the body's tissues; also called erythrocytes.
> *White blood cells (WBCs)* Blood cells that have a role in the body's immune defense mechanisms against infection; also called leukocytes.
> *Plasma* A sticky, yellow fluid that carries the blood cells and nutrients and transports cellular waste material to the organs of excretion.

Red Blood Cells

Red blood cells carry oxygen to the tissues. They are disk-shaped and are also known as erythrocytes. Erythrocytes are unable to move on their own; the flowing plasma passively propels them. Red blood cells contain a protein known as *hemoglobin*, which gives them their reddish color. Hemoglobin carries oxygen from the lungs and to the tissues by binding to it.

> *Hemoglobin* An iron-containing protein within red blood cells that has the ability to combine with and carry oxygen.

Erythropoiesis is the ongoing process by which red blood cells are made. Red blood cells have a finite lifespan of 120 days. Those cells that are destined for destruction decompose in the spleen and other tissues that are rich in cells known as *macrophages*. Macrophages protect the body against infection. The body recycles some components of hemoglobin, such as the protein, globin, and iron. The part of hemoglobin that is not recycled is converted to bilirubin, which is a waste product that undergoes further metabolism in the liver. Normally, a chemical derivative of bilirubin, urobilinogen, is excreted in the stool and in the urine.

White Blood Cells

White blood cells are also known as leukocytes. There are several different types of white blood cells, and each has a different function. The primary function of all white blood cells is to fight infection. Antibodies to fight infection may be produced or leukocytes may directly attack and kill bacterial invaders. Most leukocytes are motile and leave the blood vessels by a process known as diapedesis to move toward the tissue where they are needed most.

Platelets and Blood Clotting

Platelets are small cells in the blood that are necessary for the series of chemical reactions that occur to form a clot. The blood clotting, or coagulation, process is a complex set of events involving platelets, clotting proteins in the plasma (clotting factors), other proteins, and calcium. The process begins with platelets clumping together. Then clotting proteins produced by the liver solidify the remainder of the clot, which eventually includes red and white blood cells.

Macrophages Cells that provide the body's first line of defense in the inflammatory process.
Platelets Small cells in the blood that are responsible for clot formation; also called thrombocytes.

Following injury to a blood vessel wall, a predictable series of events takes place, resulting in *hemostasis* (cessation of bleeding) and formation of the final blood clot. Chemicals released from the vessel wall cause local vasoconstriction, as well as activation of the platelets. The combination of vessel contraction and loose platelet aggregation forms a temporary "plug." Other factors released by the tissues, known as tissue thromboplastin, activate a cascade of clotting proteins. Eventually, *thrombin* is formed. This causes the conversion of fibrinogen to *fibrin*, which binds to the platelet plug, forming the final mature clot.

Hemostasis The body's natural blood-clotting mechanism.
Thrombin An enzyme that causes the conversion of fibrinogen to fibrin, which binds to the platelet plug, forming the final mature clot.
Fibrin A white insoluble protein formed in the clotting process; forms the fibrous component of a blood clot.

The Blood Vessels

The General Scheme of Blood Circulation

Blood is transported through the body via the *arteries*, which carry blood away from the heart, and *veins*, which carry blood back to the heart. Arteries become smaller as they get farther from the heart. Eventually, they branch into many small *arterioles* that divide even further into *capillaries*, which are microscopic, thin-walled blood vessels. Oxygen and nutrients pass out of the capillaries into the cells, and carbon dioxide and waste products pass from the cells into the capillaries in a process called diffusion.

Arteries The blood vessels that carry blood away from the heart.
Veins The blood vessels that transport unoxygenated blood back to the heart.
Arterioles The smallest branches of arteries leading to the vast network of capillaries.
Capillaries The tiny blood vessels between the arterioles and venules that permit transfer of oxygen, carbon dioxide, nutrients, and waste between body tissues and the blood.

Once oxygenated blood has been delivered by the capillaries, deoxygenated blood is returned to the heart, starting from the capillaries. The capillaries eventually enlarge to form *venules*, which merge and form veins. Eventually the veins empty into the heart, then the blood is sent to the lungs to be reoxygenated and returned to the heart where the process begins again.

Venules Very small, thin-walled vessels.

The walls of the blood vessels are composed of three layers of tissue **FIGURE 11-5**. The smooth, thin, inner lining is called the tunica intima, or endothelium. The middle layer, the tunica media, is composed of elastic tissue and smooth muscle cells that allow the vessels to expand or contract in response to the demands of the body. It is the thickest of the three tissue layers. The outer layer of tissue is called the tunica adventitia and consists of elastic and fibrous connective tissue.

Circulation to the Heart

The heart, like any other muscle, requires oxygen and nutrients. These are supplied via the *coronary arteries*, which arise from the aorta shortly after it leaves the left ventricle. The coronary circulation emanates from the left and right coronary arteries **FIGURE 11-6**.

Coronary arteries Arteries that arise from the aorta shortly after it leaves the left ventricle and supply the heart with oxygen and nutrients.

The right coronary artery divides into nine important branches: the conus branch, sinus node branch, right ventricular branch, atrial branch, acute marginal branch, AV node branch, posterior descending branch, left ventricular branch, and left atrial branch. Not all branches are always present in all people. These branches supply blood to the walls of the right atrium and ventricle, a portion of the inferior part of the left ventricle, and portions of the conduction system (the SA and AV nodes). When vessels to the conduction system fail to arise from the right coronary artery, they originate from the left side instead.

The left main coronary artery is the largest and shortest of the myocardial blood vessels. It rapidly divides into two branches, the *left anterior descending (LAD) artery* and the *circumflex coronary artery*. These arteries subdivide further, supplying blood to most of the left ventricle, the interventricular septum, and, at times, the AV node.

Left anterior descending (LAD) artery One of the two branches of the left main coronary artery that is the largest and shortest of the myocardial blood vessels; this vessel and the circumflex coronary arteries supply blood to the left ventricle and other areas.
Circumflex coronary artery The two branches of the left main coronary artery.

Pulmonary Circulation

Within the body, the *pulmonary circulation* carries blood from the right side of the heart to the lungs and back to

At the level of the capillary, waste products are exchanged and the blood is reoxygenated. The reoxygenated blood travels through venules into the pulmonary veins. The four pulmonary veins empty into the left atrium, two from each lung (see Figure 11-3).

> *Pulmonary circulation* The circulatory system in the body that carries blood from the right side of the heart to the lungs and back to the left side of the heart.
> *Systemic circulation* The portion of the circulatory system outside of the heart and lungs.

Systemic Arterial Circulation

Oxygenated blood leaves the heart through the aortic valve and passes into the aorta. From the aorta, blood is distributed to all parts of the body. All arteries of the body are derived from the aorta. The aorta is divided into three portions: the ascending aorta, the aortic arch, and the descending aorta.

The *ascending aorta* arises from the left ventricle and consists of only two branches, the right and left main coronary arteries **FIGURE 11-7**. The aorta then arches posteriorly and to the left, forming the *aortic arch*. Three major arteries arise from the aortic arch: the brachiocephalic (innominate) artery, the left common carotid artery, and the left subclavian artery.

> *Ascending aorta* The first of three portions of the aorta; originates from the left ventricle and gives rise to two branches, the right and left main coronary arteries.
> *Aortic arch* One of three described portions of the aorta; the section of the aorta between the ascending and descending portions that gives rise to the right brachiocephalic (innominate), left common carotid, and left subclavian arteries.

The *descending aorta* is the longest portion of the aorta and is subdivided into the thoracic aorta and the abdominal aorta. The descending aorta extends through the thorax and abdomen into the pelvis. In the pelvis, the descending aorta divides into the two common iliac arteries, which further divide into the internal and external iliac arteries.

> *Descending aorta* One of the three portions of the aorta, it is the longest portion and extends through the thorax and abdomen into the pelvis.

▌Pathophysiology

Chest pain or discomfort that is related to the heart usually stems from cardiac cell *ischemia*, which is decreased blood flow to the heart muscle. Because of a partial or complete blockage of blood flow through the coronary arteries, heart tissue fails to get enough oxygen and nutrients. The tissue soon begins to starve and, if blood flow is not restored, eventually dies. Ischemic heart disease, then, is

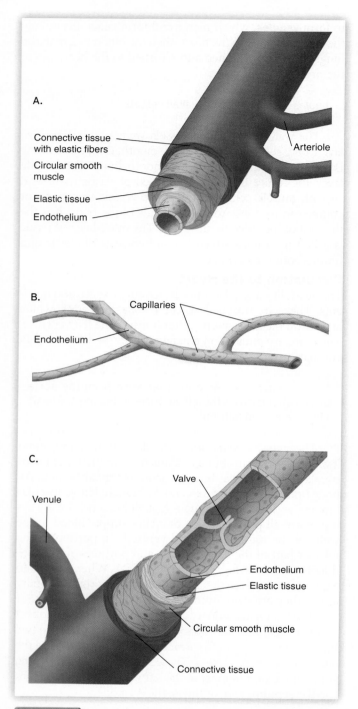

FIGURE 11-5 The walls of the blood vessels are composed of three layers of tissue: the endothelium, the elastic tissue, and the connective tissue. **A.** Artery. **B.** Capillary. **C.** Vein.

the left side of the heart, and the *systemic circulation* is responsible for blood flow to the rest of the body. Deoxygenated blood from the right ventricle is pumped through the pulmonic valve into the pulmonary artery. This artery rapidly divides into the right and left pulmonary arteries. These arteries transport the blood to the lungs. Inside the lungs, the arteries branch, becoming smaller and smaller.

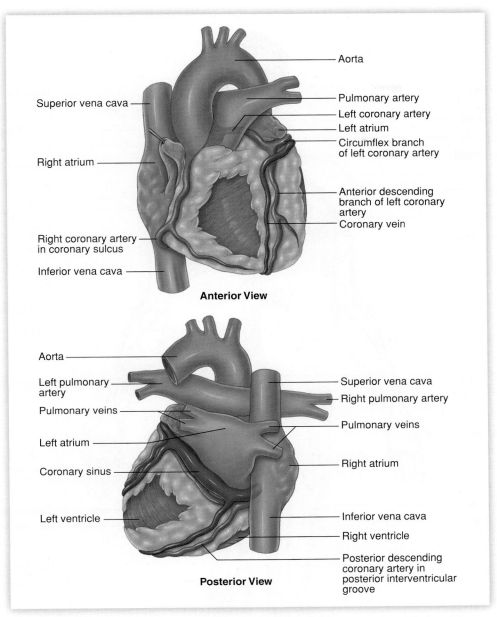

FIGURE 11-6 The coronary arteries supply oxygen and nutrients to the heart.

disease involving a decrease in blood flow to one or more portions of the heart muscle.

> *Ischemia* A lack of oxygen that deprives tissues of necessary nutrients, resulting from partial or complete blockage of blood flow; potentially reversible because permanent injury has not yet occurred.

Atherosclerosis

Most often, diminished blood flow to the myocardium is caused by coronary artery *atherosclerosis*. Atherosclerosis is a disorder in which a fatty material called cholesterol and other fatty substances build up and form a plaque inside the blood vessel walls, obstructing flow and interfering with their ability to dilate or contract. Eventually, atherosclerosis can cause complete occlusion, or blockage, of a coronary artery. Atherosclerosis usually involves other arteries of the body, as well.

> *Atherosclerosis* A disorder in which a fatty material called cholesterol and other fatty substances build up and form a plaque inside the blood vessel walls, obstructing flow and interfering with their ability to dilate or contract.

The problem begins when the first deposit of cholesterol is laid down on the inside of an artery. This may happen during the teenage years. As a person ages, more of this fatty

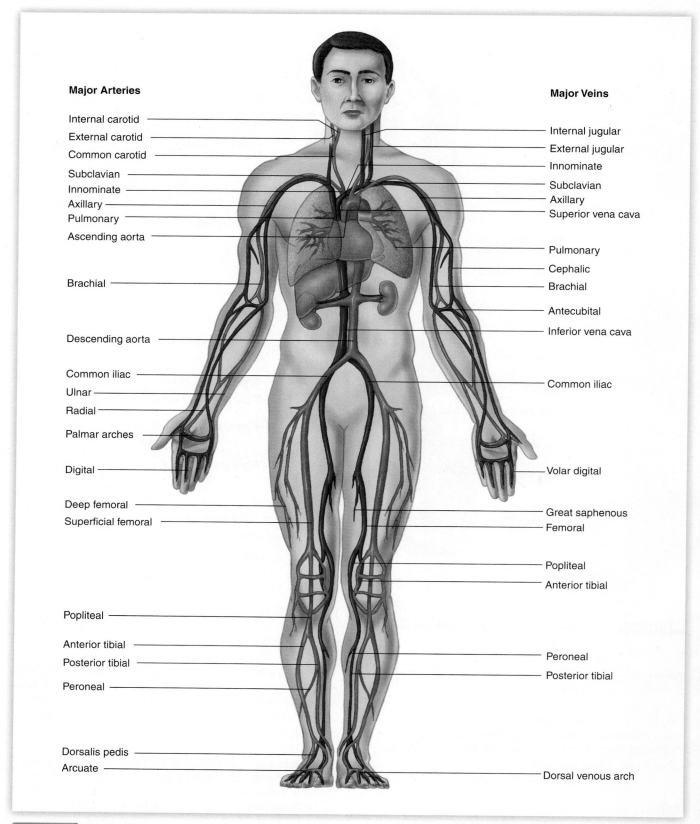

Major Arteries

Internal carotid
External carotid
Common carotid
Subclavian
Innominate
Axillary
Pulmonary
Ascending aorta

Brachial

Descending aorta

Common iliac
Ulnar
Radial
Palmar arches

Digital

Deep femoral
Superficial femoral

Popliteal

Anterior tibial
Posterior tibial

Peroneal

Dorsalis pedis
Arcuate

Major Veins

Internal jugular
External jugular
Innominate
Subclavian
Axillary
Superior vena cava

Pulmonary
Cephalic
Brachial

Antecubital

Inferior vena cava

Common iliac

Volar digital

Great saphenous
Femoral

Popliteal
Anterior tibial

Peroneal

Posterior tibial

Dorsal venous arch

FIGURE 11-7 The cardiovascular system. The systemic arterial circulation is noted in red, and the systemic venous system is noted in blue.

material is deposited; the lumen, or the inside diameter of the artery, narrows. As the cholesterol deposits grow, calcium deposits can form as well. The inner wall of the artery, which is normally smooth and elastic, becomes rough and brittle with these atherosclerotic plaques. Damage to the coronary arteries may become so extensive that they cannot accommodate increased blood flow at times of increased need, resulting in an inappropriate circulating volume.

Arteriosclerosis can also cause a reduction in blood flow. Arteriosclerosis is a thickening of the arterial walls, which causes a loss of elasticity (hardening of the arteries).

For reasons that are still not completely understood, a brittle plaque will sometimes develop a crack, exposing the inside of the atherosclerotic wall. Acting like a torn blood vessel, the jagged edge of the crack activates the blood clotting system, just as it does when an injury has caused bleeding. In this situation, however, the resulting blood clot will partially or completely block the lumen of the artery. If it does not occlude the artery at that location, the blood clot may break loose and begin floating in the blood, becoming what is known as a thromboembolism. A *thromboembolism* is a blood clot that floats through blood vessels until it reaches an area too narrow for it to pass, causing it to stop and block the blood flow at that point. Tissues downstream from the blood clot will experience a lack of oxygen (hypoxia). If blood flow is resumed in a short time, the hypoxic tissues will recover. However, if too much time goes by before blood flow is resumed, the tissues become necrotic, or die. If a blockage occurs in a coronary artery, the condition is known as an *acute myocardial infarction (AMI)*, a classic heart attack. Infarction means the death of tissue. The same sequence may also cause the death of cells in other organs, such as the brain. The death of heart muscle can lead to severe diminishment of the heart's ability to pump or cause it to stop completely (cardiac arrest).

> *Arteriosclerosis* A disease that is characterized by hardening, thickening, and calcification of the arterial walls.
> *Thromboembolism* A blood clot that has formed within a blood vessel and is floating within the bloodstream.
> *Acute myocardial infarction (AMI)* Heart attack; death of heart muscle following obstruction of blood flow to it. Acute in this context means "new" or "happening right now."

In the United States, coronary artery disease is the number one cause of death for men and women. The peak incidence of heart disease occurs between the ages of 40 and 70 years, but it can also strike teens and people in their 90s. You must be alert to the possibility that, although less likely, a 26-year-old person with chest pain could actually be having a heart attack, especially if he or she has a higher than usual risk.

Factors that place a person at higher risk for a myocardial infarction are called risk factors. The major controllable factors are cigarette smoking, high blood pressure, elevated cholesterol levels, an elevated blood glucose level (diabetes), lack of exercise, and stress. The major risk factors that cannot be controlled are older age, family history of atherosclerotic *coronary artery disease*, and male sex.

> *Coronary artery disease* The condition that results when atherosclerosis or arteriosclerosis is present in the arterial walls.

Acute Coronary Syndrome

Acute coronary syndrome (ACS) is the term used to describe any group of symptoms consistent with acute myocardial ischemia. Myocardial ischemia is a decrease in blood flow to the heart, which leads to chest pain through reduction of oxygen and nutrients to the tissues of the heart. This can be a temporary situation known as *angina pectoris*, or a more serious condition, such as an AMI. Because the signs and symptoms of these two conditions are very similar, they are treated basically the same under the designation of ACS.

> *Acute coronary syndrome (ACS)* A group of symptoms caused by myocardial ischemia that includes angina and myocardial infarction.

Angina Pectoris

Angina pectoris, or angina, is chest pain that occurs when heart tissues do not receive enough oxygen. Although angina can result from a spasm of the artery (also known as vasospastic angina or Prinzmetal's angina), it is most often a symptom of atherosclerotic coronary artery disease. Angina occurs when the heart's need for oxygen exceeds its supply, usually during periods of physical or emotional stress when the heart is working hard. A large meal or sudden fear may also trigger an attack. When the increased oxygen demand goes away (for example, the person stops exercising), the pain typically goes away.

> *Angina pectoris* Transient (short-lived) chest discomfort caused by partial or temporary blockage of blood flow to the heart muscle.

Transition Tip

Various changes in the walls of coronary arteries can result in certain disease states. Atherosclerosis is a disorder characterized by the formation of plaques of material, mostly lipids and cholesterol, on the intima of the artery. This process gradually narrows the lumen (opening or hollow part of the artery), resulting in a reduction in arterial blood flow. Arteriosclerosis is hardening of the arteries so they cannot compensate for atherosclerosis by dilating.

Angina pain is typically described as crushing, squeezing, or "like somebody standing on my chest." It is usually felt in the midchest, under the sternum (substernal). However, it can radiate to the jaw, the arms (frequently the left arm), the midback, or the epigastrium (the upper-middle region of the abdomen). The pain usually lasts from 3 to 8 minutes, rarely longer than 15 minutes. It may be associated with shortness of breath, nausea, or sweating. It disappears promptly with rest, supplemental oxygen, or nitroglycerin, all of which increase the supply of oxygen to the heart. Although angina pectoris is frightening, it does not mean that heart cells are dying; nor does it usually lead to death or permanent heart damage. It is, however, a warning that you and the patient should both take seriously. A single episode may be a precursor to a myocardial infarction. Even with angina, because oxygen supply to the heart is diminished, the electrical system can be compromised and the person is at risk for significant cardiac rhythm problems. Even though chest pain may dissipate, myocardial ischemia and injury can continue.

The first episode of angina is called initial angina. Angina is generally classified as stable or unstable. Stable angina occurs at a relatively fixed frequency and is usually relieved by rest and/or medication. Unstable angina occurs without a fixed frequency and may or may not be relieved by rest and/or medication. Progressive angina is stable or unstable angina that is accelerating in frequency and duration. Preinfarction angina presents with pain that occurs at rest when the patient is sitting or lying down. EMS usually becomes involved when stable angina becomes unstable, such as when a patient whose pain is normally relieved by sitting down and taking one nitroglycerin tablet has taken three tablets with no relief. Keep in mind that it can be very difficult even for physicians in hospitals to distinguish between the pain of angina and the pain of a myocardial infarction. For this reason, any complaint of chest pain should be treated as a myocardial infarction until proven otherwise.

Acute Myocardial Infarction

The pain of an AMI signals the actual death of cells in the area of the heart where blood flow is obstructed. Once dead, the cells cannot be revived. Instead, they will eventually turn to scar tissue and become a burden to the beating heart. This is why fast action is so critical in treating a heart attack. The sooner the blockage can be cleared, the fewer cells that may die. About 30 minutes after blood flow is cut off, some heart muscle cells begin to die. After about 2 hours, as many as half of the cells in the area can be dead; in most cases, after 4 to 6 hours, more than 90% of them will be dead. However, studies show that in many cases, opening the coronary artery with clot-busting medications, a class of medications called fibrinolytics, can prevent or minimize damage to the heart muscle if administered no later than 12 hours after the onset of symptoms. Angioplasty

or percutaneous coronary intervention (PCI), which is the mechanical clearing of the artery, has been shown to be the most effective treatment for a patient experiencing an AMI if performed promptly. Therefore, immediate treatment and transport to a hospital with cardiac catheterization capabilities is essential.

An AMI is more likely to occur in the larger, thick-walled left ventricle, which needs more blood and oxygen, than in the right ventricle.

A patient with an AMI may show any of the following signs and symptoms:

- Sudden onset of weakness, nausea, and sweating without an obvious cause
- Chest pain, discomfort, or pressure that is often crushing or squeezing and that does not change with each breath
- Pain, discomfort, or pressure in the lower jaw, arms, back, abdomen, or neck
- Irregular heartbeat and syncope (fainting)
- Shortness of breath, or dyspnea
- Pink, frothy sputum (indicating possible pulmonary edema)
- Sudden death

Transition Tip

The pain of an AMI differs from the pain of angina in three ways:

- It may or may not be caused by exertion but can occur at any time, sometimes when a person is sitting quietly or even sleeping.
- It does not resolve in a few minutes; rather, it can last between 30 minutes and several hours. It also increases in frequency and/or duration.
- It may or may not be relieved by rest or nitroglycerin.

The pain of AMI is typically felt just beneath the sternum and is variously described as heavy, squeezing, crushing, or tight. The pain may radiate to the arms (most often the left arm) and into the fingers; it may also radiate to the neck, jaw, upper back, or epigastrium. The pain of AMI is not influenced by coughing, deep breathing, or other body movements.

Not all patients who are having an AMI experience pain or recognize it when it occurs. In fact, about a third of patients never seek medical attention. This can be attributed, in part, to the fact that people are afraid of dying and do not wish to face the possibility that their symptoms may be serious. Middle-aged men, in particular, are likely to minimize or deny their symptoms. However, a few patients, particularly older people, women, and people with diabetes, do not experience any pain during an AMI but have other common complaints associated with ischemia.

This is often referred to as a "silent MI" because of the lack of pain. Others may feel only mild discomfort and call it indigestion. It is not uncommon for the only complaint, especially in older women, to be fatigue. Heart disease is the number one killer of women in the United States, and AEMTs should consider AMI even when the classic symptom of chest pain is not present. This is also true for elderly people and people with diabetes.

> **Transition Tip**
>
> More men have heart disease, but more women die of heart disease, in part because their symptoms are less clear-cut.

The physical findings of AMI vary, depending on the extent and severity of heart muscle damage. The following are common:

- **General appearance.** The patient often appears frightened. There may be nausea, vomiting, and a cold sweat. The skin is often pale or ashen gray because of poor cardiac output and loss of perfusion, or blood flow through the tissue. Occasionally, the skin will have a bluish tint, or cyanosis; this is the result of poor oxygenation of the circulating blood.
- **Pulse.** Generally, the pulse rate increases as a normal response to pain, stress, fear, or actual injury to the myocardium. Alternately, because dysrhythmias are common in an AMI, you may feel an irregularity or even a slowing of the pulse. The pulse may also be dependent on the area of the heart that has been affected by the AMI. Damage to the inferior area of the heart often presents with bradycardia.
- **Blood pressure.** Blood pressure may fall as a result of diminished cardiac output and diminished capability of the left ventricle to pump. However, most patients with an AMI will have a normal or, most likely, elevated blood pressure.
- **Respiration.** A complaint of breathing difficulty is common with cardiac compromise, so even if the rate seems normal, look at the work of breathing, and treat the patient as if respiratory compromise were present, especially in patients with a history of congestive heart failure.
- **Mental status.** Patients with AMIs sometimes experience an almost overwhelming feeling of impending doom. If a patient tells you, "I think I am going to die," pay attention.

An AMI can have three serious consequences:

- Sudden death
- Cardiogenic shock
- Congestive heart failure

Sudden Death

Approximately 40% of all patients with AMI never reach the hospital. Sudden death is usually the result of cardiac arrest, in which the heart fails to generate an effective blood flow. Although you cannot feel a pulse in someone experiencing cardiac arrest, there may still be electrical activity, though chaotic. The heart is using up energy without pumping. Such an abnormality of heart rhythm is a ventricular *dysrhythmia* (also called an *arrhythmia*), known as ventricular fibrillation.

> *Dysrhythmia* An irregular or abnormal heart rhythm.
> *Arrhythmia* An irregular or abnormal heart rhythm; also, absence of heart rhythm.

A variety of other lethal and nonlethal arrhythmias may follow an AMI, usually within the first hour. In most cases, it is premature ventricular contractions (PVCs), or extra beats from the damaged ventricle. PVCs by themselves are harmless and are common among healthy people, as well as in sick people. Other arrhythmias are much more dangerous **FIGURE 11-8**. These include the following:

- **Tachycardia:** Rapid beating of the heart, 100 beats/min or more
- **Bradycardia:** Unusually slow beating of the heart, 60 beats/min or fewer
- **Ventricular tachycardia (VT):** Rapid heart rhythm, usually at a rate of 150 to 200 beats/min. The electrical activity starts in the ventricle instead of the atrium. This rhythm usually does not allow adequate time between beats for the left ventricle to fill with blood. Therefore, the patient's blood pressure may fall. He or she may also feel weak or lightheaded or may even become unresponsive. In some cases, the patient may develop worsening chest pain or chest pain that was not there before onset of the arrhythmia. A string of three or more PVCs, back to back, can be called a "run of V-tach." Most cases of ventricular tachycardia will be more sustained and may deteriorate into ventricular fibrillation.
- **Ventricular fibrillation (VF):** Disorganized, ineffective quivering of the ventricles caused by unorganized electrical activity. No blood gets to the body, and the patient usually becomes unresponsive within seconds. The only way to treat this arrhythmia is to electrically defibrillate the heart. To defibrillate means to shock the heart with a specialized electrical current to stop all electrical activity in an attempt to restore a normal, rhythmic beat. By stopping the arrhythmia, it gives the conduction system the chance to resume its normal activity. Defibrillation is highly successful in terms of saving a life if delivered within a minute or two after the onset of ventricular fibrillation. If a defibrillator is not immediately available, CPR with compressions must be initiated

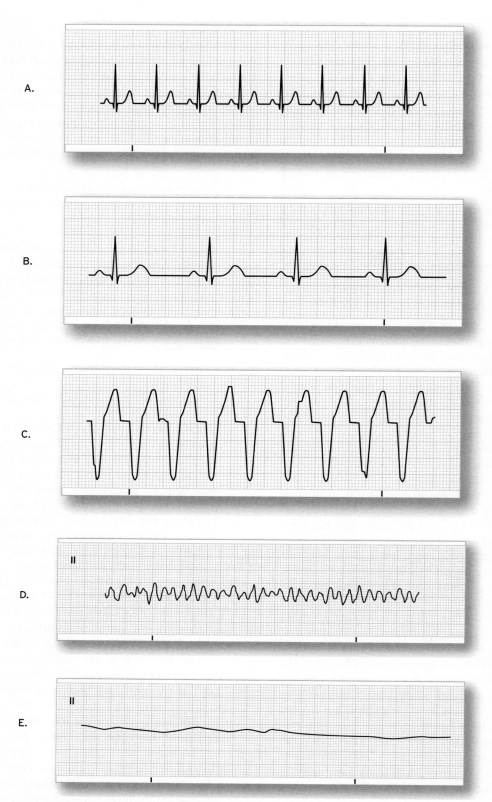

From *Arrhythmia Recognition: The Art of Interpretation*, courtesy of Tomas B. Garcia, MD

FIGURE 11-8 Common cardiac arrhythmias. **A.** Sinus tachycardia. **B.** Sinus bradycardia. **C.** Ventricular tachycardia (VT). **D.** Ventricular fibrillation (VF). **E.** Asystole.

to buy a few more minutes for arrival of an AED or manual defibrillator. Even if CPR is begun right at the time of collapse, chances of survival diminish each minute until defibrillation is accomplished.

If uncorrected, unstable ventricular tachycardia or ventricular fibrillation will eventually lead to *asystole*, the absence of all cardiac electrical and mechanical activity. Without CPR, this may occur within minutes. Because it reflects a long period of ischemia, nearly all patients you find in asystole will die.

> *Asystole* Complete absence of heart electrical activity.

Cardiogenic Shock

In *cardiogenic shock*, the problem is that the heart lacks enough power to force the proper volume of blood through the circulatory system. Cardiogenic shock can occur immediately or as late as 24 hours after the onset of an AMI. The various signs and symptoms of cardiogenic shock are produced by the improper functioning of the body's organs. The challenge for you is to recognize shock in its early stages, when treatment is likely to be more successful.

> *Cardiogenic shock* Shock caused by inadequate function of the heart, or pump failure.

Cardiogenic shock may be differentiated from hypovolemic shock by one or more of the following:

- Chief complaint (chest pain, dyspnea, tachycardia)
- Heart rate (bradycardia or excessive tachycardia)
- Signs and symptoms of congestive heart failure
- Arrhythmias

A patient with suspected cardiogenic shock should receive the same initial evaluation and treatment as any patient who is reporting chest pain. Pay particular attention to respiratory effort and the presence of peripheral or pulmonary edema. It is imperative to recognize the urgency of transport and to make sure the patient is taken to the closest, most appropriate facility.

A patient in cardiogenic shock may have the following signs and symptoms:

- Anxiety or restlessness as the brain becomes relatively starved for oxygen. The patient may report "air hunger." Think of the possibility of shock when the patient is yelling, "I can't breathe." The patient's brain is sensing that it is not getting enough oxygen.
- Pale, clammy skin. As the shock continues, the body shunts blood to the most important organs such as the brain and heart, and away from less important organs such as the skin.
- An increased pulse rate. As the shock gets worse, the body will attempt to compensate by increasing the amount of blood pumped through the heart. In

severe shock, the heart rate will often be more than 120 beats/min.

- Rapid and shallow breathing, nausea and vomiting, and a decrease in body temperature.
- Fall in blood pressure below normal. A systolic blood pressure of less than 90 mm Hg is easy to recognize, but it is a late finding that indicates decompensated shock. Do not assume that shock is not present just because the blood pressure is normal (compensated shock).

Take the following steps when treating patients with signs and symptoms of cardiogenic shock:

1. Position the patient comfortably. Most patients with heart failure will be more comfortable in the semi-Fowler's position; however, those with low blood pressure may not tolerate this position. These patients may be more comfortable and more alert in a supine position.
2. Administer high-flow oxygen.
3. Assist ventilations as necessary.
4. Cover the patient with sheets or blankets as indicated to preserve body heat. Be sure to cover the patient's head in cold weather; this is where the most heat is lost.
5. Gain IV access, and give a fluid bolus of 20 mL/kg of an isotonic crystalloid solution if the patient is hypotensive. Monitor breath sounds for the development of pulmonary edema.
6. Provide prompt transport to the closest, most appropriate emergency department.

Congestive Heart Failure

Failure of the heart occurs when the ventricular myocardium is so damaged that it can no longer keep up with the return flow of blood from the atria. *Congestive heart failure (CHF)* can occur any time after a myocardial infarction, heart valve damage, or longstanding high blood pressure, but it usually happens between the first few hours and the first few days after an AMI.

> *Congestive heart failure (CHF)* A disorder in which the heart loses part of its ability to effectively pump blood, usually as a result of damage to the heart muscle and usually resulting in a backup of fluid into the lungs.

Just as the pumping function of the left ventricle can be damaged by coronary artery disease, it can also be damaged by diseased heart valves or chronic hypertension. In any of these cases, when the myocardium can no longer contract effectively, the heart tries other ways to maintain an adequate cardiac output. Two specific changes in heart function occur: the heart rate increases and the left ventricle enlarges in an effort to increase the amount of blood pumped each minute.

When these adaptations can no longer make up for the decreased heart function, CHF eventually develops. It is called congestive heart failure because the lungs become congested with fluid once the heart fails to pump the blood effectively. Blood tends to back up in the pulmonary veins, increasing the pressure in the capillaries of the lungs. When the pressure in the capillaries exceeds a certain level, fluid (mostly water) passes through the walls of the capillary vessels and into the alveoli. This condition is called pulmonary edema. It may occur suddenly, as in an AMI, or slowly over months, as in chronic CHF. Sometimes in patients with an acute onset of CHF, severe pulmonary edema will develop, in which the patient has pink, frothy sputum and severe dyspnea.

If the right side of the heart is damaged, fluid collects in the body, often showing up as swelling in the feet and legs. The collection of fluid in the part of the body that is closest to the ground is called *dependent edema* (which may be in the sacral area of the back in a bedridden patient). *Pedal edema* is swelling specifically in the feet and legs. The swelling causes relatively few symptoms other than discomfort. However, chronic pedal edema may indicate underlying heart disease (right-sided heart failure) even in the absence of pain or other symptoms.

> **Dependent edema** Swelling in the part of the body closest to the ground or the most dependent portion, caused by collection of fluid in the tissues (typically in the sacral area in a bedridden patient); a possible sign of congestive heart failure.
>
> **Pedal edema** Swelling of the feet and ankles caused by collection of fluid in the tissues; a possible sign of congestive heart failure.

The following signs and symptoms may be present in a patient with CHF:

- Orthopnea. The patient finds it easier to breathe when sitting up. When the patient is lying down, more blood is returned to the right ventricle and lungs, causing further pulmonary congestion and shortness of breath.
- Mild or severe agitation
- Chest pain (may or may not be present)
- Distended neck veins that do not collapse even when the patient is sitting
- Swollen ankles from pedal edema. If the patient is bedridden, the edema may be seen in the sacral area.
- Hypertension, tachycardia, and tachypnea
- Use of accessory breathing muscles of the neck and ribs, reflecting the additional hard work of breathing
- Rales caused by fluid surrounding small airways, heard by listening to either side of the patient's chest, about midway down the back. In severe CHF, these soft sounds can be heard even at the top (apex) of the lung.

- A productive cough, or you may note the presence of pink, frothy sputum
- A delayed capillary refill time. With damage to the myocardium, the pumping mechanism is effectively reduced; therefore, there is a lack of perfusion in the extremities, causing delayed capillary refill time.

Treat a patient with CHF the same way as a patient with chest pain:

1. Take the vital signs, monitor heart rhythm, and administer oxygen by a nonrebreathing face mask with an oxygen flow of 10 to 15 L/min, ventilating if needed. Continuous positive airway pressure (CPAP) therapy may also be beneficial for patients who meet the requirements.
2. Allow the patient to remain sitting in an upright position with the legs down.
3. Gain IV access. Before giving any medication, you need to gain IV access. You may also give fluid if the patient becomes hypotensive.
4. Be reassuring; many patients with CHF are quite anxious because they cannot breathe.
5. Patients who have had problems with CHF before will usually have specific medications for its treatment. Gather these medications and take them along to the hospital.
6. Nitroglycerin may be of value if the patient's systolic blood pressure is above 100 mm Hg. If the patient has prescribed nitroglycerin and medical control advises you to do so, you can administer it sublingually.
7. Provide prompt transport to the closest, most appropriate emergency department.

Pulmonary Edema

Pulmonary edema is a common complication of myocardial ischemia that may or may not be the result of an AMI. Without treatment, pulmonary edema can lead to acute respiratory failure and death. Precipitating causes include heart failure (primarily left-sided), myocardial infarction, pulmonary embolism, hypertension, and cardiomegaly (enlarged heart).

Preload and afterload can greatly influence the buildup of pulmonary edema. As the left ventricle loses its ability to pump effectively, blood backs up into the pulmonary veins and subsequently into the lungs. This increased pressure causes fluid to leak from the capillaries into the interstitial tissue and the alveoli. This is common in CHF because the loss of contractile ability results in fluid overload. Pulmonary edema may be acute, as the result of an AMI, or may be chronic as a result of multiple events or chronic CHF.

Treatment is focused on maintaining the airway, breathing, and circulation, and in transporting the patient for definitive care. Obtain a thorough history from the patient and provide psychological support en route.

Hypertensive Emergencies

Aortic/Dissecting Aneurysm

An *aortic aneurysm* is a weakness in the wall of the aorta. The aorta dilates at the weakened area, which makes it susceptible to rupture. A *dissecting aneurysm* occurs when the inner layers of the aorta become separated, allowing blood (at high pressures) to flow between the layers.

Uncontrolled hypertension is the primary cause of dissecting aortic aneurysms. This separation of layers weakens the wall of the aorta significantly, making it more likely to be ruptured under conditions of continued high blood pressure. If the aorta ruptures, the amount of internal blood loss will be so large that the patient will die rapidly. Aortic aneurysms can occur in either the thrice or abdominal portion of the aorta, and symptoms will vary depending on the location. The signs and symptoms of a dissecting thoracic aortic aneurysm include very sudden chest pain located in the anterior part of the chest or in the back between the shoulder blades. It may be difficult to differentiate the chest pain of a dissecting thoracic aortic aneurysm from that of an AMI, but a number of distinctive features may help. The pain from an AMI is often preceded by other symptoms—nausea, indigestion, weakness, and sweating—and tends to come on gradually, getting more severe with time and often described as "pressure" rather than "stabbing."

By contrast, the pain of a dissecting thoracic aortic aneurysm usually comes on full force from one minute to the next with a description more consistent of "a tearing, burning sensation" originating in back or scapular area and radiating interiorly; some cases originate in front and radiate posteriorly. A patient with a dissecting thoracic aortic aneurysm also may exhibit a difference in blood pressure between the arms or diminished pulses in the lower extremities. Thoracic aortic aneurysms are almost impossible to diagnose in the prehospital setting, but you must consider them a possibility in any patient with significant hypertension. Transport the patient without delay.

> *Aortic aneurysm* A weakness in the wall of the aorta that makes it susceptible to rupture.
> *Dissecting aneurysm* A condition in which the inner layers of an artery such as the aorta become separated, allowing blood (at high pressures) to flow between the layers.

Patient Assessment of Cardiovascular Emergencies

When you are called to a scene where a patient's chief complaint is chest pain, complete a thorough assessment. Any complaint of chest pain or discomfort or other symptoms suggestive of a cardiac etiology is a serious matter. In fact, the best thing you can do is to assume the worst.

It is imperative that you recognize a sense of urgency for reperfusion when the patient receives no relief with medications or presents with hypotension or signs of hypoperfusion. Throughout the call, provide emotional support for the patient and an explanation for the family or significant others.

Scene Size-up

Do not let your guard down on medical calls. Always ensure that the scene is safe for you, your partner, your patient, and bystanders. For patients with cardiac problems, the clues often include a report of chest pain, difficulty breathing, or sudden loss of consciousness. Once you establish a preliminary nature of illness, you will be able to guide your assessment to find the important information much more effectively. Just remember not to become fixated on a specific condition at this early point in the assessment; sometimes the situation turns out to be very different from how it initially appeared.

Primary Assessment

As you approach the patient, form a general impression of his or her condition to recognize and address life threats. You will likely begin by determining whether the patient is responsive. Perform a rapid scan of the patient.

If the patient is not responsive, not breathing, and does not have a pulse, begin CPR starting with chest compressions. Consider use of an AED. Call for paramedic backup if needed.

If the patient is responsive, the airway will most likely be patent. Responsive patients should be able to maintain their own airway. Some episodes of cardiac compromise may produce dizziness or even fainting spells (syncope). If dizziness or fainting has occurred, consider the possibility of a spinal injury from a fall.

Assess the patient's breathing to determine whether it is adequate to provide enough oxygen to an ailing heart. Determine the rate, quality, and degree of distress. Listen for abnormal breath sounds at this time because these can also be important indicators of respiratory distress. Breath sounds may be affected by the presence of fluid buildup. Auscultate for rales or congestion indicative of pulmonary edema. Some patients feel short of breath even though there are no obvious signs of respiratory distress. In either situation, apply oxygen with a nonrebreathing mask at 10 to 15 L/min. If the patient is not breathing or has inadequate breathing, ensure adequate ventilations with a bag-mask device and 100% oxygen.

If available, consider the use of CPAP when needed. For example, patients experiencing pulmonary edema may require positive-pressure ventilation with a bag-mask device or CPAP. CPAP is the most effective way to assist a person with CHF to breathe effectively and to avoid the need for intubation and mechanical ventilation. You should be aware of the indications and contraindications of CPAP and be competent in using this equipment.

Determine the rate and quality of the patient's pulse. If you find abnormalities in the pulse, you should be more suspicious. Alterations in heart rate and rhythm may occur, although peripheral pulses are usually not affected.

Assess the patient's skin condition, color, moisture, and temperature, as well as the capillary refill time. The patient may present with pallor during the episode, and diaphoresis is usually present. Assess blood pressure. Blood pressure may be elevated during the episode and normalize afterwards and temperature may vary. Changes in perfusion may indicate more serious cardiac compromise. Begin treatment for cardiogenic shock early to reduce the workload of the heart. Place the patient in a comfortable position, usually sitting up and well supported.

As a general rule, patients with cardiac problems should be transported in the most gentle, stress-relieving manner possible. Very little time is saved by using the lights and siren, but you can do a lot to calm your patient and reduce the release of heart-damaging adrenaline. Limit patient exertion.

Your decision as to where to transport the patient will depend on your local protocol. Patients are generally transported to the closest appropriate facility. Some medical directors have written protocols requiring patients with suspected cardiac emergencies to be transported to medical centers with certain capabilities such as emergency angioplasty. Others require the patient to be transported to the nearest facility for stabilization before transporting to a specialty hospital. Be sure you know your local protocol.

History Taking

Remember that not all patients experiencing an AMI have the same signs and symptoms. A chief complaint of chest pain or discomfort, shortness of breath, or dizziness should be taken seriously. Many patients who suspect that something is wrong experience restlessness, appear anxious, and perhaps have a sense of impending doom. Patients often have a good idea about what is happening, so do not offer false reassurance. Begin by asking questions about the current situation. Determine whether the patient is experiencing chest pain or discomfort and whether there are any other signs and symptoms. Ask the patient about recurring events along with any increase in frequency and/or duration of an event. Remember that typical angina has a sudden onset of discomfort that is generally of brief duration, lasting only 3 to 5 minutes, not 30 minutes to 2 hours, and is usually relieved by rest and/or medication.

If the patient is experiencing dyspnea, find out whether it is related to exertion and whether it is related to the patient's position. Also determine whether the dyspnea is continuous or if it changes, especially with deep breathing. Note whether the patient has a productive cough. Ask about other signs and symptoms commonly found such as nausea and vomiting, fatigue, headache, and palpitations (a feeling of the heart skipping a beat or racing). Make sure to ask about any trauma the patient might have experienced during the last few days. Be sure to record your findings, including those that are negative (known as pertinent negatives).

If the patient is responsive, begin obtaining the SAMPLE history and asking the following questions specific to a cardiovascular emergency:

- Have you ever had a heart attack?
- Have you been told that you have heart problems?
  - Have you ever been diagnosed with angina, heart failure, or heart valve disease?
  - Have you ever had high blood pressure?
  - Have you ever been diagnosed with an aneurysm?
  - Do you have any respiratory diseases such as emphysema or chronic bronchitis?
- Do you have diabetes or have you ever had any problems with your blood sugar?
- Have you ever had kidney disease?
- Do you have any risk factors for coronary artery disease, such as smoking, high blood pressure, or high-stress lifestyle?
  - Is there a family history of heart disease?
  - Do you currently take any medications?

Determine whether the patient has taken nitroglycerin, aspirin, or any other medications before your arrival. If the patient has had a heart attack or angina before, ask whether the pain is similar.

Make sure to ask about medication allergies. If the patient is taking medications, determine whether they are prescribed, over-the-counter, and/or recreational drugs. Even when a patient may not be able to articulate his or her exact medical condition, knowing the patient's medications may give you important clues. For example, a patient may say he has heart problems. You see that he is taking furosemide (Lasix), digoxin, and amiodarone (Cordarone). Furosemide is a diuretic, digoxin increases the strength of heart contractions, and amiodarone controls certain types of dysrhythmias. These drugs are most often prescribed together for patients with CHF and may alert you to carefully evaluate the lungs for the presence of rales or crackles, which indicate fluid in the lungs and a need to increase the amount of oxygen being delivered.

Be sure to include the OPQRST-I questions when you are obtaining the symptoms as part of the SAMPLE history. Using OPQRST-I helps you to understand the details of specific complaints, such as chest pain.

Secondary Assessment

A physical examination of a patient with chest pain would focus primarily on the cardiovascular and respiratory systems. These two systems are closely related, and some problems with the respiratory system can be caused by cardiovascular issues. Assess the patient's circulation by assessing pulses at various locations. Compare the strength of the carotid to the radial. Assess skin color, temperature, and condition. Is the skin cool or moist? In addition to the cardiovascular system, examine the respiratory system for signs of inadequate ventilation. Auscultate breath sounds for depth, equality, and any adventitious sounds such as crackles or wheezing. Listen for gurgling, and look for blood-tinged or foamy froth from the mouth and/or nose. Wet-sounding lungs indicate fluid is being moved into the lungs from the circulatory system, possibly because of a problem with the heart. Are the breath sounds equal? Are the neck veins distended? Is the trachea deviated or is it midline? The answers to these questions can help determine whether a problem exists with the lungs or with the heart. Measure and record the patient's vital signs at appropriate intervals—every 5 minutes for unstable patients and every 15 minutes for stable patients.

If available, use pulse oximetry. Pulse oximetry may not give an accurate measurement if the patient has poor circulation, has been exposed to a toxic chemical, or is in cardiac arrest, but it should be used and the readings noted for all patients with possible cardiac problems. Assess blood glucose levels.

Reassessment

Repeat the primary assessment by checking to see whether the patient's chief complaint and condition have improved or are deteriorating. Vital signs should be reassessed at least every 5 minutes or any time significant changes in the patient's condition occur. It is essential to monitor the patient with a suspected AMI closely because sudden cardiac arrest is always a risk. If cardiac arrest occurs, you must be ready to begin automated defibrillation or chest compressions immediately. If an AED is immediately available, use it; if not, perform CPR until the AED is available. Reassess your interventions to see whether they are helping and whether the patient's condition is improving. Reassessment will also determine whether further interventions are indicated or contraindicated.

Emergency Care of Cardiovascular Conditions

Your treatment of the patient begins with proper positioning. As mentioned before, some patients will not tolerate being positioned supine, so they should be allowed to sit up (leaning back on the stretcher). Also loosen tight clothing to try to make the patient as comfortable as possible.

You should be giving the patient oxygen by this time, but if you are not, then you should do it now. For patients with mild dyspnea, a nasal cannula may be all that is needed, whereas patients with more serious respiratory difficulty will respond better to a nonrebreathing mask. A patient who is unresponsive or in obvious respiratory distress may need assistance with breathing. Use a bag-mask device or a positive-pressure ventilation device such as positive end-expiratory pressure, CPAP, bilevel positive airway pressure, or a manual or automatic transport ventilator if available and you have been approved to use one of these methods in your service.

Gain IV access. A saline lock is sufficient unless the patient is hypotensive. If so, consider a 20 mL/kg bolus of an isotonic crystalloid solution such as normal saline.

Depending on local protocol, prepare to administer aspirin and assist with prescribed nitroglycerin. Aspirin (acetylsalicylic acid) prevents clots from forming or becoming larger. Administer aspirin according to local protocol. Low-dose aspirin comes in 81 mg chewable tablets. The recommended dose is 162 mg (two tablets) to 324 mg (four tablets). Be sure you have verified that the patient is not allergic to aspirin before you give it. Also, ask the patient if he or she has any history of internal bleeding such as stomach ulcers, and, if so, contact medical control before giving the patient aspirin.

Nitroglycerin helps to relieve the pain of angina by relaxing the muscle of blood vessel walls, dilating coronary arteries, increasing blood flow and the supply of oxygen to the heart muscle, and decreasing the workload of the heart. Nitroglycerin also dilates blood vessels in other parts of the body and can sometimes cause hypotension and/or a severe headache. Other side effects include changes in the patient's pulse rate, including tachycardia or bradycardia. For this reason, you should take the patient's blood pressure within 5 minutes after each dose. If the patient is hypertensive, do not give more nitroglycerin. Other contraindications include the presence of a head injury, use of erectile dysfunction drugs within the previous 24 hours, and if the maximum prescribed dose has already been given (usually three doses). If the patient has a nitroglycerin patch on when you arrive, be sure to carefully remove it if the patient is hypotensive or in cardiac arrest (before use of AED).

After you obtain permission from medical control, administer prescribed nitroglycerin to the patient. Nitroglycerin works in most patients within 5 minutes. Most patients who have been prescribed nitroglycerin carry a supply with them. Patients take one dose of nitroglycerin under the tongue whenever they have an episode of angina that does not immediately go away with rest. If the pain is still present after 5 minutes, patients are typically instructed by their physicians to take two subsequent doses as needed, up to a total of three doses. Follow local protocols for administration of additional doses of nitroglycerin.

Early, prompt transport to the emergency department is critical so that treatments such as clot-busting medications or angioplasty can be initiated. To be most effective, these treatments must be started as soon as possible after the onset of the attack. Therefore, alert the emergency department about the status of your patient and your estimated time of arrival. Do not delay transport to assist with administration of nitroglycerin. The drug can be given en route.

Cardiac Arrest

Cardiac arrest may be the result of trauma or numerous medical conditions, such as end-stage renal disease, hyperkalemia with renal disease, or hypothermia, among others. Cardiac arrest is the cessation of functional cardiac activity—electrical, mechanical, or both. It is identified in the field by the absence of a carotid pulse.

Emergency Medical Care for Cardiac Arrest

When dispatch reports an unresponsive patient with CPR being performed, the AED is probably one of the first pieces of equipment you will obtain from the ambulance. As the operator of the AED, you are responsible for making sure that the electricity injures no one, including yourself. Remote defibrillation using pads allows you to distance yourself safely from the patient. As long as you place the pads in the correct position and make sure no one is touching the patient, you should be safe. Be sure to consult local protocols for issues such as pad placement and preparation of the pad site.

If a defibrillator is not readily available, initiate CPR beginning with chest compressions and try to obtain as much history as possible. In a witnessed event, a precordial thump can potentially work like a very low powered defibrillator. Provide a single blow to the center of the sternum with the heel of a closed fist. This should be a solid strike originating no farther than 6 to 12 inches above the patient's chest. However, this should be used only if you actually witness the arrest, if an AED is not immediately available, and only tried once. If you are in a tiered system and the patient is in cardiac arrest, call for ALS assistance.

Indications for not initiating resuscitative techniques include rigor mortis, dependent lividity, and decapitation. Local protocols may also dictate other circumstances such as advance directives (that is, living wills) and do not resuscitate (DNR) orders.

Performing Defibrillation

Prepare with standard precautions en route to the scene. On arrival at the scene, make sure that the scene is safe for you and your partner to enter. Ask any bystanders or first responders who are performing CPR to continue while you apply the AED and prepare to defibrillate the patient, if needed. Take the following steps to use the AED **SKILL DRILL 11-1**:

1 Assess responsiveness while continuing to perform CPR if it is already in progress (it is important to limit the amount of time compressions are interrupted). If the patient is responsive, do not apply the AED.

2 If the patient is unresponsive and CPR has not been started yet, begin providing chest compressions and rescue breaths at a ratio of 30 compressions to two breaths, continuing until an AED arrives and it is ready for use (**Step 1**). It is important to start chest compressions and use the AED as soon as possible. Compressions provide vital blood flow to the heart and brain, improving the patient's chance of survival.

3 Turn on the AED. Remove clothing from the patient's chest area. Apply the AED pads to the chest: one just to the right of the breastbone (sternum) just below the collarbone (clavicle), the other on the left lower chest area with the top of the pad 2 to 3 inches below the armpit. Do not place the pads on top of breast tissue. If necessary, lift the breast out of the way and place the pad underneath. Ensure that the pads are attached to the patient cables (and that they are attached to the AED in some models). Plug in the pad's connector to the AED.

4 Stop CPR (**Step 2**).

5 State aloud, "Clear the patient," and ensure that no one is touching the patient.

6 Push the *Analyze* button if there is one, and wait for the AED to determine whether a shockable rhythm is present.

7 If a shock is not advised, perform five cycles (about 2 minutes) of CPR beginning with chest compressions and then reanalyze the cardiac rhythm. If a shock is advised, reconfirm that no one is touching the patient and push the *Shock* button.

8 After the shock is delivered, immediately resume CPR, beginning with chest compressions (**Step 3**).

9 After five cycles (about 2 minutes) of CPR, reanalyze the cardiac rhythm (**Step 4**). Do not interrupt chest compressions for more than 10 seconds.

10 If the AED advises a shock, clear the patient, push the *Shock* button, and immediately resume CPR compressions. If no shock is advised, immediately resume CPR, beginning with chest compressions.

11 Gather additional information about the arrest event.

12 After five cycles (2 minutes) of CPR, reanalyze the cardiac rhythm.

13 Repeat the cycle of 2 minutes of CPR, one shock (if indicated), and 2 minutes of CPR.

14 Transport, and contact medical control as needed (**Step 5**).

If the AED advises no shock and the patient has a pulse, check the patient's breathing. If the patient is breathing adequately, administer 100% oxygen via a nonrebreathing mask and transport. If the patient is not breathing adequately, provide artificial ventilation with a bag-mask device or pocket mask device attached to 100% oxygen and transport. Ensure that proper airway techniques are used at all times.

If the patient has no pulse, perform five cycles (approximately 2 minutes) of CPR beginning with chest compressions. After 2 minutes of CPR, reassess the patient's pulse and reanalyze the patient's cardiac rhythm. If the AED advises a shock, deliver one shock followed immediately by CPR, beginning with chest compressions. Repeat these steps if needed.

SKILL DRILL 11-1

AED and CPR

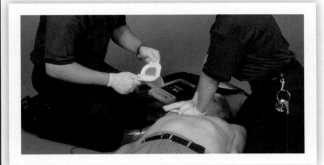

1 Assess responsiveness while continuing to perform CPR if it is already in progress. If the patient is unresponsive and CPR has not been started yet, begin providing chest compressions and rescue breaths at a ratio of 30 compressions to two breaths, continuing until an AED arrives and is ready for use.

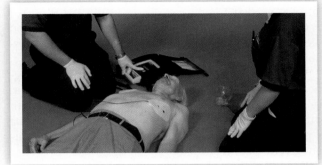

2 Turn on the AED. Apply the AED pads to the chest and attach the pads to the AED. Stop CPR.

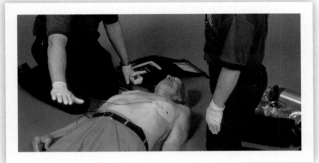

3 Verbally and visually clear the patient. Push the *Analyze* button, if there is one. Wait for the AED to analyze the cardiac rhythm. If no shock is advised, perform five cycles (2 minutes) of CPR and then reassess the cardiac rhythm. If a shock is advised, recheck that all are clear, and push the *Shock* button. After the shock is delivered, immediately resume CPR beginning with chest compressions.

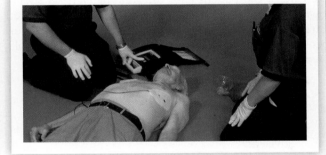

4 After five cycles (2 minutes) of CPR, reanalyze the cardiac rhythm. Do not interrupt chest compressions for more than 10 seconds.

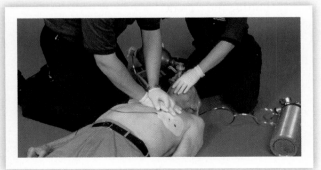

5 If shock is advised, clear the patient, push the *Shock* button, and immediately resume CPR compressions. If no shock is advised, immediately resume CPR compressions. After five cycles (2 minutes) of CPR, reanalyze the cardiac rhythm. Repeat the cycle of five cycles (2 minutes) of CPR, one shock (if indicated), and 2 minutes of CPR. Transport, and contact medical control as needed.

If the patient has no pulse and the AED advises no shock, perform five cycles (approximately 2 minutes) of CPR beginning with chest compressions. After five cycles (2 minutes) of CPR, reassess the patient's pulse, and reanalyze the patient's cardiac rhythm. If no shock is advised, continue CPR. Transport the patient, and contact medical control as needed.

Gain IV access, and initiate fluid therapy based on patient status. Give a 20 mL/kg bolus of an isotonic crystalloid solution if hypovolemia is suspected.

Provide psychological support for the family and significant others. On arrival at the emergency department, give a full report to the attending staff, including length of time since resuscitation efforts were initiated, how long the patient was "down" before EMS arrival, and any treatment given.

It is imperative to assess the glucose level of any patient with an altered mental status. This includes those in cardiac arrest. If a glucose level cannot be obtained, consider administration of $D_{50}W$. Contact medical control or follow local protocols.

Patient Care After Automated External Defibrillator Shocks

The care of the patient after the AED delivers its shock depends on your location and the EMS system; therefore, you should follow your local protocols. After the AED protocol is completed, the patient will have had one of the following occur:

- Pulse is regained.
- No pulse, and the AED indicates that no shock is advised.
- No pulse, and the AED indicates that a shock is advised.

Commonly, patients who are successfully defibrillated by an AED will develop a normal heart rhythm for a while. However, because the heart still is not receiving optimal amounts of oxygen, ventricular fibrillation will often recur.

Patients who do not regain a pulse on the scene of the cardiac arrest usually do not survive. Follow your EMS system's protocols to determine the patient's treatment. If paramedics are not responding to the scene, you should begin transport, if local protocols allow, when one of the following occurs:

- The patient regains a pulse.
- Six to nine shocks are delivered (or as directed by local protocol).
- The machine gives three consecutive messages (separated by 2 minutes of CPR) that no shock is advised (or as directed by local protocol).

If you transport a patient while performing CPR, you need a plan for managing the patient in the ambulance. Ideally, you should have two EMS providers in the patient compartment while a third provider drives. You may deliver additional shocks at the scene or en route with the approval of medical control. *Keep in mind that AEDs cannot analyze rhythm while the vehicle is in motion;* nor is it as safe to defibrillate in a moving ambulance. Therefore, you should come to a complete stop if more shocks are needed. Be sure to memorize the protocol of your EMS service **FIGURE 11-9**.

Cardiac Arrest During Transport

If you are traveling to the hospital with an unresponsive patient, check the pulse at least every 30 seconds. If a pulse is not present, take the following steps:

1. Stop the vehicle.
2. If the AED is not immediately ready, perform CPR, beginning with chest compressions, until it is available.
3. Analyze the rhythm.
4. Deliver one shock if indicated and immediately resume CPR.
5. Continue resuscitation according to your local protocol.

If you are en route with a conscious adult patient who is having chest pain and becomes unresponsive, take the following steps:

1. Check for a pulse.
2. Stop the vehicle.
3. If the AED is not immediately ready, perform CPR beginning with chest compressions, until it is ready.
4. Analyze the rhythm.
5. Deliver one shock if indicated and immediately begin CPR.
6. Begin compressions and continue resuscitation according to your local protocol, including transporting the patient.

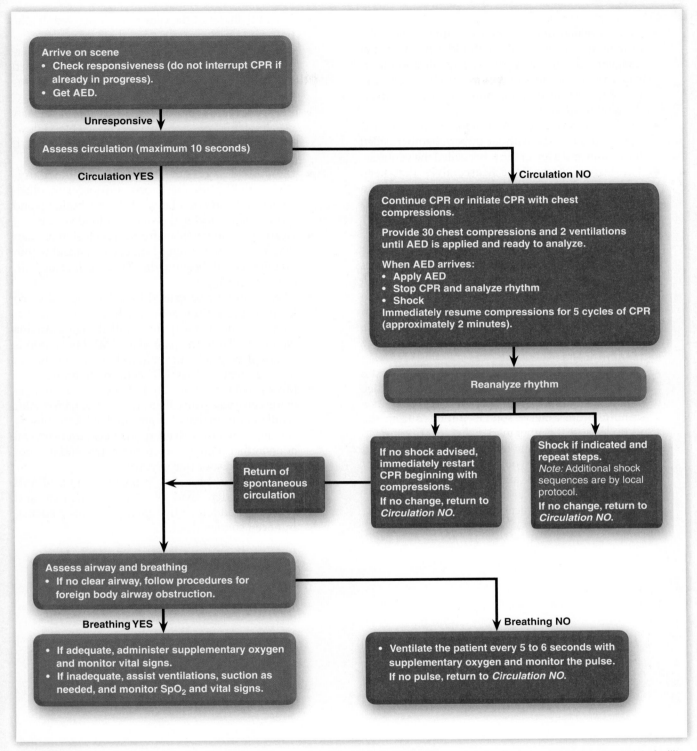

FIGURE 11-9 AED algorithm. Follow procedures for return of spontaneous circulation for your region (ie, transport to the appropriate facility; monitor ETCO$_2$ and vital signs; consider hypothermia; consider obtaining a 12-lead ECG; etc.).

PREP KIT

Ready for Review

- Cardiovascular diseases are the number one killer of men and women. Although older people are at a higher risk, such a sweeping generalization overlooks a large number of younger people. For these reasons, early recognition and early treatment are the keys to survival.

- The heart is divided down the middle into two sides, right and left, each with an upper chamber called the atrium and a lower chamber called the ventricle.

- The largest of the four heart valves that keep blood moving through the circulatory system in the proper direction is the aortic valve, which lies between the left ventricle and the aorta, the body's main artery.

- The heart's electrical conduction system controls heart rate and helps to keep the atria and ventricles working together. The mechanical pumping action of the heart can occur only in response to an electrical stimulus. The electrical conduction system consists of the SA node, the AV node, the bundle of His, the right and left bundle branches, and the Purkinje fibers.

- Cardiac muscle cells have a special characteristic called automaticity. Automaticity allows a cardiac muscle cell to contract spontaneously without a stimulus from a nerve source. Impulses from the SA node cause the other myocardial cells to contract.

- Regulation of heart function is provided by the brain via the autonomic nervous system, the hormones of the endocrine system, and the heart tissue. Baroreceptors and chemoreceptors sense abnormalities in the pressure and chemical composition of the blood.

- The two phases of the cardiac cycle are systole, the pumping phase, and diastole, the resting phase.

- During periods of exertion or stress, the myocardium requires more oxygen. This is accomplished by dilation of the coronary arteries, which increases blood flow.

- Chest pain or discomfort that is related to the heart usually stems from ischemia (decreased blood flow) to the heart. The tissue soon begins to starve and, if blood flow is not restored, eventually dies.

- Diminished blood flow to the myocardium is usually caused by atherosclerosis, a disorder in which cholesterol and other fatty substances build up and form a plaque inside the walls of blood vessels.

- Heart tissue downstream from an occlusion of a cardiac artery suffers from a lack of oxygen and within 30 minutes will begin to die. This is called an AMI, or heart attack.

- Chest pain may be caused by a brief period when heart tissues do not get enough oxygen. The discomfort associated with this is called angina. Angina pain is similar to the pain of an AMI, but responds to nitroglycerin administration. However, angina can be a sign that an AMI will occur in the future.

- Myocardial tissues that are ischemic but are not yet dying can cause pain called angina. The pain of AMI is different from that of angina in that it can come at any time, not just with exertion; it lasts up to several hours rather than just a few moments; and it is not relieved by rest or nitroglycerin.

- In addition to chest pain or pressure, signs of AMI include sudden onset of weakness, nausea, and sweating; sudden arrhythmia; pulmonary edema; and even sudden death.

- Heart attacks can have three serious consequences. One is sudden death, usually the result of cardiac arrest caused by abnormal heart rhythms, or arrhythmias. These include tachycardia, bradycardia, ventricular tachycardia, and most commonly, ventricular fibrillation.
- The second consequence is cardiogenic shock. Symptoms include restlessness; anxiety; pale, clammy skin; pulse rate higher than normal; and blood pressure lower than normal. Patients with these symptoms should receive oxygen, assisted ventilation as needed, and immediate transport.
- The third consequence of AMI is CHF, in which the damaged myocardium can no longer contract effectively enough to pump blood through the system. The lungs become congested with fluid, breathing becomes difficult, the heart rate increases, and the left ventricle enlarges.

- Signs of CHF include swollen ankles from pedal edema, high blood pressure, rapid heart rate and respirations, rales, and sometimes pink sputum and dyspnea from pulmonary edema.
- Treat a patient with CHF as you would a patient with chest pain. Monitor the patient's vital signs. Give the patient oxygen via a nonrebreathing mask. Allow the patient to remain sitting up.
- If the patient is an unresponsive infant or child younger than 8 years who weighs less than 55 lb, perform automated external defibrillation with special pediatric pads if available.
- Effective CPR and early defibrillation with an AED are critical interventions to the survival of a patient in cardiac arrest. If the patient is in cardiac arrest, start CPR beginning with chest compressions and apply the AED as soon as it is available.

Case Study

You arrive at the scene of a 68-year-old man with shortness of breath. The patient tells you that he's been experiencing trouble breathing over the past 3 days that has gotten progressively worse. His wife tells you that he can no longer sleep in their bed and that he now sleeps in the living room recliner. As you apply oxygen to the patient, your partner obtains a set of vital signs. You note the patient seems to have an altered mental status and appears to be in moderate distress. His vital signs are a pulse of 108, respirations of 30, a blood pressure of 88/50, and a pulse oximetry of 88%. When examining the patient, you hear rales/crackles in the lungs, and you note distended jugular veins and pitting edema in the ankles. His wife tells you he has a history of hypertension, two heart attacks, diabetes, chronic obstructive pulmonary disease, and aortic stenosis.

1. Discuss the signs and symptoms typically seen in a patient with cardiogenic shock.

2. Explain the difference between chronic obstructive pulmonary disease (COPD) and congestive heart failure (CHF).

3. What is the pathophysiology of atherosclerosis?

4. The ability of a cardiac muscle cell to contract spontaneously without receiving a stimulus from a nerve source is referred to as:
   A. ischemia.
   B. afterload.
   C. automaticity.
   D. preload.

5. Explain the differences in symptoms of an acute myocardial infarction (AMI) and an aortic dissection.

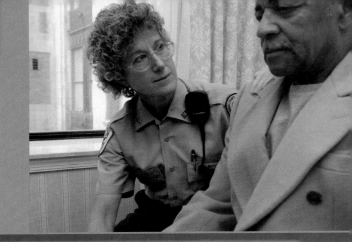

National EMS Education Standards

Anatomy and Physiology
Applies complex knowledge of the anatomy and function of all human systems to the practice of EMS.

Medicine
Applies fundamental knowledge to provide basic and selected advanced emergency care and transportation based on assessment findings for an acutely ill patient.

Review

As an EMT-I, you know about the importance of the neurologic system. You should have a good understanding of various causes of altered mental status, including hypoxia, diabetes, stroke, and seizures. Hypoglycemia associated with diabetes is a common cause of altered mental status and should be considered whenever you encounter any patient who is not completely alert and oriented. A patient experiencing a stroke or seizure or a hypoxic patient may also present with altered mental status. A complete physical assessment and patient history may help you determine the cause of the altered mental status and provide appropriate emergency medical care.

What's New

This chapter explains the pathophysiology of specific neurologic disorders including headaches, strokes, transient ischemic attacks (TIAs), seizures, and altered mental status. In addition, you will review the different types of strokes and seizures to reinforce your knowledge in these areas. The information provided will help you to better understand, communicate with, and care for patients who have experienced a neurologic emergency.

■ Introduction

According to the National Center for Health Statistics, three of the top 15 causes of death in the United States in 2003 were neurologic: stroke, neoplasms (cancer), and Alzheimer disease. In the United States someone has a stroke every 45 seconds. Clearly, AEMTs will encounter many neurologic emergencies.

This chapter describes the structure and function of the brain and the most common causes of brain disorders, including headaches, strokes, transient ischemic attacks (TIAs), seizures, and altered mental status.

■ Anatomy and Physiology Review

The brain is the body's computer. It controls breathing, speech, and all other body functions. All of your thoughts, memories, wants, needs, and desires reside in the brain. Different parts of the brain perform different functions. For example, some parts of the brain receive input from the senses, including sight, hearing, taste, smell, and touch; others control the muscles and movement; and still others control the formation of speech.

The brain is divided into three major parts: the brainstem; the cerebellum; and the largest part, the cerebrum

FIGURE 12-1 . The brainstem controls the most basic functions of the body such as breathing, blood pressure, swallowing, and pupil constriction. Located just behind the brainstem, the cerebellum controls muscle and body coordination. It is responsible for coordinating complex tasks that involve many muscles such as standing on one foot without falling, walking, writing, picking up a coin, and playing the piano.

The cerebrum, located above the cerebellum, is divided down the middle into the right and left cerebral hemispheres. Each hemisphere controls activities on the opposite side of the body. The front part of the cerebrum controls emotion and thought while the middle part controls touch and movement. The back part of the cerebrum processes sight. In most people, speech is controlled on the left side of the brain near the middle of the cerebrum.

Messages sent to and from the brain travel through nerves. The 12 cranial nerves run directly from the brain to various parts of the head, including the eyes, ears, nose, and face. All of the rest of the nerves join in the spinal cord and exit the brain through a large opening in the base of the skull called the foramen magnum **FIGURE 12-2** . At each vertebra in the neck and back, the two spinal nerves branch out from the spinal cord and carry signals to and from the body.

The complex activity of the brain is made possible by the *synapses*. Nerve cells do not actually come in direct contact with one another. Instead, a slight gap separates the cells, which allows for a far greater level of fine control. The synapse, which is present wherever a nerve cell terminates, connects to the next cell via chemicals called *neurotransmitters*. A host of neurotransmitters are present in the brain and throughout the body. Dopamine, acetylcholine, epinephrine, and serotonin are all examples of neurotransmitters. These chemicals take the electrically

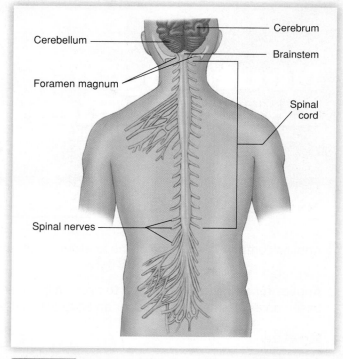

FIGURE 12-2 The spinal cord is the continuation of the brainstem. It exits the skull at the foramen magnum and extends down to the level of the second lumbar vertebra.

conducted signal from one nerve cell (a neuron) and relay it to the next cell. Nerve cells respond to these signals in an all-or-nothing manner: They fire or they do not fire. A neuron cannot fire weakly.

How do the neurotransmitters achieve a greater degree of control than that permitted by simply wiring the cells together? The answer lies in the connections made as the signal travels from the cell to the synapse **FIGURE 12-3** .

1. The first neuron fires and sends a signal along its *axon* to the axon terminal.
2. The impulse reaches the axon terminal, where neurotransmitters are released and trickle across the synapse.
3. Dendrites detect these chemicals and are triggered to send the signal to the cell's nucleus, which then transmits it down that axon, and so on.
4. Dendrites release neurotransmitter deactivators so that one impulse from cell one generates one response from cell two.

> *Synapses* The gaps between nerve cells across which nervous stimuli are transmitted.
> *Neurotransmitters* The chemicals produced by the body that stimulate electrical reactions in adjacent neurons.
> *Axon* A projection from a neuron that makes connections with adjacent cells.

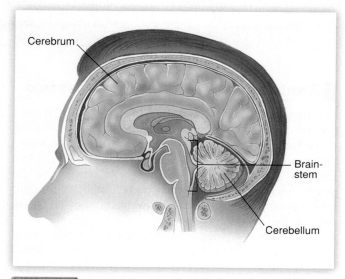

FIGURE 12-1 The three main parts of the brain are the brainstem, cerebellum, and cerebrum.

TABLE 12-1 summarizes the structures of the nervous system and their functions.

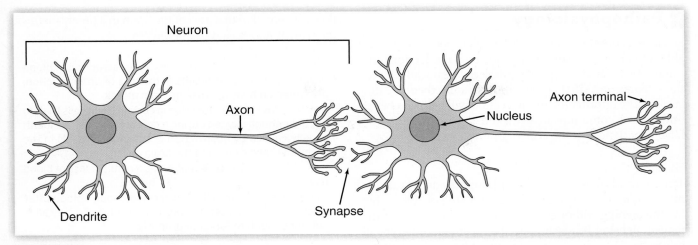

FIGURE 12-3 Neuron and synapse.

Table 12-1
Structures of the Nervous System and General Functions

Major Structure	Subdivision	General Function
Central Nervous System		
Brain	Occipital	Vision and storage of visual memories
	Parietal	Sense of touch and texture; storage of those memories
	Temporal	Hearing and smell; language; storage of sound and odor memories
	Frontal	Voluntary muscle control; storage of those memories
	Prefrontal	Judgment and predicting consequences of actions; abstract intellectual functions
	Limbic system	Basic emotions; basic reflexes (such as chewing and swallowing)
	Diencephalon (thalamus)	Relay center; filters important signals from routine signals
Brainstem	Diencephalon (hypothalamus)	Emotions; temperature control; interaction with endocrine system
	Midbrain	Level of consciousness; reticular activating system; muscle tone and posture
	Pons	Respiratory patterning and depth
	Medulla oblongata	Heart rate; blood pressure; respiratory rate
Spinal cord	Not applicable	Reflexes; relays information to and from body
Peripheral Nervous System		
Cranial nerves	Not applicable	Brain to body-part communication, including "body parts" within the skull; special peripheral nerves that connect directly to body parts
Peripheral nerves	Not applicable	Brain to spinal cord to body-part communication; receive stimuli from body; send commands to body

Pathophysiology

Stroke is a common brain disorder that is potentially treatable. Other brain disorders include coma, infection, and tumor. Although these specific problems are not addressed, the seizures or AMS that often accompanies them are discussed. The information in this section will help you better understand, communicate with, and care for patients who have experienced some type of brain disorder.

Headaches

Tension headaches, migraines, and sinus headaches are the most common types of headaches and are not considered life threatening, although they may be debilitating for the patient. Tension headaches are the most common type of headache. These headaches are caused by muscle contractions in the head and neck and are attributed to stress. The jaw, neck, or shoulders may be stiff or sore. Patients usually describe the pain as squeezing or dull or as an ache. This type of headache does not have any associated symptoms and usually does not require medical attention.

Migraine headaches are thought to be caused by changes in blood vessel size within the base of the brain. The patient may experience an aura (for example, seeing bright lights) and unilateral, focused pain that then spreads over time. The pain is throbbing, pounding, or pulsating. Nausea or vomiting may be present as well as photophobia. During a migraine headache, patients prefer dark, quiet environments. Migraines can last several days.

Two other types of headaches are cluster headaches and sinus headaches. Cluster headaches are rare vascular headaches that may recur for days and then stop entirely. They may return the next month. The pattern consists of minor pain around one eye, pain that quickly intensifies and spreads to one side of the face, and a feeling of anxiety. Sinus headaches are caused by inflammation or infection within the sinus cavities of the face. The pain is located in the superior portions of the face and increases with bending the head forward.

Stroke

A *cerebrovascular accident (CVA)*, or *stroke*, is an interruption of blood flow to the brain that often is sudden and results in the loss of function in the affected part of the brain. Without oxygen, brain cells stop working and begin to die; these dead cells are called *infarcted cells*. Once the cells are dead, medical science has little to offer. However, it may take several hours or more for cell death to occur, even when it appears that severe disability will occur. In some cases, small amounts of blood may still be getting through to the affected area of the brain. This blood may supply enough oxygen to keep a larger group of brain cells called *ischemic cells* alive, but not enough to let the cells work properly and perform their given jobs. For example, if ischemic cells are responsible for controlling the left arm, the patient will experience a decreased ability to move that arm or may not be able to move it at all. If normal blood flow is restored to that area of the brain in a timely manner, the patient may regain use of the arm.

> *Cerebrovascular accident (CVA)* An interruption of blood flow to the brain that results in the loss of brain function; also referred to as a stroke or brain attack.
>
> *Stroke* A loss of brain function in certain brain cells that do not get enough oxygen during a cerebrovascular accident; usually caused by obstruction of the blood vessels in the brain that feed oxygen to the brain cells.
>
> *Infarcted cells* The cells that die as a result of loss of blood flow.
>
> *Ischemic cells* The cells that receive enough blood after an event, such as a cerebrovascular accident, to stay alive but not enough to function properly.

> ### Transition Tip
> A stroke is also called a "brain attack." This phrase is used with the general public to emphasize that rapid recognition of the signs and symptoms and prompt transport to an appropriate facility can mean the difference between the patient regaining function and needing lifetime care.

Interruption of cerebral blood flow may result from a *thrombus*, a clot that has developed locally, in this case, *in a cerebral artery;* an *arterial rupture*, *rupture of a cerebral artery;* or a *cerebral embolism*, *obstruction of a cerebral artery* caused by a clot that was formed elsewhere, detached, and traveled to the brain.

> *Thrombus* In terms of neurologic emergencies, the local clotting of blood in the cerebral arteries that may result in the interruption of cerebral blood flow and subsequent stroke.
>
> *Arterial rupture* The rupture of an artery. Involvement of a cerebral artery may contribute to interruption of cerebral blood flow.
>
> *Cerebral embolism* Obstruction of a cerebral artery caused by a clot that was formed elsewhere in the body and traveled to the brain.

There are two main types of stroke: *ischemic* (from an embolism or thrombus) and *hemorrhagic* (from arterial rupture).

Ischemic Stroke

When blood flow to a particular part of the brain is cut off by a blockage inside a cerebral artery, the result is an *ischemic stroke*. This can be from a thrombus or an embolism that obstructs blood flow. As with coronary artery disease, atherosclerosis in the blood vessels is usually the cause. *Atherosclerosis* is a disorder in which calcium and cholesterol build up, forming a plaque inside the walls of blood vessels. This plaque obstructs blood flow, interfering with the

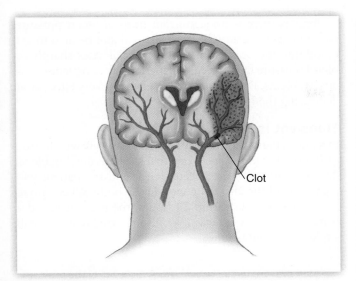

FIGURE 12-4 Atherosclerosis can damage the wall of a cerebral artery, producing narrowing or a clot. When the vessel is narrowed or completely blocked, blood flow to that part of the brain may be blocked and the cells begin to die.

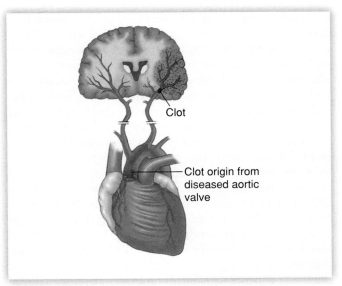

FIGURE 12-5 An embolus, a blood clot usually formed on a diseased heart valve, can travel through the body's vascular system, lodge in a cerebral artery, and cause a stroke.

vessels' ability to dilate. Eventually, atherosclerosis can cause complete occlusion (blockage) of an artery **FIGURE 12-4**. In other cases, an atherosclerotic plaque in a carotid artery will rupture. A blood clot will form over the rupture in the plaque, sometimes growing big enough to completely block all blood flow through that artery. Deprived of oxygen, the parts of the brain supplied by the artery will become ischemic. Patients with an ischemic stroke will have dramatic symptoms including loss of movement on the opposite side of the body, confusion, and the inability to speak.

> *Ischemic stroke* One of the two main types of stroke; occurs when blood flow to a particular part of the brain is cut off by a blockage (for example, a clot) inside a blood vessel.
> *Atherosclerosis* A disorder in which cholesterol and calcium build up inside the walls of blood vessels, forming plaque, which eventually leads to partial or complete blockage of blood flow; a plaque can become a site where blood clots can form, detach, and travel elsewhere in the circulatory system (embolize).

If the blockage in the carotid artery is incomplete, smaller pieces of the clot may embolize (detach and travel) deep into the brain. There, a piece of clot will lodge in a branch of a cerebral artery. This cerebral embolism then obstructs blood flow **FIGURE 12-5**. Depending on the location of the obstruction, the patient may experience anything from few symptoms to an inability to move one side of the body or complete paralysis.

Hemorrhagic Stroke

A *hemorrhagic stroke* occurs as a result of bleeding within the brain, typically when a cerebral artery ruptures. The severity of the hemorrhagic stroke depends on the location and size of the ruptured cerebral vessel. As bleeding continues within the brain, intracranial pressure (ICP) increases and compresses brain tissue. When brain tissue is compressed, oxygenated blood cannot get into the area and the surrounding cells begin to die.

> *Hemorrhagic stroke* One of the two main types of stroke; occurs as a result of bleeding inside the brain.

Certain patients are at higher risk for hemorrhagic stroke. The patients at highest risk are those who have chronic, poorly controlled hypertension. After many years of high pressure, the blood vessels in the brain weaken, making them prone to rupture. Proper treatment of hypertension can help prevent this long-term damage to the blood vessels.

Cerebral hemorrhages are often fatal although proper treatment of high blood pressure can help prevent this long-term damage to the blood vessels, reducing morbidity and mortality.

People who have been born with weaknesses, called aneurysms, in the walls of the arteries are also at increased risk for hemorrhagic stroke. Aneurysms occur in the following way:

1. A small tear or defect occurs within the wall of an artery.
2. Blood penetrates between the layers of the artery.
3. Pressure builds up and the initial small tear increases in size.
4. If the buildup continues, the wall will become so damaged that it can no longer withstand the normal pressure of blood within it. A bulge may then develop. If the weakness is severe, the bulge may leak or fail catastrophically, causing an intracranial hemorrhage.

Many people with a hemorrhagic stroke caused by a ruptured aneurysm have a sudden onset of a severe headache, frequently described as "the worst headache of my life," which signals the rupture of the aneurysm. Shortly after experiencing the severe headache, it is common for the patient's level of consciousness (LOC) to rapidly decrease, indicating increased ICP. When a hemorrhagic stroke occurs in an otherwise healthy young person, it is often the result of a berry aneurysm. This type of aneurysm resembles a tiny balloon (or berry) that protrudes from a cerebral artery. When the aneurysm is overstretched and ruptures, bleeding occurs in the subarachnoid space—the area between the coverings (meninges) of the brain. Therefore, these types of strokes are called subarachnoid hemorrhages. With prompt care, surgical repair of the aneurysm is possible. Continued bleeding within the brain will cause the ICP to increase further, thus decreasing cerebral perfusion pressure. Eventually the brain, which is significantly compressed, will be forced out of the cranial vault through the foramen magnum in a process called herniation. With herniation, pressure on the medulla oblongata located directly above the spinal cord can result in rather bizarre vital signs and other findings, including slowed heart and erratic respiratory rates, eventually leading to death.

Intracranial Pressure

Hemorrhagic strokes that cause bleeding into the brain place patients at risk for increased *intracranial pressure (ICP)*. Treatment is directed at providing some degree of control over this potentially deadly effect.

> *Intracranial pressure (ICP)* The pressure within the cranial vault.

The skull (cranial vault) is filled with three substances: brain, blood, and cerebrospinal fluid. These substances exert a pressure (ICP) against the skull and the skull in turn exerts a reflected pressure. This balanced exchange allows the brain to fit snugly within the skull without permitting any voids. If the skull contained empty spaces, the brain would slam into the skull and cause damage with head movement.

When the pressure within the cranial vault begins to climb and remains high, it creates two major problems. The brain may become ischemic as a result of lack of blood supply or herniate (push through the ligaments that compartmentalize the brain).

As the ICP rises, the amount of blood available to the brain decreases. Cerebral perfusion pressure, the pressure of blood within the cranial vault, then begins to fall.

The ICP changes constantly. Coughing, vomiting, and bearing down, for example, will increase the ICP. These momentary spikes in ICP are not harmful. By contrast, if there is blood, swelling, pus, or a tumor within the cranial vault, the ICP will increase and remain high. Because the volume of the cranial vault is limited and inflexible, pressure increases as more substances squeeze into this space.

As long as there is no significant drop in blood pressure or significant rise in ICP, the heart will still be able to get blood into the brain. However, if the ICP rises sharply or blood pressure falls critically, patients may experience serious problems. Prehospital treatment is not very effective at decreasing the ICP.

Transient Ischemic Attack

In some patients, normal processes in the body will destroy a blood clot in the brain. When that happens quickly, blood flow is restored to the affected area, and the patient will regain use of the affected region of the body. When stroke symptoms subside within 24 hours, the event is called a *transient ischemic attack (TIA)*, also referred to as a "small stroke" or a "ministroke."

> *Transient ischemic attack (TIA)* A disorder of the brain in which brain cells temporarily stop working because of insufficient oxygen, causing strokelike symptoms that resolve completely within 24 hours of onset.

Although most patients with TIAs do well, they still represent a neurologic emergency. A TIA may be a warning sign that a larger, full stroke is imminent. For this reason, all patients with a TIA should be evaluated by a physician to determine whether preventive action can be taken.

Signs and Symptoms of Stroke

Left Hemisphere Problems If the left cerebral hemisphere has been affected, the patient may have a speech disorder called *aphasia* (an inability to produce or understand speech). Speech problems vary widely. Patients may have trouble understanding speech but can speak clearly. This condition is called receptive aphasia. You can detect aphasia by asking the patient a question such as "What day is today?" In response, a patient with aphasia may say, "Green." The speech is clear, but the answer does not make sense. Other patients will be able to understand the question but cannot produce the right sounds to answer. Only grunts or other incomprehensible sounds emerge. This type of aphasia is expressive. Strokes that affect the left side of the brain cause paralysis on the right side of the body and vice versa.

> *Aphasia* The inability to understand or produce speech.

Right Hemisphere Problems If the right cerebral hemisphere of the brain is not getting enough blood, patients will have trouble moving the muscles on the left side of the body. Usually, they will understand language and be able to speak, but their words may be slurred and difficult to understand. Slurred speech is one characteristic of *dysarthria*.

> *Dysarthria* The inability to pronounce speech clearly, often due to loss of the nerves or brain cells that control the small muscles in the larynx.

Meningitis is a consideration when dealing with pediatric patients exhibiting signs of increased intracranial pressure. A patient with bacterial meningitis can progress rapidly from appearing mildly ill to coma and even death.

The symptoms of meningitis vary depending on the age of the child and the infectious agent. In general, the younger the child, the more vague the symptoms. A newborn with early bacterial meningitis may have a fever as the only symptom. Young infants will often have fever and perhaps localized signs such as lethargy, irritability, poor feeding, and a bulging fontanelle. They rarely show typical signs such as nuchal rigidity until they are older. Verbal children will often complain of headaches and neck pain. An altered level of consciousness and seizures are ominous signs at any age.

Children with meningococcal sepsis and meningitis get very sick very fast, so move quickly through your assessment. Form a general impression and perform a primary assessment as usual, keeping in mind that symptoms may be quite varied. Look for fever, altered mental status, bulging fontanelle, photophobia, nuchal rigidity, irritability, petechiae (small, pinpoint red spots), purpura (larger purple or black spots), and signs of shock. Assess glucose levels because hypoglycemia may result from the hypermetabolic state. Treat symptomatically and provide prompt transport to the closest, most appropriate facility.

It is interesting that patients with right hemisphere strokes may be completely oblivious to their problem. If you ask the patients to lift the left arm and they cannot, they will lift the right arm instead. They seem to have forgotten that the left arm even exists. This symptom is called neglect. Patients with a problem affecting the posterior aspect of the cerebrum (occiput) may neglect certain parts of their vision. Generally, this is difficult to detect in the field, but you should be aware of the possibility. Try to sit or stand on the patient's unaffected side, because he or she may be unable to see things on the affected side.

Neglect causes many patients who have had large strokes to delay seeking help. Unless caused by a ruptured cerebral artery, in which case the patient will complain of a severe headache, strokes are typically not painful. Therefore, a patient may be unaware that there is a problem until a family member or friend points out that some part of the patient's body is not working correctly.

Bleeding in the Brain Patients who have bleeding in the brain (intracerebral hemorrhage) may present with hypertension. Sometimes this is the cause of the bleeding, but many times it is a response to the bleeding; hypertension may be a response of the body to shunt more oxygenated blood to the injured portion of the brain. Remember, the brain is located inside a box (skull) with only a few openings. When bleeding occurs inside the brain, the pressure inside the skull increases. The body must increase the blood pressure to get blood to the brain's tissues.

High blood pressure in stroke patients should not be treated in the field. However, monitoring the blood pressure and watching for a trend of increasing blood pressure is important. Blood pressure may return to normal or drop significantly on its own. Significant drops in blood pressure may also occur as the patient's condition worsens.

Conditions That May Mimic Stroke

The following three conditions may present similarly to stroke:

- *Hypoglycemia* (a condition characterized by a low blood glucose level)
- A *postictal state* (the reset period of the brain after a seizure)
- Subdural or epidural bleeding (bleeding within the skull that compresses the brain)

Hypoglycemia A condition characterized by a low blood glucose level.
Postictal state The period following a seizure that lasts between 5 and 30 minutes, characterized by labored respirations and some degree of altered mental status.

Because oxygen and glucose are needed for brain metabolism, a patient with hypoglycemia may look like a patient who is having a stroke. You should check the patient's blood glucose level and find out whether the patient has diabetes and takes insulin or a glucose-lowering medication.

A patient in the postictal state may appear to be having a stroke; however, in most cases a patient in a postictal state will recover spontaneously whereas a patient having a stroke will not.

Subdural bleeding and epidural bleeding usually occur as a result of trauma. The dura is a leathery covering over the brain, next to the skull. A fracture near the temporal region of the skull may cause an artery (usually the middle meningeal artery) to bleed on top of the dura, resulting in pressure on the brain **FIGURE 12-6A**. Because the source of bleeding is from an artery, the onset of symptoms from epidural bleeding is usually very rapid after the injury. In other cases, the veins just below the dura may be torn and bleed, which is known as subdural bleeding **FIGURE 12-6B**. Because veins tend to bleed slowly, the onset of symptoms occurs more slowly, sometimes over several days.

With subdural bleeding, the onset of strokelike signs and symptoms may be subtle. The patient or family may not even remember the original injury that is causing the bleeding.

Seizures

Seizures involve sudden, erratic firing of neurons. Patients who have epilepsy commonly have seizures, for example. Patients may experience a wide array of signs and symptoms when having seizures, ranging from one hand shaking

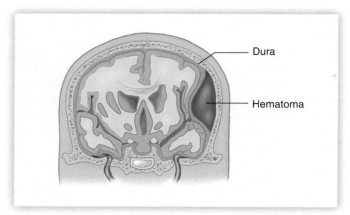

A.

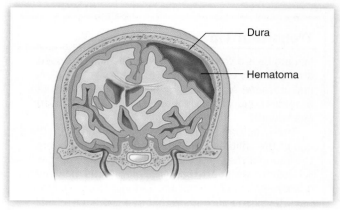

B.

FIGURE 12-6 Trauma to the head can result in intracranial bleeding. **A.** Bleeding outside the dura but under the skull is epidural. **B.** Bleeding beneath the dura but outside the brain is subdural.

or having a taste of pennies in the mouth to movement of every limb or the complete loss of consciousness. They may be aware of the seizure or they may wake up afterward not knowing what happened.

> *Seizures* Episodes often characterized by generalized, uncoordinated muscular activity associated with loss of consciousness; a convulsion.

Types of Seizures

Seizures can be classified as generalized (affecting large portions of the brain) or partial (affecting a limited area of the brain). The classification of seizures is outlined in **TABLE 12-2**.

Within the category of generalized seizures are the tonic-clonic (formerly grand mal) and absence (formerly petit mal) types. *Tonic-clonic seizures* present AEMTs with

Table 12-2
Seizure Classification

Generalized Seizures	Characteristics
Absence (formerly called petit mal) seizure	<ul><li>Staring episodes or "absence spells," during which the patient's activity ceases; loss of motor control uncommon; eye blinking or lip smacking possible</li><li>Most common in children between 4 and 12 years; rarely occurs after age 20 years</li><li>Typically lasts less than 15 seconds, after which the person's level of consciousness immediately returns to normal</li></ul>
Tonic-clonic (formerly called grand mal) seizure	<ul><li>Characterized by a loss of consciousness, followed by generalized (entire-body) muscle contraction (tonic phase) alternating with rhythmic, jerking movements (clonic phase)</li><li>Often preceded by an aura—a strange taste, smell, or other abnormal sensation—that warns the patient of the impending seizure</li><li>Can occur at any age</li><li>Often lasts several minutes; may progress to status epilepticus—a prolonged seizure or two consecutive seizures without an intervening lucid interval</li><li>Typically followed by a postictal phase, during which the patient is confused, appears sleepy, and may be agitated or combative</li></ul>
Partial (Focal) Seizures	**Characteristics**
Simple partial seizure	<ul><li>Also referred to as focal motor seizure</li><li>Characterized by tonic-clonic activity localized to one part of the body; may spread and progress to a generalized tonic-clonic seizure</li><li>No aura or associated loss of consciousness</li></ul>
Complex partial seizure	<ul><li>Also referred to as temporal lobe or psychomotor seizure</li><li>Manifests as changes in behavior (mood changes, abrupt bouts of rage)</li><li>Often preceded by an aura</li><li>Usually lasts less than 1 to 2 minutes, after which the patient quickly regains normal mental status (no postictal phase)</li></ul>

the most challenges. Most tonic-clonic seizures follow a pattern, traveling through each of the following steps in order, although sometimes skipping a step:

1. *Aura.* A sensation the patient experiences before the seizure occurs (for example, muscle twitch, odd taste, seeing lights, hearing a high-pitched noise)
2. **Loss of consciousness**
3. *Tonic phase.* Bodywide rigidity
4. **Hypertonic phase.** Arched back and rigidity
5. *Clonic phase.* Rhythmic contraction of major muscle groups; arm, leg, head movement; lip smacking; biting; teeth clenching
6. **Postseizure.** Major muscles relax; nystagmus (rhythmic shaking of the eyes) may still occur; eyes possibly rolled back
7. **Postictal.** Reset period of the brain. The reset can take several minutes to hours before the patient gradually returns to the preseizure LOC **FIGURE 12-7**. During this time, patients are often initially aphasic (unable to speak), confused or unable to follow commands, very emotional, or tired or sleeping, and may be incontinent of urine and/or feces. They may present with a headache. Gradually the brain will begin to function normally.

> *Tonic-clonic seizures* The seizures characterized by severe twitching of all of the body's muscles that may last several minutes or more; formerly known as a grand mal seizure.
> *Aura* Sensations experienced before an attack occurs; common in seizures and migraine headaches.
> *Tonic phase* In a seizure, the steady, rigid muscle contractions with no relaxation.
> *Clonic phase* Seizure movement marked by repetitive muscle contractions and relaxations in rapid succession.

In contrast to tonic-clonic seizures, *absence seizures* present with little or no movement. The typical patient with absence seizures is a child. Classically, the child will simply

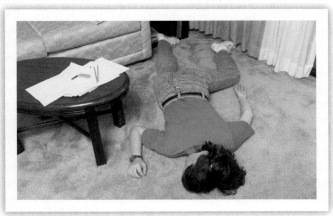

Courtesy of AAOS
FIGURE 12-7 A patient who has had a seizure may be found in the postictal state when you arrive. In such a case, ask family members or bystanders to verify that a seizure has occurred by asking them to tell you about the movements of the patient's body and body parts.

stop moving; he or she may be walking and just stop, may be speaking and stop midsentence, or may be playing and freeze with a toy in the hand. The child will rarely fall. These seizures usually last no more than several seconds. There is no postictal period and no confusion. These may be brought on by flashing lights or hyperventilation.

Partial seizures may be classified as simple partial or complex partial. Such seizures involve only a limited portion of the brain. They may be localized to just one spot within the brain or they may begin in one spot and move in a wavelike manner to other locations.

Simple partial seizures involve movement of one part of the body (when originating in the frontal lobe) or altered sensations in one part of the body (when originating in the parietal lobe). This movement may stay in one body part or spread from one part to another in a wave. *Complex partial seizures* involve subtle changes in the LOC. The patient may become confused, lose alertness, have hallucinations, or be unable to speak. The head or eyes may make small movements. Patients typically do not become unresponsive.

> *Absence seizures* The seizures that may be characterized by a brief lapse of attention in which the patient may stare and does not respond; formerly known as a petit mal seizure.
> *Partial seizures* The seizures affecting a limited portion of the brain.
> *Simple partial seizures* The seizures involving the movement of one part of the body or altered sensations in one part of the body; the movement may stay in one body part or spread from one part to another in a wave.
> *Complex partial seizures* The seizures that involve subtle changes in the level of consciousness that may include confusion, less alertness, hallucinations, and inability to speak.

Status Epilepticus

Status epilepticus is a seizure that lasts for longer than 4 or 5 minutes or consecutive seizures that occur without the return of consciousness between seizure episodes. This time frame is arbitrary, however, and some authors suggest that status epilepticus does not occur until 20 minutes of uninterrupted seizures. Refer to your local protocols for guidelines on how long a seizure can continue before you should intervene.

> *Status epilepticus* A condition in which seizures recur every few minutes without a lucid interval or last more than 4 or 5 minutes.

During a seizure, neurons are in a hypermetabolic state (using huge amounts of glucose and producing lactic acid). For a short period, this state does not produce long-term damage. If the seizure continues, however, the body cannot remove waste products effectively or ensure adequate glucose supplies. Such a hypermetabolic state can result in neurons being damaged or killed. The goals of prehospital care are to stop the seizure and ensure adequate ABCs.

Causes of Seizures

There are various reasons why a patient may have a seizure, ranging from a congenital disorder to a diabetic emergency to fever (a possible cause if the patient is an infant). Knowing the cause will help direct management.

Some seizure disorders such as epilepsy are congenital, meaning the patient was born with the condition. Other types of seizures may be caused by a high fever, structural problems in the brain, or metabolic or chemical problems in the body **TABLE 12-3**. Epileptic seizures can usually be controlled with medications such as phenytoin (Dilantin), phenobarbital (for example, Solfoton), carbamazepine (for example, Tegretol), gabapentin (Gabarone, Neurontin), or lamotrigine (Lamictal). Patients with epilepsy often have seizures if they stop taking their medications or if they do not take an adequate dose. In fact, most seizures are the result of medication noncompliance. In the emergency department, blood analysis will frequently show a subtherapeutic level of the antiepileptic drug.

Seizures may also be caused by an area of abnormality in the brain such as a benign or cancerous tumor, an infection (brain abscess), or a scar from a previous injury. These seizures are said to have a structural cause; in other cases the seizures are metabolic. Metabolic causes include abnormal levels of certain blood chemicals (for example, an extremely low sodium level), hypoglycemia (low blood glucose level), poisons, drug overdoses, or sudden withdrawal from routine and heavy alcohol or sedative drug use or even from prescribed medications. Phenytoin (Dilantin), a drug that is used to control seizures, can cause seizures itself if the person takes too much. In some cases, seizures are idiopathic (of unknown cause).

Seizures can also result from sudden high fevers, particularly in infants and small children. Such seizures, known as *febrile seizures*, are usually unnerving for parents to observe but are generally well tolerated by the child. Nevertheless, you must transport a child who has had a febrile seizure because this condition needs to be evaluated in the hospital. The fact that a second seizure may occur is worrisome, and if it occurs the patient requires rapid evaluation in a hospital to identify possible causes such as serious inflammation in the brain or tissues covering the brain (conditions known as encephalitis and meningitis, respectively; infection also may be present). Febrile seizures result from a rapid increase in body temperature. In other words, it is not necessarily how high the fever gets, but how quickly it gets there.

> *Febrile seizures* The seizures that result from sudden high fever, particularly in children.

Transition Tip

Use the mnemonic **FACTS** to obtain pertinent history for patients having a seizure:

F—Focus (Generalized or focal?)

A—Activity (Type of movements?)

C—Color or Cocaine (Cyanosis? Indications of cocaine use?)

T—Time (How long did the seizure last?)

S—Secondary information (Medications? Events leading up to the seizure? Incontinence? Tongue biting?)

The Importance of Recognizing Seizures

Regardless of the type or cause of a seizure, it is extremely important for you to recognize when a seizure is occurring or whether one has already occurred. You must also determine whether this episode differs from any previous ones. For example, if a previous seizure occurred on only one side of the body and this seizure occurred over the entire body, some additional or new problem may be involved. In addition to recognizing that seizure activity has occurred and/or that something different may now be occurring, you must also recognize the postictal state and the complications of seizures.

Because most seizures involve vigorous twitching of the muscles, they use a lot of oxygen. This excessive demand consumes oxygen that was being delivered by the circulation to support the vital functions of the body. It is similar to a situation in which you exercise vigorously without giving your body a chance to rest. As a result, there is a buildup of acids in the bloodstream, and the patient may turn cyanotic (bluish lips, mucous membranes, and skin) from the lack of oxygen. Often the seizures themselves prevent the patient from breathing normally, making the problem worse.

Recognizing seizure activity also means looking at other problems associated with the seizure. For example, the patient may have fallen during the seizure episode and injured some part of the body; head injury is the most

Table 12-3 Common Causes of Seizures	
Type	**Cause**
Epileptic	Congenital
Structural	Tumor (benign or cancerous) Infection (brain abscess) Scar from previous injury Head trauma Degenerative cerebral diseases
Metabolic	Abnormal blood chemical levels Hypoglycemia Poisoning Eclampsia Drug overdose Sudden withdrawal from alcohol or medications
Febrile	Sudden high fever

serious possibility. Patients having a generalized seizure may experience *incontinence*, meaning that they may lose bowel and/or bladder control. Therefore, one clue that unresponsive or confused patients may have had a seizure is to find that they were incontinent. Although incontinence is possible with other medical conditions, sudden incontinence is likely a sign that a seizure has occurred.

> *Incontinence* Loss of bowel and bladder control; can be the result of a generalized seizure and other conditions.

Transition Tip

Be on the lookout for patients who may behave violently during the postictal phase. The patient might not know what has happened and might be frightened by strangers providing care or trying to move him or her into the ambulance. Most patients who have had a seizure pose no threat to EMS providers. Alcohol and/or drugs are not always associated with violent behavior during the postictal phase, but signs of their use or abuse should heighten your awareness of the potential for dangerous behavior.

The Postictal State

Once a seizure has stopped, the patient's muscles relax, becoming almost flaccid, or floppy, and breathing becomes labored (fast and deep) in an attempt to compensate for the buildup of acids in the bloodstream. By breathing faster and more deeply, the body can balance the pH in the bloodstream. With normal circulation and liver function, the acids clear away within minutes, and the patient will begin to breathe normally. The longer the seizure was, the longer it will take for this imbalance to correct itself. Likewise, longer and more severe seizures will result in a longer postictal phase.

In some situations, the postictal state may be characterized by *hemiparesis*, or weakness on one side of the body, resembling a stroke. Unlike the typical stroke, hypoxic hemiparesis spontaneously resolves within a short period. Most commonly, the postictal state is characterized by lethargy and confusion to the point that the patient may be combative and appear angry. You must be prepared for these circumstances in your approach to scene control and in your treatment of the patient's symptoms. If the patient's condition does not improve, you should consider other possible underlying problems including hypoglycemia and infection.

> *Hemiparesis* Weakness on one side of the body.

Altered Mental Status

Aside from stroke and seizures, the most common type of neurologic emergency that you will encounter is a patient with altered mental status. Simply put, altered mental status means that the patient is not thinking clearly or is incapable of being aroused. In some cases, patients will be unresponsive; in others, they may be responsive but confused. The range of problems is wide and the causes are many including common problems such as hypoglycemia (low blood glucose level), hypoxemia, intoxication, drug overdose, unrecognized head injury, brain infection, body temperature abnormalities; and uncommon conditions such as brain tumors, glandular abnormalities, and poisonings.

Transition Tip

Physician evaluation of a patient who has had a seizure depends heavily on reports of the seizure pattern and changes in that pattern. Record all pertinent information about the seizure in terms of duration, areas of body movement, and possible precipitating factors (such as recent trauma, fever, and medication noncompliance). Effective interviewing of available witnesses, family members, or caregivers is needed to obtain the required information.

Transition Tip

Besides recognizing that a seizure has occurred, it is important to learn whether the pattern has changed. Was this seizure different from previous ones? If so, how?

Hypoglycemia

The clinical picture of patients with altered mental status due to hypoglycemia is complex. Patients might have signs and symptoms that mimic stroke and seizures. Patients may have hemiparesis, similar to what occurs as a result of a stroke. The principal difference, however, is that a patient who has had a stroke may be alert and attempting to communicate normally, whereas a patient with hypoglycemia almost always has an altered mental status.

Patients with hypoglycemia commonly, but not always, take medications that lower the blood glucose level. Thus, if the patient appears to have signs and symptoms of stroke and an altered mental status, you should report your findings to medical control and treat the patient accordingly. Check for and report medications but remember that not all patients who have diabetes take insulin or other medications to lower the blood glucose level. Remember also that patients with a decreased LOC should not be given anything by mouth. Local protocols should guide your actions.

Patients with hypoglycemia can also experience seizures, and you may arrive at the scene to find a patient in a postictal state: confused and disoriented or unresponsive. The mental status of a patient who has had a typical seizure is likely to improve; however, in a patient with hypoglycemia, the mental status is not likely to improve even after several minutes. Therefore, you should consider the possibility of hypoglycemia in a patient who has had a seizure, especially if the blood glucose reading is low.

Likewise, you should consider hypoglycemia in a patient who has altered mental status after an injury such as a motor vehicle crash, even when there is the possibility of an accompanying head injury. As with any other patient, you should look for medical identification bracelets or medications that might confirm your suspicions.

Other Causes of Altered Mental Status

In addition to hypoglycemia, three other possible causes of altered mental status include hypoxia (regardless of the cause), unrecognized head injury, and severe alcohol intoxication. Your consideration of these and other possibilities becomes important because a patient with altered mental status may be combative and refuse treatment and transport. You should be prepared for difficult patient encounters and follow local protocols for dealing with these situations, recognizing the potential for serious underlying problems.

A patient who appears intoxicated may be intoxicated; however, the patient might have other problems as well. People with alcoholism can have abnormalities in liver function, blood clotting, and the immune system, which can predispose them to intracranial bleeding, brain and bloodstream infections, and hypoglycemia.

Psychological problems and adverse effects of medications are also possible causes of altered mental status. In addition, a person who appears to have a psychological problem may also have an underlying medical condition.

Infections are another possible cause, particularly those involving the brain or bloodstream. Infections in these areas are obviously life threatening and need immediate attention. Patients may not demonstrate typical signs of infection such as fever, particularly if they are very young or very old or have an impaired immune system.

Altered mental status can also be caused by drug overdose and poisonings; therefore, you should monitor patients closely for accompanying cardiac and respiratory problems.

The presentation of altered mental status varies widely from simple confusion to coma. Regardless of the cause, you should consider altered mental status to be an emergency that requires immediate attention, even when it appears that the culprit may be alcohol intoxication or a minor car crash or fall.

Syncope

Syncope (fainting) is the sudden and temporary loss of consciousness with accompanying loss of postural tone. It affects mainly adults and accounts for nearly 3% of all emergency department visits. The brain uses glucose at a high rate and has no ability to store glucose, so even a 3- to 5-second interruption in blood flow can cause loss of consciousness. The question then becomes: "What caused the sudden decrease in cerebral perfusion?" Potential causes include problems with cardiac rhythm or conduction, problems with cardiac muscle, myocardial infarction, dehydration, hypoglycemia, and a vasovagal episode.

> *Syncope* Fainting, often caused by an interruption of blood flow to the brain.

A patient with syncope is usually in a standing position before the event occurs and then passes out. This is why you should always seat a patient before drawing blood or inserting an intravenous (IV) line.

Patient Assessment

Many different disorders can cause brain or other neurologic symptoms and thus can affect the patient's LOC, speech, and voluntary muscle control. The key to identifying a neurologic problem is to look for obvious changes and subtle changes. Without any blood flow (cardiac arrest), the patient will go into a coma and can have permanent brain damage within minutes even if cardiopulmonary resuscitation is performed immediately. If there is poor blood supply to the middle part of the left cerebral hemisphere, the patient may not be able to move some parts of the right side of the body such as the right arm or the right leg. Facial muscles may also be affected on one side (one side of the face may appear to droop), the tongue may deviate to one side, or the patient may be unable to swallow.

Scene Size-up

Ensure that the scene is safe and follow standard precautions.

Scene considerations for a patient with a suspected neurologic emergency include an evaluation of the patient's environment, assessing for any signs of potential trauma (mechanism of injury), indications of a previous medical condition such as diabetic supplies or medical alert tags, and evidence of a seizure. Be aware of indications of the nature of illness. Most patients with a neurologic emergency have a change in LOC and their ability to interact with their environment and others.

> ### Transition Tip
>
> When you are assessing a patient with altered mental status, consider the mnemonic **AEIOU-TIPS**.
>
> A–Alcohol, acidosis
>
> E–Encephalitis, epilepsy
>
> I–Insulin
>
> O–Overdose
>
> U–Uremia
>
> T–Trauma
>
> I–Infection
>
> P–Psychiatric
>
> S–Seizures

Primary Assessment

As you approach the patient, note the patient's body position and LOC. Observe for seizure activity. Most seizures will be over by the time you arrive. If the seizure is still occurring, the potentially life-threatening condition of status epilepticus may be present. If the patient is in a postictal state, he or she may be unresponsive or starting to regain awareness of the surroundings. Determining the patient's LOC should be first in the list of assessment actions for anyone with an altered mental status.

Note the patient's posture. Decorticate or decerebrate posturing indicates the patient has severe brain dysfunction and is in critical condition. In *decorticate posturing*, the patient flexes the arms and curls them toward the chest. At the same time, he or she points his or her toes. Finally, the wrists are flexed **FIGURE 12-8** . You can easily remember the meaning because with decorticate posturing, the patient's hands are flexed toward his or her core. In *decerebrate posturing*, the patient again points the toes, but now extends the arms outward and rotates the lower arms in a palms-down manner (called *pronation*). The wrists are again flexed **FIGURE 12-9** . This posture is a more severe finding than decorticate posturing.

> *Decorticate posturing* A body position in which the patient flexes the arms and curls them toward the chest, flexes the wrists, and points his or her toes; indicates severe brain dysfunction from pressure on the brainstem.
> *Decerebrate posturing* A body position in which the patient extends the arms outward and rotates the lower arms in a palms-down manner, and points the toes; indicates severe brain dysfunction from pressure on the brainstem.
> *Pronation* The act of extending the arms outward and turning the palms downward.

Ensure the patient's airway is clear and respirations are adequate. The greater the breathing rate deviates from normal, the more severely the nervous system is affected. Strokes affect how the body functions in many ways. Patients may have difficulty swallowing and are at risk for choking on their own saliva. Evaluate the airway of an unresponsive patient to make sure it is patent and will remain that way during transport. Continually reassess the patient closely for depressed respirations. If the patient requires assistance maintaining an airway, consider an oropharyngeal

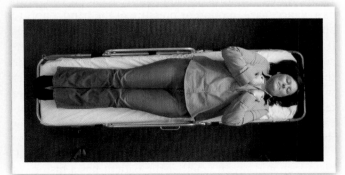

Courtesy of Chuck Sowerbrower, MED, NREMT-P
FIGURE 12-8 Decorticate posturing.

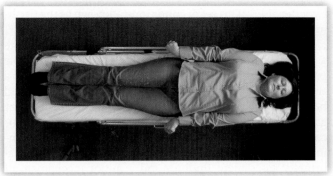

Courtesy of Chuck Sowerbrower, MED, NREMT-P
FIGURE 12-9 Decerebrate posturing.

or nasopharyngeal airway. Provide suction, and position the patient to prevent aspiration. If you determine that the patient cannot protect his or her airway, place the patient in the recovery position to help prevent secretions from entering the airway. Suction as necessary.

Unless you are concerned about possible cervical spine fracture, elevate the head 30°. Provide ventilatory support at 16 to 20 breaths/min. Do not increase the rate any higher than 30 breaths/min because hyperventilation will cause vasoconstriction and decrease perfusion to the brain. Do not suction vigorously. Stimulating the cough and gag reflexes will increase ICP.

A patient who has had or is having a seizure may have been eating or chewing gum at the time of the seizure so there may be a foreign body obstruction. Bystanders may have tried to put objects in the patient's mouth to keep the person from swallowing the tongue, even though this practice is not advised. A seizure patient may clench his or her teeth (*trismus*) and require sedation. Call early for paramedic backup if dealing with a difficult airway.

> *Trismus* The involuntary contraction of the mouth resulting in clenched teeth; occurs during seizures and head injuries.

Check the patient's pulse if he or she is unresponsive. If no pulse is found, immediately begin CPR beginning with chest compressions and attach an automated external defibrillator. If the patient is responsive, determine whether the pulse is fast or slow and weak or strong. Evaluate the peripheral and central pulse pressures. The absence of a peripheral pulse with a central pulse present should cause you to suspect shock. Remember, shock is rarely caused solely by a neurologic problem. Oxygen administration is helpful for limiting the effects of hypoperfusion to the brain.

Evaluate the patient quickly for external bleeding. It is unlikely a patient with a stroke has sustained trauma, but it is possible with a patient who has had a seizure.

If a patient has increased pressure within the cranium, the vital signs may provide evidence of this problem. With increased ICP, the blood pressure rises, the heart and respiratory rates fall, and the pulse pressure widens (systolic hypertension). This set of conditions—known as the Cushing reflex—is the opposite of what is expected in shock.

At this point in the examination, an AEMT may make a broad decision about whether to "load and go." Unstable patients—those with inadequate or deteriorating ABCs or a significant mechanism of injury or nature of illness—should be transported urgently to an emergency department. Defer gathering very detailed information about patients in critical condition; instead, focus on stabilizing and maintaining the ABCs. With stable patients—that is, with normal primary assessment findings and a minor mechanism of injury or nature of illness—you have more time to gather detailed information at the scene. Rapidly transport any patient whom you suspect has increased ICP.

If you suspect the patient is experiencing a stroke, you should rapidly transport the patient to an appropriate facility to ensure that every chance is available to reduce the disability caused by an ischemic stroke. New therapies, such as fibrinolytic drugs, commonly referred to as "clot busters," have been shown to reverse symptoms, thus aborting the stroke, if given within 3 hours after the onset of symptoms. It is also essential that they be taken to a stroke center or appropriate facility with a stroke team on duty. Your local protocols should address this or you should contact medical control to help choose the most appropriate destination. The sooner the treatment is initiated, the better the chance for a positive patient outcome. If you suspect the patient may have had a stroke, place him or her in a comfortable position, usually on one side, with the paralyzed side down and well protected with padding. The patient's head should be elevated about 6 inches.

Transition Tip

When you are working with geriatric patients, take their medical history into account. Patients with a history of dementia could be complicated to manage. The primary question is: "How much change has occurred in the patient's level of consciousness (LOC)?" Do not assume that the patient's baseline LOC is what you would consider normal; speak to the family, friends, or other caregivers to determine the patient's baseline LOC and document that level clearly.

After you begin transport, you should relay the information you have obtained to the receiving hospital. Be sure to include the time that the patient was last seen to be normal, the findings of your neurologic examination, and the time you anticipate arriving at the hospital. This information will allow the emergency department staff to allocate the appropriate resources for the patient's arrival.

History Taking

Obtain a history from patients who are in stable condition and have minor complaints. If the patient is unresponsive, you will need to gather any history of the present illness from family or bystanders. If no one is around, quickly look for explanations for the altered mental status (for example, signs of trauma, medical alert tags, track marks, and environmental clues such as empty alcohol or medication containers).

To determine the chief complaint in a responsive patient, begin by asking the patient what happened. Look for signs and symptoms that may indicate a cause for his or her altered mental status, such as a stroke, and determine whether there is any evidence of a seizure (such as incontinence or a bitten tongue). Evaluate the patient's speech. Is the patient making any sense? Is speech slurred?

If you know that the patient has had a seizure and is now in a postictal state, you will not be able to obtain a history from the patient. Look for any obvious trauma or explanations as to why the patient may have had a seizure.

If the patient has a headache, try to determine the patient's level of stress, possible infections, and history of headaches. Stroke patients can also experience headaches. If you suspect a more complicated problem, perform a rapid scan to ensure that you give the patient the best possible care.

If the patient is responsive and breathing, obtain a SAMPLE history. Also try to speak with family or friends who may be able to explain the events leading up to the altered mental status, remembering that time can be critical in a neurologic emergency. Make a special effort to determine when the patient last appeared to be healthy. This information will help physicians in the emergency department decide whether it is safe to begin certain treatments (for example, fibrinolytic therapy) that must be given within a narrow time frame after the onset of symptoms.

History taking from a patient with a potential neurologic complaint should follow the same process as for any other medical or trauma patient. The physical examination for this complaint should investigate potential cardiac, neurologic, respiratory, metabolic, and infectious causes.

Although a patient who has had a stroke may appear to be unresponsive and unable to speak, the patient may still be able to hear and understand what is taking place. Therefore, you should treat the patient as if he or she is able to hear. Try to communicate with the patient by looking for indications that the patient can understand you, such as a glance, gaze, motion or pressure of the hand, effort to speak, or head nod. Allow the patient to write responses if he or she is able. Reassure your patient that you understand that communication between the two of you may be difficult at this point but that you will provide him or her with continuous information as to what you and the other team members are doing. Establishing effective communication can help you to calm the patient and lessen the fear that accompanies an inability to communicate.

For patients who have had a seizure, your SAMPLE history should reveal whether the patient has a history of seizures. If so, it is important to find out how the patient's seizures typically occur and whether this episode differs in some way from previous episodes. You should also ask what medications the patient has been taking. If the patient takes phenytoin (Dilantin) and phenobarbital (for example, Solfoton), he or she most likely has a seizure disorder. You might find that the patient ran out of medication or stopped taking the medication for a time. Patients who have a history of seizures *and* diabetes may use up all the glucose in the body to fuel the seizure.

If the patient does not have a history of seizures and suddenly has a seizure, a serious condition such as a brain tumor, intracranial bleeding, or serious infection should be suspected. You should also determine whether the patient takes medications that lower the blood glucose level such as insulin and oral hypoglycemic agents. In other situations, you may want to inquire about drug use or exposure to poisons.

Secondary Assessment

As soon as possible, perform a secondary assessment. Look for potential causes of neurologic signs and symptoms such as trauma not previously noticed. Does the patient have any complaints related to the abdomen? Signs of nausea and vomiting are common with some neurologic conditions such as headaches and increased ICP. Note whether the patient is incontinent; urinary and fecal incontinence are common findings with seizures or syncope. The patient should also be assessed for injuries including head lacerations, shoulder dislocation, bitten tongue, and long bone fractures.

You should perform at least three key physical tests on patients you suspect of having had a stroke: tests of speech, facial movement, and arm movement. If any one of the three

tests is positive (abnormal), the patient should be assumed to be having (or to have had) a stroke.

During the assessment phase, use a stroke assessment tool—the Cincinnati Prehospital Stroke Scale TABLE 12-4 or the Los Angeles Prehospital Stroke Screen TABLE 12-5. All patients with altered mental status (stroke, TIA, seizure, of unknown cause) should also have a Glasgow Coma Scale score calculated TABLE 12-6.

Blood pressure must be closely monitored in any patient with a potential ICP problem. Frequent assessment becomes

Table 12-4
Cincinnati Prehospital Stroke Scale

Test	Normal	Abnormal
Facial droop (Ask patient to show teeth or smile.)	Both sides of face move equally well.	One side of face does not move as well as the other.
Arm drift (Ask patient to close eyes and hold both arms out with palms up.)	Both arms move the same, or both arms do not move.	One arm does not move, or one arm drifts down compared with the other side.
Speech (Ask patient to say, "The sky is blue in Cincinnati.")	Patient uses correct words with no slurring.	Patient slurs words, uses inappropriate words, or is unable to speak.

Table 12-5
Los Angeles Prehospital Stroke Screen

Criteria	Yes	Unknown	No
1. Age > 45	☐	☐	☐
2. History of seizures or epilepsy absent	☐	☐	☐
3. Symptoms < 24 hours	☐	☐	☐
4. At baseline, patient is not wheelchair-bound or bedridden	☐	☐	☐
5. Blood glucose between 60 and 400 mg/dL	☐	☐	☐
	Equal	Right Weak	Left Weak
6. Obvious asymmetry (right vs. left) in any of the following three exam categories (must be unilateral)*:			
Facial smile/grimace	☐	☐ Droop	☐ Droop
Grip	☐	☐ Weak grip ☐ No grip	☐ Weak grip ☐ No grip
Arm strength	☐	☐ Drifts down ☐ Falls rapidly	☐ Drifts down ☐ Falls rapidly

Interpretation: If criteria 1–6 are marked yes, the probability of a stroke is 97%.
*Patients with strokes may have weakness or paralysis (hemiplegia) on one side of the body.

Table 12-6 Glasgow Coma Scale		
Test	**Response**	**Score**
Eye opening	Spontaneous	4
	Voice	3
	Pain stimulation	2
	None	1
Verbal	Oriented conversation	5
	Confused conversation	4
	Inappropriate words	3
	Incomprehensible sounds	2
	None	1
Motor	Obeys commands	6
	Localizes pain	5
	Withdraws from pain	4
	Abnormal flexion (decorticate)	3
	Abnormal extension (decerebrate)	2
	None	1

Score: 15 indicates no neurologic disabilities.
Score: 13–14 may indicate mild dysfunction.
Score: 9–12 may indicate moderate dysfunction.
Score: 8 or less is indicative of severe dysfunction.

even more essential when a decrease in blood pressure is also present. For any patient at risk for increased ICP, AEMTs need to ensure a systolic blood pressure of at least 110 to 120 mm Hg.

Changes in pupil size and reactivity indicate significant bleeding and pressure on the brain. If the patient has an altered mental status (regardless of the cause), you should check the blood glucose level if you have the equipment available and your local protocol allows.

During most active seizures, it is impossible to evaluate vital signs nor is this the priority when a patient is having a seizure. Unless the situation is unusual, vital signs in a postictal state will approximate normal. Obtain pulse rate, rhythm, and quality; respiratory rate, rhythm, and quality; blood pressure; skin color, temperature, and condition; and pupil size and reactivity.

Reassessment

Reassessment is intended to monitor ABCs, vital signs, and interventions and to monitor patients for changes. Talk with them. Casual conversation will allow you to closely monitor brain functions. If the patient is nonverbal, keep a close eye on respiratory patterns and eye and body movements, and monitor for seizure activity.

Routine monitoring should include heart rate, blood pressure, respiratory rate and pattern, pulse oximetry, repeated glucose level (if the level was low and glucose was given to the patient), and Glasgow Coma Scale scores. Continue oxygenation and ventilation support. Monitor the IV fluids closely to ensure that accidental fluid overload does not occur. If the patient's condition undergoes a sudden dramatic change, repeat the assessment as if this were a new patient and modify your care.

Observe for recurrent seizures. If another seizure occurs, note whether it starts at a focal part of the body (for example, one arm or one leg) and then progresses to the rest of the body. Most important, evaluate the patient's mental status and monitor it frequently to verify progressive improvement.

When your patient shows signs and/or symptoms of stroke, seizure, hypoglycemia, or hypoxia, these conditions typically can be relatively easily identified, and treatment options are readily available. With other neurologic emergencies, the cause of the patient's symptoms will not always be obvious and you may not be able to determine the cause. It is possible that hospital staff will need more time and diagnostic testing to determine the cause. This may make it difficult for you to provide definitive treatment in the field. Most of your interventions will be based on your assessment findings. For example, if the blood glucose level is low, you may give oral glucose according to protocol, or if a patient is unresponsive, you may need to position him or her in the recovery position to protect the airway. Remember, never give anything orally to a patient with decreased mental status or a patient who is unable to swallow normally because doing so may result in aspiration. Your best treatment in these situations is to perform a thorough assessment and maintain the ABCs.

If you suspect the patient of having a stroke, continue giving 100% oxygen, or if needed, assisted ventilations en route. Establish IV access and obtain blood samples for analysis. Only give 50% dextrose if the patient's blood glucose level is low. Consider the administration of glucagon for hypoglycemia as an alternative. Use an isotonic crystalloid solution at a keep-vein-open rate unless the patient is hypovolemic. If the patient is hypotensive, give a fluid bolus of 20 mL/kg to maintain adequate perfusion (for example, to maintain the radial pulses). Excessive fluids will increase bleeding in patients with hemorrhagic strokes as well as increase ICP.

If you cannot check the patient's blood glucose level for some reason, you need to be more cautious in administering dextrose. In a situation in which the patient is unresponsive or has a decreased LOC and no blood glucose monitor is available, administer 12.5 g (½ syringe) and then reassess the response. Proceed with additional dextrose cautiously, based on responses to previous doses. Hyperglycemia can increase the morbidity rate among stroke patients.

In most patients with a suspected stroke, physicians in the emergency department need to determine whether there is bleeding in the brain. The only reliable way to determine bleeding in the brain is with advanced diagnostic imaging techniques such as CT scan or MRI. Blood is usually easy to see on either of these studies.

In most situations, patients who have had a seizure require definitive evaluation and treatment in the hospital. Unless the patient has a well-established history of seizures and is completely alert and oriented, supplemental oxygen is strongly advised, not only to provide extra oxygen but also to reduce the possibility of a recurrent seizure. It is never wrong to administer supplemental oxygen to a patient who has had a seizure.

For patients who are having a seizure, protect them from harm, maintain a clear airway by suctioning as necessary, and provide oxygen as quickly as possible. If trauma is suspected, provide spinal immobilization. With recurrent seizures, protect the patient from further injury and manage the airway once the seizure ceases.

For patients who continue to have a seizure, as in status epilepticus, suction the airway, provide positive-pressure ventilations, and transport quickly to the hospital. If you have the option to rendezvous with paramedics, you should do so. Paramedics can administer medications that can stop a prolonged seizure.

Notify the receiving facility of your patient's chief complaint and your assessment findings. Most designated stroke centers will want you to call a stroke alert for patients you have assessed and found to be having a stroke (check local protocol). This will alert the stroke team members at the hospital and give them time to assemble their resources to treat the patient without delay. If anything changes en route to the hospital, manage the situation and document any changes or additional treatment.

Emergency Medical Care

Management for all patients who experience a change in LOC is directed at ensuring that the body has an adequate internal environment to allow for optimal brain function.

Provide emotional support for the patient and family. Neurologic emergencies can produce confusion, fear, anger, and helplessness. Use a calm, reassuring voice to show that you are there to help.

Consult your local protocol to determine whether the blood glucose reading is considered low. One guideline states that if the blood glucose level is below 60 mg/dL, glucose is needed. Two medications are available for pre-hospital treatment of hypoglycemia: dextrose 50% (D_{50}) and glucagon.

Oral glucose administration is another option for patients with a decreased LOC who can swallow safely. Alternatives to oral glucose include cake icing, a plain chocolate bar, and orange juice with sugar added. Administration of sugar by mouth will take longer to raise the blood glucose level. Constantly supervise patients as they consume the sugar. To the extent possible, make sure they do not

aspirate. Never administer anything by mouth to a patient you believe to be at risk for aspiration because of a decreased level of consciousness.

Transition Tip

When you are assessing an infant for increased ICP, consider the quality of the cry. As the ICP increases, the pitch of the cry will increase until a shriek similar to that of a cat can be heard. At the same time, the shape of the pupils can change from round to more oval. These two findings lead to the saying related to infants and increased ICP: "cat's eyes and cat's cries."

Transition Tip

You may be the only provider to witness some patient activity, so accurate and complete documentation is critical to ensure continuity of care.

There is currently no safe way to lower a high blood glucose level in the field. For patients with hyperglycemia, provide standard care and ensure adequate blood pressure. Hyperglycemic patients are often dehydrated and usually need volume support. Of course this only corrects the dehydration, not the blood glucose level.

Headaches

Be cautious because headaches can indicate a more serious problem. Give standard care. Ask which medications the patient has taken. Many patients will appreciate a darkened, quiet environment, so do not use lights and sirens if transporting.

Stroke

Because it is often impossible to differentiate the symptoms of a TIA from a stroke, assume that a patient with TIA or stroke symptoms is having a stroke. Administer 100% supplemental oxygen, obtain IV access, and transport the patient to the closest appropriate facility for evaluation.

Most treatments for stroke must be started as soon as possible after the onset of the event TABLE 12-7 . Few if any current treatments are effective if they are started more than 3 hours after the stroke begins. Even if 3 hours have passed since the onset of symptoms, prompt action on your part is essential.

As mentioned, fibrinolytic drugs need to be administered within 3 hours of stroke onset. Do not administer aspirin in the field; it will help in an ischemic CVA but hurt in a hemorrhagic CVA. Aspirin should be administered only after a CT scan or MRI has been completed in the hospital.

> ### Table 12-7
> ### Tips on Patient Care for a Possible Stroke Patient
>
> Patients who experience a TIA typically have the same signs and symptoms as patients who have a stroke. These signs and symptoms can last from minutes up to 24 hours. Therefore, the signs of stroke that you note on arrival may gradually resolve. Patients who appear to have had a TIA should be transported for further evaluation.
>
> Place the patient's affected or paralyzed extremity in a secure and safe position during patient movement and transport.
>
> Some patients who have had a stroke may be unable to communicate but they can often understand what is being said around them. Be aware of this possibility.
>
> New therapies for stroke must be used shortly after the onset of symptoms. Minimize time on the scene, and notify the receiving hospital as soon as possible.

Transient Ischemic Attack

As with strokes, management of TIAs begins with standard care. Follow the same management guidelines as for CVA. Close neurologic assessment is needed. Patients may experience multiple TIAs in a short time frame.

Strongly encourage the patient to be transported. If the patient refuses transportation, appeal to the patient's family for assistance. Encourage the patient to seek medical care very soon. Offer to return and tell the patient to call 9-1-1 again if he or she wants. It is important to reinforce the message that the TIA is a warning sign of a serious and potentially deadly problem with the blood vessels in the brain.

Seizures

During the seizure, respirations may become very erratic, loud, and obviously abnormal. Alternatively, the patient may stop breathing and become cyanotic. These periods of apnea are usually very short-lived and do not require assistance. If the patient is apneic for more than 30 seconds, immediately begin ventilatory assistance.

In most situations, patients who have had a seizure require definitive evaluation and treatment in the hospital. Even a patient who has a history of chronic epilepsy that is controlled with medications may have an occasional seizure, commonly referred to as a breakthrough seizure, and also should be taken to the hospital for evaluation. Administer 100% supplemental oxygen to any patient who has experienced a seizure, whether it is the first or whether the patient has chronic seizures. This intervention will help ameliorate any associated hypoxia. Gain IV access as a medication

route even if fluid resuscitation is not needed. Note any medications the patient is currently taking and any previous seizures, the time of onset, the duration of the seizure activity, the number of seizures, and whether the patient was responsive between seizures. Provide spinal immobilization if trauma was involved or cannot be ruled out.

Depending on local protocols, you should assess and treat the patient for possible hypoglycemia (for example, a person with diabetes who has altered mental status and takes insulin or oral agents that lower the blood glucose level). Look for tongue lacerations and bleeding that may create an obstruction or lead to aspiration. With recurrent seizures, protect the patient from further injury and manage the airway as needed.

In all cases, you should be patient and tolerant because many of the patients are likely to be confused and occasionally frightened. Many patients who experience seizures are frustrated with their condition and may refuse transport. Compassion and professional behavior are required to help convince the patient that transport is necessary for definitive care.

> ## Transition Tip
>
> Children can have altered mental status caused by strokes, seizures, and other brain emergencies. However, children who have subarachnoid hemorrhages may not have a berry aneurysm; instead, they may have a congenital problem with the blood vessels in the brain known as an arteriovenous malformation. Children who have sickle cell anemia are at particularly high risk for ischemic stroke. Treat stroke in children the same way that you do in adults.
>
> As mentioned, seizures can result from sudden high fever, particularly in children. If you are treating a child whom you suspect is having a febrile seizure, you should attempt to lower the body temperature by removing the child's clothing and cooling the child with tepid water, particularly around the head and neck, and then fanning the moistened areas. Be careful not to make the patient shiver, which will further increase temperature and precipitate another seizure.
>
> Remember that although febrile seizures are generally well tolerated by children, you must transport them to the hospital. The possibility of a second seizure makes transport mandatory so that if other problems develop, the child is in the hospital and can receive immediate, definitive care.
>
> If you suspect that a patient with altered mental status has hypoglycemia, you should test for it and treat the patient according to local protocols. Patients with hypoglycemia require close monitoring, particularly of the airway, en route to the hospital.

Syncope

Begin with standard care. Determine whether the patient may have experienced trauma during the fall, and take cervical spine precautions as needed. Focus on the blood glucose level and likely cardiac causes. Obtain orthostatic vital signs, if possible. Provide supplemental oxygen and gain IV access.

Provide emotional support because syncope can be embarrassing. Transport the patient to the hospital. Syncope can be a sign of life-threatening cardiac arrhythmias, stroke, and other serious medical conditions. Call early for paramedic backup if needed.

PREP KIT

Ready for Review

- The nervous system is the most complex organ system within the human body and consists of the brain and spinal cord and thousands of nerves. The system is responsible for fundamental functions such as controlling breathing, heart rate, and blood pressure and higher-level activities. Many disorders can cause neurologic symptoms.
- The cerebrum—the largest part of the brain—is divided into right and left hemispheres, each controlling the opposite side of the body.
- Different parts of the brain control different functions. The front part of the cerebrum controls emotion and thought; the middle part controls touch and movement; and the back part is involved with vision. In most people, speech is controlled on the left side of the brain, near the middle of the cerebrum.
- A CVA, or stroke, is an interruption of blood flow to the brain that is often sudden and results in loss of function in the affected part of the brain.
- The two types of stroke are hemorrhagic and ischemic. Ischemic stroke occurs when blood flow to part of the brain is cut off by a blockage inside a cerebral artery. Hemorrhagic stroke occurs as a result of bleeding within the brain, typically when a cerebral artery ruptures.
- Rapidly transport patients in critical condition and patients in whom you suspect stroke.
- Seizures are characterized by unresponsiveness and generalized twitching of all or part of the body. There are types of seizures that you should learn to recognize: generalized, partial, and febrile.
- Most seizures last between 3 and 5 minutes and are followed by a postictal state in which the patient may be unresponsive, have labored breathing and hemiparesis. Seizures are occasionally associated with incontinence.
- Altered mental status is a neurologic problem commonly caused by hypoglycemia, intoxication, drug overdose, and poisoning.
- When you are assessing a patient with an altered mental status, do not always assume intoxication.
- Interventions will be based on assessment findings and may include providing 100% oxygen, assisting ventilations, providing spinal immobilization, administering oral glucose, establishing IV access, obtaining blood samples, administering dextrose 50%, administering glucagon, and administering fluid.

Case Study

You are providing EMS service at a local fair. It's a hot summer day and you are doing your best to stay cool. Just as you are ready to go eat lunch, a fair official comes running over to you. He tells you that someone is unconscious in the midway tent. You grab your gear and follow the man toward the tent. When you arrive, you find a man in his 60s lying supine on the ground. Bystanders tell you that the patient was complaining of a headache for the past hour and then suddenly passed out. As you examine the patient, you note that he is responsive to verbal stimuli and appears confused. On further exam you note that he is flaccid on his left side and appears to be incontinent. His wife is present and tells you the patient has a history of TIAs and hypertension.

1. If this patient had a seizure, explain the reasoning behind the flaccidness on his left side.

2. This patient initially complained of a headache. Explain the difference between a tension headache and a migraine headache.

3. Perhaps this patient has experienced a hemorrhagic stroke. How does an epidural hematoma differ from a subarachnoid hemorrhage?

4. The bystanders report that just prior to your arrival the patient was shaking all over while unconscious. This most likely describes a:
   A. generalized seizure.
   B. simple partial seizure.
   C. complex partial seizure.
   D. restless leg syndrome.

5. This patient currently is responsive to verbal stimuli, appears confused, and localizes to pain. On the basis of this information, the patient's Glasgow Coma Scale score is:
   A. 15.
   B. 14.
   C. 13.
   D. 12.

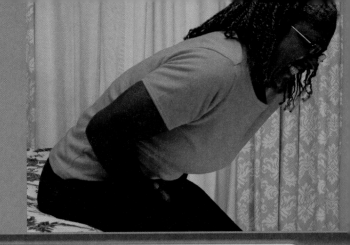

CHAPTER 13

Gastrointestinal and Urologic Emergencies

Introduction

Abdominal pain is a common complaint, but its cause is often difficult to identify. For the AEMT, it is not essential to determine the exact cause of acute abdominal pain, but it is helpful to understand the pathophysiology and signs and symptoms associated with common illnesses. The key is to be able to recognize a life-threatening problem and act quickly in response. Remember that the patient is in pain and is probably anxious, requiring your skills of rapid assessment and emotional support.

Anatomy and Physiology

The Gastrointestinal System
The gastrointestinal (GI) system is also known as the digestive tract. It consists of the mouth and many organs **FIGURE 13-1** and **FIGURE 13-2**.

The digestive process begins with saliva, which is secreted into the mouth to help lubricate food. The combination of pulverizing and lubrication creates a substance that can be easily moved. Saliva also contains enzymes that begin the chemical breakdown of foods—in particular, starches. These complex carbohydrates can be disassembled into simple sugars that are more easily absorbed. In addition, some initial breakdown of triglycerides occurs.

Once food is swallowed, it moves through the esophagus. This muscular tube is typically collapsed (that is, closed in on itself), which allows for air to easily flow into the lungs but not into the stomach. This collapsed tube idea also explains how gastric dilation and impairment of lung expansion can occur during ventilation. If a person needs positive-pressure ventilation, bag-mask ventilation can push air into the lungs. If the pressure of inhalation during breathing is too high, the esophagus dilates; air then follows the path of least resistance. Given the choice between

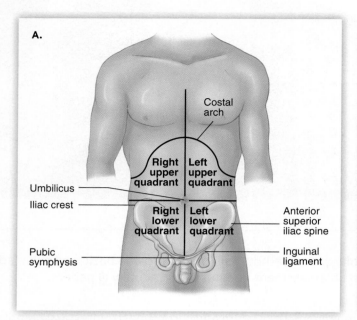

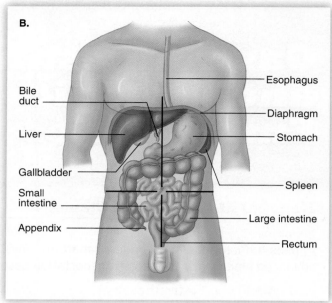

FIGURE 13-1 The anatomy of the abdomen. **A.** The four quadrants of the abdomen. **B.** Abdominal organs can lie in more than one quadrant.

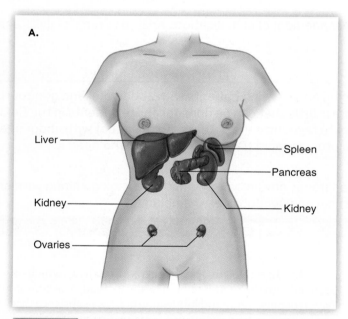

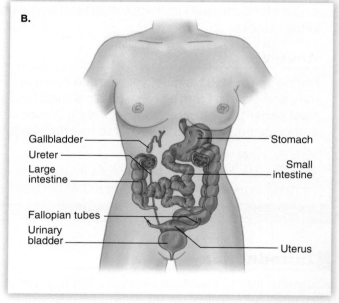

FIGURE 13-2 The solid and hollow organs of the abdomen. **A.** Solid organs include the liver, spleen, pancreas, kidneys, and in women, ovaries. **B.** Hollow organs include the gallbladder, stomach and large intestine, and urinary bladder.

moving through a large tube into a large open space (the stomach) or moving down a series of progressively smaller tubes (through the trachea into the right or left mainstem bronchus), air will flow into the stomach.

Intertwined around the esophagus are veins that drain into an even more complex series of veins that ultimately join together to form the portal vein. The portal vein transports venous blood from the GI tract directly to the liver for processing of the nutrients that have been absorbed. If blood flow through the liver slows for any reason, the blood may

back up throughout the entire GI system because this series of veins lacks any valves. The veins surrounding the stomach and esophagus then become dilated. Even a low amount of pressure may cause leaking or rupture of these vessels.

The esophagus does not absorb nutrients but rather pushes the food along using rhythmic contractions called *peristalsis*. The food travels through the diaphragm and comes to a doorway—namely, the sphincter—located at the junction of the esophagus and the stomach. The cardiac sphincter (which earns its name because people who have regurgitated acid out of the stomach into the esophagus often felt they were having a heart attack) is designed to prevent food from backing up into the esophagus.

> *Peristalsis* The wavelike contraction of smooth muscle by which the ureters or other tubular organs propel their contents.

When empty, the stomach is rather small, but it is capable of stretching many times beyond its normal size to accommodate meals. As the food enters this muscular organ, the stomach begins to secrete hydrochloric acid to help to break down the food. To mix the acid with the food more evenly, the stomach also contracts, churning the acid and food mixture together until a relatively smooth consistency is achieved. The material that exits the pyloric sphincter, the doorway at the inferior portion of the stomach, is called chyme.

The stomach absorbs some materials, such as water and fat-soluble substances (for example, alcohol). Alcohol is absorbed slowly within the stomach, but it is rapidly absorbed within the duodenum. The longer the alcohol remains within the stomach, the slower the rate of its absorption into the bloodstream. Drinking alcohol with a fatty meal will delay gastric emptying as the stomach works to digest the difficult fats.

The real purpose of the digestive system is revealed in the next portion of the GI system, the duodenum. The main function of the GI system is to absorb resources for use by other cells in the body.

The duodenum is the first part of the small intestine. It is where the pancreas, liver, and gallbladder connect to the digestive system. It is where the active stage of absorption begins. The stomach is designed to release only small amounts of the food into the duodenum at a time, thereby enabling the small intestine to better manage digestion. The exocrine portion of the pancreas secretes several enzymes into the duodenum that assist with digestion of fats, proteins, and carbohydrates. In addition, pancreatic juice helps neutralize gastric acids.

The liver creates bile, which is then stored in the gallbladder. Bile is an enzyme used by the body to help break down fats. Bile is released into the duodenum where it helps to emulsify (that is, dissolve into solution) the fats.

The liver also affects the GI system indirectly through carbohydrate metabolism. Brain cells can burn only one fuel source—glucose. If the blood glucose level falls, the liver can convert glycogen into glucose. Dramatic drops in sugar glucose will cause the liver to convert fats and proteins into sugar. As blood flows through the liver, fat and protein metabolism continues. Without a functioning liver, a person would soon die because he or she would not be able to use any of the proteins absorbed from the GI system. In addition, the liver detoxifies drugs, completes the breakdown of dead red and white blood cells, and stores vitamins and minerals.

The real workhorse of the digestive system is the small intestine; 90% of all absorption occurs there. This 22-ft-long structure is divided into three sections: the duodenum (the last section of the upper GI system), the jejunum (the first part of the lower GI system), and the ileum. The small intestine produces enzymes that work with the pancreatic enzymes to turn chyme into substances that can be directly absorbed by the capillaries of the small intestine and thereby move into the bloodstream.

Blood filled with these nutrients exits the intestinal circulation and heads to the liver, where additional metabolism of fats takes place, and then returns to the heart. The blood then leaves the liver and enters the subclavian vessels. Water-soluble vitamins are absorbed into the bloodstream for use by cells.

The large intestine, or colon, is the next destination. The substance that arrives in this 5-ft-long structure is no longer called chyme, but rather feces. The first portion of the large intestine is called the cecum. Between the terminal portion of the ileum and the cecum is the ileocecal valve, which prevents fecal matter from reentering the small intestine. Immediately after this valve is a blind pouch called the appendix. This blind pouch is able to hold small amounts of material. If the feces contains too much bacteria, indigestible foreign bodies are present, or the appendix becomes compressed or twisted, it can become inflamed, resulting in appendicitis.

Rising up from the cecum is the ascending colon. It attaches to the transverse colon, which runs from right to left. After a 90° turn, the descending colon begins. The end of the colon is therefore found near the left lower quadrant. The sigmoid colon then takes an "S" turn, which aligns its most inferior portion in the center of the pelvis. Attached to the sigmoid colon is the rectum, the last portion of the colon. The colon terminates at a sphincter called the anus, where the feces are expelled from the body.

The primary role of the large intestine is to complete the reabsorption of water. Although the majority of water is reabsorbed in the small intestine, the osmotic function within the colon helps to solidify the digested material into a formed stool. Failure of this portion of the bowel can lead to a soft, watery stool, and eventual dehydration.

The colon is also the site of bacterial digestion. Bacteria normally found within the colon help to finish the breakdown of the chyme. This breakdown produces gas as a byproduct. Flatulence may be considered impolite, but it is also a sign of normal digestive function.

The entire digestion process takes 8 to 72 hours. At this pace, bowel movements normally range between three movements per day and one movement every 3 days. Of course, this number varies based on the types of food a person eats, the amount of water consumed, exercise level, stress level, and genetics.

The Genital System

The pelvis also holds the male and female reproductive organs. The male reproductive system consists of the testicles, epididymis, vasa deferentia, seminal vesicles, prostate gland, and penis. The female reproductive system includes the ovaries, fallopian tubes, uterus, cervix, and the vagina.

The Urinary System

The urinary system performs two main functions for the body. It acts as the body's accounting firm, keeping track of the electrolytes, water content, and acids of the blood; and it acts as the blood's sewage treatment plant, removing metabolic wastes, drug metabolites, and excess fluids. The kidneys perform these functions continuously, filtering 200 liters of blood each day.

The urinary system consists of the *kidneys*, which filter the blood and produce *urine*; the *urinary bladder*, which stores the urine until it is released from the body; the *ureters*, which transport the urine from the kidneys to the bladder; and the *urethra*, which transports the urine from the bladder out of the body. The bean-shaped kidneys are found in the retroperitoneal space (behind the peritoneum), which extends from the 12th thoracic vertebra to the third lumbar vertebra. The right kidney is slightly lower than the left because of the position of the liver. The medial side of the kidney is concave, forming a cleft called the *hilus*, where the ureters, renal blood vessels, lymphatic vessels, and nerves enter and leave the kidney.

Kidneys Two retroperitoneal organs that excrete the end products of metabolism as urine and regulate the body's salt and water content.

Urine Liquid waste products filtered out of the body by the urinary system.

Urinary bladder A hollow, muscular sac in the midline of the lower pelvis that stores urine until it is released from the body.

Ureters Small, hollow tubes that carry urine from the kidneys to the bladder.

Urethra The canal that conveys urine from the bladder to outside the body.

Hilus When used in the context of the kidneys, a cleft where the ureters, renal blood vessels, lymphatic vessels, and nerves enter and leave the kidney.

A fibrous capsule covers the kidney and protects it against infection. Surrounding this capsule is a fatty mass of adipose tissue that cushions the kidney and holds it in place in the abdomen. A layer of dense fibrous connective tissue called the *renal fascia* anchors the kidney to the retroperitoneal flank.

Renal fascia Dense, fibrous connective tissue that anchors the kidney to the retroperitoneal flank.

Once the urine enters the collecting ducts, it passes through the minor calyx, into the major calyx, and then into the renal pelvis. From there, the urine moves through the ureter (one ureter from each kidney) and is stored in the urinary bladder. Most of the bladder sits in the anterior pelvis immediately adjacent to the abdominal peritoneum, but the dome of the bladder sits in the posterior abdominal cavity, or retroperitoneum, where the ureters and kidneys reside. When empty, the bladder collapses, and the muscular walls fold over onto themselves. In contrast, as urine accumulates, the bladder expands and becomes pear-shaped. Normally, the brain exerts control over the urge to void, keeping the external urinary sphincter contracted until conditions are favorable for urination. At this point, the inhibition of the external urinary sphincter is reduced and the urine passes from the urinary bladder into the urethra.

The beginning of the urethra, through which urine is expelled, sits at the inferior aspect of the bladder. In both men and women, the urethra exits at the site of the external genitalia. The female urethra is shorter than the male urethra (4 cm versus 20 cm).

▪ Pathophysiology

Causes of Acute Abdomen

Many organs in the abdominal cavity are covered by visceral peritoneum; parietal peritoneum covers the inside aspect of the abdominal wall that forms the abdominal cavity. The entire abdominal cavity normally contains a very small amount of peritoneal fluid to bathe the organs. Any condition that allows pus, blood, feces, urine, gastric juice, intestinal contents, bile, pancreatic juice, amniotic fluid, or other foreign material to lie within or adjacent to this cavity can cause peritonitis and, thus, an acute abdomen. Technically, organs such as kidneys, ovaries, and other genitourinary structures are *retroperitoneal* (behind the peritoneum). However, because they lie next to the peritoneum, problems in these organs can lead to irritation of the peritoneum and symptoms of an acute abdomen.

Therefore, nearly every kind of abdominal problem can cause an acute abdomen.

Ulcers

The stomach and duodenum are subjected to high levels of acidity. To prevent damage to these organs, protective layers of mucus line the inside cavity of both organs. In peptic ulcer disease, the protective layer is eroded, allowing the acid to eat into the organ itself over a period of weeks, months, or even years.

Most peptic *ulcers* are the result of infection of the stomach with *Helicobacter pylori*. Another major cause is long-term use of nonsteroidal anti-inflammatory drugs. Alcohol and smoking can also affect the severity of peptic ulcer disease by increasing gastric acidity.

Ulcers Abrasions of the inner lining of the stomach or small intestine.

Peptic ulcer disease affects men and women equally but tends to occur more often in the older population. As people age, the immune system's ability to fight infection decreases, making infection more likely. The geriatric population, in general, also uses nonsteroidal anti-inflammatory drugs frequently for arthritis and other musculoskeletal conditions.

Patients with peptic ulcers experience a classic sequence of burning or gnawing pain in the stomach that subsides or diminishes immediately after eating and then reemerges 2 to 3 hours later. The pain usually presents in the upper part of the abdomen but sometimes may be found below the sternum. With some patients, the pain occurs immediately after eating. Nausea, vomiting, belching, and heartburn are common symptoms. If the erosion is severe, gastric bleeding can occur, resulting in hematemesis and melena (black, tarry stools containing blood).

Some ulcers will heal without medical intervention, but often complications can occur from bleeding or perforation (a hole through the wall of the stomach). More serious ulcerative conditions can cause severe peritonitis and an acute abdomen.

Gallstones

The gallbladder is a storage pouch for bile, digestive juices produced by the liver. Gallstones can form and block the outlet from the gallbladder, causing pain. Sometimes the blockage will pass, but if not, it can lead to severe inflammation of the gallbladder, called cholecystitis. This is a condition in which the wall of the gallbladder becomes inflamed. In severe cases, the gallbladder may rupture, causing inflammation to spread and irritate surrounding structures such as the diaphragm and bowel. This condition presents as a constant, severe pain in the right upper or midabdominal region and may refer to the right upper part of the back, shoulder area, or flank. The pain may steadily increase for hours or may come and go. Cholecystitis commonly produces symptoms about 30 minutes after a particularly fatty meal and usually at night. Other symptoms include general GI distress such as nausea and vomiting, indigestion, bloating, gas, and belching.

Pancreatitis

The pancreas forms digestive juices and is also the source of insulin. Inflammation of the pancreas is called pancreatitis. *Pancreatitis* can be caused by an obstructing gallstone, alcohol abuse, and other diseases. Severe pain may present in the upper left and right quadrants and may often radiate to the back. Other signs and symptoms accompanying the pain are nausea and vomiting, abdominal distention, and tenderness. Complications such as sepsis or hemorrhage can occur, in which case assessment may also reveal fever or tachycardia.

> *Pancreatitis* Inflammation of the pancreas.

Appendicitis

The appendix is a small blind pouch attached to the large intestine. Inflammation or infection in the appendix is called appendicitis and is a frequent cause of acute abdomen. This inflammation can eventually cause the tissues to die and/or rupture, causing an abscess, peritonitis, or shock. Initially, the pain caused by appendicitis is more generalized, dull, and diffuse and may center in the umbilical area. The pain later localizes to the right lower quadrant of the abdomen. Appendicitis can also cause referred pain. The patient may also report nausea and vomiting, anorexia (lack of appetite for food), fever, and chills. A classic symptom of appendicitis is *rebound tenderness*. Rebound tenderness is a result of peritoneal irritation. This can be assessed by pressing down gently and firmly on the abdomen. With rebound tenderness, the patient will feel increased pain when the pressure is released as opposed to when the pressure is initially applied. Women who are pregnant may not exhibit this symptom.

> *Rebound tenderness* Pain that the patient feels when pressure is released as opposed to when pressure is applied; characteristic of appendicitis.

Gastrointestinal Hemorrhage

Bleeding within the GI tract is a symptom of another disease, not a disease itself. GI hemorrhage can be acute, which may be shorter term and more severe, or chronic, which may be of longer duration and less severe. All complaints of bleeding should be considered serious.

A GI hemorrhage can occur in the upper or lower GI tract. Bleeding in the upper GI tract occurs from the esophagus to the upper part of the small intestine. In the esophagus, problems might include esophagitis, esophageal varices, or Mallory-Weiss syndrome.

Lower GI bleeding occurs between the upper part of the small intestine and the anus. Bowel inflammation, diverticulitis, cancer, and hemorrhoids are common causes of bleeding in the lower GI tract.

Esophagitis

Esophagitis occurs when the lining of the esophagus becomes inflamed by infection or from the acids in the stomach (gastroesophageal reflux disease). The patient may report pain with swallowing and complain of feeling like an object is stuck in his or her throat. Additional symptoms include heartburn, nausea, vomiting, and sores in the mouth. In the worst cases, bleeding can occur from the small capillary vessels within the esophageal lining or larger blood vessels.

> *Esophagitis* Inflammation of the lining of the esophagus.

Esophageal Varices

Esophageal varices occur when the amount of pressure within the blood vessels surrounding the esophagus increases. The esophageal blood vessels eventually deposit their blood into the portal system. If the liver becomes damaged and blood cannot flow through it easily, blood begins to back up into these portal vessels, dilating the vessels and causing the capillary network of the esophagus to begin leaking. If pressure continues to build, the vessel walls may fail, causing bleeding.

> *Esophageal varices* A condition in which the amount of pressure within the blood vessels surrounding the esophagus increases, eventually causing the capillary network of the esophagus to leak, which in turn leads to severe hematemesis.

In industrialized countries, alcohol is the main cause of portal hypertension. Long-term alcohol consumption damages the tissue of the liver (cirrhosis), leading to slower blood flow. In developing countries, viral hepatitis is the main cause of liver damage.

Presentation of esophageal varices takes two forms. Initially, the patient shows signs of liver disease—fatigue, weight loss, jaundice, anorexia, edema in the abdomen, abdominal pain, nausea, and vomiting. This very gradual disease process takes months to years before the patient reaches a state of extreme discomfort.

By contrast, the rupture of the varices is far more sudden. The patient will complain of sudden-onset discomfort in the throat. He or she may have severe difficulty swallowing, vomiting of bright red blood, hypotension, and signs of shock. If the bleeding is less dramatic, hematemesis (vomiting blood) and melena (black, tarry stools) are likely. Regardless of the speed of bleeding, damage to these vessels can be life threatening. Spontaneous rupture is often life threatening, and significant blood loss at the scene may be evident. Major ruptures can lead to death in a matter of minutes.

Mallory-Weiss Syndrome

Mallory-Weiss syndrome may lead to severe hemorrhage. In this condition, the junction between the esophagus and the stomach tears, causing severe bleeding and, potentially, death. This typically occurs in the context of severe prolonged cases of forceful vomiting or retching. Primary risk factors include alcoholism and eating disorders. Mallory-Weiss syndrome affects men and women equally but is more prevalent in older adults and older children.

> *Mallory-Weiss syndrome* A condition in which the junction between the esophagus and the stomach tears as a result of prolonged forceful vomiting or retching, causing severe bleeding and, potentially, death.

Vomiting is the principal cause. In women, this syndrome may be associated with severe vomiting related to pregnancy. The extent of the bleeding can range from very minor bleeding, resulting in very little blood loss, to severe bleeding and extreme fluid loss. In extreme cases, patients may experience signs and symptoms of shock, upper abdominal pain, hematemesis, and melena.

Gastroenteritis

Acute infectious *gastroenteritis* comprises a family of conditions revolving around a central theme of infection combined with diarrhea, nausea, and vomiting. Bacterial and viral organisms can cause this condition. These organisms typically enter the body through contaminated food or water. Patients may begin to experience an upset stomach and diarrhea as soon as several hours or several days after contact with the contaminated matter. The disease can then run its course in 2 to 3 days or continue for several weeks.

> *Gastroenteritis* A family of conditions resulting from diarrhea, nausea, and vomiting; some have infectious causes.

Other types of gastroenteritis are not infectious but have all of the hallmarks of acute infectious gastroenteritis. Patients with this condition experience nausea, vomiting, and diarrhea from a noninfectious cause, such as medications, toxins from shellfish, or chemotherapy.

Diarrhea is the principal symptom in both types of gastroenteritis. Patients may experience large dumping-type diarrhea or frequent small liquid stools. The diarrhea may contain blood and/or pus, and it may have a foul odor or be odorless. Abdominal cramping is frequently reported. Nausea, vomiting, fever, and anorexia are also present. If the diarrhea continues, dehydration will result. As the volume of fluid loss increases, the likelihood of shock increases.

Diverticulitis

Diverticulitis was first recognized around 1900, when the types of foods people ate began to change dramatically. In particular, the amount of fiber within the United States diet plummeted as the amount of processed foods eaten increased.

As the amount of fiber consumed as part of the diet decreases, the consistency of the normal stool becomes more solid. This hard stool requires more intestinal contractions, subsequently increasing pressure within the colon. In this environment, small defects within the colonic wall that would otherwise never pose a problem now fail, resulting in bulges in the wall. These small outcroppings eventually turn into pouches called diverticula. As feces travel through the colon, some may become trapped within these pouches. When bacteria grow there, they cause localized inflammation and infection.

The main symptom of diverticulitis is abdominal pain, which tends to be localized to the left side of the lower abdomen. Classic signs of infection include fever, malaise, body aches, chills, nausea, and vomiting. Bleeding is rare with this condition. Because of the local infections of these pouches, adhesions may develop, narrowing the diameter of the colon and resulting in constipation and bowel obstruction.

Hemorrhoids

Hemorrhoids are created by swelling and inflammation of the blood vessels surrounding the rectum. They are a common problem, with almost half the population having at least one hemorrhoid by age 50 years. Hemorrhoids may result from conditions that increase pressure on the rectum or irritation of the rectum. Pregnancy, straining at stool, and chronic constipation cause increased pressure. Diarrhea can cause irritation.

Hemorrhoids often result in bright red blood noted during defecation. This bleeding tends to be minimal and is easily controlled. In addition, patients may experience itching and a small mass on the rectum. Typically, this mass is a clot formed in response to the mild bleeding.

Urinary System

Diseases and problems of the renal and urologic system can cause acute abdominal pain. These conditions range from mild (urinary tract infections) to true emergencies (acute renal failure). Although the prehospital care for many urologic diseases is supportive, your ability to recognize the signs and symptoms of the true emergencies is critical to providing your patients with the best chance of a positive outcome.

Urinary tract infections (UTIs) usually develop in the lower urinary tract (urethra and bladder) when normal flora bacteria, which exist naturally on the skin, or other bacteria enter the urethra and grow. These infections are more common in women owing to the relatively short urethra and the proximity of the urethra to the vagina and rectum. A UTI in the upper urinary tract (ureters and kidneys) occurs most often when a lower UTI goes untreated. Upper UTIs can lead to *pyelonephritis* (inflammation of the kidney and renal pelvis) and abscesses, which eventually reduce kidney function. In severe cases, untreated UTIs can lead to sepsis.

> *Urinary tract infections (UTIs)* Infections, usually of the lower urinary tract (urethra and bladder), which occur when normal flora bacteria or other bacteria enter the urethra and grow.
> *Pyelonephritis* Inflammation of the kidney and renal pelvis.

Common symptoms in patients with a lower UTI include painful urination, frequent urges to urinate, and difficulty in urination. The pain usually begins as a *visceral discomfort* but then converts to an extreme burning pain, especially during urination. The pain, which remains localized in the pelvis, is often perceived as bladder pain in women and prostate pain in men. Sometimes the pain may be referred to the shoulder or neck. In addition, the urine may have a foul odor and may appear cloudy.

> *Visceral discomfort* Crampy, aching pain deep within the body, the source of which is usually difficult to pinpoint; common with urologic problems.

Renal System

Kidney stones originate in the renal pelvis and result when an excess of insoluble salts or uric acid crystallizes in the urine. This excess of salts is typically the result of water intake that is insufficient to dissolve the salts. The stones consist of different types of chemicals, depending on the precise imbalance in the urine.

> *Kidney stones* Solid crystalline masses formed in the kidney, resulting from an excess of insoluble salts or uric acid crystallizing in the urine; may become trapped anywhere along the urinary tract.

The most common stones—calcium stones—occur more frequently in men than in women and may have a hereditary component. These stones also occur in patients with metabolic disorders such as gout or with hormonal disorders.

Patients who have kidney stones will almost always be in pain. (Many rate kidney stone pain as 11 on a scale of 1 to 10.) The pain usually starts as a vague discomfort in the flank but becomes very intense within 30 to 60 minutes. It may migrate forward and toward the groin as the stone passes through the system.

Some patients will be agitated and restless as they walk and move in an attempt to relieve the pain. Others will attempt to remain motionless and guard the abdomen. Either behavior makes palpation of the abdomen difficult. Vital signs will vary, depending on the severity of pain. The greater the pain, the higher will be the blood pressure and pulse.

If a stone has become lodged in the lower part of the ureter, signs and symptoms of a UTI (frequency and urgency of urination, painful urination, and/or *hematuria*) may be present, but the patient will not have a fever. If a kidney stone is suspected, be sure to obtain a patient history and a family history; both can supply important information.

> *Hematuria* The presence of blood in the urine.

Acute renal failure (ARF) is a sudden (possibly during a period of days) decrease in kidney filtration. It is accompanied by an increase of toxins in the blood. Patients with ARF have an overall mortality rate of 50%, but the disease is reversible if diagnosed and treated early.

> *Acute renal failure (ARF)* A sudden decrease in filtration through the glomeruli of the kidneys.

If the urine output drops to less than 750 mL/day, the condition is called *oliguria*. If urine production stops completely, the condition is called *anuria*. Whenever ARF occurs, the patient may experience generalized edema, acid buildup, and high levels of waste products in the blood. If left untreated, ARF can lead to heart failure, hypertension, and metabolic acidosis.

> *Oliguria* A decrease in urine output to the extent that total urine output drops to less than 750 mL/day.
> *Anuria* A complete stop in urine production.

Chronic renal failure (CRF) is progressive and irreversible inadequate kidney function. This disease develops over months or years. More than half of all cases are caused by systemic diseases such as diabetes or hypertension. In addition, CRF can be caused by congenital disorders such as polycystic kidney disease or prolonged pyelonephritis, or can be a secondary complication of some infections such as strep throat.

> *Chronic renal failure (CRF)* Progressive and irreversible inadequate kidney function as a result of permanent loss of nephrons.

As the *nephrons* of the kidney become damaged and cease to function, scarring occurs. The tissue begins to shrink and waste away as the scarring progresses, leading to a loss of nephrons and renal mass. As kidney function diminishes, waste products and fluid build up in the blood. Systemic complications can develop, such as hypertension, congestive heart failure, anemia, and electrolyte imbalances.

> *Nephrons* The structural and functional units of the kidney that form urine; composed of the glomerulus, the glomerular (Bowman) capsule, the proximal convoluted tubule, loop of Henle, and the distal convoluted tubule.

Patients with CRF exhibit several signs and symptoms, beginning with an altered level of consciousness. In the late stages, seizures and coma are possible. The patients may also present with lethargy, nausea, headaches, cramps, and signs of anemia.

In a case of CRF, the patient's skin will be pale, cool, and moist, and the patient may appear jaundiced because of the buildup of wastes. A powdery accumulation of uric acid, called *uremic frost*, may also be present, especially on the face. The skin may appear bruised, and muscle twitching may be present.

> *Uremic frost* A powdery buildup of uric acid, especially on the face.

Patients with CRF exhibit edema in the extremities and face as a result of fluid imbalances; they will also be hypotensive and have tachycardia. Pericarditis and pulmonary edema are also common and should be considered during auscultation of the chest.

Patient Assessment

Scene Size-up

Ensure that the scene is safe and follow standard precautions. Consider donning a gown and covering your shoes with disposable, protective covers because there may be feces and urine on the floor and some patients may have active projectile vomiting. Examples of additional resources for a GI patient include extra gloves, masks, gowns, change of uniform, suction equipment, extra linens, blankets, washcloths, towels, and adult and child diapers.

Acute abdomen can be the result of violence, such as blunt or penetrating trauma, so always be vigilant. Note that most calls for GI problems will not involve multiple patients. However, a call for assistance at an office building where several people are complaining about GI symptoms should lead you to suspect release of an agent. Biologic or chemical agents, for example, can cause people to have abdominal pain, nausea, vomiting, diarrhea, and other GI signs and symptoms.

Primary Assessment

The following is a checklist of common signs and symptoms of irritation or inflammation of the peritoneum that you can use to determine whether a patient may have an acute abdomen:

- Local or diffuse abdominal pain and/or tenderness
- A quiet patient who is guarding the abdomen
- Rapid and shallow breathing
- Referred (distant) pain
- Anorexia, nausea, and vomiting
- Hematemesis (bright red or "coffee-ground" emesis)
- Tense, often distended, abdomen
- Sudden constipation or bloody diarrhea
- Dark, tarry stool (melena)
- Painful or frequent urination
- Tachycardia
- Hypotension
- Fever

A patient with urologic or renal problems may exhibit extremes of activity. Is the patient constantly changing positions in an attempt to find a comfortable position ("the kidney stone dance")? Or is the patient sitting very still with the knees drawn to the chest? Is the abdomen distended or rigid? If you find any life-threatening conditions, take immediate steps to correct them.

Remember, it is not critical for an AEMT to determine the cause of acute abdomen but to recognize potential causes and provide the correct supportive care.

One aspect of the general impression that is different for GI patients is odor. What is the smell of the room or location of the patient? There are few EMS calls that rise to the level of noxious odor more than those that involve upper GI bleeding. The foul-smelling stool that accompanies these calls can make even an experienced AEMT nauseous. When dealing with these strong odors, the key is to hold your ground. The sense of smell is the most acute for about 1 minute, but then more than 50% of the intensity of an odor is lost because the olfactory nerve becomes tired of sending the same signal. If you are faced with a strong odor on a call, stay in the environment. After 2 to 5 minutes, the smell may be barely noticeable.

Airway patency becomes a pertinent concern with a GI patient. A patient who is vomiting has a greater chance to aspirate. In patients who are awake and responsive, positioning is key to maintaining a patent airway. In patients who have an altered mental status, open the airway using the appropriate maneuvers and closely inspect it for foreign bodies. Remove or suction any obstructions found. While evaluating the airway, notice any unusual odors emanating from the mouth. Patients who have extremely advanced bowel obstructions can have feculent breath, smelling of stool.

GI problems rarely affect breathing directly. If a breathing problem is encountered, it typically stems from a severe complication. Ensure that the airway is clear. In particular, if the patient has aspirated, it can affect his or her ability to oxygenate and ventilate. Also, as a result of the abdominal pain, the patient may show shallow or inadequate respirations because deep breaths often intensify the pain.

The assessment of the circulatory system is essential in understanding how the GI issue is affecting the body. As with all patients, assess skin color, temperature, and condition (that is, moist or dry and turgor). Determine the heart rate. Evaluate the peripheral pulses and compare them with the central pulses. Remember to assess for major bleeding. The patient's pulse rate and quality, as well as skin condition, may indicate shock. Check the pulses in both arms because a difference in pulse strength may be a sign of a thoracic aortic aneurysm.

Many GI diseases involve pain and/or hemorrhage. As blood volume begins to drop, the body tries to compensate for this change by releasing catecholamines in the form of epinephrine and norepinephrine. These agents attempt to stabilize blood pressure through vasoconstriction, increased heart rate, and increased force of left ventricular contraction. Pain stimulates similar body responses. Either problem can leave the patient with tachycardia, diminished peripheral pulses, diaphoresis, and pale, cool, clammy skin.

Shock may be caused by hypovolemia or may be the result of a severe infection (sepsis). If evidence of shock (inadequate perfusion) is present, interventions should include high-flow oxygen, elevating the patient's legs 6 to 12 inches by placing a pillow or blanket under the knees and lower legs or to a position of comfort, and keeping the patient warm. Ensure that you provide prompt treatment for life threats, and do not delay in providing transport.

Check the patient's blood pressure. To ensure the accuracy of this measurement, obtain a manual pressure before you use one of the automated blood pressure machines. *Orthostatic vital signs* will help you determine the extent of bleeding that has occurred.

> *Orthostatic vital signs* Assessing vital signs in three different patient positions (for example, from a lying position, to a sitting position, then to a standing position) to determine the degree of hypovolemia; also called a tilt test.

When you examine a patient with a GI problem for gross bleeding, it is not unusual to find large amounts of blood. Take note of the amount of blood lost, focusing on being accurate. The emotional effects of seeing large amounts of blood could lead people to overestimate the volume lost. The amount of blood in a toilet is particularly difficult to estimate owing to dilution. To practice volume estimation, measure the amount of water in a glass, and then spill it on a carpet; note the size of the puddle. Spill another volume of water on a hard surface such as a tile floor; again note the size of the puddle.

When making your transport decision, integrate the information obtained in the primary assessment. If the patient has positive orthostatic vital signs (that is, serial vital signs change with a change in position), thoughtfully consider how the patient will be moved. Ensure that the ride during transport is as gentle as possible for the patient. Drive smoothly and steadily. Rapid driving can result in increased vehicle movement, potentially aggravating and possibly worsening the patient's abdominal pain.

History Taking

Pain is often a finding of importance in patients with GI problems because it can indicate trauma, hemorrhage, infection, or obstruction. As with the primary assessment, use OPQRST (**O**nset, **P**rovocation/palliation, **Q**uality, **R**egion/radiation, **S**everity, and **T**iming of pain) to elaborate on the chief complaint. **TABLE 13-1** describes the types of pain that may be experienced with an abdominal problem.

In patients with a urologic problem, the patient history and physical examination will provide important information. Determining that the pain actually started in the flank and not in its present location of the lower right quadrant could mean the difference between a correct field diagnosis of a kidney stone and an incorrect field diagnosis of appendicitis. Similarly, determining that the patient has a history of diabetes and hypertension along with signs of uremia can help confirm your impression of CRF.

The SAMPLE history will help elicit the relevant current and past medical history. Ask the following questions specific to the signs and symptoms of a GI or urologic emergency:

- **Nausea and vomiting.** Do you feel nauseous? Have you vomited? How many times? In what period of time? Was there red blood? Did it look like coffee grounds?
- **Changes in bowel habits.** Has there been any change in your bowel habits? Have you been constipated? Did the stool look dark and tarry? Have you had diarrhea? Was there any red blood in it?
- **Urination.** Have you been urinating more or less often than usual? Is there pain when you urinate? Is the color of the urine dark or unusual? Is there an unusual odor?
- **Weight loss.** Have you lost weight recently? How many pounds?
- **Belching or flatulence.** Have you experienced belching or flatulence? For how long?
- **Pain.** What does the pain feel like? How long have you had this pain? Is the pain constant or intermittent?
- **Other.** Ask about any other signs or symptoms related to this complaint, such as "Are there any changes you have noted recently that may be contributing to your pain?"
- **Concurrent chest pain.** If the patient reports chest pain, use OPQRST.

Table 13-1
Types of Abdominal Pain

Abdominal Pain Type	Origin	Description	Cause
Visceral discomfort	Hollow organs	Difficult to localize; described as burning, cramping, gnawing, or aching; usually felt superficially	Organ contracts too forcefully or is distended (stretched)
Parietal pain/rebound pain	Peritoneum	Steady achy pain; easier to localize than visceral; increases with movement	Inflammation of the peritoneum (caused by blood and/or infection)
Somatic pain	Peripheral nerve tracts	Well localized pain; usually felt deeply	Irritation or injury to tissue causing activation of peripheral nerve tracts
Referred pain	Peripheral nerve tracts	Pain originating in the abdomen and causing "pain" in distant locations; usually occurs after initial visceral, parietal, or somatic pain	Similar paths for the peripheral nerves of the abdomen and the distant location

The SAMPLE history may not affect the interventions you perform, but it will help provide needed information for the physician in the emergency department to aid in determining the cause of the acute abdomen.

Secondary Assessment

In some situations, patients with an acute abdomen are comfortable only when lying in one particular position, which tends to relax muscles adjacent to the inflamed organ and thus lessen the pain. Therefore, the position of the patient may provide you with an important clue. For example, a patient with appendicitis may draw up the right knee. A patient with pancreatitis may lie curled up on one side.

A healthy or normal abdomen should be soft and should not be tender. An acute abdomen is characterized by abdominal pain and tenderness. The pain may be sharply localized or diffuse (widespread) and will vary in severity. Localized pain gives a clue to the problem organ or area causing it. Tenderness may be minimal or so great that the patient will not allow you to touch the abdomen. In some cases, the muscles of the abdominal wall become rigid in an involuntary effort to protect the abdomen from further irritation. This boardlike muscle spasm, called *guarding*, can be seen with major problems such as a perforated peptic ulcer or pancreatitis.

Guarding Involuntary muscle contractions (spasms) of the abdominal wall in an effort to protect an inflamed or injured abdomen; may be a sign of peritonitis.

Remember, a patient with peritonitis usually has abdominal pain, even when lying quietly. The patient can be quiet but have difficulty breathing and may take rapid, shallow breaths because of the pain. Usually, you will find tenderness on palpation of the abdomen or when the patient moves. The degree of pain and tenderness is usually related directly to the severity of peritoneal inflammation.

Findings of a high respiratory rate with a normal pulse rate and blood pressure may indicate the patient is unable to ventilate properly because deep breathing causes pain. A high respiratory rate and pulse rate with signs of shock, such as pallor and diaphoresis (profuse sweating), may indicate septic or hypovolemic shock.

Use pulse oximetry and noninvasive blood pressure devices when these monitoring devices are available. It is recommended that you always assess the patient's first blood pressure manually with a sphygmomanometer (blood pressure cuff) and stethoscope.

Reassessment

Because it is often difficult to determine the cause of an acute abdominal emergency, it is extremely important to reassess your patient frequently to determine whether the patient's condition has changed. Remember, the condition of a patient with an acute abdomen can change rapidly from stable to unstable.

Vital signs must be reassessed and compared with the patient's baseline vital signs. If anything changes en route to the hospital, manage the problem and document any changes or additional treatment.

Routine monitoring should include heart rate, blood pressure, respiratory rate, and pulse oximetry. If the patient has GI bleeding, continue to assess for signs of shock. Equally important, you should determine what effect your treatment is having. Before giving additional fluid boluses, listen to the patient's lung sounds to determine whether acute pulmonary edema is developing. If the patient wants to lie on his or her side, try to make that possible. Be sure that you can observe and maintain the patient's airway because vomiting is common.

Remember to call for paramedic backup if the patient's condition is unstable. If transport time is extended and rapid transport is needed, consider air medical transport if available.

Patients with urologic emergencies, especially patients with signs and symptoms of renal failure, need reassessment. The electrolyte imbalances caused by the buildup of toxins can cause major, rapid changes in the functioning of the body's organs. Serial vital signs should be obtained and documented on the prehospital care report, at least every 5 minutes in cases of possible renal failure. Note any trends in the vital signs and level of consciousness because they can be indicators of disease progression. Patients with possible urologic disease should not be given anything by mouth because this may induce vomiting or complicate surgical procedures.

If the patient's condition undergoes a sudden, dramatic change, repeat the rapid and detailed assessments as if this were a new patient. This will give you the best chance of modifying your care appropriately to manage this new development.

Emergency Medical Care

The signs and symptoms of an acute abdomen signal a serious medical or surgical emergency. Ensure that you provide prompt, gentle transport for the patient; do not delay transport. Carry out the following steps as quickly as possible before transport.

1. Do not attempt to diagnose the cause of the acute abdomen.
2. Clear and maintain the airway.
3. Anticipate vomiting. Place the patient in the recovery position or position of comfort. Most patients feel better in a lateral recumbent position with the knees pulled in toward the chest.
4. Administer 100% supplemental oxygen and be prepared to assist ventilation if the patient has a reduced tidal volume (shallow breathing).
5. Do not give the patient anything by mouth. Food or fluid will only aggravate many of the symptoms because intestinal paralysis will prevent it from passing out of the stomach. In addition, the stomach will have to be emptied before surgery if it is required.
6. Document all pertinent information. Use OPQRST. Note the presence of abdominal tenderness, distention, or guarding.
7. Anticipate the development of hypovolemic shock. Monitor blood pressure. Treat the patient for shock when it is evident. Elevate the patient's legs 6 to 12 inches (shock position).
8. Establish IV access, and give a 20-mL/kg bolus of an isotonic crystalloid if the patient presents with signs of hypovolemia. Otherwise, maintain fluid at a keep-vein-open rate. If kidney function is present, administer a bolus of fluid to the patient with a UTI and to a patient with a kidney stone. The fluid will rehydrate the patient, and an increased volume of urine will help flush any infection from the system. For a patient with renal calculi, the increased urine formation will help move the stone though the system.
9. Make the patient as comfortable as possible for transport. Place in a position of comfort, usually with the legs bent. Patients are more comfortable with their legs pulled up toward the abdomen because this position takes the pressure off the abdominal wall and diminishes pain. Conserve body heat with blankets, as needed. Provide gentle but rapid transport and constant psychological support.
10. Monitor vital signs; these may change quickly.
11. Consider calling for additional paramedic backup if the patient's condition shows any signs of instability.

Remember that with pelvic inflammatory disease (PID), acute pain and tenderness in the lower part of the abdomen may be intense and accompanied by a high fever. If you suspect PID, promptly transport the patient to the emergency department for treatment.

The combination of acute abdominal pain and hypovolemic shock mandates immediate transport to the hospital. Consider an ectopic pregnancy in any female of childbearing age who presents with acute abdominal distress, especially in the presence of hypotension.

Pneumonia, especially in the lower parts of the lung, may cause both ileus and abdominal pain. In this case, the problem lies in an adjacent body cavity, but the intense inflammatory response can affect the abdomen. Treat and transport this patient as you would any patient with abdominal pain.

The association of acute abdominal signs and symptoms with shock could also signify an aneurysm and requires prompt transportation. Because this is a fragile situation with a large, leaking artery, avoid unnecessary and vigorous palpation of the abdomen. Remember to handle the patient gently during transport. Avoid maneuvers that result in sudden spikes in blood pressure, as these could potentially cause rupture of an aneurysm.

Finally, ARF and CRF can lead to life-threatening emergencies. Support of the ABCs is imperative. Be alert for the possibility of hypotension or pulmonary edema. Because of possible toxic buildup and electrolyte problems, medications to regulate acidosis and electrolyte imbalance and fluids for volume regulation may be required. Emergency transport and supportive care are often preferred over aggressive management in these cases.

Renal Dialysis

The only definitive treatment in cases of CRF is *renal dialysis*. This is a technique for filtering toxic wastes from the blood, removing excess fluid, and restoring the normal balance of electrolytes. Renal dialysis and problems associated with it may require prehospital interventions.

> *Renal dialysis* A technique for filtering the blood of its toxic wastes, removing excess fluids, and restoring the normal balance of electrolytes.

There are two types of dialysis—peritoneal dialysis and hemodialysis. In peritoneal dialysis, large amounts of specially formulated dialysis fluid are infused into (and back out of) the abdominal cavity. This fluid stays in the cavity for 1 to 2 hours, allowing equilibrium to occur. Peritoneal dialysis is very effective but carries a high risk of peritonitis; consequently, aseptic technique is essential. With proper training, however, peritoneal dialysis can be performed in the home.

In hemodialysis, the patient's blood circulates through a dialysis machine that functions in much the same way (albeit not as elegantly) as the normal kidneys. Most patients undergoing long-term hemodialysis have some sort of shunt, that is, a surgically created connection between a vein and an artery that is usually located in the forearm or upper arm. The patient is connected to the dialysis machine through this shunt, which allows blood to flow from the body into the dialysis machine and back to the body.

There are many adverse effects and complications that can occur with dialysis. These include hypotension, muscle cramps, nausea and vomiting, hemorrhage, infection at the access site, altered mental status, loss of consciousness, air embolism, electrolyte imbalance, and/or myocardial ischemia.

A sudden drop in blood pressure is not uncommon during or immediately after dialysis, but it can lead to cardiac arrest if not promptly detected and treated. The patient may feel lightheaded or become confused, and often he or she yawns more than usual. Because dialysis alters the blood's chemistry, an electrolyte imbalance may develop. For this reason, you should consider the possibility of cardiac dysrhythmias and the need for advanced life support backup. Shock secondary to bleeding is also possible from any number of causes. Patients with CRF, for example, are very prone to duodenal ulcers; bleeding from those ulcers is not unusual. Bleeding may also occur from the dialysis cannula.

Also, if a patient misses a dialysis treatment, he or she may experience weakness, pulmonary edema, or excesses of electrolytes. If your call involves a patient receiving dialysis, start with the ABCs: assess and manage the airway, breathing, and circulation. Provide high-flow oxygen and manage any bleeding from the access site. Position the patient sitting up in cases of pulmonary edema or supine if the patient is in shock and transport promptly.

When you find a shunt leaking during the dialysis cycle, see if you can tighten the connection. If it has become disconnected at the vein, clamp the cannula and disconnect the patient from the machine. In a suicide attempt, the patient may open up the cannula and allow himself or herself to exsanguinate. Keep in mind that patients receiving dialysis have often endured numerous medical interventions to simply survive. If you encounter this situation, immediately clamp off the cannula and apply direct pressure.

During transport, unless there is a life-threatening event, make all attempts to deliver the patient to a hospital with dialysis capability.

PREP KIT

Ready for Review

- The GI system is also known as the digestive tract. It consists of the mouth and many organs and is divided into four quadrants.
- The genitourinary system includes the kidneys, urinary bladder, ureters, urethra, male and female reproductive organs, and specific structures within the kidneys.
- Many kinds of abdominal problem can cause an acute abdomen.
- Acute abdominal pain be caused by GI or renal sources, diverticulitis, cholecystitis, appendicitis, perforated gastric ulcer, aortic aneurysm, hernia, cystitis, kidney infection, kidney stone, pancreatitis, UTI, and in women, ectopic pregnancy and pelvic inflammation.
- Gynecologic problems are a common cause of acute abdominal pain. Always consider that a woman with lower abdominal pain and tenderness may have a problem related to her ovaries, fallopian tubes, or uterus.
- Remember that GI complaints often involve body substances. Take extra gloves, masks, gowns, and other protective equipment and supplies with you to the scene.
- Pain is commonly located directly over the inflamed area of the peritoneum, or it may be referred to another part of the body.
- A healthy or normal abdomen should be soft and not tender. The pain in the abdomen may be sharply localized or diffuse and will vary in severity.
- Renal dialysis is a procedure for removing toxic wastes and excess fluids from the blood. Patients receiving dialysis are vulnerable to problems such as hypotension, potassium imbalance, disequilibrium syndrome, and air embolism.

Case Study

You are dispatched to a local apartment complex for a person with abdominal pain. The dispatcher informs you the patient is a 38-year-old woman with abdominal pain, nausea, and vomiting. When you arrive on scene, you find the patient lying on her left side with her knees pulled up to her chest. The patient tells you that she had a sudden onset of abdominal pain that began approximately 1 hour after eating dinner. She describes the pain as a "stabbing" sensation and rates the severity of pain as 10 out of 10. She vomited twice prior to your arrival and points to her pain in the upper right quadrant. She says this happened once before, but the pain went away without treatment. She denies any past medical history and reports that she finished her menstrual cycle last week.

1. What is the pathophysiology behind cholecystitis?

2. In terms of upper GI bleeding, compare and contrast esophageal varices with Mallory-Weiss syndrome.

3. Explain how hemodialysis differs from peritoneal dialysis.

4. Which of the following conditions will have pain located in the right upper quadrant?
  A. Diverticulitis
  B. Appendicitis
  C. Cholecystitis
  D. Cystitis

5. What are the signs and symptoms of a serious hernia problem?

CHAPTER 14

Endocrine and Hematologic Emergencies

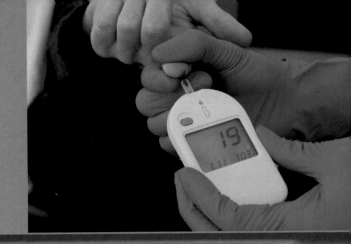

National EMS Education Standards

Anatomy and Physiology
Applies fundamental knowledge of the anatomy and function of all human systems to the practice of EMS.

Pharmacology
Applies fundamental knowledge of the medications that the AEMT may assist or administer to a patient during an emergency.

Medicine
Applies fundamental knowledge to provide basic and selected advanced emergency care and transportation based on assessment findings for an acutely ill patient.

Review

As you learned in your EMT-I course, diabetes is a disorder affecting the endocrine system, in which the body is unable to effectively utilize glucose. You have most likely encountered many diabetic patients. Treatment of these patients primarily consists of administering glucose or intravenous fluid and providing transport to the hospital for further evaluation.

Blood is made up of erythrocytes (red blood cells), which carry oxygen; leukocytes (white blood cells), which are responsible for fighting infection; platelets, which are responsible for clot formation; and plasma, which is the liquid portion of the blood responsible for carrying blood cells and nutrients and also for carrying cellular waste to the organs of excretion.

What's New

This chapter provides an in-depth look at diabetes, including the signs and symptoms that allow you to differentiate between hypoglycemia and hyperglycemia. New terminology—hyperglycemic crisis and hypoglycemic crisis—is presented to describe conditions that were previously referred to as diabetic coma and insulin shock, respectively. Glucagon is also introduced as a treatment for hypoglycemia.

Hematology is new in its entirety to the AEMT. This chapter describes the pathophysiology of blood, including sickle cell anemia and hemophilia and appropriate assessment and emergency management techniques.

Introduction

The endocrine system directly or indirectly influences almost every cell, organ, and function of the body. Consequently, patients with an endocrine disorder often are seen with a multitude of signs and symptoms that require a thorough assessment and immediate treatment. This chapter also discusses hematologic emergencies, which rarely occur in most EMS systems. Although hematologic disorders can be difficult to assess and treat in a prehospital setting, your actions may not only offer support but may save the patient's life.

Anatomy and Physiology of the Endocrine System

The *endocrine system* is a complex message and control system that integrates many body functions. Each *endocrine gland* produces one or more hormones, which it releases directly into the bloodstream **FIGURE 14-1**. A hormone is a chemical substance produced by an endocrine gland that has special regulatory effects on other organs and tissues **TABLE 14-1**. Epinephrine, norepinephrine, and insulin are examples of hormones. The main function of the endocrine system and its hormone messengers is to maintain homeostasis—that is, stability in the body's internal environment. Endocrine disorders can be caused by either hypersecretion (overproduction) or hyposecretion (underproduction) of hormones by a gland.

> *Endocrine system* The body system that regulates metabolism and maintains homeostasis.
> *Endocrine gland* Any of the glands that secrete or release hormones—that is, chemicals that are used inside the body.

Transition Tip

The brain controls the release of hormones by the endocrine glands.

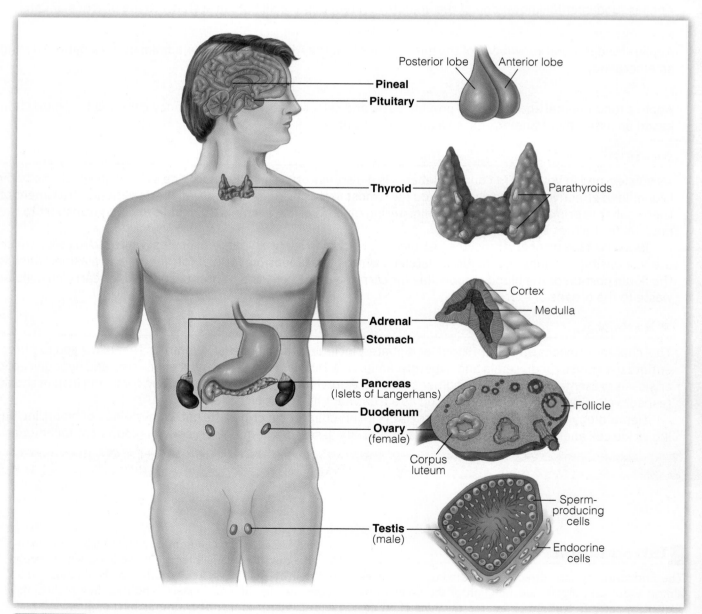

FIGURE 14-1 The endocrine system uses the various glands to deliver chemical messages to organ systems throughout the body.

Table 14-1
Endocrine Glands

Gland	Location	Function	Hormone Produced
Adrenal	Above the kidneys	Stress response, "fight or flight"	Epinephrine, norepinephrine, and others
Ovary	Female pelvis (two glands)	Regulates sexual function, characteristics, and reproduction	Estrogen and others
Pancreas	Retroperitoneal space	Regulates glucose metabolism and other functions	Insulin and others
Parathyroid	Neck (behind and beside the thyroid) (three to five glands)	Regulates serum calcium	Parathyroid hormone
Pituitary	Base of skull	Regulates all other endocrine glands	Multiple hormones; controls other endocrine glands
Testes	Male scrotum (two glands)	Regulates sexual function, characteristics, and reproduction	Testosterone and others
Thyroid	Neck (over the larynx)	Regulates metabolism	Thyroxine and others

Pathophysiology

Endocrine disorders can be caused by either hypersecretion or insufficient secretion of a gland. Hypersecretion presents as overactivity of the target organ regulated by the gland. Insufficient secretion (hyposecretion) results in underactivity of the organ controlled by the gland. Hyperthyroidism and hypothyroidism are two serious illnesses of the endocrine system. Most of the endocrine emergencies you will encounter will be related to diabetic emergencies.

Hypothyroidism and Hyperthyroidism

Thyroid hormone is secreted in response to the stimulation of the thyroid gland by the anterior pituitary gland. The anterior pituitary gland secretes thyroid-stimulating hormone (TSH) in response to the hypothalamus' secretion of thyrotropin-releasing hormone (TRH). **TABLE 14-2** summarizes the major effects of hypothyroidism and hyperthyroidism. Although millions of Americans suffer from some kind of thyroid disorder, many are unaware of their condition. Treatment of these patients should be symptomatic with transport to the closest, most appropriate facility.

Pathophysiology of Diabetes

Excesses or deficiencies in hormone levels cause many different diseases. In such cases, specific body functions are increased, decreased, or absent.

Table 14-2
Comparison of Major Effects of Hypothyroidism and Hyperthyroidism

	Hypothyroidism	Hyperthyroidism
Cardiovascular effects	Slow pulse, reduced cardiac output	Rapid pulse, increased cardiac output
Metabolic effects	Decreased metabolism, cold skin, weight gain	Increased metabolism, skin hot and flushed, weight loss
Neuromuscular effects	Weakness, sluggish reflexes	Tremor, hyperactive reflexes
Mental, emotional effects	Mental processes sluggish, personality placid	Restlessness, irritability, emotional lability
Gastrointestinal effects	Constipated	Diarrhea
General somatic effects	Cold, dry skin	Warm, moist skin

"Diabetes mellitus" means "sweet diabetes"—a reference to the presence of glucose in the urine. This disease is characterized by an inability to sufficiently metabolize glucose. Glucose (also known as dextrose) is one of the basic sugars used in the body and, in conjunction with oxygen, serves as the primary fuel for cellular metabolism.

The central problem in diabetes is the lack of or ineffective action of insulin. This hormone, which is normally produced by the endocrine glands in the pancreas, enables glucose to enter cells. Without insulin, cells begin to "starve," because the glucose is not able to get into the cells FIGURE 14-2 .

If left untreated, diabetes leads to a wasting of body tissues and death. Even with medical care, some patients with particularly aggressive forms of diabetes will die relatively young of one or more complications of the disease. Most diabetics live a normal life span. Nevertheless, diabetes is a life-altering disease that requires patients to make adjustments in their eating habits and activities.

Types of Diabetes

As you know, there are two distinct types of diabetes. In type 1 diabetes, patients cannot produce insulin and, therefore, need daily injections of supplemental, synthetic insulin to control their blood glucose levels. This type of diabetes typically develops during childhood and in the past was referred to as "juvenile-onset diabetes," or insulin-dependent diabetes mellitus (IDDM). It is now recognized that type 1 diabetes also may develop later in life, so those terms are no longer used. Patients with type 1 diabetes are more likely to have metabolic problems and to experience organ damage, such as blindness, heart disease, kidney failure, and nerve disorders.

In type 2 diabetes, which usually appears later in life, patients can produce insulin, but either the amount is too small or the insulin does not function effectively. Although some patients with type 2 diabetes may require supplemental insulin, many of these patients can be treated with diet, exercise, and non–insulin-type oral medications (hypoglycemic agents) TABLE 14-3 .

Hypoglycemic agents stimulate the pancreas to produce more insulin, which in turn lowers blood glucose levels. In some patients, however, these medications can lead to hypoglycemia (an abnormally low level of blood glucose), particularly when patient activity and exercise levels are too vigorous or excessive, causing the patient to use up more glucose. In the past, type 2 diabetes was called non–insulin-dependent diabetes mellitus (NIDDM), or adult (maturity)-onset diabetes. Because some patients with type 2 diabetes may, in fact, require insulin, those terms are no longer used.

Both types of diabetes are equally serious, although type 2 diabetes is often easier to regulate. Both can affect

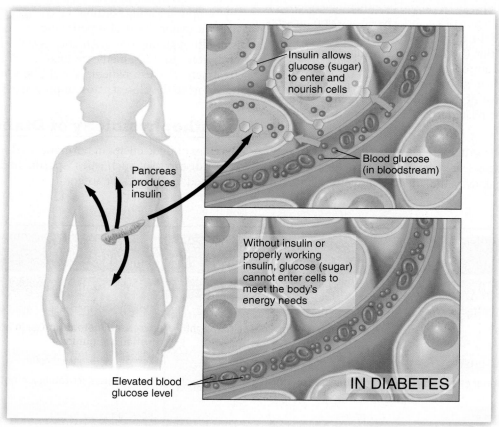

FIGURE 14-2 Diabetes results from the lack of or ineffective action of insulin. Without insulin, cells begin to "starve," because insulin is needed to allow glucose to enter and nourish the cells.

Table 14-3 Common Hypoglycemic Agents	
Generic Name	**Trade Name**
Chlorpropamide	Diabinese
Tolbutamide	Orinase
Glyburide	Micronase
Glipizide	Glucotrol
Metformin	Glucophage
Rosiglitazone	Avandia

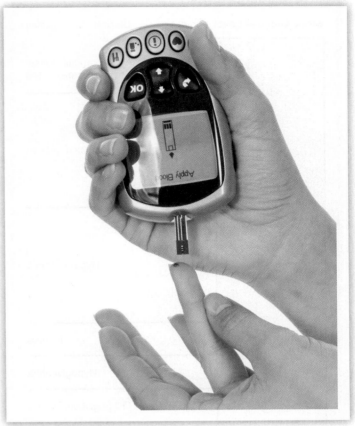

© Dmitry Lobanov/ShutterStock, Inc.

FIGURE 14-3 The blood glucose self-monitoring kit with a digital meter is a device used by patients at home and by AEMTs in some areas.

many body tissues and functions, and both require lifelong medical management. Type 1 diabetes is considered an auto-immune problem, in which the body becomes allergic to—and, therefore, destroys—the insulin-producing cells of the endocrine glands in the pancreas. The severity of diabetic complications reflects how high the average blood glucose level is and how early in life the diabetes begins.

Type 2 diabetes is much more common than type 1 diabetes and is becoming more prevalent in today's society. Approximately 90% of all diabetics in the United States suffer from type 2 diabetes. Obesity is one risk factor that has become more widespread in the population, leading to more cases of type 2 diabetes.

Whereas diabetes mellitus is treatable, treatment must be tailored for each individual patient. The patient's need for glucose must be balanced with the available supply of insulin by testing either the blood or the urine. Patients with type 1 diabetes are typically instructed to monitor their blood glucose levels several times a day with a glucometer **FIGURE 14-3**.

The Role of Glucose and Insulin

Glucose is the major source of energy for the body. All cells need glucose to function properly, and some cells will even cease to function without it. In fact, for the brain, having a constant supply of glucose is as important as having a constant supply of oxygen. Without glucose, brain cells rapidly suffer permanent damage.

Without insulin, glucose from food remains in the blood, so that glucose levels gradually become extremely high (hyperglycemia). Once the blood glucose level reaches 200 mg/dL or more (twice the usual amount), excess glucose is excreted by the kidney. This process requires a large amount of water. The loss of water in such large amounts causes the classic symptoms of uncontrolled diabetes, which are known as the "three Ps":

- Polyuria: frequent and plentiful urination
- Polydipsia: frequent drinking of liquid to satisfy continuous thirst (following the loss of excessive amounts of body water)
- Polyphagia: excessive eating as a result of cellular "hunger"

Hyperglycemia and Hypoglycemia

The two conditions that can lead to a diabetic emergency are hyperglycemia, in which excessive blood glucose is present in the blood, and hypoglycemia, in which not enough glucose is available in the blood. Extremes of hyperglycemia and hypoglycemia can lead to diabetic emergencies **FIGURE 14-4**.

The signs and symptoms of hyperglycemia and hypoglycemia are often similar **TABLE 14-4**. For example, staggering, an intoxicated appearance, and complete unresponsiveness are signs and symptoms of both types of endocrine emergencies.

> **Transition Tip**
>
> Do not waste time at the scene determining which type of diabetic crisis the patient is having. You should, however, gather as much information as possible to relay to hospital staff, so they can provide definitive care.

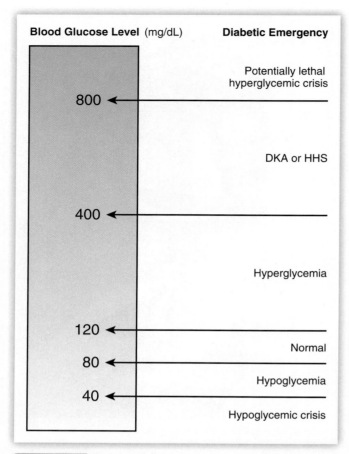

Blood Glucose Level (mg/dL)   **Diabetic Emergency**

800 — Potentially lethal hyperglycemic crisis

— DKA or HHS

400 —

— Hyperglycemia

120 —

80 — Normal

— Hypoglycemia

40 —

— Hypoglycemic crisis

FIGURE 14-4 The two most common diabetic emergencies—hyperglycemic crisis and hypoglycemic crisis—develop when the patient has either too much or too little glucose in the blood, respectively.

Hyperglycemic Crisis

Hyperglycemic crisis is a potentially life-threatening condition in which there is an excessive level of glucose in the blood. It includes diabetic ketoacidosis (DKA) and hyperosmolar hyperglycemic state (HHS).

> *Hyperglycemic crisis* Acute and potentially life-threatening complication of diabetes resulting from a combination of problems.

When glucose is not available to supply energy for cells because of lack of insulin, the body uses fat and other alternative fuel sources for this purpose. When fat is broken down, chemicals called ketones and fatty acids are formed as waste products. These substances build up because they require insulin to break down. As ketones accumulate in the bloodstream, they cause the blood to become more acidic (acidosis), resulting in a toxic condition.

In uncontrolled diabetes, when insulin is not available and the body uses fat for fuel, the form of acidosis seen is called *diabetic ketoacidosis (DKA)*. DKA is a type of hyperglycemic crisis; it is more commonly found in type

Table 14-4 Characteristics of Diabetic Emergencies		
	Hyperglycemia	**Hypoglycemia**
History		
Food intake	Excessive	Insufficient
Insulin dosage	Insufficient	Excessive
Onset	Gradual (hours to days)	Rapid, within minutes
Skin	Warm and dry	Pale, cool, and moist
Infection	Common	Uncommon
Gastrointestinal Tract		
Thirst	Intense	Absent
Hunger	Variable	Intense
Vomiting	Common	Uncommon
Respiratory System		
Breathing	Rapid, deep (Kussmaul respirations)	Normal or rapid
Odor of breath	Sweet, fruity	Normal
Cardiovascular System		
Blood pressure	Normal to low	Normal to low
Pulse	Rapid, weak, and thready	Rapid, weak
Nervous System		
Consciousness	Restlessness possibly progressing to coma; abnormal or slurred speech; unsteady gait	Irritability, confusion, seizure, fainting or coma; unsteady gait; changes in mental status
Treatment		
Response	Gradual, within 6 to 12 hours following medical treatment	Immediately after administration of glucose

1 diabetes because no insulin is produced in this form of the disease. One sign of DKA is a deep, rapid breathing pattern called Kussmaul respirations, which help the body "blow off" excess acids. Another symptom is a fruity odor of ketones on the breath. When the acid levels in the body become too high, individual cells cease to function. If the patient is not given proper fluid and insulin to reverse fat metabolism and restore the use of glucose as a source of

energy, ketoacidosis will progress to hyperglycemic crisis, coma, and eventually death.

> *Diabetic ketoacidosis (DKA)* A form of hyperglycemia in uncontrolled diabetes in which certain acids accumulate when insulin is not available.

Type 2 diabetes more often results in *hyperosmolar hyperglycemic state (HHS)*. HHS is less common than DKA and carries a higher mortality rate (approximately 10% to 20%). The onset of HHS is typically slower and occurs over a longer period than DKA. Because the body is producing some insulin, the body does not burn fat for energy. Therefore, ketones are not produced, and the sweet smell is not present on the breath. Instead, the body tries to rid the excess glucose in the urine. Because fluid follows the glucose, dehydration results.

A hyperglycemic crisis may occur in patients who are not under medical treatment, take an insufficient amount of insulin, markedly overeat, or experience stress in the form of an infection, illness, overexertion, fatigue, or alcohol consumption. Ketoacidosis usually develops over a period of time, from hours to days.

Hypoglycemic Crisis

When insulin levels remain high, glucose is rapidly taken out of the blood to fuel the cells. If glucose levels fall too low, an insufficient amount may be available to supply the brain. In this circumstance, the mental status of the patient declines (*hypoglycemic crisis*), and he or she may become aggressive or display unusual behavior. If blood glucose remains low, unresponsiveness and permanent brain damage can quickly follow.

> *Hyperosmolar hyperglycemic state (HHS)* A metabolic derangement that occurs principally in patients with type 2 diabetes; it is characterized by hyperglycemia, hyperosmolarity, and an absence of significant ketosis. HHS was previously called hyperosmolar hyperglycemia nonketotic coma (HHNC). The term was changed because coma occurs in fewer than 20% of patients with HHS.
> *Hypoglycemic crisis* Severe hypoglycemia resulting in changes in mental status.

A hypoglycemic crisis (also known as insulin shock) occurs when an imbalance in the body of the patient with diabetes arises for any of several reasons:

- The patient takes too much insulin.
- The patient takes a regular dose of insulin but does not eat enough food.
- The patient engages in an unusual amount of activity or vigorous exercise that uses up all available glucose.
- The patient is sick, which causes the body to use more glucose than usual, or vomits after eating, thereby depleting the body of nutrients.

Sometimes, however, hypoglycemia may occur with no identifiable predisposing factor.

Hypoglycemia develops much more quickly than hyperglycemia. In some instances, it can become evident in a matter of minutes.

> **Transition Tip**
>
> Both hyperglycemia and hypoglycemia may produce unresponsiveness and, in some instances, death. They call for very different treatment, however. Hyperglycemia is a complex metabolic condition that usually develops over time and involves all tissues of the body. Correcting this condition may take many hours in a well-controlled hospital setting. Hypoglycemia, in contrast, is an acute condition that can develop rapidly and is just as quickly reversed by giving the patient glucose. Without the glucose, the patient can suffer permanent brain damage.

> **Transition Tip**
>
> Although most patients with diabetes understand and manage their disease well, emergencies can occur. In addition to hyperglycemic and hypoglycemic crises, patients with diabetes may have "silent" (painless) heart attacks, which is a possibility that should always be considered. Their only symptom in this situation may be "not feeling so well." Don't automatically assume that a patient with diabetes is suffering from a diabetic emergency.

Complications of Diabetes

Because diabetes affects all body systems, over time a diabetic patient may develop many different complications:

- Damage to blood vessels in the eyes may result in vision problems or blindness. Diabetics are at increased risk for cataracts, diabetic retinopathy, and glaucoma.
- Damage to nerves (diabetic neuropathy) may cause pain or numbness in the feet as well as other problems with the stomach, intestines, heart, and other organs.
- Kidney damage (diabetic nephropathy) may result in the need for kidney dialysis.
- Blood vessel damage puts the diabetic patient at greater risk for developing circulatory disorders such as heart attack, stroke, peripheral vascular disease, hypertension, and high cholesterol. In addition, skin sores are often slow to heal, increasing the chance of infection. Furthermore, because nerve damage often decreases feeling in the legs, the patient may have a deep skin ulcer and not even know it. If not treated properly, even a small break in the skin can progress to deep sores in a diabetic patient, which may ultimately require amputation of the affected limb.

Special Populations

Pediatric Patients

Type 1 diabetes usually presents itself in children by age 5 years. It is possible that you might encounter a pediatric patient with type 1 diabetes who has not yet been diagnosed. Pediatric diabetic patients are prone to seizures and dehydration. In addition, hyperglycemia in a pediatric patient can cause cerebral edema (swelling of the brain)—the number one cause of diabetic-related death in children.

Glucose levels in children with diabetes may be difficult to regulate. Youngsters' high levels of activity cause them to use up circulating glucose more quickly than adults, even after a normal injection of insulin. In addition, children do not always eat nutritious foods or eat on a regular schedule. As a result, hypoglycemic crises may develop more often and more severely in children compared with adults.

> **Transition Tip**
>
> A pregnant woman may develop diabetes during pregnancy, a variant called gestational diabetes. According to the American Diabetes Association, gestational diabetes affects approximately 4% of all pregnant women.

Elderly Patients

As an AEMT, you may occasionally encounter a geriatric patient who has undiagnosed diabetes. Such a patient is likely to report that he or she has not been feeling well for a while but has not seen a physician. A patient with undiagnosed diabetes or one who is in denial or ignores the advice of his or her physician may call 9-1-1 when the signs and symptoms become annoying. Nonhealing wounds (which can lead to infection), blindness, renal failure, atypical (silent) myocardial infarction presentation, and other complications are associated with poorly controlled or uncontrolled diabetes in elderly patients.

Elderly diabetic patients are prone to dehydration and infections. In addition, the signs and symptoms of diabetes can mask the signs and symptoms of myocardial infarction. Always suspect AMI in a diabetic patient who presents with atypical symptoms.

Patient Assessment of Diabetic Emergencies

Scene Size-up

Assess each situation quickly and make sure the necessary personal protective equipment is used. Remember that diabetic patients often use syringes to administer insulin—be careful to ensure that you do not get stuck by a used needle that was not disposed of properly. Insulin syringes on the bed stand, insulin bottles in the refrigerator, a plate of food, or glass of orange juice are important clues that may help you decide what is possibly wrong with your patient.

Although your report from dispatch may be for a patient with an altered mental status, be open to the possibility that trauma may have occurred because of a medical incident. Determine the mechanism of injury and/or nature of illness. Do not let your guard down even on what appears to be a routine call.

> **Transition Tip**
>
> Managing problems related to diabetes and altered mental status poses minimal risk to you because exposure to body fluids is generally very limited. Even so, you should recognize that some patients may become confused or aggressive at times. Follow standard precautions, as you would with any other patient. Always use gloves and carefully wash your hands after obtaining and checking blood glucose levels or performing airway management techniques.

Primary Assessment

Form a general impression of the patient. Identify life threats and provide lifesaving interventions, particularly airway management. Determine the patient's level of consciousness using the AVPU scale. If a suspected diabetic patient is unresponsive, immediately call for advanced life support (ALS); an unresponsive patient may have undiagnosed diabetes. You may be able to determine whether diabetes is present in the field by assessing the patient's blood glucose level if you have the proper equipment and training. Perform cervical spine stabilization, when appropriate, and provide rapid transport to the emergency department, where diabetes and its associated complications can be quickly diagnosed.

Remember that even though a person has diabetes, this disease may not be causing the current problem. Heart attack, stroke, or another medical emergency may be the cause of the presenting symptoms. In addition, a diabetic patient may appear confused and is often mistakenly perceived as being intoxicated.

A patient who is hyperglycemic may have rapid, deep respirations (Kussmaul respirations) and sweet, fruity breath. In contrast, a patient who is hypoglycemic will have normal or shallow to rapid respirations. If the patient is not breathing or is having difficulty breathing, open the airway and insert an airway adjunct, administer oxygen, and assist ventilations. Continue to monitor the airway as you provide care.

If the patient is unresponsive, immediately assess for a pulse while determining whether the patient is breathing or has agonal respirations. If no pulse is evident, immediately begin CPR.

A diabetic patient with dry and warm skin may have hyperglycemia, whereas a diabetic patient with moist and pale skin may have hypoglycemia. The patient in hypoglycemic crisis will have a rapid, weak pulse.

Patients with an altered mental status and impaired ability to swallow should be transported promptly. Patients who have the ability to swallow and are conscious enough to maintain their own airway may be further evaluated on scene, with additional interventions performed there.

History Taking

Alert patients are usually able to provide their own medical history. If the patient has eaten but not taken insulin, it is more likely that hyperglycemia is developing. If the patient has taken insulin but has not eaten, the problem is more likely to be hypoglycemia. A patient with diabetes will often know what is wrong. Obtain a SAMPLE history from the patient, and ask the following questions specific to a patient with known diabetes:

- Do you take insulin or any pills that lower your blood glucose?
- Have you taken your usual dose of insulin (or pills) today?
- Have you eaten normally today?
- Have you had any illness, especially fever or vomiting, or had an unusual amount of activity, or stress?

If the patient is not thinking or speaking clearly (or is unresponsive), ask family members or bystanders about the patient's history.

If no one else is present and you know that the unresponsive patient has diabetes, you must use your knowledge of the signs and symptoms to decide whether the problem is hypoglycemia or hyperglycemia. A patient in hypoglycemic crisis (rapid onset of altered mental status, hypoglycemia) needs sugar immediately. A patient in hyperglycemic crisis (acidosis, dehydration, hyperglycemia) needs insulin and IV fluid therapy. If you are uncertain, it is best to treat for hypoglycemia and provide transport to the hospital. Severe hypoglycemia can be rapidly fatal if untreated. Conversely, hyperglycemic patients will not be severely harmed by treatment for hypoglycemia unless it somehow results in delay in treatment for their hyperglycemia. Both types of patients need prompt transport to the hospital for appropriate medical care.

> **Transition Tip**
>
> Diabetes is a systemic disease affecting all tissues of the body, especially the kidneys, eyes, small arteries, and peripheral nerves. As an AEMT, you will likely encounter patients with a variety of complications of diabetes, such as heart disease, visual disturbances, renal failure, stroke, and ulcers or infections of the feet or toes. With the exception of heart attack and stroke, most of these conditions will not be acute emergencies. Because diabetes is a major risk factor for cardiovascular disease, however, patients with diabetes—and particularly older patients—should always be suspected of having a potential for heart attack, even when they do not present with classic symptoms such as chest pain and shortness of breath.

Secondary Assessment

Assess unresponsive patients from head to toe with a full-body scan. The patient may have experienced trauma resulting from dizziness or from changes in level of consciousness. Physical signs such as tremors, abdominal cramps, vomiting, a fruity breath odor, or a dry mouth may guide you in determining whether the patient is hypoglycemic or hyperglycemic. Look for emergency medical identification devices—for example, a wallet card, a necklace, or a bracelet.

Although an altered mental status may be caused by a blood glucose level that is either too high or too low, the patient may also have sustained trauma or have another metabolic problem or unrelated condition, such as intoxication, poisoning, or a head injury. When a diabetes-related problem is suspected, the secondary assessment should focus on the patient's mental status and ability to swallow and protect the airway. Obtain a Glasgow Coma Scale score to track the patient's neurologic status.

> **Transition Tip**
>
> Although diabetes and alcoholism can coexist in a patient, it is important to be alert to the similarity in symptoms of acute alcohol intoxication and diabetic emergencies. Likewise, hypoglycemia and head injury can coexist, but the potential for hypoglycemia exists even when the head injury is obvious.

Obtain a complete set of vital signs, including a measurement of the patient's blood glucose level using a glucometer, if available and if local protocols allow. Some glucometers indicate a low (Lo) reading when they detect a glucose level of less than 20 mg/dL, whereas others display Lo when they detect a level of less than 30 mg/dL. A high (Hi) reading may be indicated by some glucometers when they detect a glucose level of 550 mg/dL and others at 600 mg/dL. It is important to know both the upper and lower ranges for your specific glucometer functions.

The normal range for glucose levels in blood in non-fasting adults and children is 80 to 120 mg/dL; the blood glucose level in neonates should be greater than 70 mg/dL.

> **Transition Tip**
>
> A diabetic patient may have abnormal vital signs and a normal blood glucose value. In this case, something else is most likely the cause of the patient's altered mental status and other complaints. Just because a patient has a history of diabetes, it does not mean that the diabetes is always the cause of the current problem.

By using pulse oximetry, you will be able to determine the percentage of oxygen saturation in the bloodstream. In general, unless the patient is suffering from an altered level of consciousness or difficulty breathing, oxygen administration should be titrated to an SpO_2 of 95% based on local protocols. The decision of how much oxygen to administer should be based on a careful assessment of the patient's airway and breathing, not solely on pulse oximetry readings.

Reassessment

Reassess the diabetic patient frequently to identify changes in his or her condition. In many patients with diabetes, you will note marked improvement with appropriate treatment. Document assessment findings, the times at which interventions were administered, and any changes in patient condition. Base the administration of glucose on glucose levels, if available. If a glucometer is unavailable, a deteriorating level of consciousness indicates the need to provide additional glucose.

> ### Transition Tip
>
> When there is any doubt about whether a responsive patient with diabetes is going into hypoglycemic or hyperglycemic crisis, most protocols will err on the side of giving glucose, even though the patient may have hyperglycemia or DKA. When in doubt, consult medical control.

Communication with hospital staff is important for continuity of care. Hospital personnel need to be informed about the patient's history, the present situation, assessment findings, and interventions provided and their results.

Interventions

A patient in hypoglycemic crisis needs sugar immediately. A patient in hyperglycemic crisis needs insulin and IV fluid therapy. Both of these patients need prompt transport to the hospital for appropriate medical care.

Hypoglycemic patients may experience permanent cerebral damage if blood glucose levels are not restored rapidly. If the hypoglycemic patient is alert and able to swallow without the risk of aspiration, administer oral glucose or sugar by mouth. The patient will usually become more alert within minutes. Remember that even when the patient responds after receiving glucose, he or she may still need additional treatment and should be transported to the hospital for further evaluation.

If the hypoglycemic patient is unresponsive, or if there is any risk of aspiration, do not give anything by mouth! Instead, administer IV glucose or intramuscular (IM) glucagon.

When there is any doubt about whether a responsive patient with diabetes is going into hypoglycemic or hyperglycemic crisis, most protocols will err on the side of giving glucose. The risk of increasing the glucose level of a patient who is already hyperglycemic is minimal compared with the benefit of increasing the glucose level of one who is hypoglycemic. When in doubt, consult medical control.

When treating the patient, place him or her in a position of comfort. Obtain IV access for all patients experiencing a diabetic emergency and obtain a blood glucose analysis. For patients presenting with signs of dehydration, administer a 20-mL/kg bolus of an isotonic crystalloid solution such as normal saline or lactated Ringer's. Reassess the patient after the initial bolus and repeat if needed.

Document clearly your assessment findings as the basis for your treatment. Patients who refuse transport because you "cured" them with oral glucose may require even more thorough documentation. Follow local protocols for patients who refuse treatment or transport.

Emergency Medical Care of Endocrine Emergencies

Management of Hypoglycemia

The first treatment for patients with hypoglycemia is to administer oral glucose, assuming the patient is responsive and there is no risk of aspiration. If this is not possible, you should administer D_{50} via the IV route. Finally, if IV access cannot be obtained, you should administer glucagon via the IM route.

> ### Transition Tip
>
> D_{50} is usually supplied in a prefilled container called a "bristojet" containing 25 g of dextrose dissolved in 50 mL of water. Doses of D_{50} are as follows:
>
> - Adults: 25 g (50 mL) of D_{50} (or follow local protocol)
> - Children 3 months to 7 years old: D_{25} (empty half of the bristojet of D_{50} and draw up normal saline to fill the tube; this will give a concentration of 25% if your service does not carry the prefilled syringes of D_{25})
> - Newborns to 3 months old: D_{10} solution (put 2 mL of D_{50} into a syringe and add 8 mL of normal saline)

Administering Glucagon

Glucagon is supplied in 1-mg ampules and requires reconstitution with the provided diluent. The dosage for an adult is 0.5 to 1 mg IM and may be repeated in 7 to 10 minutes. The pediatric dosage is 0.5 mg or 20 to 30 µg/kg IM for children who weigh less than 20 kg. For children who weigh greater than 20 kg, the dose is the same as for adults. Glucagon should be used in conjunction with D_{50} whenever possible. If the patient does not respond to the second dose of glucagon, D_{50} must be administered.

Management of Hyperglycemia and DKA

Patients in DKA will generally present with a markedly elevated glucose level (greater than 300 mg/dL) and signs and symptoms consistent with severe hyperglycemia. The goals of prehospital treatment of DKA are to begin rehydration and correct the patient's electrolyte and acid–base abnormalities.

Maintain the patient's airway and administer oxygen. Start an IV line and infuse a 20 mL/kg bolus of normal saline over the first half an hour or at the rate suggested by local protocol or online medical control. Remember, a patient with DKA is severely dehydrated, often to the point of shock, and needs volume replacement, usually at a rate of about 1 L/h for at least the first few hours.

Hyperglycemic patients who have not reached the stage of DKA may not need large quantities of fluid. Treat the patient symptomatically, providing oxygen and IV fluid as needed. Specific treatment with insulin will occur upon the patient's arrival at the hospital.

Management of HONK/HHNC

Hyperosmolar nonketotic coma (HONK), also called *hyperosmolar hyperglycemic nonketotic coma (HHNC)*, is a metabolic derangement that may occur, usually in patients with type 2 diabetes. This condition is characterized by hyperglycemia, hyperosmolarity, and an absence of significant ketosis. The clinical features of HONK/HHNC and DKA tend to overlap and are often observed simultaneously, but the sweet, fruity smell associated with DKA is not present on the breath.

> *Hyperosmolar nonketotic coma (HONK)* Condition characterized by severe hyperglycemia, hyperosmolality, and dehydration but no ketoacidosis; also called hyperosmolar hyperglycemic nonketotic coma (HHNC) or HONK/HHNC.
> *Hyperosmolar hyperglycemic nonketotic coma (HHNC)* A metabolic derangement characterized by hyperglycemia, hyperosmolality, dehydration, and an absence of significant ketosis; occurs principally in patients with type 2 diabetes; also called hyperosmolar nonketotic coma (HONK) or HONK/HHNC.

Airway management is a top priority in prehospital treatment of HONK/HHNC. Large-bore IV access should be gained as soon as possible, but do not delay patient transfer while initiating the IV line. If necessary, obtain IV access during transport to the emergency department. Also obtain a blood glucose level as soon as possible.

Once you have initiated the IV line, a bolus of 20 mL/kg 0.9% normal saline is appropriate for nearly all adults who are clinically dehydrated. In patients with a history of congestive heart failure and/or renal insufficiency, you may be directed to give fluid more sparingly. Fluid deficits in patients with HONK/HHNC may amount to 10 L or more. These patients may receive 1 to 2 L within the first hour. If the glucose level is less than 60 to 80 mg/dL, then (depending on your local protocols), administer 25 g of D_{50} as soon as possible.

■ Hematologic Emergencies

Hematology is the study and prevention of blood-related diseases, such as sickle cell disease or hemophilia. To understand how hematologic disorders affect the body, you should have a basic understanding of the *hematopoietic system* (the blood components and the organs involved in their development and production) and hematologic disorders, and should know how to respond appropriately to these kinds of emergencies.

> *Hematology* The study and prevention of blood-related disorders.
> *Hematopoietic system* The system that includes all blood components and the organs involved in their development and production.

■ Anatomy and Physiology of Blood and Plasma

Blood is made up of two main components: cells and plasma. Red blood cells (RBCs), also known as erythrocytes, make up approximately 47% of the blood volume in males and 42% in females of childbearing age. Within the RBCs, hemoglobin is responsible for carrying oxygen to the tissues. White blood cells (WBCs), also called leukocytes, serve as the "cleaners" of the body, traveling throughout all of its parts to rid the body of infection and dead cells. Platelets are small cells in the blood that are essential for clot formation. When damage occurs to a blood vessel, platelets respond to the site of injury to assist in creating a blood clot to stop the bleeding. All of these components—erythrocytes, leukocytes, and platelets—are suspended in a straw-colored, protein-filled fluid called plasma, which helps to transport cells throughout the body.

Blood performs the following functions:

- **Respiratory function.** Transports oxygen from the lungs to the tissues and carbon dioxide from the tissues to the lungs
- **Nutritional function.** Carries nutrients (glucose, proteins, and fats) from the digestive tract to cells throughout the body
- **Excretory function.** Ferries the waste products of metabolism from the cells where they are produced to the excretory organs
- **Regulatory function.** Transports hormones to their target organs and transmits excess internal heat to the surface of the body to be dissipated
- **Defensive function.** Carries defensive cells and antibodies, which protect the body against foreign organisms

Table 14-5 Blood Types			
Blood Type	**ABO Antigens**	**ABO Antibodies**	**Acceptable Blood Donor Types**
A	A	Anti-B	A, O
B	B	Anti-A	B, O
AB	A, B	None	A, B, AB, O
O	None	Anti-A Anti-B	O

Blood-Forming Organs and RBC Production

Although many parts and organs of the human body can alter or affect the hematologic system, the major players are the bone marrow, liver, and spleen. The bone marrow is the primary site for blood cell production within the human body. Bone marrow may be found in most of the long bones plus the pelvis, skull, and vertebrae.

The liver produces the **clotting factors** found in the blood. It filters the blood, removing toxins, and is essential to normal metabolism and homeostasis. As old RBCs enter the liver, they are broken down into bile. The liver is a highly vascular organ that also stores some blood within itself.

The spleen is also quite vascular. It stores platelets, is involved with the filtering and breakdown of RBCs, assists with the production of WBCs, and has an important role in providing infection control and maintaining homeostasis.

> **Clotting factors** Substances in the blood that are necessary for clotting; also called coagulation factors.

Blood Classifications

To ensure compatibility and prevent medical problems during blood component replacement, blood type classifications have been developed **TABLE 14-5**. Some patients may be receiving or may have recently received a blood transfusion. It is important to determine a patient's blood type and the type of blood received. Blood reactions are similar to an anaphylactic reaction—they can cause severe circulatory collapse and even death. When a patient receives a blood transfusion, it is important to monitor the patient very closely for the first 30 to 60 minutes because transfusion reactions typically begin within this time frame.

Pathophysiology of Hematologic Emergencies

Sickle Cell Disease

Sickle cell disease is a leading inherited blood disorder. In the United States, about 1,000 newborns are born with this disease each year. The disease primarily affects African American, Puerto Rican, and European populations, but it can occur in anyone. Mortality at younger ages is common, with the average life expectancy being 45 years in men. Women with this disease tend to live slightly longer than men.

> **Sickle cell disease** A hereditary disease that causes normal, round red blood cells to become oblong, or sickle shaped.

Sickle cell disease starts with a genetic defect of the adult-type hemoglobin (HbA). When the RBCs are first developing their membranes, they may become rigid and deformed. The defective RBCs have an oblong shape instead of a smooth, round shape **FIGURE 14-5**. This shape makes the RBC a poor oxygen carrier, which means a patient with this disease is highly susceptible to hypoxia. Because sickle cells also have a much shorter life span than normal erythrocytes, the patient is more prone to developing anemia.

The odd shape may also cause RBCs to lodge in small blood vessels, leading to thrombosis. Defective RBCs may

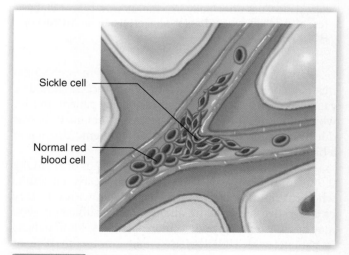

FIGURE 14-5 Normal RBCs and sickle cells.

migrate to the spleen, causing the organ to swell and rupture, which can lead to death.

There are four main types of sickle cell crises:

- A *vasoocclusive crisis* results from blood flow to an organ becoming restricted, causing pain, ischemia, and often organ damage. Most vasoocclusive crises last between 5 and 7 days. Frequently, circulation to the spleen becomes obstructed as a result of its narrow vessels and function of removing damaged RBCs. Vasoocclusion in the brain may result in a cerebrovascular accident or stroke.
  - *Acute chest syndrome* is a vasoocclusive crisis that results from sickling in the lung and can be confused with pneumonia. Common signs and symptoms include chest pain, fever, and cough.
- An *aplastic crisis* is a worsening of the patient's baseline anemia (lack of circulating functional RBCs in the body), which causes tachycardia, pallor, and fatigue. This may be caused by the parvovirus B19, which affects the production of RBCs, nearly stopping new production for 2 to 3 days.
- A *hemolytic crisis* is an acute accelerated drop in the patient's hemoglobin level. Caused by RBCs breaking down at a faster than normal rate, this type of crisis is common in patients with glucose-6-phosphate dehydrogenase deficiency (a common enzyme deficiency).
- A *splenic sequestration crisis* is caused by painful, acute enlargement of the spleen, causing the abdomen to become very hard and bloated.

Vasoocclusive crisis Ischemia and pain caused by sickle-shaped red blood cells that obstruct blood flow to a portion of the body.

Acute chest syndrome A vasoocclusive crisis that can be confused with pneumonia; common signs and symptoms include chest pain, fever, and cough.

Aplastic crisis A condition in which the body stops producing red blood cells; typically caused by infection.

Hemolytic crisis A rapid destruction of red blood cells that occurs faster than the body's ability to create new cells.

Splenic sequestration crisis An acute, painful enlargement of the spleen caused by sickle cell disease.

Transition Tip

Acute splenic sequestration syndrome is generally a childhood condition that is the result of mutated cells causing blood to become trapped in the spleen. As the organ enlarges (splenomegaly), serious damage or death may occur.

In acute crises, patients may have significant pain resulting from congested vessels that do not allow for the passage of oxygen and nutrients into tissues and joints. They may experience frequent infections, which can lead to sepsis and death. Over time, various organs may be destroyed as circulation is impeded. Patients often may have signs of mild dehydration, splenomegaly, cardiomegaly, and many other complaints.

Patients with chronic sickle cell attacks are prone to severe, life-threatening complications which you must recognize. Although some of these complications take days to weeks to develop, some complications are acute and life threatening. Some of the problems that patients with sickle cell disease frequently experience are as follows:

- Cerebral vascular attack
- Gallstones
- Jaundice
- Osteonecrosis
- Splenic infections
- Osteomyelitis
- Opiate tolerance
- Leg ulcers
- Retinopathy
- Chronic pain
- Pulmonary hypertension
- Chronic renal failure

Clotting Disorders

A clotting disorder is a condition in which there is an abnormality in clotting of the blood. The development of a blood clot is called *thrombosis* and can occur in either arterial or venous blood vessels. The patient's symptoms are related to the part of the vascular system in which the clot occurs, the size of the clot, and whether the clot becomes dislodged and travels to another part of the body.

Thrombosis A blood clot, either in the arterial or venous system.

Thrombophilia

Thrombophilia, or the tendency to develop blood clots, affects a large number of people around the world and affects approximately 5% to 7% of the Caucasian population of European descent in the United States.

Thrombophilia A tendency toward the development of blood clots as a result of an abnormality of the coagulation system.

Thrombosis is a common medical problem. Currently, an estimated 2 million people experience a deep venous thrombosis, or the formation of a clot in a deep vein, each year in the United States. In addition, nearly 50% of the patients experience long-term health consequences.

Thrombosis may manifest itself as the formation of a blood clot in a blood vessel or in one of the chambers of the heart. Deep venous thromboses are a leading cause of death in hospitalized patients. This form of clot develops for the first time in 200,000 to 300,000 patients annually during hospitalization because of their lack of mobility. Nearly 40% of the patients have pulmonary embolism (a clot that travels to the lung and obstructs a significant amount of blood flow to the organ) as a complication.

Many patients with thrombophilia receive anticoagulant medications that thin the blood, which helps decrease the tendency to form a clot. Examples of these medications include aspirin, heparin, and warfarin (Coumadin). Typically, pediatric patients do not experience blood clots.

The following are some risk factors for increased clotting:

- Recent surgery
- Impaired mobility
- Congestive heart failure
- Cancer
- Respiratory failure
- Infectious diseases
- Age older than 40 years
- Being overweight/obesity
- Smoking
- Oral contraceptive use

Hemophilia

Hemophilia is a genetic bleeding disorder in which clotting does not occur or occurs insufficiently (von Willebrand disease). In people with hemophilia, the body is not able to control bleeding by developing clots normally, resulting in an increased bleeding tendency. This condition occurs predominately in males and occurs in approximately 1 in every 5,000 to 10,000 births. The disease is classified into two primary types:

- **Hemophilia A.** The most common type, hemophilia A is caused by low levels of factor VIII.
- **Hemophilia B.** This second most common type is associated with a deficiency of factor IX.

> *Hemophilia* A congenital abnormality in which the body's ability to clot is impaired, resulting in uncontrollable bleeding.

The levels of factors VIII and IX determine the severity of the disease. Both type A and type B have the same signs and symptoms. Acute and chronic bleeding can occur at any time and may or may not be life threatening. Any injury or illness that can cause bleeding should not be taken lightly in a person with hemophilia. Spontaneous intracranial bleeding is common in patients with hemophilia and is a major cause of death. Patients with significant acute bleeding episodes require hospitalization for transfusion and often

require infusion of factors VIII and IX. If a patient has just had or needs surgery, these factors should be at 100% at the beginning of the procedure and should be maintained to a level up to 50% for several weeks thereafter.

Patient Assessment of Hematologic Emergencies

Assessment of a patient suspected of having a hematologic disorder should be no different from assessment of any other patient, albeit with a few additional items to consider and questions to ask. In addition, be very supportive of the patients and their families—some patients with a blood disorder may not be willing to disclose the condition because they may feel that they will be treated differently.

Scene Size-up

Although your report from dispatch may be for a patient with an unknown medical problem, most patients presenting with a sickle cell crisis have had a crisis before and will relay that information to the dispatcher. Patients experiencing a vasoocclusive crisis are often in extreme pain and would benefit from administration of analgesics. Call for paramedic backup early. Remember to maintain an index of suspicion that trauma may have occurred because of a medical incident.

Primary Assessment

An African American patient or any patient of Mediterranean descent who complains of severe pain may have undiagnosed sickle cell disease.

Perform cervical spine stabilization, if necessary. Remember that even though a person has a history of sickle cell disease, sickle cell disease may not be causing the current problem; trauma or another type of medical emergency may be the cause. For this reason, you must always perform a thorough, careful primary assessment, paying attention to the ABCs and immediately correcting any life-threatening issues.

Patients showing signs of inadequate breathing or altered mental status should receive high-flow oxygen at 12 to 15 L/min via nonrebreathing mask or ventilation via bag-mask as needed. A patient who is experiencing a sickle cell crisis may have increased respirations as a result of severe pain or exhibit signs of pneumonia. Continue to monitor the airway as you provide care.

An increased heart rate represents a compensatory mechanism, in an attempt to "force" the sickled cells through smaller vasculature.

In patients with suspected hemophilia, be alert for signs of acute blood loss such as pallor, weak pulse, and hypotension. Note any bleeding of unknown origin, such as nosebleeds, bloody sputum, and blood in the urine or stool. Owing to blood loss, patients with hemophilia may exhibit signs of hypoxia or shock.

Whether you decide to rapidly transport the patient will depend on the severity of the patient's pain and the patient's wishes. Patients with a history of sickle cell disease, but who have not had a crisis in some time, may require emotional support and refuse transport. However, transport to an emergency department should always be recommended to any patient who is experiencing a sickle cell crisis or hemophilia.

History Taking

Responsive medical patients are usually able to provide their own medical history to help you identify a cause for their severe pain. Do not take a call for a person having a sickle cell crisis lightly. Patients can present with life-threatening conditions, characterized by shortness of breath and signs of pneumonia. Their skin will show signs of inadequate perfusion, accompanied by hypotension. Physical signs, such as swelling of the fingers and toes, priapism, and jaundice may also guide you in determining whether the patient is experiencing a sickle cell crisis.

Has the patient experienced muscle pain or stiffness for unknown reasons? Ascertain whether the pain is isolated to a single location or if pain is felt throughout the entire body. Be alert for signs of acute blood loss (pallor, weak pulse, and hypotension). Look for changes in level of consciousness and symptoms such as vertigo, feelings of fatigue, or syncopal episodes. Ask if the patient has had skin changes such as color changes, burning, or itching. Is the patient having any visual disturbances? Note any bleeding of unknown origin, such as nosebleeds, bloody sputum, and blood in the urine or stool. Is the patient experiencing any gastrointestinal problems, such as nausea, vomiting, or abdominal cramping? Is the patient reporting any chest pain or shortness of breath?

Transition Tip

Many anti-inflammatory drugs (aspirin, ibuprofen) and some herbals (ginkgo, garlic, ginger, ginseng, feverfew) decrease platelet aggregation. Although this effect may be beneficial (such as in myocardial infarction or stroke prevention), these drugs may also increase the tendency to bleed. Always ask patients about medications, including over-the-counter and herbal medications.

In a patient with known sickle cell disease, ask the following questions in addition to obtaining a SAMPLE history:

- Have you had a crisis before?
- When was the last time you had a crisis?
- How did your last crisis resolve?
- Have you had any illness, unusual amount of activity, or stress lately?

Secondary Assessment

The secondary assessment may be performed on scene, en route to the emergency department, or not at all. This will depend on transport time and the patient's condition.

Systematically examine the patient and obtain your patient's baseline vital signs. Evaluate and document mental status using the AVPU scale. **TABLE 14-6** shows common findings in patients with blood disorders.

Obtain a complete set of vital signs, including a measurement of the patient's oxygen saturation level. In patients experiencing a sickle cell crisis, respirations are normal to rapid, the pulse is weak and rapid, and the skin is typically pale and clammy with a low blood pressure.

Use pulse oximetry, if available. However, keep in mind that the oxygen saturation reading you obtain may be inaccurate as a result of the patient's anemic state.

Reassessment

It is important to reassess the patient frequently to determine if there have been changes in his or her condition. For example, are there changes in the patient's mental status? Are the ABCs still intact? How is the patient responding to the interventions performed? Should you adjust or change the interventions? In many patients, you will note marked improvement with appropriate treatment. Document each assessment, your findings, the time of the interventions, and any changes in the patient's condition.

Interventions

Supplemental oxygen should be administered via nonrebreathing mask at 12 to 15 L/min in an attempt to hypersaturate the remaining hemoglobin and increase the level of perfusion that has been decreased by the sickled cells or

---

Table 14-6
Common Findings With Blood Disorders

System	Common Findings
Skin	Uncontrolled bleeding, unexplained or chronic bruising, itching, pallor or jaundice (yellow appearance usually indicates liver problems)
Gastrointestinal	Epistaxis (bloody nose), bleeding or infected gums, ulcers, melena (blood in the stool), and liver failure (causes jaundice)
Skeletal	Chronic joint or bone pain or rigidity
Cardiovascular	Dyspnea, tachycardia, chest pain, hemoptysis (coughing up blood)
Genitourinary	Hematuria, menorrhagia, chronic or recurring infections

hemophilia. Ventilation should be provided when respirations are insufficient.

Place the patient in a position of comfort and cover to maintain body temperature. Administer IV fluid for hydration and nitrous oxide for pain as allowed by local protocol. At the hospital, the patient may receive a transfusion of blood or plasma.

Clearly document your assessment findings as the basis for your treatment. Follow your local protocols for patients who refuse treatment or transport.

Emergency Medical Care of Hematologic Emergencies

Emergency medical care for any patient with problems related to a blood disorder should include the following:

- **Oxygen.** The amount needed and how it is given (that is, bag-mask ventilation, nonrebreathing mask) depends on the severity of the patient's condition and respiratory status.
- **Fluids.** Initiate IV fluid replacement as indicated for the specific disorder or chief complaint.
- **Transport.** Transport to the closest, most appropriate facility.
- **Pharmacology.** Pain management is often necessary, especially in the case of a sickle cell crisis. Follow local protocols.

- **Psychological support.** Be supportive and communicate with the patient.

High levels of oxygen are recommended for patients with sickle cell disease to prevent further tissue damage as a result of hypoxia. Besides providing oxygen therapy and rapid transport to an appropriate facility, you may need to give IV fluid therapy to counter the patient's dehydration. Remember that patients may have lived with the disease for a long time and, thus, may have a very high pain threshold. As a consequence, they often require a higher level of analgesia. Nitrous oxide may provide a measure of relief. Follow local protocols for pain management and consider requesting paramedic support for administration of narcotics if available and appropriate.

Although patients with hemophilia may require IV therapy in cases of unstable hypotension, understand that the patient actually needs a transfusion and/or administration of clotting factors. The patient may also exhibit worsening signs of hypoxia as IV fluid dilutes the blood, further diminishing oxygen levels. Some patients will have significant pain, so analgesics may be appropriate. Although you may be called to treat someone with bleeding of unknown cause only to find that the bleeding stopped before you arrive on scene, you should suggest that the patient receive immediate transport to the hospital.

PREP KIT

Ready for Review

- The endocrine system comprises a network of glands that produce and secrete hormones.
- The major components of the endocrine system are the hypothalamus, pituitary, thyroid, parathyroid, adrenal glands, reproductive organs, and pancreas.
- The main function of the endocrine system is to maintain homeostasis.
- Diabetes is a metabolic disorder caused by a lack of insulin, a hormone that enables glucose to enter the cells.
- There are two types of diabetes. Type 1 diabetes usually starts in childhood and requires daily insulin to control, and type 2 diabetes usually develops in middle age and can often be controlled with diet and oral medications.
- Acute complications of blood glucose imbalance in diabetic patients include hyperglycemia (excess blood glucose) and hypoglycemia (insufficient blood glucose).
- Symptoms of hypoglycemia include confusion, rapid respirations, pale moist skin, diaphoresis, dizziness, fainting, coma, and seizures.
- Hyperglycemia is usually associated with dehydration and DKA.
- HONK/HHNC may occur in patients with type 2 diabetes.
- Either too much or too little blood glucose can result in altered mental status.
- Be prepared to give oral glucose to a conscious patient who is confused or has a slightly decreased level of consciousness, and D_{50} to an unresponsive patient.
- You may administer glucagon intramuscularly when you cannot obtain IV access for D_{50}.
- Hematology is the study and prevention of blood-related diseases.
- Blood is made of two main components: plasma and formed elements (cells), which include RBCs, WBCs, and platelets.
- RBCs carry oxygen to the tissues. WBCs provide immunity, fight infection, and remove dead cells. Platelets help form clots.
- The bone marrow is the primary site for blood cell production within the human body. The liver produces clotting factors and breaks down old RBCs, and the spleen is involved in the breakdown of RBCs, the production of WBCs, and storing platelets.
- Sickle cell disease is an inherited blood disorder that inhibits the ability of RBCs to carry oxygen effectively.
- Symptoms of sickle cell disease include pain in the joints, fever, respiratory distress, and abdominal pain.
- Patients with sickle cell disease have chronic complications that place them at risk for other problems such as heart attack, stroke, and infection.
- Thrombophilia is a tendency to develop blood clots, whereas hemophilia is the inability to develop clots to stop bleeding.
- Emergency care for sickle cell disease or a clotting disorder includes administering oxygen and fluids, pain management, psychological support, and transport.

Case Study

You arrive at the scene of a 32-year-old African American woman complaining of severe abdominal pain. The patient tells you that she has sickle cell disease and that this has happened in the past. The husband tells you that in addition to her sickle cell disease, the patient also has a history of hypertension and diabetes. The patient's abdominal pain is accompanied with nausea and vomiting. The husband says he's concerned about dehydration because of his wife's dark urine. He is aware that dehydration can trigger a sickle cell pain crisis. On examination you notice the patient has deep, rapid breathing, dry mucous membranes, poor skin turgor, an altered mental status, and tachycardia with a pulse of 110 beats/min. Your partner places the patient on oxygen as you obtain a list of medications. During transport to the hospital, the patient tells you that her pain is starting to improve with the oxygen therapy.

1. Explain the pathophysiology of diabetes.

2. Discuss the complications associated with diabetes.

3. Compare and contrast DKA with HHNC.

4. What is the pathophysiology of sickle cell disease?

5. What are some of the potential complications associated with sickle cell disease?

CHAPTER 15

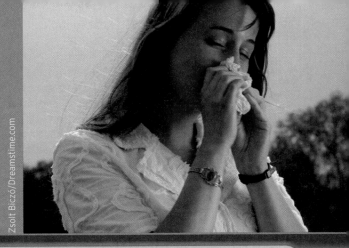

Zsolt Biczó/Dreamstime.com

Infectious Diseases

Introduction

The personal health, safety, and well-being of all AEMTs are vital to an EMS operation. As a part of your training, you will learn how to recognize possible hazards and protect yourself from them. These hazards vary greatly, ranging from personal neglect to environmental and human-made threats to your health and safety.

Infectious Diseases

As an AEMT, you will be called on to treat and transport patients with a variety of communicable or infectious diseases.

An *infectious disease* is a medical condition caused by the growth and spread of small, harmful organisms within the body. A *communicable disease* is a disease that can be spread from one person or species to another. This chapter covers protection of the AEMT against such diseases and the treatment of patients who may have a communicable disease.

> **Infectious disease** A disease caused by infection or one that is capable of being transmitted with or without direct contact.
> **Communicable disease** Any disease that can be spread from person to person or from animal to person.

Immunizations, protective techniques, and simple handwashing can dramatically minimize the health care provider's risk of *infection*. When these protective measures are used, the risk of the health care provider contracting a serious communicable disease is smaller. Proper cleaning and disinfecting of the ambulance and equipment will help to prevent transfer of illnesses from one patient to another.

> **Infection** The invasion of a host or host tissues by organisms such as bacteria, viruses, or parasites, with or without signs or symptoms of disease.

Along with personal protection, it is necessary to inform other health care workers who may come into contact with the patient of the potential risk. Discretion is imperative when communicating with other providers. Sensitive patient history should not be given out over the radio during your patient report. However, during your transfer of care, provide a complete patient history for the receiving facility. Also include all patient history in your written documentation.

Routes of Transmission

Many people confuse the terms *infectious* and *contagious*. In fact, all contagious diseases are infectious, but only some infectious diseases are contagious. For example, pneumonia caused by pneumococcus bacteria is an infectious process, but it is not contagious. In other words, it will not be transmitted from one person to another. However, other infectious agents, such as the hepatitis B virus, are contagious because they can be transmitted from one person to another. An infection is an abnormal invasion of a host or host tissue by organisms such as bacteria, viruses, or parasites. A *pathogen* is a microorganism that is capable of causing disease in a host. A *host* is simply the person invaded by the pathogen. An infectious disease, then, is a disease that is caused by an infection. For example, Lyme disease is an infectious disease caused by the *Borrelia burgdorferi* bacterium, which lives in deer ticks. However, Lyme disease is not contagious. Again, a contagious or communicable disease can be transmitted from one person to another. The only way to get Lyme disease is to be bitten by a deer tick.

> **Pathogen** A microorganism that is capable of causing disease in a susceptible host.
> **Host** The organism or person attacked by the infecting agent.

While all infections result from an invasion of body spaces and tissues by germs, different germs use different means of attack. These means are known as the mechanisms of transmission. *Transmission* is the way an infectious agent

is spread. There are several ways infectious diseases can be transmitted, consisting of contact (direct or indirect), airborne, foodborne, and vector-borne (transmitted through insects or parasitic worms) transmission.

> **Transmission** The way in which an infectious agent is spread: contact, airborne, by vehicles (for example, food or needles), or by vectors.

Contact transmission is the movement of an organism from one person to another through physical touch. There are two types of contact transmission: direct and indirect. *Direct contact* occurs when an organism is moved from one person to another through touching without any intermediary **FIGURE 15-1**.

> **Direct contact** Exposure to or transmission of a communicable disease from one person to another by physical contact.

The scenario of a vehicle crash can help you understand how transmission occurs through direct contact. The driver of the vehicle has *hepatitis* B and is bleeding from an arm injury. The AEMT caring for the patient is not wearing gloves and has a small unnoticed cut on his hand. As he handles a bloody dressing, the hepatitis virus can move from the victim's blood on the dressing into the AEMT's body through the cut on his hand, thus infecting him. This is an example of direct contact where blood is the vehicle. *Bloodborne pathogens* are microorganisms that are present in human blood and can cause disease in humans. Another example of direct contact is sexual transmission. Patients who are infected with the *human immunodeficiency virus (HIV)* can transfer the virus to their partners during sex.

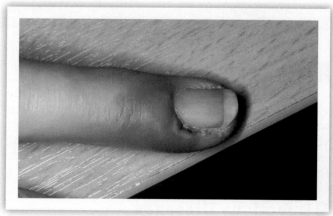

© Hercules Robinson/Alamy Images

FIGURE 15-1 Finger infection resulting from not wearing gloves during patient contact.

Hepatitis Inflammation of the liver, usually caused by a virus, that causes fever, loss of appetite, jaundice, fatigue, and altered liver function.

Bloodborne pathogens Pathogenic microorganisms that are present in human blood and can cause disease in humans. These pathogens include, but are not limited to, hepatitis B virus and human immunodeficiency virus.

Human immunodeficiency virus (HIV) The virus that causes acquired immunodeficiency syndrome (AIDS), which infects the cells in the body's immune system rendering them unable to fight certain types of infection.

Indirect contact involves the spread of infection between the patient with an infection to another person through an inanimate object. The object that transmits the infection is called a fomite. Using the same patient from the previous example, the AEMT wore gloves. As the AEMT was caring for the patient, blood got onto the ambulance stretcher. If the stretcher is not correctly cleaned afterwards, the virus remains on the stretcher and can be transmitted to someone else days later. Needlesticks are another example of the spread of infection through indirect contact. In this case, the virus moves from the patient to the needle to the health care provider. This route of transmission was common many years ago before the advent of safety equipment such as needleless IV systems.

Indirect contact Exposure or transmission of disease from one person to another by contact with a contaminated object.

Airborne transmission involves spreading an infectious agent through mechanisms such as droplets or dust. The common cold is moved from person to person by coughing and sneezing. Interestingly, when a person sneezes, the moisture from the airway moves forcefully and quickly through a narrow opening. If the moisture droplets are large, they travel short distances and can be involved in direct contact transmission. If the moisture droplets are very small, they are turned into an aerosol and can now float in the air for long distances. Sneezing actually can transmit disease through direct contact and airborne routes.

Airborne transmission The spread of an organism in aerosol form.

Because of airborne transmission, it is unsanitary to use your hands to cover a cough or sneeze because the organism travels onto your hands. If you then touch a telephone, doorknob, or a patient, the organisms will travel. Using a tissue when coughing or sneezing is better for controlling the spread of organisms, but you then have a piece of paper full of organisms. One of the best techniques to avoid contaminating your hands is to cough or sneeze into your arm/sleeve. Because you do not touch objects with your

inner arms, the risk of moving the organism to an object or person is reduced. The organisms are trapped in the fabric and will eventually die.

Foodborne transmission involves the contamination of food or water with an organism that can cause disease. When food is prepared, it is important to ensure that raw meats do not come into contact with other foods to prevent the spread of bacteria. It is also important that food is prepared and stored properly at all times to minimize the possibility of illness. Proper cleaning of food preparation surfaces, as well as good handwashing techniques, before and after use also helps to decrease the likelihood of transmitting foodborne bacteria.

Foodborne transmission The contamination of food or water with an organism that can cause disease.

Transmission of some illnesses involves the fecal-oral route, from ingestion of food or water contaminated by infected feces. One example of contamination is the use of human waste as fertilizer. Crops such as onions that have multiple layers are particularly susceptible.

Vector-borne transmission involves the spread of infection by animals or insects that carry an organism from one person or place to another. The Black Death in Europe and Asia in the Middle Ages killed more than 25 million people. This disease is thought to have been caused by a flea that lived on rats. As the rats moved, so did their fleas, carrying the bubonic plague. Other vector-borne diseases include rabies and Lyme disease.

Vector-borne transmission Spread of a disease-causing organism by an animal or insect to human hosts.

Transition Tip

Other potentially infectious materials include cerebrospinal fluid, pericardial fluid, amniotic fluid, synovial fluid, peritoneal fluid, and any fluid containing visible blood.

■ Risk Reduction and Prevention

Although the risk of contracting a communicable disease is real, it should not be exaggerated and certainly should not be a source of fear and stress. Fear comes from lack of proper education and training, and there is no reason an AEMT should not be properly educated about disease issues.

Standard Precautions

The *Occupational Safety and Health Administration (OSHA)* develops and publishes guidelines concerning reducing risk in the workplace. It is also responsible for enforcing these guidelines. All EMS personnel are required by OSHA to be trained in handling bloodborne pathogens and in approaching a patient who may have a communicable or infectious disease. Training must also be provided for issues including blood and body fluid precautions and *contamination* precautions.

> *Occupational Safety and Health Administration (OSHA)* The federal regulatory compliance agency that develops, publishes, and enforces guidelines concerning safety in the workplace.
>
> *Contamination* The presence of infective organisms or foreign bodies on or in objects such as dressings, water, food, needles, wounds, or a patient's body.

Because health care workers are exposed to so many different kinds of infections, the *Centers for Disease Control and Prevention (CDC)* developed a set of *standard precautions* for health care workers to use when providing patient care. These protective measures are designed to prevent workers from coming in direct contact with germs carried by patients. The CDC recommendation from 2007 is to assume that every person is potentially infected or can spread an organism that could be transmitted in the health care setting; therefore, you must apply infection control procedures to reduce infection in patients and health care personnel. **TABLE 15-1** summarizes the CDC recommendations. You must also notify your *designated officer* if you are exposed.

> *Centers for Disease Control and Prevention (CDC)* The primary federal agency that conducts and supports public health activities in the United States. The CDC is part of the US Department of Health and Human Services.
>
> *Standard precautions* Protective measures that have traditionally been developed by the Centers for Disease Control and Prevention for use in dealing with objects, blood, body fluids, and other potential risks of communicable disease.
>
> *Designated officer* The person in the department who is charged with the responsibility of managing exposures and infection control issues.

> ### Transition Tip
> One of the most effective ways to control disease transmission is by washing your hands thoroughly with soap and water after any patient contact.

Proper Hand Hygiene

Proper handwashing is perhaps one of the simplest yet most effective ways of controlling disease transmission.

You should always wash your hands before and after contact with a patient, regardless of whether you wore gloves. The longer the germs remain with you, the greater their chance of getting through your barriers. Although soap and water are not protective in all cases, in certain cases their use provides excellent protection against further transmission from your skin to others (cross-contamination).

If no running water is available, you may use waterless handwashing substitutes. If you use a waterless substitute in the field, make sure that you wash your hands as soon as possible. The proper procedure for handwashing is as follows:

1. Use soap and warm water.
2. Rub your hands together for at least 10 to 15 seconds to work up a lather.
3. Rinse your hands and dry them with a paper towel.
4. Use the paper towel to turn off the faucet.

Gloves

Gloves and eye protection are the minimum standard for all EMS personnel. Both vinyl and latex gloves provide adequate protection. Your department may prefer one type of glove over the other, or you may choose the glove. You should evaluate each situation and choose the glove that works best. Some people are allergic to latex. If you suspect that you are, consult your supervisor for options. Vinyl gloves may be best for routine procedures, and latex gloves may be best for invasive procedures. Change latex gloves if they have been exposed to motor oil, gasoline, or any petroleum-based product. Do not perform tasks such as using a radio, driving, writing a patient care report, or using any monitoring device such as a cardiac monitor or pulse oximeter when wearing contaminated gloves. Wear double gloves if there is substantial bleeding. You may also wear double gloves if you will be exposed to large volumes of other body fluids. Be sure to change gloves as you move from one patient to another. For cleaning and disinfecting the unit, you should use heavy-duty utility gloves. You should never use lightweight latex or vinyl gloves for cleaning.

Removing used latex or vinyl gloves requires a methodical technique to avoid contaminating yourself with the materials from which the gloves have protected you.

Gloves are the most common type of *personal protective equipment (PPE)*. In many EMS rescue operations, you must also protect your hands and wrists from injury. You may wear puncture-proof leather gloves with latex gloves underneath. This combination will allow you free use of your hands with added protection from blood and body fluids. Remember that latex or vinyl gloves are considered medical waste and must be disposed of properly. Leather gloves must be treated as contaminated material until they can be properly decontaminated.

Table 15-1
Standard Precautions for the Care of All Patients in All Health Care Settings, Centers for Disease Control and Prevention, 2007

Component	Recommendation
Hand hygiene	After touching blood, body fluids, secretions, excretions, or contaminated items Immediately after removing gloves Between patient contacts
Personal Protective Equipment	
Gloves	For touching blood, body fluids, secretions, excretions, or contaminated items For touching mucous membranes and nonintact skin
Gown	During procedures and patient care activities when contact of the AEMT's clothing/exposed skin with blood, body fluids, secretions, excretions, or contaminated items is anticipated
Mask, eye protection, face shield	During procedures and patient care activities likely to generate splashes or sprays of blood, body fluids, secretions, or excretions. Examples include suctioning or endotracheal intubation.
HEPA respirator	Use when working with a patient with tuberculosis
Patient Care Environment	
Soiled patient care equipment	Handle in a manner that prevents transfer of microorganisms to others and to the environment. Wear gloves if visibly contaminated. Hand hygiene
Environmental controls	Have procedures for the routine care, cleaning, and disinfection of environmental surfaces. Special attention to frequently touched surfaces within the ambulance (handrails, seats, cabinets, doors) Have patients with tuberculosis wear a surgical mask.
Textiles and laundry	Handle in a manner that prevents transfer of microorganisms to others and to the environment.
Needles and other sharp objects	Do not recap, bend, break, or hand-manipulate used needles. Use safety features when available (needleless IV systems). Place sharps in puncture-resistant containers.
Special Circumstances	
Patient resuscitation	Use mouthpiece, resuscitation bag, or other ventilation devices to prevent contact with mouth and oral secretions.
Respiratory hygiene/cough etiquette	Instruct symptomatic patients to cover mouth and nose when sneezing or coughing. Use tissues and dispose in no-touch receptacle. Perform hand hygiene after touching tissues. Place surgical mask on patient and provider. If mask cannot be used, maintain special separation (>3 ft) if possible.

Personal protective equipment (PPE) Clothing or specialized equipment that provides protection to the wearer.

Eye Protection

Eye protection is important in case blood splatters toward your eyes. If this is a possibility, wearing goggles is your best protection. EMS personnel who wear prescription glasses will also need additional protection for their eyes. Prescription glasses offer little side protection. Obviously, contact lenses offer no added protection from splashing. Face shields will also provide good eye protection.

Gowns

Occasionally, you may need to wear a mask and gown. A mask and gown provide protection from extensive blood splatter. Gowns may be worn in situations such as field delivery of an infant or major trauma. However, wearing a gown may not be practical in many situations. In fact, in some instances, a gown may pose a risk for injury. Your department will likely have a policy regarding gowns. Be sure you know your local policy. There are times when a change of uniform is preferred because trying to clean off contaminants is difficult and sometimes impossible without professional cleaning and disinfection or disposing of the uniform entirely.

Masks, Respirators, and Barrier Devices

The use of masks is a complex issue, especially in light of OSHA and CDC requirements regarding protection from tuberculosis. You should wear a standard surgical mask if blood or body fluid splatter is a possibility. If you suspect that a patient has an airborne disease, you should place a surgical mask on the patient. However, if you suspect that the patient has tuberculosis, place a surgical mask on the patient and a HEPA respirator on yourself **FIGURE 15-2**. If the patient needs oxygen, apply a nonrebreathing mask with an oxygen flow rate of 10 to 15 L/min instead of a surgical mask. Do not place a HEPA respirator on the patient; it is unnecessary and uncomfortable. A simple surgical mask will reduce the risk of transmission of germs from the patient into the air. Use of a HEPA respirator should comply with OSHA standards, which state that facial hair, such as long sideburns or a mustache, will prevent a proper fit.

Although there are no documented cases of disease transmission to rescuers as a result of performing unprotected mouth-to-mouth resuscitation on a patient with an infection, you should use a pocket mask with a one-way valve or bag-mask device. Mouth-to-mouth resuscitation is rarely necessary in a work situation.

Remember that the outside surfaces of these items are considered contaminated after they have been exposed to the patient. You must ensure that gloves, masks, gowns, and all other disposable items that have been exposed to infectious processes or blood are properly disposed of according to local guidelines. If you are stuck by a needle, get blood or other body fluid in your eye, or have contact with any body fluid from the patient, seek medical care as soon as it is feasible and report the incident to your supervisor.

Proper Disposal of Sharps

Be careful when handling needles, scalpels, and other sharp items. The spread of HIV and hepatitis in the health care setting can usually be traced to careless handling of sharps.

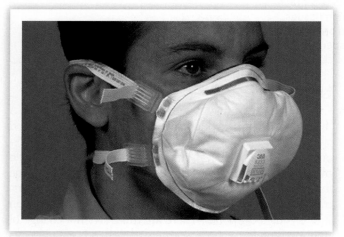

FIGURE 15-2 Wear a high-efficiency particulate air respirator if you treat a patient whom you suspect has tuberculosis.

- Do not recap, break, or bend needles. Even the most careful people may stick themselves accidentally.
- Dispose of all sharp items that have been in contact with human secretions in approved, closed, puncture-proof containers. Such containers are typically red and are labeled with a biohazard insignia.

Employer Responsibilities

Your employer cannot guarantee a 100% risk-free environment. Taking the risk of *exposure* to a communicable disease is a part of your job. You have a right to know about diseases that may pose a risk to you. Remember, though, that your risk for infection is not high; however, OSHA regulations, especially for private and federal agencies, require that all employees be offered a workplace environment that reduces the risk for exposure. Note that in some states that have their own OSHA laws, state and municipal employees must also be covered.

> *Exposure* A situation in which a person has had contact with blood, body fluids, tissues, or airborne particles that increases the risk of disease transmission.

In addition to OSHA guidelines, other national guidelines and standards, including those from the CDC and National Fire Protection Association (NFPA) 1581, *Standard on Fire Department Infection Control Program*, address reducing risk for exposure to bloodborne pathogens (disease-causing organisms) and airborne diseases. These agencies set a standard of care for all fire and EMS personnel and apply whether you are a full-time paid employee or a volunteer. It is your responsibility to know your department's infection control plan and to use it **TABLE 15-2**.

Establishing an Infection Control Routine

Infection control, or the use of procedures to reduce infection in patients and health care personnel, should be an important part of your daily routine. These steps should be followed to manage potential exposure situations:

1. En route to the scene, make sure that PPE is out and available.
2. Upon arrival, make sure the scene is safe to enter, then do a quick visual assessment of the patient, noting whether any blood is present.
3. Select the proper PPE according to the tasks you are likely to perform. Typically, gloves will be used for all patient contacts.
4. Change gloves and wash hands between patients; do not unnecessarily delay treatment for use of PPE, thereby potentially putting patients at risk. Remove gloves and other gear after contact with the patient, unless you are in the patient compartment. Remember that good hand hygiene is always necessary. Just

Table 15-2
Components of an Infection Control Plan

Determination of Exposure	▪ Determines who is at risk for ongoing contact with blood and other body fluids ▪ Creates a list of tasks that pose a risk for contact with blood or other body fluids ▪ Includes PPE required by OSHA
Education and Training	▪ Explains why a qualified person is required to answer questions about communicable diseases and infection control, rather than relying on packaged training materials ▪ Includes availability of an instructor able to train AEMTs regarding bloodborne and airborne pathogens, such as hepatitis B and C viruses, HIV, and the bacteria that cause diseases such as syphilis and tuberculosis ▪ Ensures that the instructor provides appropriate education, which is the best means for correcting many myths surrounding these issues
Hepatitis B Vaccine Program	▪ Spells out the vaccine offered, its safety and efficacy, record keeping, and tracking ▪ Addresses the need for postvaccine antibody titers to identify people who do not respond to the initial three-dose vaccination series
Personal Protective Equipment	▪ Lists the PPE offered and why it was selected ▪ Lists how much equipment is available and where to obtain additional PPE ▪ States when each type of PPE is to be used for each risk procedure
Cleaning and Disinfection Practices	▪ Describes how to care for and maintain vehicles and equipment ▪ Identifies where and when cleaning should be performed, how it is to be done, that PPE is to be used, and what cleaning solution is to be used ▪ Addresses medical waste collection, storage, and disposal
Tuberculin Skin Testing/ Fit Testing	▪ Addresses how often employees should undergo tuberculin skin testing (PPD) ▪ Addresses how often fit testing should be done to determine the proper size HEPA mask to protect the AEMT from tuberculosis ▪ Addresses all issues dealing with HEPA respirator masks
Postexposure Management	▪ Identifies whom to notify when exposure may have occurred, forms to be filled out, where to go for treatment, and what treatment is to be given
Compliance Monitoring	▪ Addresses how the service or department evaluates employee compliance with each aspect of the plan ▪ Ensures that employees understand what they are to do and why it is important ▪ States that noncompliance should be documented ▪ Indicates what disciplinary action should be taken in the face of noncompliance
Record Keeping	▪ Outlines all records that will be kept, how confidentiality will be maintained, and how records can be accessed and by whom

Abbreviations: HEPA, high-efficiency particulate air; HIV, human immunodeficiency virus; OSHA, Occupational Safety and Health Administration; PPD, purified protein derivative; PPE, personal protective equipment.

because you were wearing gloves during patient contact does not mean you do not need to wash your hands after.

5. If you or your partner is exposed while providing care, try to relieve one another as soon as possible so that you can seek care. Notify the designated officer and report the incident. This will also help to maintain confidentiality.

> *Infection control* Procedures to reduce transmission of infection among patients and health care personnel.

Be sure to routinely clean the ambulance after each run and on a daily basis. Cleaning is an essential part of the prevention and control of communicable diseases and will remove surface organisms that may remain in the unit. You should clean your unit as quickly as possible so that it can be returned to service. Address the high-contact areas, including surfaces that were in direct contact with the patient's blood or body fluids or surfaces that you touched while caring for the patient after having contact with the patient's blood or body fluids.

Whenever possible, cleaning should be done at the hospital. If you clean the unit back at the station, make sure you have a designated area with good ventilation and a floor drain. Any medical waste should be put in a red bag and disposed of at the hospital whenever possible. Any contaminated equipment that is left with the patient at the hospital should be cleaned by hospital staff or bagged for transport and cleaned at the station.

You can use a bleach and water solution at a 1:10 dilution to clean the unit. The solution you mix should not have a strong odor of bleach if mixed correctly. A hospital-approved disinfectant that is effective against *Mycobacterium tuberculosis* can also be used. Use the cleaning solution in a bucket or pistol-handled spray container. Do not use alcohol or aerosol spray products to clean the unit. Pay attention to disinfectant directions.

Remove contaminated linen and place it into an appropriate bag for handling. Each hospital may have a different system for handling contaminated linen; you should learn hospital or department protocols.

Any reusable medical equipment should be properly cleaned and sanitized or sterilized per your department's standard operating procedures. Keep in mind that in hospitals entire departments are devoted to sterilizing medical instruments. Proper sterilization requires the right tools and the right skills, so always carefully follow your department's procedures.

Learn the regulations defining medical waste in your area. The procedures for disposal of infectious waste such as needles and heavily soiled dressings may vary from hospital to hospital and from state to state.

Immunity

Even if germs do reach you, they may not infect you because you may have *immunity*, or resistance, to those particular germs. Immunity is a major factor in determining which hosts become ill from which germs TABLE 15-3. One way to gain immunity from many diseases today is to be immunized, or vaccinated, against them. Vaccinations have almost eliminated some childhood diseases, such as measles and polio.

> **Immunity** The body's ability to protect itself from acquiring a disease.

Another way in which the body becomes immune to a disease is to recover from an infection from that germ. Afterward, the body recognizes and repels that germ when it shows up again. Once exposed, healthy people will develop lifelong immunity to many common pathogens. For example, a person who contracts and becomes infected with the

Table 15-3 Immunity to Infectious Diseases

Type of Immunity	Characteristics	Examples	Comments
Lifelong	The illness will not recur.	Measles Mumps Polio Rubella Hepatitis A Hepatitis B	Infection or vaccination provides long-term immunity to new infection. A live vaccine is required for measles only.
Partial	The person who has recovered from a first infection is unlikely to get a new infection from another person, but may experience illness from germs that lie dormant from the initial infection.	Chickenpox Tuberculosis	Infection provides lifelong immunity to the patient from acquiring a new infection, but the original illness may recur, or it may recur in a different way. In the case of chickenpox, which is caused by the varicella virus, an infection may recur years later in the form of shingles.
None	Exposure confers no protection from reinfection. The infection may wear down the patient's resistance to other pathogens.	Gonorrhea Syphilis HIV infection	No vaccine is available. Repeated infections are common. For example, there is effective immediate treatment for gonorrhea, and the germs may be eradicated; however, reinfection is likely if the high-risk practices (eg, unprotected sex) continue. For syphilis and HIV infection, the lack of immunity allows the germs to continue to cause damage within the host.

Abbreviation: HIV, human immunodeficiency virus.

hepatitis A virus may be ill for several weeks, but because immunity will develop, he or she will not have to worry about getting the illness again. Sometimes, however, the immunity is only partial. Partial immunity protects against new infections, but germs that remain in the body from the first illness may still be able to cause the same disease again when the body is stressed or has some impairment in its immune system. For example, tuberculosis can cause a mild, unnoticeable infection before the body builds up a partial immunity. If the infection is never treated, it may be reactivated when immunity is weakened; however, people with partial immunity are protected against a new infection from another person.

Humans seem unable to mount an effective immune response to some infections, such as HIV infection, which can progress to AIDS. HIV is a virus that attacks the immune system and weakens the body's ability to fight infections. Because the immune system is our natural defense, the body is unable to fight off disease if it is not strong.

Although OSHA does not require hepatitis A immunization, you may want to be vaccinated as a preventive measure. Hepatitis A vaccination is not necessary if you have had hepatitis A in the past. All these vaccines are effective and rarely cause side effects. Many EMS systems require you to show proof that you are up-to-date with your immunizations.

Remember, germs that cause no symptoms in one person may cause serious illness in another.

General Postexposure Management

The likelihood of becoming infected during your performance of routine patient care is low. In the event that you are exposed to blood or other body substances despite all of your precautions, there are still preventive measures that you can take to protect your health. If you are exposed to a patient's blood or body fluids, first turn over patient care to another EMS provider. When it is safe to do so, clean the exposed area with soap and water. If your eyes were exposed, rinse them with water for at least 20 minutes as soon as possible.

Next, activate your department's infection control plan. This usually involves contacting a supervisor or your department's infection control officer to assist you. This person will help you to navigate the infection control process.

You will need to be screened to determine if there was a significant exposure to possible bloodborne pathogens. Just because you were exposed to a patient's blood or body fluids does not mean that there is a risk of infection. Typically, you will need a follow-up evaluation by a physician to determine if a significant exposure occurred. If the exposure was significant, blood may need to be drawn from both you and the patient to determine if any infectious agents were present.

You will have to complete an exposure report. Questions in the report may include: When did the event happen?

What were you doing when you were exposed? What did you do after you were exposed? Completion of this paperwork will help relay critical information to the right people, resulting in help for you and possibly new protocols in the future to help prevent another incident.

Transition Tip

In the event of exposure involving the eyes, immediately flush with sterile water or saline for at least 20 minutes.

Time is important! If you are exposed, let your supervisor or infection control officer know immediately. Some diseases will act quickly whereas others may lie dormant for a long time. The best way to reduce your risk of contracting a work-related disease is through early activation of your department's infection control plan.

Transition Tip

The ability of your EMS system to support you in case of exposure to a communicable disease depends on your understanding of how exposure can occur and your immediate report of exposure to potentially infectious materials. Document the event as soon as possible to ensure that you remember all pertinent information, and report immediately after the exposure, following your service's guidelines.

Ambulance Cleaning and Disinfection

The AEMT has an obligation to protect patients from nosocomial infections (infections acquired from a health care setting—in this instance, the ambulance). One way to protect patients is by complying with work restriction guidelines: Reporting for work when you have a sore throat or the flu is not in the best interests of your patients or your coworkers.

Another way to protect patients from nosocomial infections is to keep the ambulance interior and its equipment clean and disinfected. When you are cleaning equipment, select cleaning solutions to fit the equipment category:

- **Critical equipment:** Items that come in contact with mucous membranes; laryngoscope blades, endotracheal tubes, Combitubes. High-level disinfection—that is, use of Environmental Protection Agency (EPA)-registered chemical "sterilants"—is the minimum level for this equipment.
- **Semicritical equipment:** Items that come in direct contact with intact skin; stethoscopes, blood pressure cuffs, splints, pneumatic antishock garments. Clean with solutions that have a label claiming to

kill the hepatitis B virus. Bleach and water at 1:100 dilution fits this requirement.

- **Noncritical equipment:** Cleaning surfaces, floors, ambulance seats, work surfaces. EPA-registered hospital-grade cleaner or bleach and water mixture is effective for this equipment.

General cleaning routines need to be listed in the department's Exposure Control Plan. A basic rule is to do the following after every call:

1. Strip used linens from the stretcher immediately after use and place them in a plastic bag or in the designated receptacle in the emergency department.
2. In an appropriate receptacle, discard all disposable equipment used for care of the patient that meets your state's definition of medical waste. Most items will be considered general trash.
3. Wash contaminated areas with soap and water. For disinfection to be effective, cleaning must be done first.
4. Disinfect all nondisposable equipment used in the care of the patient. For example, disassemble the bag-mask device and place the components in a liquid sterilization solution as recommended by the manufacturer.
5. Clean the stretcher with an EPA-registered germicidal/virucidal solution or bleach and water at 1:100 dilution.
6. If any spillage or other contamination occurred in the ambulance, clean it up with the same germicidal/virucidal or bleach/water solution.
7. Create a schedule for routine full cleaning for the vehicle, as required by the Exposure Control Plan. Name the brands of solution to be used.
8. Have a written policy/procedure for cleaning each piece of equipment. Refer to the manufacturer's recommendations as a guide.

Pathophysiology of Infectious Diseases

General Assessment Principles

The assessment of a patient suspected to have an infectious disease should be approached much like any other medical patient. First, the scene must be sized up and standard precautions taken. Once you can determine that the scene is safe, proceed with the primary assessment by assessing the patient's mental status and airway, breathing, and circulation and by prioritizing treatment of the patient. With most patients who have a potentially infectious disease in the prehospital setting, the next step is to gather patient history, using OPQRST to elaborate on the patient's chief complaint. Typical chief complaints include fever, nausea, rash, pleuritic chest pain, and difficulty breathing. Obtain a SAMPLE history and a set of baseline vital signs, paying

particular attention to medications the patient is currently taking and the events leading up to the current problem.

Also ask whether the patient has recently traveled. Always show respect for the feelings of the patient, family members, and others at the scene.

General Management Principles

The general management of the patient with a suspected infectious disease first focuses on any life-threatening conditions that were identified in the primary assessment (airway maintenance, oxygen and ventilatory assistance, bleeding control, and circulatory support). Remember to be empathetic. Because most of these patients will have a fever of unexplained origin or mild breathing problems, place the patient in the position of comfort on the stretcher to keep warm. Remember to use standard precautions for your own safety. Always follow your agency's exposure control plan in cleaning equipment and properly discard any disposable supplies as well as linens.

> ### Transition Tip
>
> An infectious disease is a medical condition caused by the growth and spread of small harmful organisms within the body. A communicable disease is a disease that can be spread from one person or species to another. Most of these diseases are much harder to be infected with than is commonly believed. In addition, there are many immunizations, protective techniques, and devices that can be used to minimize your risk of infection. When these protective measures are used, the risk of your contracting a serious infectious disease is negligible.

Common or Serious Communicable Diseases

Human Immunodeficiency Virus Infection

HIV type 1 was first identified in the late 1970s. Today, an estimated 60 million people worldwide are infected with this virus. In the United States, HIV infection is not a reportable disease in all states.

Exposure to the virus that causes AIDS is the most feared infection risk for AEMTs. This potential exposure led to the development of standard precautions. There is no vaccine to protect against HIV infection, and despite great progress in drug treatments, AIDS is still often fatal. Fortunately, it is not easily transmitted in your work setting. Furthermore, the overwhelming majority of cases of HIV infection can be managed effectively with antiretroviral drug therapy and therefore do not progress to AIDS.

HIV is primarily a sexually transmitted disease, but is also bloodborne. It can also be transmitted from a pregnant woman to her infant in the delivery process. HIV is also transmitted through blood transfusions, but this is no longer as common because donated blood is now tested for a protein indicating HIV.

In HIV infection, the entire immune system begins to fail, allowing for life-threatening opportunistic infections. The HIV pathogen invades infected cells and attacks the immune system and other body organs. The immune system is then unable to assist in protecting the infected person from other diseases. It takes about 7 days for the virus to invade a cell, and this process may occur 4 to 6 weeks after the exposure event.

Transition Tip

Causes of Infectious Disease

Type of Organism	Description	Example
Bacteria	Grow and reproduce outside the human cell in the appropriate temperature and with the appropriate nutrients	*Salmonella*
Viruses	Smaller than bacteria; multiply only inside a host and die when exposed to the environment	Influenza
Fungi	Similar to bacteria in that they require the appropriate nutrients and organic material to grow	Mold
Protozoa (parasites)	One-celled microscopic organisms, some of which cause disease	Amoebas
Helminths (parasites)	Invertebrates with long, flexible, rounded, or flattened bodies	Worms

---

Often patients with HIV infection are asymptomatic. For those who are symptomatic, signs and symptoms of acute infection may include acute febrile illness, malaise, fatigue, sore throat, swollen spleen and lymph glands, headache, weight loss, and possibly rash. Following initial infection, most patients present with enlargement of the lymph nodes and appear healthy. However, the immune system ultimately becomes weakened in the absence of treatment. Because of the availability of effective treatment, most cases of HIV infection do not progress to AIDS in the United States. However, as these treatments do not represent cures, lifelong treatment is necessary to prevent late development of AIDS.

Acquired immunodeficiency syndrome (AIDS) is the end-stage disease process caused by HIV infection. A patient with AIDS is extremely vulnerable to numerous bacterial, viral, and fungal infections that would not affect a person with an intact immune system. These opportunistic infections include pneumonia in infants or people with compromised immune systems, loss of vision because of cytomegalovirus, reddish/purple skin lesions, atypical tuberculosis, and cryptococcal meningitis.

> **Acquired immunodeficiency syndrome (AIDS)** The end-stage disease process caused by the human immunodeficiency virus (HIV). A person with this is extremely vulnerable to numerous infections.

Prehospital management is supportive. Support the airway and respiratory status, assisting ventilations as needed. Establish IV access and give a fluid bolus of an isotonic crystalloid solution if the patient is hypovolemic. Use a nonrebreathing mask or other mask for respiratory isolation if the patient is coughing.

HIV infection is a potential hazard only when deposited on a mucous membrane or directly into the bloodstream. This can occur via sexual contact or exposure to blood or body fluids, meaning your risk of infection is limited to exposure to an infected patient's blood and body fluids. Exposure can take place in the following ways:

- The patient's blood is splashed or sprayed into your eyes, nose, or mouth or into an open sore or cut, however tiny; even a microscopic opening in the skin is an invitation for infection with a virus.
- You have blood from the infected patient on your hands and then touch your own eyes, nose, mouth, or an open sore or cut.
- A needle used to inject the patient breaks your skin. The risk to you from a single injection, even with a hollow-bore needle, is small, probably less than 1 in 1,000. However, this is by far the most dangerous form of exposure.
- Broken glass at a motor vehicle crash or other incident may penetrate your glove (and skin), which may have already been covered with blood from an infected patient.

Because many patients infected with HIV do not show any symptoms, the government requires health care workers to wear certain types of gloves any time they are likely to come into contact with secretions or blood from any patient. You should always put on the proper type of gloves before leaving the ambulance to care for a patient. You must take great care in handling and disposing of needles and scalpels so that you and others are not inadvertently exposed to them. You should cover any open wounds that you have whenever you are on the job. Finally, as always, good handwashing technique and routine ambulance cleaning after transport are critical.

If you have any reason to think that a patient's blood or secretions may have entered your system, especially through inoculation with a patient's blood, you should seek medical advice urgently. If you know that the patient is infected with HIV, your physician may suggest immediate treatment to try to prevent you from becoming infected. This type of treatment is known as postexposure prophylaxis. Such treatment has been shown to significantly decrease the risk of ultimate conversion to HIV infection, particularly when started within 72 hours of exposure. It is therefore critical to inform your infection control officer immediately upon sustaining exposure or possible exposure to the virus. However, if the patient is unlikely to be infected with HIV, your physician may recommend that you and the patient be tested before you undergo therapy. As scientists learn more about HIV infection, testing and treatment recommendations change. The most recent version of the US Public Health Service Guidelines for the Management of Occupational Exposures to HIV and Recommendations for Postexposure Prophylaxis are always available online at http://aidsinfo.nih.gov/guidelines. It is important that you immediately see your physician (or your program's designated physician or infection control officer) any time you are potentially exposed to a communicable or infectious disease. Know the policy for your system, and take time now to consider what you would do in the event of exposure.

> ### Transition Tip
> An AEMT with a cold or flu can be extremely hazardous to a patient who is immunocompromised.

Hepatitis

The term hepatitis refers to an inflammation (and often infection) of the liver. Hepatitis is the leading cause of liver cancer and the most common reason for liver transplantation. Complications of hepatitis include scarring of the liver, liver cancer, and liver failure. Populations most at risk include those with STDs, HIV/AIDS, men who have sex with men, and IV drug users. Hepatitis can be caused by a number of different viruses. It can also be caused by toxins such as medications, drugs, or alcohol. The severity of toxin-induced hepatitis depends on the amount of agent absorbed and the duration of exposure. Toxin-induced hepatitis is not contagious. Mortality rates without supportive management and/or liver transplantation are in excess of 70%.

Depending on the severity of the infection, patients may be asymptomatic or may have a variety of signs and symptoms. Early signs of viral hepatitis include loss of appetite, nausea and vomiting, fever, fatigue, sore throat, cough, headache, and muscle and joint pain. Several weeks later, jaundice (yellow eyes and skin), right upper quadrant abdominal pain, diarrhea, dark urine, and light-colored stools develop. Acute liver failure, also known as fulminant hepatitis, is a rare but potentially fatal disease.

Management of patients with any type of hepatitis is strictly supportive. Maintain a patent airway, give 100% oxygen, and assist ventilations as needed. Establish IV access, and if fluid resuscitation is needed, give a 20 mL/kg bolus of an isotonic crystalloid solution. If no trauma is suspected, transport in a position of comfort to the closest, most appropriate facility.

There is no sure way to tell which patients with hepatitis have a contagious form of the disease and which do not. **TABLE 15-4** shows the characteristics of different types of hepatitis, from which you can assess your risk of exposure. Hepatitis A can be transmitted only from a patient who has an acute infection, whereas hepatitis B and hepatitis C can be transmitted from long-term carriers with no signs of illness. A carrier is a person (or animal) in whom an infectious organism has taken up permanent residence and may or may not cause any active disease. Carriers may never know that they harbor the organism; however, they can infect others.

Hepatitis A is transmitted orally through oral or fecal contamination. This means that, generally, you must eat or drink something contaminated with the virus in order to become exposed. The organisms that cause hepatitis B, C, and G are transmitted through vehicles other than food or water. For example, these organisms may enter the body through a transfusion or needlestick with infected blood, which puts health care workers at high risk for contracting hepatitis B, the more contagious and virulent form. *Virulence* is the strength or ability of a pathogen to produce disease. Hepatitis B is far more contagious than HIV. For this reason, vaccination with hepatitis B vaccine is highly recommended for AEMTs. Unfortunately, not everyone who is vaccinated develops immediate immunity to the virus. Sometimes, but not always, an additional dose will provide immunity. You should be tested after vaccination to determine your immune status.

> *Virulence* The strength or ability of a pathogen to produce disease.

If you are stuck with a needle or injured in some other way while caring for a patient who might have hepatitis, see your physician immediately.

Herpes Simplex

Herpes simplex is a common virus strain carried by humans. Eighty percent of persons carrying the virus are asymptomatic, but symptomatic infections can be serious and are on the rise, especially in immunocompromised patients. The primary mode of infection is through close personal contact, so standard precautions are generally sufficient to prevent spread to or from health care workers.

Table 15-4
Characteristics of Hepatitis

Type	Route of Infection	Incubation Period	Chronic Infection	Vaccine and Treatment	Comments
Viral Hepatitis					
Hepatitis A (infectious)	Fecal-oral, infected food or drink	2–6 wk	Chronic condition does not exist.	Vaccine is available; no treatment is available.	Mild illness, approximately 2% of patients die; after acute infection, the patient has lifelong immunity.
Hepatitis B	Blood, sexual contact, saliva, urine, breast milk	4–12 wk	Chronic infection affects up to 10% of patients and up to 90% of newborns who have the disease.	Vaccine is available; treatment is minimally effective.	Up to 30% of patients may become chronic carriers. Patients are asymptomatic and without signs of liver disease, but they may infect others. Approximately 1% to 2% of patients die.
Hepatitis C	Blood, sexual contact	2–10 wk	Chronic infection affects 90% of patients	No vaccine is available; treatment is minimally effective.	Cirrhosis of the liver develops in 50% of patients with chronic hepatitis C. Chronic infection increases the risk of cancer of the liver.
Hepatitis D	Blood, sexual contact	4–12 wk	Chronic infection is common	No vaccine is available; no treatment is available.	Occurs only in patients with active hepatitis B infection; fulminant disease may develop in 20% of patients.
Hepatitis E (AKA epidemic non-A, non-B hepatitis)	Fecal-oral, contaminated water or food	15–60 day	Hepatitis E usually resolves on its own over several weeks to months.	No vaccine is available; no treatment is available.	Mild illness; fatal in about 2% of all cases; elevated mortality rate of approximately 20% for pregnant women, especially in third trimester
Hepatitis G (AKA hepatitis GB)	Blood, sexual contact, breast milk	Possibly 15–50 day	Mild and usually short-lived	No vaccine is available; no treatment is available.	It is possible that HGV can cause severe liver damage resulting in liver failure; often seen in conjunction with hepatitis B, C, or both.
Toxin-Induced Hepatitis					
Medication, drugs, and alcohol	Inhalation, skin or mucous membrane exposure, oral ingestion, or IV administration	Within hours to days following exposure	Some chemicals may initiate an inflammatory response that continues to cause liver damage long after the chemical is out of the body.	No vaccine is available; treatment is to stop exposure. In patients with an overdose of acetaminophen, certain drugs may minimize liver injury if given early enough.	This type of hepatitis is not contagious. Patients with toxin-induced hepatitis may have liver damage, such as jaundice. Not every exposure to a toxin will cause liver damage.

> *Herpes simplex* Virus caused by human herpes viruses 1 and 2, characterized by small blisters whose location depends on the type of virus. Type 2 results in blisters on the genital area, while type 1 results in blisters in nongenital areas.

Syphilis

Although syphilis is commonly thought of as a sexually transmitted disease, it is also a bloodborne disease. There is a small risk for transmission through a contaminated needlestick injury or direct blood-to-blood contact. If treated with penicillin, the patient is considered noncommunicable within 24 to 48 hours.

The initial infection with syphilis produces a lesion called a chancre. Chancres are most commonly located in the genital region.

Meningitis

Meningitis is an inflammation of the meningeal coverings of the brain and spinal cord. Patients with meningitis will have signs and symptoms such as fever, headache, stiff neck, and altered mental status. It is an uncommon but frightening infectious disease. Meningitis can be caused by viruses or bacteria, most of which are not contagious. However, one form, meningococcal meningitis, is highly contagious. The meningococcus bacterium colonizes the human nose and throat and only rarely causes an acute infection. When it does, it can be rapidly lethal. Patients with this infection often have red blotches on their skin; however, many patients with forms of meningitis that are not contagious also have red blotches.

> *Meningitis* Inflammation of the meninges that cover the spinal cord and the brain.

Only laboratory tests can sort out the different forms of meningitis; therefore, you should take standard precautions with any patient who is suspected of having meningitis. Gloves and a mask will go a long way to prevent the patient's secretions from getting into your nose and mouth. Again, the risk of infection is small, even if the organism is transmitted. For this reason, vaccines, which are available for most types of meningococci, are rarely used. Meningitis can be treated at the emergency department with antibiotics.

After treating a patient with meningitis, you should contact your infection control officer. Many states consider meningitis "reportable" and will notify you that one of your patients was diagnosed with meningitis. Prophylactic treatment is then in order for you.

> ### Transition Tip
> Place a surgical mask on the patient suspected of having tuberculosis and a HEPA mask on yourself.

Tuberculosis

Most patients infected with *Mycobacterium tuberculosis* (the tubercle bacillus) are well most of the time. If the disease involves the brain or kidneys, the patient is only slightly contagious. In the United States, however, *tuberculosis* is a chronic mycobacterial disease that usually strikes the lungs. Disease that occurs shortly after infection is called primary tuberculosis. Except in infants, this infection is not usually serious. After the primary infection, the tubercle bacillus is rendered dormant by the patient's immune system. However, even after decades of lying dormant, this germ can reactivate. Reactive tuberculosis is common and can be much more difficult to treat, especially because an increasing number of tuberculosis strains have grown resistant to most antibiotics.

> *Tuberculosis* A chronic bacterial disease caused by *Myobacterium tuberculosis* that usually affects the lungs but also can affect other organs such as the brain or kidneys.

> ### Transition Tip
> Everyone has body defenses that help protect against becoming ill, but the aging process can pose a threat to the body's natural defense mechanisms against invading microorganisms. As a person ages, his or her physical defenses weaken or are eliminated. The thinning and loss of supportive collagen in the skin and a reduction in the number of blood vessels allow bacteria or viruses to enter the body with less resistance. The respiratory system cannot trap and eliminate bacteria and viruses in the airways as efficiently as it previously did. Finally, the gastrointestinal system allows easier entry for bacteria or viruses through the intestines. As the body ages, physical barriers to entry weaken, the immune system deteriorates, and invading organisms are not as easily identified as abnormal. Infectious agents can take hold in elderly patients much more easily because of reduced defenses.
>
> When transporting an elderly patient, protect the patient from the environment because extremes in heat or cold can further reduce the body's defenses. If your patient has a cold or the flu, protect yourself. However, remember that your defense system is probably much stronger than that of the patient.

Although tuberculosis is often hard to distinguish from other diseases, patients who pose the highest risk almost invariably have a cough. Therefore, for your safety, you should consider respiratory tuberculosis to be the only contagious form because it is the only one that is spread by airborne transmission. The droplets produced by coughing are not the real problem. The real problem is the droplet nuclei, which are the remnants of the droplets after the excess water has evaporated. These particles are tiny enough to be totally invisible and can remain suspended in the air for a long time. In fact, as long as these particles are shielded from ultraviolet light, they can remain alive for decades. Particles the size of droplet nuclei are not stopped by routine surgical masks. Inhaled, they are carried directly to the alveoli of the lungs, where the bacteria may begin to grow. High-efficiency particulate air masks, or HEPA masks, are required to stop droplet nuclei.

Why is tuberculosis not more common than it is? After all, absolute protection from infection with the tubercle bacillus does not exist. Everyone who breathes is at risk. According to the CDC, one third of the world's population is infected with tuberculosis. The vaccine for tuberculosis, BCG, is only rarely used in the United States. Under normal circumstances, however, the mechanism of transmission used by *M. tuberculosis* is not very efficient. Infected air is easily diluted with uninfected air. *M. tuberculosis* is one of those germs that typically causes no illness in a new host. In fact, many patients with tuberculosis do not even transmit the infection to family members. However, in crowded environments with poor ventilation, the disease spreads more easily.

If you are exposed to a patient who is found to have pulmonary tuberculosis, you will be given a tuberculin skin test. This simple skin test determines whether a person has been infected with *M. tuberculosis*. A positive result means that exposure has occurred; it does not mean that the person has active tuberculosis. It takes at least 6 weeks for the bacteria to show up in the laboratory test. If you are tested for the disease within a few weeks of the exposure and your results are positive, this means that you had already acquired the infection at an earlier time from somebody else. You will probably never identify the source. Most transmissions occur silently, so it is necessary that you have tuberculin skin tests regularly. If the infection is found before you become ill, preventive therapy is almost 100% effective. Usually, a daily dose of the medication isoniazid will prevent the development of active infection.

Whooping Cough

Whooping cough, also called pertussis, is an airborne disease caused by bacteria that mostly affects children younger than 6 years. Signs and symptoms include fever and a "whoop" sound that occurs when the patient tries to inhale after a coughing attack.

> **Whooping cough** An airborne disease caused by bacteria that mostly affects children younger than 6 years and presents with fever and a "whoop" sound that occurs when the patient tries to inhale after a coughing attack; also called pertussis.

The best way to prevent exposure to whooping cough is to place a mask on the patient and on yourself.

Methicillin-Resistant *Staphylococcus aureus*

Methicillin-resistant Staphylococcus aureus *(MRSA)* is a bacterium that causes infections and is resistant to most antibiotics. In health care settings, MRSA is believed to be transmitted from patient to patient via unwashed hands of health care providers. Studies have shown that 5% to 15% of health care providers carry MRSA in their nares; the pathogen can subsequently be transferred to skin and other areas of the body through a break in the skin. Surfaces contaminated with MRSA do not seem to be important in transmission. Factors that increase the risk for developing MRSA include antibiotic therapy, prolonged hospital stays, a stay in an intensive care or burn unit, and exposure to an infected patient.

> **Methicillin-resistant** Staphylococcus aureus *(MRSA)* A bacterium that causes infections in different parts of the body and is often resistant to commonly used antibiotics; can be found on the skin, in surgical wounds, in the bloodstream, lungs, and urinary tract.

The incubation period for MRSA appears to be between 5 and 45 days. The communicable period varies, because patients who have active infection may carry MRSA for months. MRSA results in soft-tissue infections. Its signs and symptoms may involve localized skin abscesses, and sepsis may be found in older patients with the infection.

To prevent MRSA transmission, use standard precautions (gloves and good handwashing technique) when in contact with patient wounds and nonintact skin. If you are in direct contact with wound drainage but your skin is intact, no exposure will occur. If you have a true exposure, no postexposure treatment is recommended. The incident must still be documented, however.

New and Emerging Diseases

Hantavirus

Newly recognized diseases, such as those caused by hantavirus (a rare but deadly virus transmitted through rodent urine and droppings) and enteropathogenic *Escherichia coli* (a common cause of pediatric diarrhea in developing countries), are being reported. These diseases are not transmitted from person to person directly; rather, they are carried by a vehicle, such as food, or a vector, such as rodents.

West Nile Virus

Although not a newly discovered illness, West Nile virus has caused some concern in the past. The virus vector, the mosquito, affects humans and birds. The virus is tracked by tests done on birds suspected of being killed by the virus. These diseases are not communicable and do not pose a risk to you during patient care.

Severe Acute Respiratory Syndrome

A virus that has caused significant concern in the recent past is known as *SARS (severe acute respiratory syndrome)*.

SARS is a serious, potentially life-threatening viral infection caused by a recently discovered family of viruses. SARS usually starts with flulike symptoms, which may progress to pneumonia, respiratory failure, and in some cases, death. The SARS virus strain probably spread from Guangdong province in southern China to Hong Kong, Singapore, and Taiwan. Canada experienced a significant outbreak in the Toronto area between 2002–2003. SARS is thought to be primarily transmitted by close person-to-person contact. Most cases have involved persons who lived with or cared for a person with SARS or who had exposure to contaminated secretions from a patient with SARS. Travel history should be a routine part of patient assessment.

> **SARS (severe acute respiratory syndrome)** Potentially life-threatening viral infection that usually starts with flulike symptoms.

Avian Flu

Avian (bird) flu is caused by a virus that occurs naturally in the bird population. This virus is carried in the intestinal tract of wild birds and does not usually cause illness.

Transition Tip

Travel history should be a routine part of patient assessment.

However, in domestic bird populations (eg, chickens, ducks, and turkeys), it is very contagious. Birds acquire the illness from contact with contaminated excretions or surfaces that are contaminated with excretions. If an infected bird is used for food and is cooked, it does not pose a risk to those who eat it.

The first case of this flu was reported in Hong Kong in 1997; 18 people became infected and six died in the outbreak. In the cases that have occurred since then, the death rate is approximately 25%. No cases involving human-to-human transmission of this disease have been reported. Instead, the cases occurring involving humans have involved close contact with infected birds. The transmission risk for humans is low.

H1N1 Virus

Another virus of recent concern is the H1N1 virus that was initially identified as the "swine flu." This virus is not new, having been present for years in animals. H1N1 is contagious. Whereas this virus is new to humans, it is only one type of influenza among the hundreds of other strains of influenza that exist and infect humans regularly. Many deaths have been caused by the H1N1 virus, although deaths caused by other influenza viruses also have occurred. The most positive effect of the outbreak of H1N1 virus has been a greater awareness on the part of the general public of the routes of transmission of contagious diseases. This increased awareness could result in a reduction of all communicable diseases, not only H1N1.

Transition Tip

The ability of your EMS service to support you in the event of exposure to a communicable disease depends on your understanding of how an exposure can occur and your immediate reporting of exposure to potentially infectious materials. Make notes right away to ensure that you remember all pertinent information, and report the possible exposure immediately after the response, following your local protocol.

PREP KIT

Ready for Review

- A communicable disease is an infectious disease that can be passed from one person to another.
- An infectious disease is a medical condition caused by the growth and spread of harmful organisms within the body.
- Contact transmission is the movement of an organism from one person to another through physical contact. Two types of contact transmission are possible: direct and indirect. Transmission of communicable diseases can also occur through airborne, bloodborne, foodborne, vector-borne, or sexually transmitted mechanisms.
- The term "standard precautions" describes infection control practices that reduce the opportunity for an exposure to occur in the daily care of patients. It replaces the older terms "universal precautions" and "body substance isolation" (BSI).
- Standard precautions suggest that all moist (with the exception of sweat) body substances may transmit bacterial or viral infections. Because it is often impossible to tell which patients have infectious diseases, AEMTs should avoid direct contact with the moist body substances of all patients.

- AEMTs are responsible for maintaining the ambulance so that it is safe and available on a moment's notice.
- Be especially compliant with wearing of PPE when infectious disease is a possibility. Follow standard precautions. Place a surgical mask on patients with suspected or confirmed respiratory disease.
- Emergency care for a patient with an infectious disease depends on presentation. If the patient is suffering from severe dyspnea, administer oxygen. Be prepared to suction—but never suction a patient with suspected croup or epiglottitis.
- If you think you may have been exposed to an infectious disease, contact your designated infection control officer (DICO). This person is charged with ensuring that proper postexposure medical treatment and counseling are provided to the exposed person.
- Infection control should be an important part of your daily routine. Be sure to follow the proper steps when dealing with potential exposure situations.

Case Study

You are called to the scene of an old apartment complex for a 67-year-old man with respiratory distress. The patient tells you that he has been ill for the past several days. He reports coughing up bloody mucus, has been experiencing night sweats, and has a fever. His past medical history is significant for hypertension, chronic obstructive pulmonary disease, and alcoholism. You and your partner take the necessary standard precautions and place the patient on oxygen. During your exam, you notice that the patient is breathing rapidly at 28 breaths/min and is very warm to touch; you also hear wheezing when listening to his lung sounds. The patient states that he has lived in this apartment for more than 10 years and rarely goes out.

1. This scenario states that "standard precautions" were used. Describe the meaning of this term, and discuss the various methods used to achieve standard precautions.

2. Discuss the prevention and treatment of pertussis.

3. Both croup and epiglottitis can present with stridor. What are some of the differences between the two illnesses?

4. Which of the following infections may initially cause no symptoms or may produce a lesion called a chancre, most commonly located in the genital region?
   A. Herpes simplex
   B. Tuberculosis
   C. Syphilis
   D. HIV

5. Which type of hepatitis infection causes a chronic liver infection in 90% of patients, does not have a vaccine available for its prevention, and is typically spread by blood and sexual contact?
   A. Hepatitis A
   B. Hepatitis B
   C. Hepatitis C
   D. Hepatitis D

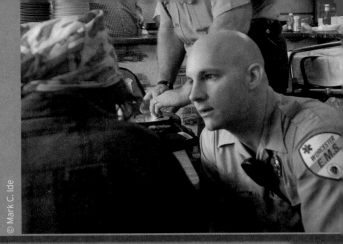

© Mark C. Ide

National EMS Education Standards

Anatomy and Physiology
Applies complex knowledge of the anatomy and function of all human systems to the practice of EMS.

Medicine
Applies complex knowledge to provide advanced emergency care and transportation based on assessment findings for an acutely ill patient.

Pharmacology
Applies complex knowledge of the medications that an AEMT may assist/administer to a patient during an immunologic or toxicologic emergency.

Review

An allergic reaction or poisoning can be a life-threatening event. Your ability to recognize and manage the many signs and symptoms of allergic reactions or poisoning may be the only thing standing between life and imminent death for a patient. Allergens and poisons have the same possible routes of entry into the body—ingestion, injection, absorption, and inhalation. A patient suspected of having an allergic reaction is treated with 100% oxygen, and you may be allowed to administer epinephrine. Patients who have ingested poisons are generally treated with activated charcoal. Those who have received poisons through injection may be treated with antitoxins. Poisoning through absorption is treated based on the patient's signs and symptoms. Patients who have inhaled poisons are generally treated with high-flow oxygen.

What's New

Although you were taught about allergic reactions and poisoning in your EMT-I course, the new National EMS Education Standards suggest that AEMTs should have a more in-depth knowledge of the ways in which allergens and poisons affect the body. The differences between an allergic reaction and anaphylaxis are discussed, and the specific poisons you may encounter in your patients are described.

▌Introduction

Every year, at least 1,500 Americans die of acute allergic reactions. As much as 15% of the US population is at risk for experiencing an anaphylactic reaction, which can be fatal for approximately 1% of the people exposed. On an almost daily basis, AEMTs also treat patients who have taken drugs of abuse, including alcohol. You will probably encounter these patients frequently.

▌Anatomy and Physiology of the Immune System

The *immune system* protects the human body from substances and organisms that are considered foreign to the body. Given the right person and the right circumstances, almost any substance can trigger the body's immune system and cause an allergic reaction: animal bites, food, latex gloves, and even semen. The most common *allergens*, however, fall into the following general categories:

- Insect bites and stings
- Medications
- Plants
- Foods
- Chemicals

Allergens enter the body through oral ingestion, injection or envenomation, inhalation, or topical absorption.

> **Immune system** The system that protects the body from foreign substances.
> **Allergen** A substance that causes an allergic reaction; also referred to as an antigen.

When a foreign substance invades, the body goes on alert and initiates a series of responses. The first encounter with the foreign substance begins the primary response and mainly involves the white blood cells, the cells that fight infection in the body. Cells immediately greet, confront, and engulf the invaders to determine whether they are allowed in the body. These cells record one or two of the proteins on the surface of the invading substance and then design specific proteins, called antibodies, to match each substance. Antibodies are intended to match up with the antigen—the invader—and inactivate it.

Through the primary response, the body develops sensitivity, or the ability to recognize the foreigner the next time it is encountered. The body records enough details to assist in future identification of the substance and production of antibodies to perfectly fit the invading antigen. These details are distributed by placing the specific antibodies on two types of cells: basophils and mast cells. Basophils are stationed in specific sites within the tissues. Mast cells are on patrol through the connective tissues, bronchi, gastrointestinal mucosa, and other vulnerable border areas that act as barriers to foreign invaders.

The basophils and mast cells produce the body's **chemical mediators**. These cells release chemical mediators into the bloodstream, causing degranulation—the process in which granules filled with a host of powerful substances burst, releasing their contents to fight the invading forces of antigens. As long as the body is not invaded by one of the previously identified foreign substances, the granules are kept encapsulated in their protective walls and remain inactive. If an antigen invades the body and combines with one of the antibodies, however, the granules are ejected from the mast cells and detonated. The chemical mediators are then released into the surrounding tissue and the bloodstream FIGURE 16-1 .

The chemical mediators launch and maintain the immune response. They summon more white blood cells to the area to battle the invading force. They also increase the blood flow to the area under attack by dilating the blood vessels and increasing capillary permeability. These actions are useful when a small invasion occurs to a limited area but can be extremely dangerous when they spread throughout the body. Chemical mediators cause the local effects of an allergic reaction seen in the body. When they have systemic effects, the chemical mediators cause the signs and symptoms of anaphylactic reactions.

> **Chemical mediators** Chemicals that work to cause the immune or allergic response, for example, histamines.

Pathophysiology of the Immune System

Contrary to what many people might think, an *allergic reaction*, an exaggerated immune response to any substance, is not caused directly by an outside stimulus, such as a bite or sting. Rather, it is a reaction by the body's immune system, which releases chemicals to combat the stimulus. An allergic reaction may be mild and localized—the body limits its response to a specific area after being exposed to a foreign substance, involving only hives, itching, or tenderness. The swelling around an insect bite would be an example. Alternately, the reaction may be anaphylactic (severe and systemic), resulting in shock and respiratory failure. An allergic reaction occurs following contact with a specific allergen to which the patient has been previously exposed and sensitized. The patient may also experience hypersensitivity, an abnormal sensitivity in which there is an exaggerated response by the body to the stimulus or antigen.

When the invading substance enters the body, the mast cells recognize it as potentially harmful and begin releasing chemical mediators. Histamines, one of the primary chemical weapons, cause the blood vessels in the local area to dilate and the capillaries to leak. Leukotrienes, which are even more powerful, are released and cause additional dilation and leaking. White blood cells are called to the area to help engulf and destroy the enemy, and platelets begin to collect (aggregate) and clump together. The release of histamines and leukotrienes may result in any or all of the following:

- Urticaria
- Pruritis
- Vasodilation
- Hypotension
- Hypoperfusion
- Laryngospasm
- Bronchospasm
- Narrowing of the airway
- Fluid in the airway
- Myocardial irritability
- Coronary artery constriction
- Increased vascular permeability
- Abdominal cramping, bloating, and diarrhea
- Tachycardia
- Flushing
- Headache, dizziness, confusion, and anxiety

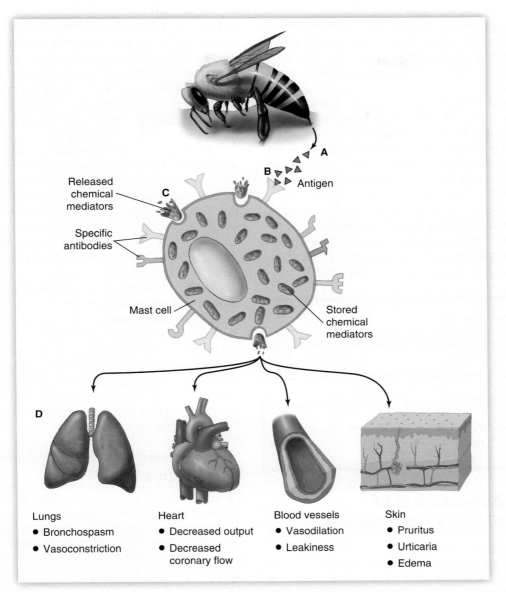

FIGURE 16-1 The sequence of events in anaphylaxis. **A.** The antigen is introduced into the body. **B.** The antigen-antibody reaction at the surface of a mast cell. **C.** Release of mast cell chemical mediators. **D.** Chemical mediators exert their effects on end organs.

- Stridor
- Runny, itchy nose
- Swollen eyes
- Angioedema
- Dyspnea

Anaphylaxis is an extreme allergic reaction that is not always life threatening, but it typically involves multiple organ systems. In severe cases, anaphylaxis can rapidly result in death. Two of the most common signs of anaphylaxis are wheezing, a high-pitched, whistling breath sound resulting from bronchospasm and typically heard on expiration, and widespread urticaria, or hives. Urticaria consists of small areas of generalized itching or burning that appear as multiple, small, raised areas on the skin.

> *Allergic reaction* The body's exaggerated immune response to an internal or surface antigen.
>
> *Anaphylaxis* An extreme, possibly life-threatening systemic allergic reaction that may include shock and respiratory failure.

The most common complaints are usually respiratory symptoms, which often present as shortness of breath or dyspnea and tightness of the throat and chest. You may also note stridor and/or hoarseness. The signs and symptoms are often caused by upper airway swelling in the laryngeal and epiglottic areas. Affected patients may complain of a lump in the throat. The lower airway is often involved as well. Bronchoconstriction and increased airway secretions may result in wheezes and crackles. It is not uncommon for the patient to cough or sneeze as the body tries to clear the airway. These symptoms may progress slowly or alarmingly fast. You may have only 1 to 3 minutes to halt this rapid, life-threatening process.

Cardiovascular symptoms are serious complications of anaphylaxis, as are gastrointestinal symptoms such as abdominal cramping, nausea, bloating, vomiting, abdominal distention, and profuse, watery diarrhea. Patients may also present with central nervous system (CNS) symptoms such as headache, dizziness, confusion, and anxiety in response to decreased cerebral perfusion and hypoxia.

Anaphylaxis may affect two or more body systems, so the picture can be confusing at times. You will need to use your assessment skills to identify the potential for anaphylaxis and take aggressive action to manage the patient and stop the anaphylactic process as rapidly as possible.

Transition Tip

Think of a patient with anaphylaxis as experiencing three types of shock:

1. Cardiogenic shock due to decreased cardiac output
2. Hypovolemic shock due to fluids leaking into the tissues
3. Neurogenic shock due to inability of the blood vessels to constrict

---

Patient Assessment of Immunologic Emergencies

Scene Size-up

Ensure that the scene is safe and follow standard precautions. The patient's environment or the activity he or she was performing may indicate the source of the reaction, such as a sting or bite from an insect, a food allergy at a restaurant, or a new medication regimen. Note that many anaphylactic reactions occur in the summer. Therefore, an anaphylactic reaction can present in conjunction with signs and symptoms of heat emergencies.

Although your report from dispatch may be for a patient with an allergic reaction, keep in mind the possibility that trauma may have occurred because of a medical incident. Determine the mechanism of injury and/or nature of illness. Look for bee stingers or contact with chemicals and other indications of a reaction. Do not let your guard down, even on what appears to be a routine call.

Primary Assessment

Next, perform your primary assessment. A patient may have bite or sting marks that may accompany other signs and symptoms of an allergic reaction. Allergic symptoms are almost as varied as the allergens themselves. Your assessment

of a patient experiencing an allergic reaction should include evaluations of the level of consciousness, the respiratory system, the circulatory system, mental status, and the skin. As mentioned earlier, allergic reactions can range from local to systemic. They can be categorized as mild, moderate, or severe. Mild reactions usually have only cutaneous involvement. **TABLE 16-1** compares signs and symptoms of allergic reactions with those of anaphylaxis.

You may have only a few minutes to assess the airway and provide lifesaving measures; however, not all allergic reactions are anaphylactic reactions. Work quickly to assess the patient to determine the severity of the symptoms. Position a responsive patient in a tripod position leaning forward. This position will help to facilitate air entry into the lungs and may help the patient to relax. Quickly listen to the lungs on each side of the chest. If wheezing or a "silent chest" is heard, the lower airways are closing, preventing oxygen from entering the circulatory system. Do not hesitate to initiate high-flow oxygen therapy. You may have to assist with ventilations for a patient in severe respiratory distress with a severe allergic reaction. Assisted ventilation can be done in a semiresponsive or an unresponsive patient. The positive-pressure ventilations you provide will force air through the swelling in the throat and into the lungs while you are waiting for more definitive treatment. In severe situations such as these, the definitive care needed is an injection of epinephrine.

Transition Tip

In some areas you may be allowed to administer or assist the patient with epinephrine. Whether naturally occurring in the body (endogenous) or made by a drug manufacturer, epinephrine works rapidly to raise the blood pressure by constricting the blood vessels and increasing the strength of cardiac contractions. Epinephrine also dilates the bronchioles, thus improving the patient's breathing. To review the steps of epinephrine administration, refer to your EMT-I textbook.

Palpating a radial pulse will help you to identify how the circulatory system is responding to the reaction. If the patient is unresponsive and pulseless, begin basic life support measures or use an automated external defibrillator if necessary. Assess for a rapid pulse rate; pale, cool, cyanotic or moist skin; and delayed capillary refill times that indicate hypoperfusion. Your initial treatment for shock should include oxygen, placing the patient in the position dictated by local protocol for shock patients, and maintaining normal body temperature. The definitive treatment for anaphylactic shock is epinephrine. Trauma is unlikely with allergic reactions, but if trauma has occurred, bandage all bleeding sites, and take spinal precautions when appropriate.

Always provide prompt transport for any patient who may be having an allergic reaction. Take with you all

Table 16-1
Common Signs and Symptoms of Allergic Reactions and Anaphylaxis*

	Allergic Reaction	Anaphylaxis
Respiratory system	<ul><li>Sneezing or an itchy, runny nose (initially)</li><li>Tightness in the chest or throat</li><li>Irritating, persistent, dry cough</li><li>Hoarseness</li><li>Rapid, labored, or noisy respirations</li><li>Wheezing, stridor, or both</li></ul>	<ul><li>Sneezing</li><li>Tightness in the chest or throat</li><li>Coughing</li><li>Stridor</li><li>Hoarseness</li><li>Lump in throat</li><li>Dyspnea</li><li>Wheezes</li><li>Crackles</li></ul>
Circulatory/cardiovascular system	<ul><li>Increase in pulse rate (initially)</li><li>Decrease in blood pressure</li><li>Pale skin and dizziness</li></ul>	<ul><li>Tachycardia</li><li>Hypotension (can be profound)</li><li>Arrhythmias</li></ul>
Skin	<ul><li>Flushing, itching, or burning skin</li><li>Hives (urticaria)</li><li>Swelling, especially of the face, neck, hands, feet, and tongue</li><li>Swelling and cyanosis or pallor around the lips</li><li>Warm, tingling feeling in the face, mouth, chest, feet, and hands</li></ul>	<ul><li>Flushed</li><li>Itching (pruritis)</li><li>Hives (urticaria)</li><li>Swollen, red eyes</li><li>Swelling of the face, neck, hands, feet, and tongue</li></ul>
Other findings	<ul><li>Anxiety; a sense of impending doom</li><li>Headache</li><li>Decreasing mental status</li><li>Abdominal cramps</li><li>Itchy, watery eyes</li></ul>	<ul><li>Anxiety and restlessness</li><li>Sense of impending doom</li><li>Headache</li><li>Altered mental status</li><li>Dizziness</li><li>Confusion</li><li>Loss of consciousness and coma</li></ul>

*Signs and symptoms of anaphylaxis include the signs and symptoms of allergic reactions, plus additional signs and symptoms, and anaphylaxis is a systemic reaction, whereas allergic reactions are usually mild and localized.

medications and auto-injectors the patient has at the time. Make your transport decision based on findings in the primary assessment. If the patient has signs of respiratory distress or shock, treat those conditions and transport. If the patient is calm and has no signs of respiratory distress or shock after contact with a substance that causes an allergic reaction, continue with the assessment.

History Taking

The patient history will help to identify problems specific to the allergic reaction. Identify any associated signs and symptoms such as wheezing or a rash. Identify the pertinent negatives, such as lack of nausea or vomiting or no chest pain.

When assessing the patient with an allergic reaction, determine the following:

- Is the patient able to speak?
- Is the patient restless or agitated?

- What is the level of consciousness using the AVPU scale (**A**lert; responsive to **V**erbal stimuli; responsive to **P**ainful stimuli; **U**nresponsive)? Has the patient experienced any confusion?
- Is there any hoarseness, stridor, or wheezing?
- What is the rate and quality of the patient's breathing? What is the degree of respiratory distress? Remember that these findings are the most troubling because a patient's condition can rapidly deteriorate from respiratory distress to arrest.
- Does the patient have adequate tidal volume?
- Is there any accessory muscle use or decrease in breath sounds?
- What is the patient's skin color, condition, and temperature?
- Is there any redness, rashes, itching, hives, pallor, bite or sting marks, or edema noted?
- Are the baseline vital signs abnormal (for example, hypotension or tachycardia)?

Ask whether the patient has a history of allergies or asthma, what the patient was exposed to, when the previous exposure occurred, how the patient was exposed, and whether he or she was hospitalized for that exposure. Determine the onset of symptoms, what the effects of the exposure have been, and how they have progressed. A severe reaction may occur at the second exposure to an antigen, so the patient might not know about the allergy.

Ask the patient what he or she last ate. This information may help you determine the cause of the reaction. For example, peanuts, chocolate, and shellfish can be potent allergens. Also ask what the patient was doing or what he or she was exposed to before the onset of symptoms. This information may be key to effective treatment.

In some cases, you may not be able to identify the offending antigen. When in doubt, in the presence of a severe reaction, intervention takes precedence over identifying the antigen. To identify where you are in the process, ask when the symptoms began. Because the airway is a major concern, ask about feelings of dyspnea.

You should also determine whether the patient or emergency medical responders have administered any treatment before your arrival. This treatment may include using an epinephrine auto-injector, taking an antihistamine such as chlorpheniramine (Chlor-Trimeton) or diphenhydramine (Benadryl), or using an inhaler that contains a bronchodilator (such as albuterol or metaproterenol) or aerosolized epinephrine (such as Primatene Mist or racemic epinephrine).

Secondary Assessment

The secondary assessment may help direct treatment. As in all emergencies, your assessment of a patient experiencing an allergic reaction should include a systematic head-to-toe or focused assessment to determine hidden trauma or other unrelated medical problems. Perform evaluations of the respiratory system. Thoroughly assess breathing, including increased work of breathing, use of accessory muscles, head bobbing, tripod positioning, nostril flaring, and grunting. Carefully auscultate the chest. Assess the circulatory system. Remember, the presence of hypoperfusion (shock) or respiratory distress indicates that the patient is having a severe enough allergic reaction that death can result.

Carefully assess the skin for swelling, rash, hives, and signs of the source of the reaction: bite, sting, or contact marks. A rapidly spreading rash can be concerning because it may indicate a systemic reaction. Red, hot skin may also indicate a systemic reaction as the blood vessels lose their ability to constrict and blood moves to the extremities. If this reaction continues, the body will have difficulty supplying blood and oxygen to the vital organs, and one of the first signs will be altered mental status as the organs are deprived of oxygen and glucose.

Assess baseline vital signs, including pulse, respirations, blood pressure, skin, pupils, and oxygen saturation. Rapid, labored breathing indicates possible airway obstruction. Rapid respiratory and pulse rates may indicate respiratory

distress or systemic shock. Fast pulse rates and hypotension are ominous signs, indicating systemic vascular collapse and shock. Skin signs may be an unreliable indicator of hypoperfusion because of rashes and swelling.

Monitoring by pulse oximetry may alert you to low oxygen saturation, which will assist in identifying the degree of respiratory distress. However, it is important to remember that pulse oximetry is just another tool in your toolbox. Factors such as decreased circulation and exposure to carbon monoxide can alter pulse oximetry readings. The decision to administer oxygen to a patient experiencing an allergic reaction should be based on a careful assessment of the patient's airway, and overall level of distress, not solely on the pulse oximetry readings. Never withhold oxygen from a patient who appears to be in distress regardless of pulse oximetry values.

Reassessment

Reassessment is conducted typically en route to the emergency department. A patient experiencing a suspected allergic reaction should be monitored with vigilance because deterioration of the patient's condition can be rapid and fatal. Special attention should be given to any signs of airway compromise, including increasing work of breathing, stridor, and wheezing. The patient's anxiety level should be monitored because increased anxiety is a good indication that the reaction may be progressing. Also, watch the skin for signs of shock, including pallor and diaphoresis, as well as for flushing because of vascular collapse. Serial vital signs are important indicators when evaluating your patient's status. Any increase in the respiratory or pulse rate or decrease in blood pressure should be noted. Finally, reassess the chief complaint.

Some allergic reactions will produce severe signs and symptoms in a matter of minutes and threaten the patient's life. Other allergic reactions have a slower onset and cause less severe distress. Epinephrine and ventilatory support are required for severe reactions. Milder reactions, without respiratory or cardiovascular distress, may require only supportive care, such as oxygen and placing the patient in a position of comfort. In either situation, the patient should be transported to a medical facility for further evaluation. Be complete in your documentation of the care provided, including not only assessment findings and treatment, but also the patient's response to your treatment.

Emergency Care of Allergic Reactions

Not all signs and symptoms are present in every allergic reaction. Maintain a high index of suspicion if a reaction has occurred previously and the patient has been exposed to the same substance. If the patient appears to be having an allergic reaction, perform a primary assessment and give 100% oxygen by nonrebreathing mask or assist ventilation with a bag-mask device if the patient is breathing inadequately. Place the patient in an upright position to assist with breathing, and protect the airway. If the patient cannot sit up, have suction readily available to maintain a clear airway. Also, maintain a high index of suspicion for developing airway occlusion because of swelling or edema. Consider calling early for advanced life support (ALS) backup.

Remove the allergen if possible. Find out what interventions have been completed before your arrival. Determine whether the patient has any prescribed, preloaded medications for allergic reactions (such as an epinephrine auto-injector), and then inform medical control of the patient's condition. Follow local protocols if epinephrine auto-injectors (such as EpiPens) are carried on your unit. If necessary, be prepared to use standard airway procedures and positive-pressure ventilation.

If the patient appears to be having a severe allergic (or anaphylactic) reaction, you should begin basic life support measures at once and provide prompt transport to the hospital. In addition to providing oxygen, you should be prepared to maintain the patient's airway or initiate cardiopulmonary resuscitation (CPR) and administer epinephrine. If necessary, treat for shock by placing the patient in the position dictated by local protocol for shock patients, maintain body heat with a blanket, and initiate intravenous (IV) therapy. Placing ice over the injury site has been thought to slow absorption of the toxin and diminish swelling, but ice packs placed directly on the skin may freeze it and cause tissue and cellular damage. Like any other attempt to reduce swelling with ice, you should be careful not to overdo the icing. However, it is contraindicated to place ice over a site of an envenomation, because constricting the vessels can push the venom into central circulation.

Types of Toxicologic Emergencies

Toxicology is the study of toxic or poisonous substances. A *poison* is any substance whose chemical action can damage body structures or impair body function. It can be introduced into the body through a variety of means. Poisons act by changing the normal metabolism of cells or by actually destroying them. Poisoning can be acute, as in an overdose of heroin, or chronic, as with years of alcohol or other substance abuse. *Substance abuse* is the misuse of any substance to produce a desired effect (eg, cocaine intoxication). A common complication of substance abuse is *overdose*, which occurs when a patient takes a toxic dose of a drug.

Toxicology The study of toxic or poisonous substances.
Poison A substance whose chemical action could damage structures or impair function when introduced into the body.
Substance abuse The misuse of any substance to produce some desired effect.
Overdose An excessive quantity of a drug that, when taken or administered, can have toxic or lethal consequences.

Excessive doses can turn even an otherwise helpful remedy into a poison. Consider a common substance such as aspirin. When taken in recommended doses, it is a safe and effective analgesic. Too much aspirin, however, can result in death.

Childhood poisonings are common, especially in younger children who may put anything into their mouths, such as colorful berries on a house or garden plant that draw their attention. A parent's prescription medication may be mistaken for candy.

Nature is fraught with toxicologic perils. For example, wild mushrooms, once in the body, can produce a wide spectrum of reactions—from nausea to death.

The workplace also harbors its share of toxic hazards. Unfortunately, some of these hazards are not identified until after the exposure has occurred. For example, cancer developed later in life in countless people who worked with polychlorinated biphenyls, or PCBs, on a daily basis in the electric energy field. Similarly, asbestosis developed in thousands of people after prolonged workplace exposure.

Unintentional toxicologic emergencies can also occur from simple neglect or oversight. For example, a geriatric person with diabetes, possibly combined with early onset dementia or Alzheimer disease, may take his or her insulin in the morning and later cannot remember whether the dose was taken and takes another dose. The result: a call to 9-1-1 for an unresponsive person in need of assistance.

Biologic warfare has drawn increasing attention in recent years owing to the heightened awareness of bioterrorism, but intentional poisoning or overdose may also commonly occur during more intimate crimes. In recent years, "date rape" drugs such as flunitrazepam (Rohypnol) have been used to facilitate sexual assault. Chloral hydrate (knockout drops) has been used to commit assault for decades, and pharmacologic agents are used in homicides as well.

Pathophysiology: Routes of Absorption

Poisoning by Ingestion

Medications around the home and household chemicals (such as cleaning agents) are the most common sources of poisoning by ingestion. Ingested poisons may produce immediate damage to tissues, or their toxic effects may be delayed for several hours. Ingestions of a caustic substance (that is, a strong acid or alkali) cause immediate damage. By contrast, some poisons must be absorbed into the bloodstream before they can produce toxic effects.

Assessment clues pointing toward ingestion can be as obvious as a plant with partially chewed leaves or a section of plant with berries missing. Stained fingers, lips, or tongue are also indicators of ingestion. Any patient complaining of a sudden onset of stomach cramps with or without nausea, vomiting, or diarrhea may have an ingestion-related problem. Empty pill bottles are another obvious clue, as is the date on which the prescription was filled. The bottle for a prescription filled 6 months ago is not likely to be full today; an empty bottle for a prescription filled yesterday is a far more ominous sign.

A toxin that enters the body by the oral route generally provides a more forgiving time frame for treatment. Little absorption occurs in the stomach; indeed, the ingested substance may stay there for a variable period, with the majority of absorption actually taking place in the small intestine. As a consequence, much of the management of poisoning by ingestion aims to remove or neutralize the poison before it gains access to the intestines.

In the past, syrup of ipecac was used to induce vomiting, but today it is recommended in only a few situations in which the risk of losing consciousness is clearly low. Today, many EMS systems allow you to carry activated charcoal on the unit. Activated charcoal comes as a suspension that binds to the poison in the stomach and carries it out of the system. Therefore, it is more effective and safer than syrup of ipecac.

> ### Transition Tip
> Always consult medical control before treating a poison victim.

Poisoning by Inhalation

Home medications and household chemical products (such as bleach and cleaning agents) are responsible for the most common types of inhalation emergencies. A person can be poisoned by inhalation only if the poison is present in the surrounding atmosphere. That fact has important implications. First, so long as the patient remains in the toxic environment, he or she will keep inhaling the poison—and so will you. Therefore, you should not enter that environment; instead, call for additional resources with specialized protective equipment. Second, when poisoning occurs because of a toxic environment, you are likely to encounter more than one patient at the emergency scene.

> ### Transition Tip
> Never pull a shirt over the head of a patient who may have been exposed to a toxin. Doing so may introduce the toxin into the eyes, nose, or mouth of the patient. Instead, unbutton or cut the shirt to remove it. Pulling clothing over a patient's head could also introduce it into the air, causing a hazard for the AEMT.

When you are dealing with an inhalation emergency, the first general management consideration is that of scene safety. Specialty personnel will likely need to access the

patient, and the patient may need to be decontaminated after removal from the toxic environment. The patient's clothing should be removed in this process because it may contain trapped gases that can be released, exposing you to the toxin. You cannot administer emergency care until this step has been completed and there is no danger of the poison contaminating you.

Inhaled toxins produce a wide range of signs and symptoms, many of which are unique to the toxin involved. The patient may complain of burning eyes, sore throat, cough, chest pain, hoarseness, wheezing, respiratory distress, dizziness, confusion, headache, or stridor in severe cases. The patient may also experience seizures or an altered mental status.

> ### Transition Tip
> Distraught people often use inhaled poisons to commit suicide. A common technique is for the patient to sit inside a vehicle with the engine running in an enclosed garage. The exhaust fumes from the vehicle contain high levels of carbon monoxide that will cause the patient to lose consciousness and eventually stop breathing.
>
> A recent variation on the use of automobiles for suicide involves people using a tightly sealed vehicle as a type of gas chamber. These people mix fairly common household chemicals inside the vehicle to produce hydrogen sulfide gas, which is quickly fatal. When responders approach the vehicle and open the door, they may be overcome by the gas as well. If you suspect this type of scenario has taken place, contact hazardous materials responders and have them remove the victim.

Poisoning by Injection

Poisoning by injection is usually the result of drug abuse, such as use of heroin or cocaine. Injection of poisons can also occur via insect or animal bites.

Poisoning by injection may result in patients having a multitude of presentations, with potential signs and symptoms including excitability, weakness, dizziness, fever, chills, and unresponsiveness.

In general, injected poisons are impossible to dilute or remove because they are usually absorbed quickly into the body or cause intense local tissue destruction. If you suspect that rapid absorption has occurred, monitor the patient's airway, provide high-flow oxygen, and be alert for nausea and vomiting. Remove rings, watches, and bracelets from areas around the injection site in case swelling occurs. Prompt transport to the emergency department is essential. Transport all suspicious containers, bottles, and labels with the patient.

Poisoning by Absorption

Some poisons gain access to the body by being absorbed through the skin. Of the poisonings that occur by absorption, those caused by pesticides such as organophosphates and similar substances are often the most serious.

Many corrosive substances have the potential to damage the skin, mucous membranes, or eyes, causing chemical burns, telltale rashes, or lesions. Notably, acids, alkalis, and some petroleum (hydrocarbon) products are very destructive. Other substances, such as poison ivy or poison oak, may cause an itchy rash without being dangerous to the patient's health. Others are absorbed into the bloodstream through the skin and have systemic effects, just like medications or drugs taken via the oral or injectable route. As such, it is important to distinguish between contact burns and contact absorption.

Signs and symptoms of absorbed poisoning include the following:

- History of exposure
- Liquid or powder on the patient's skin
- Burns, itching, irritation, or redness of the skin in light-skinned people
- Odors of the substance

> **Transition Tip**
>
> Absorption of toxic substances through the skin is a common problem in agriculture and manufacturing. Most solvents and "cides"—such as insecticides, herbicides, and pesticides—are toxic and can be readily absorbed through the skin.

Pathophysiology of Specific Poisons

Over time, a person who routinely misuses a substance may need increasing amounts of it to achieve the same result—a phenomenon known as developing a tolerance to the substance. A person with an *addiction* has an overwhelming desire or need to continue using a substance, at whatever cost, with a tendency to increase the dose. Almost any substance can be abused. The list of potential candidates for abuse includes not only the classic drugs of abuse, such as cocaine, but laxatives, nasal decongestants, vitamins, and food as well.

> *Addiction* A state of overwhelming obsession or physical need to continue the use of a drug or agent.

Alcohol

The most commonly abused drug in the United States is alcohol. It affects people from all walks of life and kills more than 200,000 people each year. More than 40% of all traffic fatalities or injuries, 67% of murders, and 33% of suicides in the United States are related to alcohol. Alcoholism is one

of the greatest health problems on a national scale, along with heart disease, cancer, and stroke.

> **Transition Tip**
>
> The importance of safety awareness and standard precautions when caring for victims of drug abuse cannot be stressed strongly enough. Known drug abusers have a fairly high incidence of serious and undiagnosed infections, including human immunodeficiency virus (HIV) and hepatitis. These patients, when intoxicated, may bite, spit, hit, or otherwise injure you, causing you to come into contact with their blood and other body fluids. Always wear appropriate protective equipment when faced with a scenario involving drug abuse.
>
> A calm, professional approach on your part can defuse frightening situations, but you must always keep your safety and that of your team uppermost in mind. Expect the unexpected. Remember—the drug user, not the drug, typically poses the greatest threat. This is especially true when dealing with a patient who is suffering from a narcotic overdose. When paramedics administer a narcotic antagonist (Narcan), the effect of the drug of abuse is negated, and the patient who previously demonstrated altered consciousness or loss of consciousness will awaken in a sudden and fierce manner. Such patients are often violent and difficult to control. In addition, they are usually angry at EMS personnel for taking away the "high" they spent a lot of money to get. Use extreme caution in these situations.

In many states, a person with a blood alcohol content (BAC) of 0.08% is considered legally under the influence. Alcoholics, however, may have a BAC as high as 0.40%, meaning that 40% of the patient's circulating blood is alcohol. This high concentration has a significant effect on the body's systems and can even prove lethal.

Alcohol abuse can result in many long-term effects on health, because it alters the functioning of all body systems. The most commonly noted effects consist of damage to the liver. In fact, an estimated 90% of heavy drinkers have hepatitis, and 10% to 20% of alcoholics develop cirrhosis. Other long-term effects of alcohol abuse include an increased incidence of pancreatitis, development of erosive gastritis, and an increased risk for breast and colorectal cancer. The long-term abuse of alcohol also leads to atrophy of the cerebrum, possibly resulting in permanently reduced mental function. Although alcohol is often seen as a substance to promote sexual activity, it actually decreases the ability to respond to sexual stimulation, and its long-term use can lead to impotence and sterility.

Alcohol is a powerful CNS depressant. It is both a sedative (it decreases activity and excitement) and a hypnotic (it induces sleep). In general, alcohol dulls the sense of awareness, slows reflexes, and reduces reaction time. It impairs the capacity to think and function rationally, and it may also cause aggressive and inappropriate behavior and lack of coordination. Of course, a person who appears intoxicated may have other medical problems as well. Look for signs of head trauma, toxic reactions, or uncontrolled diabetes. Severe acute alcohol ingestion may cause hypoglycemia, which may contribute to these symptoms. At the very least, assume that all intoxicated patients are experiencing a drug overdose and require a thorough examination by a physician. In most states, patients under the influence of drugs or alcohol cannot legally refuse transport. Because their mental status is altered, they cannot make such a refusal, and the law of implied consent takes over.

The effects of many other drugs increase when they are used in combination with alcohol. Even over-the-counter (OTC) medications, including antihistamines and diet medications, can cause serious problems when taken in conjunction with alcohol.

If an intoxicated patient exhibits signs of serious CNS depression, you must provide respiratory support. This may be difficult, however, because depression of the respiratory system can also cause emesis. The vomiting may be very forceful or even bloody because large amounts of alcohol irritate the stomach. Internal bleeding should also be considered if the patient appears to be in shock (hypoperfusion)—blood might not clot effectively in a patient who has a prolonged history of alcohol abuse.

A patient in alcohol withdrawal may experience frightening hallucinations, or delirium tremens (DTs). Such a condition may develop when a patient no longer has his or her daily source of alcohol. Alcoholic hallucinations tend to come and go, and a patient with an otherwise fairly clear mental state may see fantastic shapes or figures or hear odd voices. Such auditory and visual hallucinations often precede DTs, which are a much more severe complication.

Approximately 1 to 7 days after a person stops drinking or when alcohol consumption levels are decreased suddenly, DTs may develop. Patients may experience one or more of the following signs and symptoms:

- Agitation and restlessness
- Fever
- Sweating
- Tremors
- Confusion and/or disorientation
- Delusions and/or hallucinations
- Seizures

With a patient who is experiencing alcohol withdrawal, provide prompt transport after completing the assessment and giving necessary care. A person experiencing hallucinations or DTs is extremely ill. Complete an assessment and provide care based on signs and symptoms. Should seizures develop, treat them as you would any other seizure. The patient should not be restrained, although you must protect him or her from self-injury. Give the patient oxygen and be prepared for vomiting. Hypovolemia may develop because of sweating, fluid loss, insufficient fluid

intake, or vomiting associated with DTs. If signs of hypovolemic shock develop, consider elevating the patient's feet slightly, clear the airway, and turn the patient's head to one side to minimize the chance of aspiration during transport.

Patients in alcohol withdrawal may not respond appropriately to suggestions or conversation, and they are often confused and frightened. For this reason, your approach should be calm and relaxed. Reassure the patient and provide emotional support. Never underestimate the significance of DTs. Untreated, they are associated with a mortality of approximately 50%.

Narcotics, Opiates, and Opioids

A narcotic is a drug that produces sleep or altered mental status. Historically, narcotics have been classified into two major divisions: opiates and opioids. The term opiate is used to describe natural drugs derived from opium (that is, from poppy juice); the term opioid refers to non–opium-derived synthetics. This text uses the term *opioids* to describe licit therapeutic agents and illicit substances in this group. Abuse of narcotics remains one of the most common causes of overdose deaths reported to poison centers.

Narcotic agents include morphine, codeine, heroin, fentanyl, oxycodone, meperidine, propoxyphene, and dextromethorphan. Although these drugs share certain commonalities, they exhibit highly diverse effects and vary widely in their potency. Opioids are used primarily in clinical medicine for analgesia, whereas the illicit drug heroin is abused for the unique euphoria it produces.

Opioids produce their major effects on the CNS by binding with receptor sites in the brain and other tissues. Opioids are readily absorbed from the GI tract but can also be absorbed from the nasal mucosa (when snorted) or from the lungs (opium smoking). When taken orally, the effects of these drugs are lessened compared with their effects when given parentally. When heroin passes through the liver, it is metabolized into acetyl morphine, which continues to exert narcotic effects that may outlast the effects of naloxone (a narcotic antagonist). An AEMT who does not understand this concept can be fooled into thinking that a dose of naloxone has permanently reversed the effects of the heroin, only to have the patient lapse into unresponsiveness 15 or 20 minutes later.

Morphine is a commonly used analgesic in the prehospital setting and is a potent vasodilator. When given to young adults, its half-life is roughly 2 to 3 hours, but it typically takes longer to metabolize in older adults.

The classic presentation of opioid use features euphoria, hypotension, respiratory depression, and pinpoint pupils. Depending on the particular agent, nausea, vomiting, and constipation may occur as well. Allergic phenomena may also occur with opioid use, albeit rarely. With increased doses, coma, seizures (usually secondary to hypoxia), and cardiac arrest (usually secondary to respiratory arrest) can occur.

Morphine and heroin produce an impressive dreamlike state. Shortly after injecting heroin, a user will appear to pass out. However, the user is typically quite lucid and remains aware of what is being done or said.

Because of the CNS depressant effects, patient management initially focuses on establishing and maintaining a patent airway and providing adequate ventilation. A patient who has overdosed on opioids is almost always hypoventilating, sometimes breathing as few as 4 or 5 breaths/min, and is consequently hypoxic and hypercarbic. Place an oropharyngeal airway and provide bag-mask ventilation with 15 L/min of supplemental oxygen.

Next, establish IV access and administer 0.4 to 2 mg of naloxone. For street heroin, which can range in purity from 5% to 30%, as little as 0.4 mg of naloxone may bring a patient back to consciousness before you can remove the syringe from the injection port. This abrupt reversal of an intended high may result in a violent patient. The best approach is to draw up 2 mg of naloxone in a 10-mL syringe and fill the rest of the syringe with normal saline. Administer the naloxone just to the point that the patient's respirations improve, rather than waking the patient up completely.

If the patient doesn't respond to naloxone, it is possible that the person has a "mixed-bag overdose"—that is, the patient may have taken multiple drugs, some of which are not opioids and will therefore not respond to naloxone. Alternatively, the coma may be from another source altogether, such as a head injury. In such a scenario, insert an advanced airway (for example, endotracheal tube or laryngeal mask airway), provide other care as needed, and transport the patient to an appropriate facility.

When caring for a patient who has overdosed on opiates, it is important to remember that the patient may have other underlying chronic illnesses or conditions including hepatitis, human immunodeficiency virus/acquired immunodeficiency syndrome, malnutrition, or sepsis. Medications taken for any of these conditions may interact with the opioid, creating a myriad of signs and symptoms.

Elderly patients often take multiple medications for pain caused by arthritis, degenerative diseases, and other conditions. For those patients who have chronic pain and regularly take large doses of narcotics, dependency may become a big problem. Using a narcotic antagonist in this patient may cause withdrawal and result in seizures or other problems. Monitor the patient closely and provide prompt transport to the closest appropriate facility.

Stimulants

A stimulant is an agent that produces an excited state. Few drugs compare with stimulants in potential for abuse—particularly cocaine, amphetamines, and methamphetamine. A first-time user may become an addict to one of these substances within just a few days. If the person decides to quit using the stimulant, it is unlikely that the abstinence will be successful. The stimulants amphetamine and methamphetamine ("ice") are commonly taken by mouth, although drug abusers may take them by injection. These drugs are typically taken to make the user feel good, improve task performance, suppress appetite, or prevent sleepiness. However, they may just as easily produce irritability, anxiety, lack of concentration, or seizures.

Other widely used stimulants include phentermine hydrochloride, an appetite suppressant, and amphetamine sulfate (Benzedrine), taken for weight control, narcolepsy, and chronic fatigue syndrome. Caffeine, theophylline, and phenylpropanolamine (a nasal decongestant) are all mild stimulants. So-called designer drugs, such as ecstasy and Eve, are also frequently abused in certain areas of the United States.

Stimulant drugs are frequently called "uppers" **TABLE 16-2**. A person using one of these agents may display disorganized behavior, restlessness, and sometimes anxiety or great fear. Paranoia and delusions are common with abuse.

Cocaine (also called coke, crack, crystal, snow, freebase, rock, gold dust, blow, and lady) may be taken in a number of different ways. Classically, it is inhaled into the nose and absorbed through the nasal mucosa, damaging tissue, causing nosebleeds, and ultimately destroying the nasal septum. It can also be injected intravenously or subcutaneously (skin-popping). Cocaine can be absorbed through all mucous membranes and even across the skin. In any form, the immediate effects of a given dose last less than an hour.

Table 16-2 Street Names for Stimulants

Street Name	Drug Name
Adam	3,4-Methylenedioxymethamphetamine (MDMA)
Bennies	Amphetamines
Crank	Crack cocaine, heroin, amphetamine, methamphetamine, methcathinone
DOM	4-Methyl-2,5-dimethoxyamphetamine
Ecstasy	MDMA
Eve	MDMA
Fen-phen	Phentermine
Golden eagle	4-Methylthioamphetamine
Ice	Cocaine, crack cocaine, smokable methamphetamine, methamphetamine, MDMA, phencyclidine (PCP)
MDA	Methaqualone
Meth	Methamphetamine
Speed	Crack cocaine, amphetamine, methamphetamine
STP	PCP
Uppers	Amphetamines

Another method of abusing cocaine is by smoking it. Crack is a solid form of pure cocaine that melts at 93°F (34°C) and vaporizes at a slightly higher temperature. Given these properties, crack is easily smoked. In this form, the drug reaches the capillary network of the lungs and can be absorbed into the body in seconds. The immediate outflow of blood from the heart speeds the delivery of the drug to the brain, so its effect is felt at once. Smoked crack produces the most rapid means of absorption and, therefore, the most potent effect.

Cocaine is one of the most addicting substances known. Its immediate effects include excitement and euphoria. Acute cocaine overdose is a genuine emergency because patients are at high risk for seizures and cardiac arrhythmias. Chronic cocaine abuse may cause hallucinations; for example, patients with "cocaine bugs" think that bugs are literally crawling out of their skin.

In caring for patients who have been poisoned with sympathomimetics, be aware that their severe agitation can lead to tachycardia and hypertension. Patients may also be paranoid, putting you and other health care providers in danger. Law enforcement officers should be at the scene to restrain the patient, if necessary. Never leave the patient unattended and unmonitored during transport.

Any patient who has overdosed on stimulant drugs needs prompt transport to the emergency department because of the risk of seizures, cardiac arrhythmias, and stroke. Blood pressure measurements in these patients may be as high as 250/150 mm Hg. Request ALS assistance, administer supplemental oxygen, and be prepared to suction as necessary. If the patient is already having a seizure, protect him or her against self-injury.

Sedatives and Hypnotics

Barbiturates and benzodiazepines have been a part of legitimate medicine for a long time. They are easy to obtain and relatively inexpensive. People who abuse these medications sometimes solicit prescriptions from several physicians for either the same hypnotics or a variety of sedative-hypnotics **TABLE 16-3**. These drugs are CNS depressants, so their abuse alters the level of consciousness. When taken in excessive doses, their effects are similar to those of alcohol, with the patient appearing drowsy, peaceful, or intoxicated. By themselves, these drugs do not relieve pain, nor do they produce a specific high, although abusers often take alcohol or an opioid at the same time to boost their effects.

In general, sedative-hypnotic agents are taken by mouth. Occasionally, however, contents of capsules may be suspended or dissolved in water and injected to produce a rather sudden state of ease and contentment. Use of IV sedative-hypnotic drugs quickly induces tolerance, so the person requires increasingly larger doses to achieve the same effect. As the dose increases, the patient becomes increasingly lethargic and demonstrates an increasingly lower level of responsiveness until he or she is unresponsive.

Sedative-hypnotic drugs may also be given to unsuspecting people as a knock-out drink. More recently, agents such as flunitrazepam (Rohypnol) have been abused as date rape drugs—they cause an unwary person to become sedated and even unresponsive. The person later awakens, confused and unable to remember what happened.

Airway management is first priority in caring for a patient who has overdosed on barbiturates or benzodiazepines. Call for paramedic backup to intubate and monitor the electrocardiographic rhythm. Next, administer high-concentration oxygen and establish venous access. If shock develops, rapid infusion of 1- to 2-L boluses of normal saline may be needed. Assess breath sounds before and after each bolus, rather than infusing an entire liter and then assessing breath sounds.

Activated charcoal is an option for treatment of patients after 60 minutes has passed. Studies have shown that activated charcoal is at least as effective as gastric lavage and may

Table 16-3 Examples of Sedative-Hypnotic Drugs		
Barbiturates	**Benzodiazepines**	**Others**
Amobarbital (Amytal)	Alprazolam (Xanax)	Carisoprodol (Soma)
Butabarbital (Butisol)	Chlordiazepoxide (Librium)	Chloral hydrate ("Mickey Finn")
Pentobarbital (Nembutal)	Diazepam (Valium)	Cyclobenzaprine (Flexeril)
Phenobarbital (Luminal)	Flunitrazepam (Rohypnol)	Ethchlorvynol (Placidyl)
Secobarbital (Seconal)	Lorazepam (Ativan)	Ethyl alcohol (drinking alcohol)
	Oxazepam (Serax)	Glutethimide (Doriden)
	Temazepam (Restoril)	Hydrocarbon inhalants
		Isopropyl alcohol (rubbing alcohol)
		Meprobamate (Equagesic)

be a better option because it almost immediately reduces the patient's serum barbiturate level.

> ### Transition Tip
>
> While one provider explains the use of charcoal to the patient, the other can prepare a large plastic garbage bag to hang on the patient as a bib. This will help contain the charcoal solution if the patient vomits.

Marijuana and Cannabis Compounds

When the leaves and flower buds of the *Cannabis sativa* plant are harvested and dried, the end product is referred to as marijuana (also known as weed, pot, dope, and smoke). Marijuana is usually smoked but can be ingested (such as when baked in cookies or brownies). The onset of effects from smoking marijuana is a matter of minutes; oral ingestion slows the onset time to several hours.

Marijuana users may have a distorted sense of time and space and, occasionally, a feeling of unreality. Smoking marijuana results in bronchodilation and slight tachycardia. Other signs and symptoms of marijuana use include euphoria, drowsiness, decreased short-term memory, diminished motor coordination, increased appetite, and bloodshot eyes.

Management focuses on supportive care because there is little likelihood of a serious medical complication. A novice user may exhibit some behavioral symptoms such as paranoia and (rarely) psychosis. Reassurance generally is helpful with either issue. Demonstrating the symptoms are related to marijuana use and not to ingestion of more dangerous substances requires thorough testing. Transport to the ED for complete evaluation is therefore warranted.

Hallucinogens

Hallucinogens alter a person's sensory perceptions **TABLE 16-4**. The classic hallucinogen is lysergic acid diethylamide (LSD). Another hallucinogen, PCP (angel dust), was commonly used in the 1970s and 1980s. Phencyclidine is a dissociative anesthetic that is easily synthesized and highly potent. Its effectiveness as a hallucinogen when administered by the oral, nasal, pulmonary, and intravenous routes makes it easy to add to other street drugs. It is dangerous because it causes severe behavioral changes that lead users to inflict injury on themselves.

All hallucinogenic agents cause visual hallucinations, intensify vision and hearing, and generally separate the user from reality. The user, of course, expects that the altered sensory state will be pleasurable. Often, however, it can be terrifying. At some point, you are bound to encounter patients who are having a bad trip. They are usually hypertensive, tachycardic, anxious, and most likely paranoid.

Many hallucinogens have stimulant properties. Thus care for a patient who is having a bad reaction to a hallucinogenic agent is the same as that for a patient who has taken a stimulant. Use a calm, professional manner and provide emotional support. Do not use restraints unless you or the patient is in danger of injury. Follow the guidelines specified by local authorities. Because these patients may suddenly experience hallucinations or odd perceptions, you must watch them carefully throughout transport. Never leave a patient who has taken a hallucinogen unattended or unmonitored. Provide a great deal of reassurance and request ALS assistance as needed.

Table 16-4 Commonly Abused Hallucinogens
Bufotenine ("toad skin")
Dimethyltryptamine (DMT)
Hashish
Jimson weed
LSD
Marijuana
Mescaline
Morning glory
Mushrooms
Nutmeg
PCP
Psilocybin (mushrooms)

Cardiac Medications

The medications used to treat patients with cardiac and cardiac-related problems continue to increase in number and sophistication. The major classes of drugs used as part of these treatment regimens include antidysrhythmics, beta-blockers, calcium channel blockers, cardiac glycosides, and angiotensin-converting enzyme inhibitors. Many patients take a combination of drugs, sometimes three or more, in attempts to control hypertension, electrocardiographic rhythm disturbances, or other problems. An overdose with these drugs is usually accidental.

Signs and symptoms of overdose with cardiac drugs vary but may include hypotension, weakness or confusion, nausea and vomiting, rhythm disturbances (most commonly bradycardia or heart block), headache, and difficulty breathing. As with all emergencies, ensure a patent airway, provide adequate ventilation, and administer high-flow supplemental oxygen.

Establish vascular access in case of overdose with these agents because several therapeutic interventions and antidotes are available if the specific agent is identified. In the case of hypotension, sequential fluid boluses of normal saline will often bring the blood pressure into an acceptable range.

Because of the sophistication of cardiac drugs and the likelihood that the patient may be taking multiple cardiac and other medications, making contact with medical control to consult with a physician is prudent.

Organophosphates

Organophosphates are a major component in many insecticides (Orthene, Diazinon, and Malathion) used in agriculture and in the home. Similarly performing compounds are used as nerve gases designed for chemical warfare; like organophosphates, they are categorized as cholinergic agents. These agents overstimulate normal body functions that are controlled by the parasympathetic nerves, resulting in salivation, mucous secretion, urination, crying, and an abnormal heart rate. You are unlikely to encounter nerve gases. However, you may be called to care for patients who have been exposed to one of the organophosphate insecticides (pesticides) or certain wild mushrooms, which are also cholinergic agents.

> *Organophosphates* A class of chemicals found in many insecticides used in agriculture and in the home.

Suicide attempts account for a considerable share of organophosphate poisonings. When suicide is the goal, the poison is usually taken by mouth. Accidental agricultural exposure is another common source, and persons involved in the manufacture of organophosphates and similar compounds are at risk.

The symptoms of organophosphate poisoning are fundamentally the same regardless of route of entry—anxiety and restlessness; headache, dizziness, and confusion; tremors or seizures; dyspnea, diffuse wheezing, and respiratory depression; and loss of consciousness. A patient poisoned with organophosphates will usually present with signs and symptoms within the first 8 hours. In addition, the CNS signs and symptoms associated with cholinergic excess are often expressed; the SLUDGE mnemonic (**S**alivation, **L**acrimation, **U**rination, **D**efecation, **G**astric upset, and **E**mesis) is helpful in assessment. Never pull potentially contaminated clothing over the patient's head. This could introduce the contaminant into the eyes, nose, or mouth. Instead unbutton or cut clothing away.

Assessment and management of a patient with organophosphate poisoning start with decontamination and removal of all contaminated clothing *before* initiating care or loading the patient into the ambulance. Contaminated clothing should be placed in plastic bags and disposed of as hazardous materials. Ideally, the patient should be scrubbed with soap and water. After that, patient care includes the following measures:

- Establish and maintain the airway. Consider an advanced airway as needed.
- Suction as needed.
- Give high-flow supplemental oxygen.
- Establish vascular access.
- Call for paramedic backup for medication administration and cardiac monitoring.
- Apply the pulse oximeter.
- Transport immediately to the closest appropriate facility.

The military has developed antidotes to nerve gas agents that can be administered if they are available and indicated. The most common of these antidotes are the Mark 1 kit and the DuoDote kit. The indications for these are a known exposure to nerve agents or organophosphates with manifestation of signs and symptoms. The kits consist of an auto-injector of atropine and one of 2-PAM chloride (pralidoxime chloride). The auto-injectors are activated in the outer thigh of the patient. Removal of the patient from the source of the exposure is also critical in these cases. If your service carries these antidote kits, you should receive training on their proper use prior to being cleared to administer them.

Carbon Monoxide

Carbon monoxide (CO) is a tasteless, odorless, colorless gas produced during the incomplete combustion of organic fuels, such as in home heating devices, automobile engines, generators, and gas grills. This toxic gas is the leading cause of accidental poisoning deaths in the United States and a significant contributing factor in many deaths related to house fires. In addition, half of all successful adult suicides involve CO poisoning, resulting from the victim closing the car in the garage, turning the vehicle on, and inhaling the exhaust.

Miscellaneous Substances

Many other substances may cause toxicologic emergencies. Additional substances are discussed in this section.

Incidents involving chlorine gas are relatively common because of the widespread use of chlorine compounds in the home and occupational settings. Most cases of chlorine gas exposure occur outside the home. The signs and symptoms of chlorine gas exposure include burning sensations in the eyes, nose, and throat along with a slight cough, and for more intense exposure, chest tightness, choking, intermittent cough, headache, nausea and vomiting, diffuse wheezing, cyanosis, crackles in the chest, shock, seizures, and loss of consciousness. Remove patients from the area of exposure. Once you are in a safe environment, quickly triage the patients, prioritizing patients with breathing problems. Irrigate burning or itching eyes with water, as well as any areas of the skin that have come in contact with the chlorine.

Cyanide poisoning can occur as a result of combustion in a fire, industrial exposure, or after ingestion of products that contained cyanide. Cyanide exposure blocks the utilization of oxygen at the cellular level. The results are cellular suffocation and death of the patient within seconds if the cyanide was inhaled or within minutes to possibly an hour or two if it was ingested. A patient who has been poisoned with cyanide may have an altered mental state. The patient, if awake enough to answer questions, may complain of headache, palpitations, or dyspnea. The classic odor of bitter almonds on the patient's breath is highly suggestive of cyanide poisoning. Respirations are usually rapid and labored early on; as the poisoning progresses, they become slow and gasping. The pulse is usually rapid and thready. Vomiting, seizures, and coma are common. Treatment must be instituted as fast as possible. In the prehospital setting, amyl nitrite may be used. If given in time, the treatment is usually effective. Call for paramedic backup and a commercially available cyanide antidote kit (manufactured by Eli Lilly) if available. Notify the receiving hospital of the probable diagnosis so staff can make preparations. Transport the patient without delay to an appropriate facility.

Caustics include strong acids and strong alkalis. Both types of chemicals are commonly used in industry, agriculture (anhydrous ammonia), and the home (for example, bleach). Most cases involve accidental dermal or ocular exposure. If the patient is an adult, oral ingestion of caustics is usually an intentional suicide or homicide attempt. Most patients who have swallowed caustic substances present with severe pain in the mouth, throat, or chest. Usually the airway is not a problem and the patient is not in shock. Respiratory distress, if present, is most likely caused by soft-tissue swelling in the larynx, epiglottis, or vocal cords, which means that the patient is in immediate danger of complete airway obstruction. Establish vascular access, usually en route, because immediate transport to the ED is needed. If the patient was exposed to a strong alkali, diluting and flushing away the caustic substance is the main goal. For an eye exposure, continuously irrigate; if only one eye was exposed, be sure you do not contaminate the other eye while washing. Finally, there are a number of significant "don'ts" for caustic ingestions: *don't* give any neutralizing substances, *don't* induce vomiting, *don't* perform gastric lavage, and *don't* give activated charcoal.

> *Caustics* Chemicals that are acids or alkalis; cause direct chemical injury to the tissues they contact.

> **Transition Tip**
>
> Some chemicals react with water. Although small amounts can usually be flushed safely with large quantities of water, larger amounts of such chemicals can give off toxic fumes or explode when wet. Be sure to check the relevant warnings or placards.

Erectile dysfunction medications are the most dangerous of the drugs that improve sexual performance. These drugs, such as sildenafil (Viagra), are contraindicated for patients who take nitrates for cardiac problems. Their use by people taking nitrates may result in severe hypotension or total cardiovascular collapse, ultimately leading to death. For hypotension, repeated boluses of normal saline can bring the blood pressure up to an acceptable level. If cardiac arrest occurs, follow your standard protocols.

Drugs used to facilitate sexual assault are typically administered stealthily to victims, frequently in an alcoholic drink. These substances are called "date rape" drugs. *Gamma-hydroxybutyrate (GHB)* is a drug associated with sexual assaults. GHB is available as an odorless and colorless liquid. It has a salty taste, but this may not be noted when placed in a drink. GHB produces a pronounced hypnotic effect along with disinhibition, severe passivity, and antegrade amnesia. Treatment for GHB intoxication focuses on the CNS depression and the risks of the patient being unable to protect the airway. Establish and maintain the airway, inserting an advanced airway as needed. Carefully monitor the patient's level of consciousness. Assist breathing as necessary, and give high-flow supplemental oxygen. Establish vascular access. Apply a pulse oximeter. Finally, provide rapid transport to the ED.

> *Gamma-hydroxybutyrate (GHB)* A sedative and central nervous system depressant.

> **Transition Tip**
>
> Households have many poisonous items. Many household cleaning agents are toxic if ingested. Household plants have poisonous leaves or berries. Pesticides and herbicides used in lawn and garden care are potentially poisonous. Paint thinners and solvents can cause permanent neurologic damage or death if inhaled in the right amount; the same is true of glue fumes.

Some alcohols, including methyl alcohol and ethylene glycol, are substantially more toxic than ethyl alcohol (drinking alcohol). Methyl alcohol is found in dry gas products and Sterno; ethylene glycol is found in some antifreeze products. Both cause a drunken feeling. Left untreated, both will also cause severe complications including tachypnea, blindness (methyl alcohol), renal failure (ethylene glycol), and eventually death. Even ethyl alcohol (typical drinking alcohol) can stop a patient's breathing if taken too fast or in a dose that is too high, particularly in children. Although they may be used as a substitute by a chronic alcoholic who is unable to obtain ethyl alcohol, they are more often taken by someone attempting suicide. In either case, immediate transport to the ED is essential.

Hydrocarbons are found in a variety of products around the home, including cleaning and polishing agents, glues, spot removers, lighter fluids, paints, paint thinners and paint removers, other fuels, and pesticides. The vast majority of intentional hydrocarbon inhalations are recreational. Frequently, people who "bag" or "huff" are young—middle-school age and, occasionally, younger—children. Hydrocarbon inhalation is done by pouring the volatile material onto a rag, placing it in a trash bag, and holding the bag over the face to breathe in the fumes. Breathing fumes directly off a soaked rag or towel is termed huffing, whereas the use of a trash bag is termed bagging.

> *Hydrocarbons* Compounds made up principally of hydrogen and carbon atom mostly obtained from the distillation of petroleum.

The primary goals when dealing with a patient who has inhaled hydrocarbons are removal from the noxious environment, giving high-concentration supplemental oxygen, and prompt transport to the appropriate facility.

Hydrocarbons may also be ingested by young children who mistake them for a beverage. A single hydrocarbon substance exposure may cause life-threatening toxicity and, on occasion, sudden death. Patients who have symptoms such as coughing, choking, or vomiting within a few minutes of ingestion are likely to have aspirated and need immediate attention. Signs of respiratory distress—air hunger, intercostal retractions, tachypnea, and/or cyanosis—must be considered danger signals.

Hypoglycemia and cardiac arrhythmias may occur; call for paramedic backup if needed. The patient may have severe abdominal pain, diarrhea, and belching, sometimes lasting for hours after the incident. All symptomatic patients suspected of ingesting a hydrocarbon product should be transported immediately to the ED for further evaluation and care. Management should include the following measures:

- Remove contaminated clothing and decontaminate the patient, ideally before placing the patient in the ambulance.
- Establish and maintain the airway, and ensure adequate ventilation.
- Give high-flow supplemental oxygen.
- Establish vascular access.
- Administer sequential bolus infusions of normal saline to treat hypotension.
- Transport the patient to the most appropriate facility.

Patients taking psychiatric medications may experience toxicologic emergencies. *Tricyclic antidepressants (TCAs)* carry a high risk of intentional overdose. Also, minimal dosing errors may produce toxic effects. The signs and symptoms of TCA overdose may vary dramatically. One patient may present with only a mild symptom such as a dry mouth, whereas another may have a life-threatening or fatal dysrhythmia. The most common signs and symptoms of a TCA overdose are altered mental status (drowsy, confused, slurred speech), dysrhythmias (usually sinus tachycardia or supraventricular tachycardia), dry mouth, blurred vision or dilated pupils, urinary retention, constipation, and pulmonary edema. With a more serious toxic exposure, be alert for ventricular tachycardia, hypotension, respiratory depression, and seizures. Management of patients with a TCA overdose includes the following measures:

- Maintain the airway. If the patient's mental status suddenly deteriorates, as is often the case, insert an advanced airway.
- Call for paramedic backup as needed for cardiac monitoring, intubation, and medication administration.
- Give high-flow supplemental oxygen.
- Establish vascular access.

- Administer activated charcoal per medical control orders.
- Manage hypotension with sequential boluses of normal saline. Be alert to the possibility of pulmonary edema, which occurs frequently in cases of TCA overdose.
- Assess blood glucose levels. Give dextrose 50% in water if the patient is hypoglycemic.
- Rule out head trauma as a possible cause of decreased mental status.
- Be alert for agitation or violence. Provide rapid transport to the closest appropriate facility.

> *Tricyclic antidepressants (TCAs)* A group of drugs used to treat severe depression and manage pain; minimal dosing errors can cause toxic results.

Monoamine oxidase inhibitors (MAOIs) are sometimes used to treat depression, but have a high potential for drug interactions. MAOIs can precipitate a hypertensive crisis if taken in conjunction with tyramine-containing foods (such as beer, wine, aged cheese, chopped liver, pickled herring, sour cream, yogurt, and fava beans). Symptoms of MAOI toxicity are often delayed, occurring 6 to 12 hours after ingestion and, in some cases, as long as 24 hours later. Once signs and symptoms begin to appear, you should prepare to manage a life-threatening event. Early signs and symptoms of MAOI overdose include hyperactivity, dysrhythmias (usually sinus tachycardia), hyperventilation, and nystagmus. With increased levels of toxicity, be alert for chest pain, palpitations, hypertension, diaphoresis, agitated or combative behavior, marked hyperthermia, and hallucinations. Unfortunately, there is no antidote available for an MAOI overdose. Establish and maintain the airway, inserting an advanced airway as needed. Give high-flow supplemental oxygen. Establish large-bore vascular access. After consultation with medical control, you may administer a single dose of activated charcoal. Do *not* give syrup of ipecac. With a patient in deteriorating condition, treat hypotension with sequential fluid boluses of normal saline. If seizures occur, call for paramedic backup for medication administration.

> *Monoamine oxidase inhibitors (MAOIs)* Psychiatric medication used primarily to treat atypical depression by increasing norepinephrine and serotonin levels in the central nervous system.

Selective serotonin reuptake inhibitors (SSRIs) are among the chief medications for managing depression. Patients with an SSRI overdose may be asymptomatic. When symptoms are present, they most commonly include nausea, vomiting, dysrhythmias (usually sinus tachycardia), sedation, and tremors, and possibly dilated pupils, agitation, blood pressure changes (hypotension or hypertension), seizures, and hallucinations. Management of an

SSRI overdose follows the general approach for poisoned patients:

- Establish and maintain the airway.
- Administer high-flow supplemental oxygen.
- Establish vascular access.
- Call for paramedic backup as needed.
- Consider a single dose of activated charcoal per medical control.
- Transport to the appropriate facility.

> *Selective serotonin reuptake inhibitors (SSRIs)* A class of antidepressants that inhibit the reuptake of serotonin.

Despite the major advances made in many areas of psychiatric medicine, *lithium* remains the cornerstone drug for the treatment of bipolar disorder. Lithium is excreted from the body slowly, meaning the threat of toxic levels and overdosing is always present. Signs and symptoms of lithium overdose include nausea, vomiting, hand tremors, excessive thirst, and slurred speech, and as toxicity increases, ataxia, muscle weakness and incoordination, blurred vision, and hyperreflexia (twitching) can occur. Eventually, the patient may have seizures and become comatose. Management of a patient suspected of a lithium overdose is mostly supportive. Establish and maintain the airway, inserting an advanced airway as needed. Give high-flow supplemental oxygen, and establish vascular access. If the patient experiences hypotension, administer serial boluses of normal saline. Transport the patient to an appropriate facility.

> *Lithium* The cornerstone drug for the treatment of bipolar disorder.

Medications used for pain management make up a large part of the OTC drug market. In the OTC and prescription drug markets, nonsteroidal anti-inflammatory drugs (NSAIDs) are some of the most popular options for pain relief, fever control, and anti-inflammatory action. Most of the problems associated with NSAID use involve long-term use; patients may experience gastrointestinal bleeding and kidney dysfunction. Signs and symptoms of NSAID overdose may include headache, altered mentation, behavioral changes, seizures, bradydysrhythmias, hypotension, abdominal pain, nausea, and vomiting. For symptomatic patients, care in the prehospital setting is usually supportive. Establish and maintain the airway, inserting an advanced airway as needed. Give high-flow supplemental oxygen, and establish vascular access. If hypotension develops, administer fluid boluses of normal saline. If hypotension persists after sequential fluid boluses, consider calling for paramedic backup for medication administration. Transport the patient to an appropriate facility.

Although aspirin (acetylsalicylic acid, or ASA) can be involved in a toxic event, more typically OTC products containing *salicylates* cause toxicity (for example, Pepto-Bismol

and hot-air vaporizers). With continued use of these products for a period of days, infants or young toddlers may ingest toxic levels of the salicylate. Chief complaints are usually nausea, vomiting, abdominal pain, diaphoresis, hyperpnea, ringing in the ears, pulmonary edema, and acid-base disturbances. Severe toxicity may produce metabolic acidosis or combined respiratory alkalosis–metabolic acidosis. No salicylate antidote or antagonist is available, so field management is primarily supportive. Establish and maintain the airway, inserting an advanced airway as needed. Give high-flow supplemental oxygen and establish vascular access. If hypotension develops (from volume depletion), administer serial boluses of normal saline. Monitor carbon dioxide levels with capnometry if available. Following consultation with medical control, administer one dose of activated charcoal. Call for paramedic backup as needed. Transport the patient to an appropriate facility.

> *Salicylates* Aspirin-like drugs.

Acetaminophen is a well-tolerated drug with few side effects that is available OTC. It is important to try to accurately estimate the time of ingestion because this information drives the decision-making process for patient care in the field and the hospital. An antidote for acetaminophen toxicity exists, although not as a prehospital intervention, and should be given less than 8 hours after the ingestion. Prehospital management first focuses on establishing and maintaining the airway, with an advanced airway being inserted as needed. Give high-flow supplemental oxygen, and establish vascular access. For recent ingestions, administer activated charcoal after consulting with medical control. Transport the patient to an appropriate facility.

Patient Assessment of Toxicologic Emergencies

Generally, patients with toxicologic emergencies are considered medical patients, although toxicologic emergencies may also lead to trauma. The general assessment approach is the same as it is for all patients.

> **Transition Tip**
>
> While at the scene, make thorough (and legible) notes about the nature of the poisoning. You can then quickly state the type and amount of substance and the time and route of exposure in your radio, verbal, and written reports. Clear notes that can be handed over on arrival will be appreciated by busy hospital staff.

Scene Size-up

Dispatchers can obtain important information pertaining to a poisoning call. This background will help you anticipate the proper protection needed to ensure your safety. Make sure that the scene is safe before entering, especially if there is a suspected inhalation poison. If it is not, take steps to make it safe or call for additional resources such as the hazardous materials team.

> ### Transition Tip
>
> Never approach a contaminated patient unless you have specialized hazardous materials training and are using the appropriate specialized personal protective equipment. It is imperative that all contaminated patients be thoroughly decontaminated prior to transport to the hospital. Remember that everyone at the scene who is exposed to the hazardous material must be thoroughly decontaminated before leaving the scene. Refer to your EMT-I textbook for additional information on hazardous materials and patient decontamination.

> ### Transition Tip
>
> Some chemicals react strongly with water. Although small amounts can usually be flushed safely with large quantities of water, larger amounts of such chemicals can give off toxic fumes or explode when wet. Be sure to check the relevant warnings and placards before you apply water as a decontamination measure.

Try to determine the cause of the poison. Look around the immediate area for clues such as empty medication bottles, a needle or syringe, scattered pills, chemicals, or even an overturned or damaged plant. In particular, containers at the scene can provide critical information. In addition to the name and concentration of the drug, a pill bottle label may list specific ingredients, the number of pills that were originally in the bottle, the date the prescription was filled, the name of the manufacturer, and the dose that was prescribed. This information can help emergency department physicians determine how much of the poison has been ingested and what specific treatment may be required. The remains of any nearby food or drink may also be important. Are alcoholic beverage containers present? For certain food poisonings, a food container that lists the name and location of the maker or the vendor may be of equal importance in saving the life of the patient and possibly other people. Place any suspicious material in a plastic bag and take it with you to the hospital, along with any containers you find.

Is there a suspicious odor or are drug paraphernalia present that might indicate the presence of an illicit drug laboratory? Drug laboratories can be very volatile, so ensure scene safety whenever this suspicion arises **FIGURE 16-2**.

Keep a constant, observant eye on the surroundings, and keep an open mind when questioning the patient or

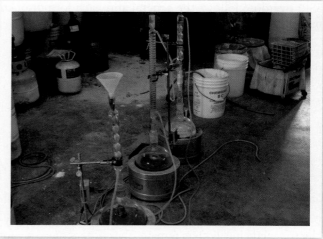

Courtesy of DEA

FIGURE 16-2 A laboratory capable of producing large quantities of methamphetamine.

bystanders to avoid coming to mistaken conclusions. If the patient vomits, examine the contents for pill fragments. Attempt to collect the vomitus in a separate plastic bag so that it can be analyzed at the hospital. Note and document anything unusual that you see.

Primary Assessment

With substance abuse and poisonings, do not be fooled into thinking that a conscious, alert, and oriented patient is in stable condition and has no apparent life threats. The patient may have a harmful or even lethal amount of poison in his or her system that has not yet had time to produce systemic reactions. A primary assessment that reveals a patient with signs of distress or an altered mental status gives you early confirmation that the poisonous substance is causing systemic reactions.

Quickly ensure that the patient has an open airway and adequate ventilation. Do not hesitate to begin oxygen therapy. If the patient is unresponsive to painful stimuli, insert an airway adjunct to ensure an open airway. Have suction available, because patients who experience any sort of poisoning are susceptible to vomiting. Given that some substances act as depressants on the body's systems, be prepared to assist ventilations with a bag-mask device.

If the patient is unresponsive, immediately assess for a pulse while determining whether the patient is breathing or has agonal gasps. If no pulse is evident, immediately begin CPR.

It is important to assess the adequacy of the patient's cardiovascular system. Palpate the pulse to determine the rate, quality, and rhythm. Evaluate skin color, temperature, and moisture to identify any circulatory compromise.

Variations in a patient's circulatory status will depend on the substance involved. Some poisons are stimulants, whereas others are depressants. Some poisons will cause vasoconstriction; others produce vasodilation. Although bleeding may not be obvious, alterations in consciousness may have resulted in traumatic injury, so always perform a gross bleeding check.

Patients with obvious alterations in the ABCs or patients with a poor general impression should be considered candidates for immediate transport. Consider the need for decontaminating the patient prior to transport depending on the poison exposure, especially if the substance poses a risk to the crew during transport. Decontamination is especially important when transporting exposed patients in a helicopter. Some industrial settings may have specific decontamination stations and antidotes available at the site. (An antidote is a substance that will counteract the effects of a particular poison.) The majority of the time, however, decontamination and antidote administration will have been initiated by the industrial response team before your arrival and should not delay rapid transport.

> ### Transition Tip
>
> In general, the SAMPLE history suggests an area of focus as you continue to assess the patient's complaints, the physical examination helps to explain what is happening outside the patient's body, and the vital signs tell you what is happening inside the body. These three assessments are important in that they suggest a direction for the interventions your patient might need.

History Taking

Investigate the chief complaint or history of present illness, and obtain the patient's medical history. If the patient is responsive and can answer questions, begin with an evaluation of the exposure and the SAMPLE history. In addition, determine the following:

- What is the substance involved? If you know the substance involved, it becomes easier to determine lethal doses, time before harmful effects begin, effects of the substance at toxic levels, and appropriate interventions.
- When did the patient become exposed to the substance? This information will help identify if and when the harmful effects will begin. It also lets the emergency department physician know which harmful effects can be reversed and which ones cannot because of the length of time that the patient has been exposed to the substance.
- What was the level of exposure? With this information, the poison center can determine whether the patient has had a harmful or lethal dose.
- Over what period of time did the patient take the substance—that is, all at once or over minutes or hours?
- Has any intervention been taken to relieve the situation (cold shower, medication, coffee, etc.)? If so,

has the intervention helped or caused additional complications?
- How much does the patient weigh? The antidote or neutralizing agent given by the emergency department physician may be based on the patient's weight as well.

If the patient is not responsive, attempt to obtain the history from other sources, such as friends, family members, or bystanders. Medical identification jewelry and cards in wallets may also provide critical information about the patient's medical history.

Secondary Assessment

Management of the ABCs during the primary assessment is the highest-priority assessment and treatment goal. Thus these interventions take precedence over a thorough physical examination. A thorough physical examination, however, often provides additional information on the exposure the patient experienced. In particular, a general review of all body systems may help to identify systemic problems. This review should be performed, at a minimum, on patients with extensive chemical burns or other significant trauma and on patients who are unresponsive.

If the poisoning is isolated, the physical examination should focus on the area of the body involved with the poisoning or the route of exposure. For example, if a person has ingested a poison, inspect the mouth for indications of poisoning. Are there burns from caustic chemicals? Are plant or pill fragments evident? If the person's skin came in contact with a poison, is there a rash or burns? How large an area is involved? If a respiratory exposure occurred, auscultate the lungs. Is good air movement in and out of the lungs apparent? Do you hear any wheezing or crackles? Much of what you should focus on in your physical examination is based on the route of exposure and the particular drug or chemical to which the patient was exposed.

A complete set of baseline vital signs is an important tool for determining the patient's status. Many poisons have no outward signs to indicate the seriousness of the exposure. Alterations in level of consciousness, pulse, respirations, blood pressure, and skin are more sensitive indicators that something serious is wrong. Keep in mind that exposure to CO may produce false pulse oximetry readings.

Reassessment

The condition of patients exposed to poisons may change suddenly and without warning. Continually reassess the adequacy of the patient's ABCs and compare them with the baseline set obtained. Evaluate the effectiveness of any interventions provided. If the assessment identified specific information about the poisonous substance, it may be possible to anticipate changes in the patient's condition. If the patient has ingested a harmful or lethal dose of a poisonous substance, repeat the assessment of vital signs every 5 minutes or constantly if needed. If the patient is in stable condition and no life threats are apparent, reassess the patient every 15 minutes. If the poison or the level of exposure is unknown, careful and frequent reassessment is mandatory.

Report to the hospital as much information as you have about the poison or chemical to which the patient was exposed. If a material safety data sheet (MSDS) is immediately available, transport it with the patient. If this information is not immediately available, ask the company or relevant entity to fax it to the receiving hospital while you are en route. The MSDS will help to identify specific interventions and potential antidotes.

Transition Tip

Children younger than 6 years have frequent iron exposures, usually secondary to ingesting chewable vitamins. Children typically remain asymptomatic when they have a low-level iron exposure. However, children who ingest a large dose of iron are at risk of dying unless aggressive and timely interventions take place. Unfortunately, little can be done in the prehospital environment for iron poisoning, other than providing basic attention to the ABCs and transporting the patient to the hospital for further evaluation and laboratory studies.

Food Poisoning

Whenever you encounter two or more people sick at the same time and at the same scene, think food poisoning or carbon monoxide poisoning—your hunch will likely be correct. Almost half of food poisonings take place in restaurants, cafeterias, and delicatessens.

Three toxins—*Salmonella*, *Listeria*, and *Toxoplasma*—produce roughly 35% of all food-related deaths. Poisoning with *Clostridium botulinum*, an extremely deadly toxin, is usually the result of improper food storage or canning. In addition, the toxins produced by dinoflagellates in "red tides" may contaminate bivalve shellfish such as oysters, clams, and mussels and produce life-threatening or fatal paralytic shellfish poisoning. Cooking does not kill these toxins.

Depending on the toxin, onset of signs and symptoms can range from several hours after ingestion to days or weeks. The longer the time until symptom onset, the more difficult it will be to link the patient's problem to the event at which the toxin was ingested. Gastrointestinal complaints are the most common and include abdominal pain and cramping, nausea, vomiting, and diarrhea. With prolonged episodes of vomiting or diarrhea, hypotension secondary to fluid loss and electrolyte imbalance becomes likely. Respiratory distress or arrest can occur with toxins such as *C. botulinum* or those found in paralytic shellfish poisoning.

Management for patients with food poisoning is usually supportive. Most of the cases you will encounter will not be life threatening, and the signs and symptoms of acute gastroenteritis are typically self-limiting. Establish and maintain the airway, inserting an advanced airway as needed. Give high-flow supplemental oxygen and establish vascular access. For hypotension secondary to fluid loss, administer fluid boluses of normal saline. Call for paramedic backup as needed. Finally, transport the patient to an appropriate facility.

Poisonous Plants

Several thousand cases of poisoning from plants occur each year, some of which prove severe. Many household plants are poisonous if ingested, and children have been known to nibble on the leaves of some of these plants TABLE 16-5. Some poisonous plants cause local irritation of the skin. Others can affect the circulatory system, the gastrointestinal tract, or the CNS. It is impossible for you to memorize every plant and poison, let alone their effects FIGURE 16-3.

Regardless of the cause of plant poisoning, emergency care includes the following steps:

1. Assess the patient's airway and vital signs.
2. Notify the regional poison center for assistance in identifying the plant.
3. Take the plant (if available) to the emergency department.
4. Provide prompt transport.

Table 16-5 Common Toxic Plants

Scientific Name	Common Name
Abrus precatorius	Jequirity bean/rosary pea
Cicuta species	Water hemlock/wild carrot
Colchicum autumnale	Autumn crocus
Conium maculatum	Poison hemlock
Convallaria majalis	Lily of the valley
Datura species	Jimson weed/stinkweed
Dieffenbachia	Dumbcane
Digitalis purpurea	Foxglove
Nerium oleander	Oleander or rose laurel
Nicotiana glauca	Tree tobacco
Phoradendron	Mistletoe
Phytolacca americana	Pokeweed
Rhododendron	Rhododendron or azalea
Ricinus communis	Castor bean
Solarium nigrum	Nightshade
Zygadenus species	Death camas

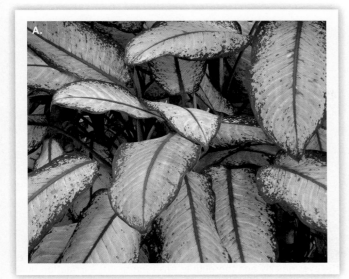

© Andriy Doriy/ShutterStock, Inc.

© MaxFX/ShutterStock, Inc.

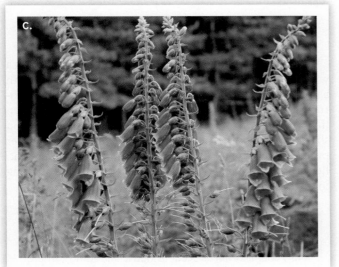

© Jean Ann Fitzhugh/ShutterStock, Inc.

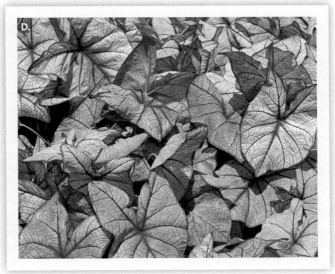

© Hatem Eldoronki/ShutterStock, Inc.

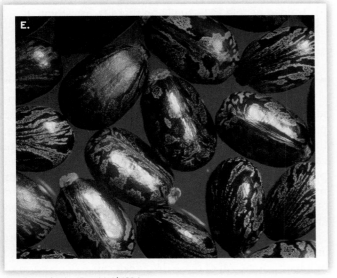

Courtesy of Brian Prechtel/USDA

FIGURE 16-3 The toxins in these common poisonous plants are often ingested or absorbed through the skin. **A.** Dieffenbachia. **B.** Lantana. **C.** Foxglove. **D.** Caladium. **E.** Castor bean.

Irritation of the skin and mucous membranes is a problem with ingestion of the common houseplant called dieffenbachia, a green plant with broad, variegated leaves. When chewed, a single leaf may irritate the lining of the upper airway enough to cause difficulty swallowing, breathing, and speaking. For this reason, dieffenbachia has been called "dumbcane." In rare circumstances, the airway may become completely obstructed. Emergency medical treatment of dieffenbachia poisoning includes maintaining an open airway, giving oxygen, and transporting the patient promptly to the hospital for respiratory support. You should continue to assess the patient for airway difficulties throughout transport, and if necessary, provide positive-pressure ventilation.

Emergency Care of Poisonings

Whenever inhalation is suspected as the route of entry, always use a self-contained breathing apparatus to protect yourself from the potentially poisonous fumes. If you are not specifically trained in the use of this apparatus or do not have appropriately fit-tested equipment available, do not enter the toxic environment or hot zone. In such cases, your patients may need to be removed from the toxic environment and decontaminated by specially trained personnel prior to your evaluation of them. The patient's clothing should be removed in this process, as it may contain trapped gases that can be released later, exposing you (and others in the vicinity) to the toxin. You cannot administer emergency care until decontamination has been completed and there is no danger of the poison contaminating you.

Patients who have inhaled poisons, including natural gas, sewer gas, certain pesticides, carbon monoxide, chlorine, or other gases, should be moved into fresh air immediately. Be prepared to give supplemental oxygen via nonrebreathing mask and/or to provide ventilatory support with a bag-mask device, if necessary, and have a suctioning unit available in case the patient vomits.

If absorbed or surface contact poisons are suspected, avoid contaminating yourself or others.

While protecting yourself from exposure, remove the irritating or corrosive substance from the patient as quickly as possible.

Remove all clothing that has been contaminated with poisons or irritating substances, thoroughly brush off any dry chemicals, flush the patient's skin with running water, and then wash the skin with soap and water. When a large amount of material has been spilled on a patient, flooding the affected part for at least 20 minutes may be the fastest and most effective treatment.

If the patient has a chemical agent in the eyes, irrigate them quickly and thoroughly. Avoid contaminating the other eye as you irrigate the affected eye, by running water from the bridge of the nose outward **FIGURE 16-4**. This action should be initially started at the scene and continued during transport.

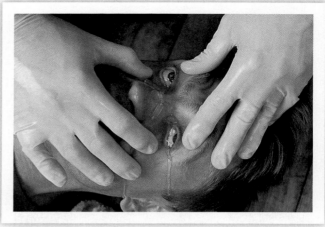

Courtesy of AAOS

FIGURE 16-4 If chemical agents are in the patient's eyes, irrigate the eyes quickly and thoroughly, ensuring that the irrigation fluid runs from the bridge of the nose outward. (Use of a nasal cannula is pictured.)

The only time you should not irrigate a contact area with water is when a patient has been contaminated with a poison that reacts violently with water, such as phosphorus or elemental sodium. These substances ignite when they come into contact with water. In such a scenario, you should wear appropriate protective gloves and the proper protective clothing and brush the chemical off the patient. Remove contaminated clothing, and apply a dry dressing to the burn area.

Transition Tip

Many chemical burns occur in industrial settings, where showers and specific protocols for handling surface burns are available. If you are called to such a scene, trained people will usually be there to assist you. If protocol documents are available, obtain the relevant material safety data sheets from the industrial site and transport them with the patient.

For ingested poisons, your goal as an AEMT is to rapidly remove as much of the poison as possible from the patient's gastrointestinal tract. For most poisoned patients, this emergency treatment will be sufficient until further care can be provided at the emergency department. If your local protocols permit you to take this step, the best method for removal of ingested poisons is administration of activated charcoal; this substance binds to the poison in the stomach and carries it out of the system.

Be prepared to provide aggressive ventilatory support and CPR to a patient who has ingested an opiate, a sedative, or a barbiturate. All of these drugs can cause depression of the CNS and slow breathing.

Poison Control Centers

Poison centers are located throughout the United States. The phone number of your local poison center is typically found on the inside cover of your local phone book. The telephone number for the nationally available Poison Help hotline is 1-800-222-1222. Specially trained nurses, doctors, and pharmacists at these centers have access to information about almost all of the commonly used medications, chemicals, and substances that could possibly be poisonous. These resources are available 7 days per week, 24 hours per day. They know the appropriate emergency treatment for each potential poison, including the antidote, if there is one.

If you believe that a patient has been poisoned, call the poison center and provide the relevant information, including the following items: the date and time when the poisoning occurred; evidence found at the scene; a description of the suspected poison, including the amount involved; and the patient's size, weight, and age.

Transition Tip

A medical toxicologist is a physician who specializes in caring for patients who have been poisoned. Approximately 100 of these specialists work in special hospitals called medical toxicology treatment centers, located throughout the United States. At times, your local protocols or online medical direction may divert a patient who meets certain poisoning criteria to one of these centers instead of to the closest hospital.

Ready for Review

- An allergic reaction is a response to chemicals the body releases to combat certain stimuli, called allergens. Almost any substance can trigger the body's immune system and cause an allergic reaction. Allergic reactions occur most often in response to five categories of stimuli: insect bites and stings, medications, foods, plants, and chemicals.

- An allergic reaction may range from mild and local, involving itching, redness, and tenderness, to severe and systemic, including shock and respiratory failure.

- Anaphylaxis is a life-threatening allergic reaction mounted by multiple organ systems that must be treated with epinephrine. Wheezing and skin wheals can be signs of evolving anaphylaxis.

- When a foreign substance first invades the body, the primary response begins. If the body is unable to identify the substance, immune cells record the features of the outside substance and produce antibodies to inactivate the foreign substance. This process is called development of sensitivity.

- Basophils and mast cells contain antibodies and can recognize the foreign substance should it enter the body again. Basophils are stationed in specific sites within the tissues. Mast cells are on patrol throughout the body.

- Chemical mediators are essentially the body's weapons against foreign substances. They release substances when an antigen invades the body and combines with one of the antibodies.

- Always provide prompt transport to the hospital for any patient who is having an allergic reaction or has been bitten by a poisonous insect. Remember that the patient's condition can deteriorate rapidly. Carefully monitor the patient's vital signs en route, especially for airway compromise.

- Poisons may act either acutely or chronically to destroy or injure body cells.

- If you believe a patient may have taken a poisonous substance, take steps to support the ABCs and notify medical control or the poison control center (1-800-222-1222).

- Management of the patient who has experienced poisoning includes the following measures:
  - Collecting any evidence of the type of poison that was used and transporting it to the hospital
  - Physically removing or diluting the poisonous agent
  - Providing respiratory support as needed
  - Providing other care as directed by medical control or the poison control center
  - Transporting the patient promptly to the hospital

- Emergency treatment may include administration of an antidote, if one exists, usually at the hospital.

- A poison can be introduced into the body in one of four ways:
  - Inhalation
  - Absorption (surface contact)
  - Ingestion
  - Injection

- It is difficult to remove or dilute injected poisons. As such, these cases are especially urgent.

- Always consult medical control before proceeding with the treatment of any poisoning victim.

- Move patients who have inhaled a poison into fresh air and provide supplemental oxygen via a nonrebreathing mask and/or ventilatory support via a bag-mask device as needed.

- Take care to avoid self-contamination when caring for a patient with absorbed or surface contact poisons. Remove all contaminated substances and clothing from the patient.

- Approximately 80% of all poisonings involve ingestion of poisonous plants, contaminated food, or some type of drug. In general, activated charcoal should be used in these patients.

- People who abuse a substance can develop a tolerance to it or develop an addiction.

- The most commonly abused drug in the United States is alcohol. Alcohol depresses the CNS and can cause respiratory depression. When caring for an intoxicated patient, be prepared for the patient to vomit and take steps to support the airway.

- Narcotics produce sleep or altered mental status and are classified as opiates and opioids. Opioids may produce euphoria. Manage the ABCs, establish vascular access, and call for paramedic backup for medication administration (naloxone) and cardiac monitoring.

- The main stimulants of concern for AEMTs include cocaine, amphetamines, and methamphetamine. The classic presentation includes excitement, delirium, tachycardia, hypertension with a fast pulse rate or hypotension with a fast pulse rate, and dilated pupils. Treatment consists of managing the ABCs, calling for paramedic backup to control anxiety and seizures as appropriate, and administering benzodiazepines per local protocol. Provide reassurance.

- A hallucinogen alters a person's sensory perception—seeing, hearing, or feeling things that are not actually present. Hallucinogenic substances include LSD, psilocybin mushrooms, PCP, ketamine, and mescaline. Treatment for a patient using hallucinogens is primarily supportive. Transport and provide psychological support.

- Sedative-hypnotic drugs may reduce anxiety and produce drowsiness and sleep. Barbiturates and benzodiazepines are the main drugs of concern in this category. Patients present similar to those with alcohol intoxication. Manage the ABCs, watch for shock, and administer fluids if needed.
- Cholinergics include organophosphates and nerve gases. These agents overstimulate normal body functions that are controlled by the parasympathetic nerves, resulting in salivation, mucous secretion, urination, crying, and an abnormal heart rate. Patients must be decontaminated before initiating care.
- Carbon monoxide causes more poisoning deaths than any other toxic substance. Exposure may occur from results of combustion in a fire, from an automobile engine, or from a home-heating device. Signs and symptoms vary and are vague, often resembling onset of the flu. Remove the patient from the environment, administer oxygen, and consider performing carbon monoxide monitoring.

- Food poisoning causes gastrointestinal complaints. Hypotension secondary to fluid loss and electrolyte imbalance becomes likely. Respiratory distress or arrest can occur. Management for patients with food poisoning is usually supportive.
- Poisonous plants may cause emergencies. Most plant-related exposures involve children younger than 6 years. Plants may irritate the skin, affect the circulatory system, or cause abdominal complaints. Most plant-related exposures require no treatment. Consult a poison center and medical control per local protocol.
- Poisoning by plants can affect the circulatory system, the gastrointestinal system, and the CNS. Ingestion of some plants, such as dieffenbachia, irritates the skin or mucous membranes and may cause airway obstruction.

Case Study

It is a warm summer day when you are dispatched to an alley in a neighborhood known for violence and drug activity; the initial report describes an unresponsive 24-year-old man. When you arrive at the scene, you are directed by police down the alley where you find the patient lying prone on the ground. You and your partner log roll the patient onto his back and begin the primary assessment. The patient's airway appears intact, but his respirations are slow and shallow. Expiratory wheezing is heard on auscultation of the chest. You insert a nasal airway and begin to assist the patient's ventilations with a bag-mask device. Bystanders tell you they found the patient in the alley just a few minutes ago. They indicate that he has a history of alcohol and drug abuse, but that he was "fine" just a little while ago. Your partner continues with the secondary assessment and informs you that the patient has pinpoint pupils and multiple track marks on his arms. While examining him, he also informs you that the patient has urticaria over his trunk and arms and what appears to be some type of insect sting on his upper arm.

1. Discuss what happens during an overdose of opioids.

2. Is epinephrine indicated for this patient? Why or why not?

Describe the proper treatment for this patient.

3. A state of overwhelming obsession or physical need to continue the use of a drug is known as:
   A. an addiction.
   B. an overdose.
   C. substance abuse.
   D. a poison.

4. Define the term "delirium tremens" and explain what happens during this process.

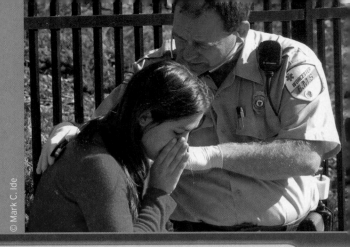

© Mark C. Ide

National EMS Education Standards

Medicine

Applies fundamental knowledge to provide basic and selected advanced emergency care and transportation based on assessment findings for an acutely psychotic patient.

Review

A psychological or behavioral crisis is any reaction to events that interferes with activities of daily living or becomes unacceptable to the patient or others. Such a crisis becomes a psychiatric emergency when the ensuing abnormal behavior threatens a person's health and safety or causes a major life interruption such as suicide attempt.

What's New

The *National EMS Education Standards* have introduced new terms to describe the state of mind of those experiencing behavioral crises and psychiatric emergencies. Psychosis is a state of delusion in which the person is out of touch with reality; its causes may include stress, delusional disorders, and, more commonly, schizophrenia. Agitated delirium is a specific behavior or condition recognized by disorientation, confusion, and possible hallucinations coupled with purposeless, restless physical activity. A psychiatric disorder (previously referred to as a mental disorder) is an illness with psychological or behavioral symptoms that may result in impaired functioning. The crisis may be the result of the emergency situation, mental illness, mind-altering substances, stress, or many other causes. This chapter discusses various types of psychiatric emergencies and mental illness.

Introduction

The most common misconception about mental illness is that if you are feeling bad or depressed, you must be sick. That is simply untrue. There are many perfectly justifiable reasons for feeling depressed including divorce, loss of a job, or the death of a relative or friend. For a teenager who just broke up with his girlfriend of 12 months, it is altogether normal to withdraw from ordinary activities and to feel blue. This is a normal reaction to a crisis situation. When a person finds that the Monday morning blues last until Friday, week after week, however, he or she may indeed have a mental health problem.

Many people believe that all individuals with mental health disorders are dangerous, violent, or otherwise unmanageable. This is also untrue. Only a small percentage of people with mental health problems fall into these categories.

Defining a Psychiatric Emergency

Behavior is what you can see of a person's response to the environment—that is, the person's actions. Most of the time, people respond to the environment in reasonable ways. Over the years, they learn to adapt to a variety of situations in daily life, including many stressors. Sometimes, however, the stress becomes so great that the normal ways of adjusting no longer work. When this happens, a person's behavior is likely to change, even if only temporarily, and the new behavior may not be appropriate or normal.

A *behavioral crisis* is the point at which a person's reactions to events interfere with activities of daily living such as bathing, dressing, and eating. If the interruption of daily routine tends to recur on a regular basis, the behavior is also considered a mental health problem.

> **Behavioral crisis** The point at which a person's reactions to events interfere with activities of daily living; the crisis becomes a psychiatric emergency when it causes a major life interruption, such as attempted suicide.

A person who experiences a panic attack after having a heart attack is not necessarily mentally ill. Likewise, you would expect a person who is fired from a job to have some sort of reaction to the event, often taking the form of sadness and depression. These problems are short-term and isolated events. In contrast, when a person reacts with a fit of rage, attacking people and property or going on a drinking binge for a week, this behavior has gone beyond what society considers appropriate or normal. Such an individual is clearly undergoing a behavioral emergency. If an abnormal or disturbing pattern of behavior lasts for at least a month, it is generally regarded as a matter of concern from a mental health standpoint.

When a *psychiatric emergency* arises, the patient may show agitation or violence or become a threat to himself or herself or to others **FIGURE 17-1** . This situation is more serious than a more typical behavioral crisis that simply causes inappropriate behavior such as interference with activities of daily living or bizarre behavior.

> **Psychiatric emergency** An emergency in which abnormal behavior threatens an individual's health and safety or the health and safety of another person—for example, when a person becomes suicidal, homicidal, or psychotic.

According to the National Institute of Mental Health, at one time or another, one in five Americans has some type of *psychiatric disorder*—that is, an illness with psychological or behavioral symptoms that may result in impaired functioning. The disorder may be the result of the emergency situation, the use of mind-altering substances, social and situational stress, a psychiatric disease such as schizophrenia, a physical illness such as a diabetic emergency, or a biologic disturbance such as an electrolyte imbalance. Sometimes these conditions can be compounded by noncompliance with prescribed medication regimens.

> **Psychiatric disorder** An illness with psychological or behavioral symptoms and/or impairment in functioning caused by a social, psychological, genetic, physical, chemical, or biologic disturbance.

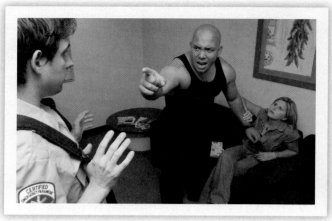

FIGURE 17-1 During a psychiatric emergency, the patient may display violence.

The mental health system in the United States provides many levels of assistance to people with psychiatric problems. Professional counselors may assist with marital conflict and parenting issues, for example, and psychologists may assist with more serious issues such as clinical depression. Some psychological conditions require the services of a psychiatrist—a physician who specializes in psychiatry and who can prescribe medication for the treatment of the most severe psychological conditions, such as schizophrenia and bipolar disorder. Most psychological problems can be handled through outpatient visits; however, some people require hospitalization in specialized psychiatric units.

Pathology of Psychiatric Emergencies

As an AEMT, you are not responsible for diagnosing the underlying cause of a behavioral crisis or psychiatric emergency. However, you should know the two basic categories of diagnoses that a physician will use: organic (physical) and functional (psychological).

Organic Brain Syndrome

Organic brain syndrome is a dysfunction of the brain caused by a disturbance in the physical or physiologic functioning of the brain tissue. This disruption can be either temporary or permanent. Causes of organic brain syndrome include sudden illness; recent trauma to the head; seizure disorders; drug and alcohol intoxication, overdose, or withdrawal; and diseases of the brain, such as Alzheimer disease and meningitis.

> **Organic brain syndrome** A temporary or permanent dysfunction of the brain, caused by a disturbance in the physical or physiologic functioning of brain tissue.

Functional Brain Syndrome

In a *functional disorder*, the abnormal operation of an organ cannot be traced to an obvious change in the actual structure or physiology of the organ or organ system. Something has gone wrong, but the root cause cannot be identified as the working of the organ itself. Schizophrenia, anxiety conditions, and depression are good examples of functional psychiatric disorders. There may be a chemical or physical cause for these functional brain syndromes, but it is not obvious or well understood.

> *Functional disorder* A disorder in which there is no known physiologic reason for the abnormal functioning of an organ or organ system.

Pathophysiology of Specific Psychiatric Emergencies

Acute Psychosis

Psychosis is a state of delusion in which the person is out of touch with reality. Affected people live in their own reality of ideas and feelings. To the person experiencing a psychotic episode, the line between reality and fantasy is blurred. That reality may make some patients belligerent and angry toward others. Other patients may become silent and withdrawn as they give all their attention to the voices and feelings within.

> *Psychosis* A mental disorder characterized by the loss of contact with reality.

Psychotic episodes may occur for many reasons. The use of mind-altering substances is one of the most common causes, in which case the experience may be limited to the duration of the substance within the body. Other causes include intense stress, delusional disorders, and more commonly, schizophrenia. Some psychotic episodes last for brief periods; others last for a lifetime.

Schizophrenia

Schizophrenia is a complex disorder that is neither easily defined nor easily treated. The typical onset occurs during early adulthood, with symptoms becoming more prominent over time. Some people diagnosed with schizophrenia display signs of this functional disorder during early childhood. Their disease may be associated with brain damage or may have other causes. People with schizophrenia interpret reality abnormally and may experience symptoms including delusions, hallucinations, a lack of interest in pleasure, and erratic speech.

Suicide

The single most significant factor that contributes to suicide is depression. Whenever you encounter an emotionally depressed patient, you must consider the possibility of suicide.

It is a common misconception that people who threaten suicide never commit it. In reality, suicide is a cry for help. Threatening suicide is an indication that someone is in a crisis that he or she cannot handle alone. Immediate intervention is necessary.

For further review of suicide, refer back to your EMT-I textbook.

Agitated Delirium

Delirium is a condition of impairment in cognitive function that can present with disorientation, hallucinations, or delusions. Agitation is a behavior that is characterized by restless and irregular physical activity. *Agitated delirium* is a condition of disorientation, confusion, and possible hallucinations coupled with purposeless, restless physical activity. Common physical symptoms include hypertension, tachycardia, diaphoresis, and dilated pupils. Although patients experiencing delirium are generally not dangerous, if they exhibit agitated behavior they may strike out irrationally. One of the most important factors to consider in these cases is personal safety.

> *Agitated delirium* A condition of disorientation, confusion, and possible hallucinations coupled with purposeless restless physical activity.

Because hallucinations are false perceptions of reality, the patient may perceive you as a threat. Agitation is recognized as a biologic attempt to release nervous tension and can produce sudden, unpredictable physical actions in the patient.

Transition Tip

Never leave a patient who may be experiencing a behavioral or psychiatric emergency unattended, unless the situation becomes unsafe for you or your partner.

Patient Assessment of Psychiatric Emergencies

Scene Size-up

Ensure scene safety and safe access to the patient. All the regular AEMT skills—assessment, providing care, patient approach, history taking, and patient communication—are used in behavioral emergencies.

Follow the general guidelines listed in **TABLE 17-1** to ensure your safety at the scene of a behavioral crisis or psychiatric emergency.

The Potentially Violent Patient

Violent patients make up only a small percentage of all patients who experience a behavioral or psychiatric crisis. Nevertheless, the potential for violence is always an important consideration in these scenarios.

While you have most likely encountered violent patients, it is important enough to review techniques for assessing and managing potentially violent patients.

- **History.** Has the patient previously exhibited hostile, overly aggressive, or violent behavior? Ask people

Table 17-1
Safety Guidelines for a Behavioral Crisis or Psychiatric Emergency
Be prepared to spend extra time.
Have a definite plan of action.
Identify yourself calmly.
Be direct.
Assess the scene.
Stay with the patient.
Encourage purposeful movement.
Express interest in the patient's story.
Do not get too close to the patient.
Respond with understanding and keep in mind that the patient is not responding to you in a normal manner.
Be honest and reassuring.
Do not judge.

Primary Assessment

Note the patient's behavior and attitude as you approach. Observe the overall appearance of the patient, including his or her age and body position. Note the patient's facial expression. Observe for tears, sweating, nervousness, or embarrassment. Assess the patient's airway, breathing, and circulation. Observe for any signs of overt behavior and give close attention to body language, such as abnormal posture or threatening gestures. While you are assessing the patient's mental status, note any evidence of rage, elation, hostility, depression, fear, anger, anxiety, confusion, or any abnormal behavior. Talk to the patient as you continue your assessment. If the patient is unresponsive, determine whether a pulse is present. If not, begin CPR and obtain an automated external defibrillator (AED). Remember that hypoxia may be the cause of changes in the patient's mental state.

Unless your patient's condition is unstable from a medical problem or trauma, prepare to spend time at the scene with your patient. Depending on your local protocol, there may be a specific facility to which patients with mental problems are transported.

> **Transition Tip**
>
> When you are assessing a patient who is having a behavioral emergency, it can be useful to obtain information separately from a relative or caregiver. Obtaining the patient's history in this way often yields valuable information and can help reduce the potential for violence when there is tension between the people involved.

at the scene, or request this information from law enforcement personnel or family.

- **Posture.** How is the patient sitting or standing? Is he or she tense, rigid, or sitting on the edge of the seat? Such physical tension is often a warning signal of impending hostility.
- **The scene.** Is the patient holding or near potentially lethal objects such as a knife, gun, glass, poker, or bat (or near a window or glass door)?
- **Vocal activity.** What kind of speech is the patient using? Loud, obscene, erratic, and bizarre speech patterns usually indicate emotional distress. Someone using quiet, ordered speech is not as likely to strike out as someone who is yelling and screaming.
- **Physical activity.** The motor activity of a person undergoing a psychiatric crisis may be the most telling factor of all. A patient who has tense muscles, clenched fists, or glaring eyes; is pacing; cannot sit still; or is fiercely protecting personal space requires careful watching. Agitation may predict a quick escalation to violence.

Other factors to consider in assessing a patient's potential for violence include the following:

- Poor impulse control
- A history of truancy, fighting, and uncontrollable temper
- Tattoos with gang identification, prison tattoos, or statements such as "Born to Kill" or "Born to Lose"
- Substance abuse
- Depression (accounts for 20% of violent attacks)
- Functional disorder (If the patient says that voices are telling him or her to kill, believe it.)

History Taking

Investigate the chief complaint. You should focus your questions on the immediate problem to avoid confusion. Establishing a good rapport with the patient will enable you to provide better care. Use therapeutic interviewing techniques by engaging in active listening, being supportive and empathetic, limiting interruptions, and respecting the patient's personal space. Take the patient seriously.

In trying to determine the reason for the patient's behavioral state, your assessment should consider three major areas as possible contributors:

- Is the patient's central nervous system functioning properly? For example, is the patient hypoglycemic or hypoxic? These conditions could cause the patient to behave in an unusual or irrational manner.
- Are hallucinogens or other drugs or alcohol a factor? Does the patient see strange things? Is everything distorted? Do you smell alcohol on the patient's breath?
- Are psychogenic circumstances, symptoms, or illness (caused by mental rather than physical factors) involved? These might include the death of a loved one, severe depression, history of mental illness, threats of suicide, or some other major interruption of activities of daily living.

A complete and careful SAMPLE history will be helpful in treating your patient and passing on information to personnel at the receiving facility. **TABLE 17-2** provides a list of questions to ask while evaluating a mental health disorder.

If time permits, use reflective listening. This technique is frequently used by mental health professionals to gain insight into a patient's thinking. It involves repeating, in question form, what the patient has said, encouraging the patient to expand on his or her thoughts.

Secondary Assessment

If the patient is unresponsive or has a poor general impression, perform a rapid systematic full-body scan beginning with the head, looking for DCAP-BTLS. Be aware that it is often difficult to perform a physical examination during a behavioral crisis or psychiatric emergency, because patients may feel threatened by your presence and actions. Obtain consent before attempting any examination or procedure, and explain what you are going to do. Observe facial expressions. Look for tears, sweating, or blushing. Note the patient's eyes and pupils; a central nervous system dysfunction may result in a blank stare or rapid eye movement. Monitor the patient's mental status for sudden changes. Hallucinations may be a sign of the patient's compromised perception of reality.

Obtain baseline vital signs if it is safe to do so, the patient allows it, and taking the measurements will not

Table 17-2 Questions for Evaluating a Behavioral Crisis
General
How is the patient dressed? Is the dress appropriate for the time of year and occasion? Are the clothes clean or dirty?
Has the patient harmed himself or herself? Is there damage to the surroundings?
Speech
How does the patient respond to you? ■ How does the patient feel? ■ Is there trauma involved? ■ Is there a medical problem?
Does the patient answer your questions appropriately?
Are the patient's vocabulary and expressions what you would expect under the circumstances? Are they in line with the patient's social and educational background?
Is the patient alert and able to speak logically and coherently?
Skin
What is the quality of the patient's skin? ■ Color? ■ Temperature? ■ Condition?
Posture/Gait
Are the patient's movements coordinated or jerky and awkward? Does he or she appear to be agitated?
Are the patient's movements purposeful? Are the movements helping to accomplish a task, such as sitting down and putting on a pair of shoes, or do they appear to be aimless, such as rocking back and forth in the chair?
Does the patient appear relaxed or stiff and guarded?
Mental Status
Does the patient understand why you are there?
Mood
Is the patient withdrawn or detached?
Is the patient hostile or friendly? Too friendly?
What are the patient's facial expressions? Are they bland and flat or expressive? Does the patient show joy, fear, or anger as appropriate? To what degree?
What is the patient's mood? Does he or she seem agitated, elated, or abnormally depressed?
Does the patient appear fearful or worried?

(continues)

Table 17-2 Questions for Evaluating a Behavioral Crisis (*continued*)
Thought
Does the patient express disordered thoughts, delusions, or hallucinations? Does he or she appear to be seeing, hearing, or responding to people or situations that are not evident to you?
Perception
Are the patient's responses to what is going on around him or her appropriate?
Judgment
Does the patient exhibit rational judgment?
Memory
Is the patient's memory intact? Check orientation to time, place, and person by asking the patient the following questions: <ul><li>Do you know what day/month/year it is?</li><li>Do you know where you are?</li><li>Do you know who I am?</li></ul>
Attention
Is the patient easily distracted? Is the patient able to concentrate?

exacerbate the patient's emotional state. Vital signs should include blood pressure by auscultation, pulse rate and quality, respiration rate and quality, and skin assessment for perfusion. Reassess the patient's level of consciousness. Use pulse oximetry, if available, to assess the patient's saturation of oxygen. Remember that if the patient has poor perfusion or cold extremities, the reading will not be accurate. Vital signs are important because the behavioral emergency may actually be the result of injury or a preexisting medical condition.

Reassessment

Be acutely aware of changes in the patient's mental state. Patients experiencing a behavioral crisis may act spontaneously and could become a danger to you and your crew. Reassess the vital signs, and chief complaint. Assist breathing as required, and administer oxygen if appropriate.

Contact medical control or the receiving department to inform personnel there about your patient's status. Many hospitals require additional personnel and a separate treatment area for patients with behavioral emergencies. Include a thorough description of the mechanism of injury (MOI)/nature of illness (NOI) and the position in which the patient was found. Describe the treatments performed, including the reason for treatment and the patient's response. Be sure to document the patient's distress, answers to questions, attitude toward emergency care providers, and any changes in patient status and the time. If restraints were used, document why and which type of restraint was used **FIGURE 17-2**. Follow local protocols.

Transition Tip

As much as your heart may go out to an emotionally distressed patient, there is often little you will be able to do for the patient during the short time you will be treating him or her. Your job is to diffuse and control the situation and to safely transport the patient to the hospital. Intervene only as much as it takes to accomplish these tasks. Be both caring and careful. If you have determined that it is necessary to restrain the patient, release the restraints only if necessary to provide patient care.

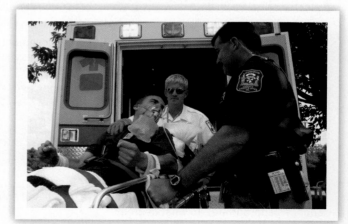

FIGURE 17-2 If the patient poses a threat to self or to others, he or she may require restraints.

Medicolegal Considerations

As an AEMT, you have limited legal authority to require or force a patient to undergo emergency medical care when no life-threatening emergency exists. Patients have the right to refuse care. However, most states have legal statutes regarding the emergency care of mentally ill and drug-impaired people. These statutory provisions permit law enforcement personnel to place the person in protective custody so that emergency care can be given. You should be familiar with your local and state laws pertaining to these situations.

Always try to transport a disturbed patient without restraints if possible. Once the decision has been made to restrain a patient, however, you should carry it out quickly. Be aware of standard precautions. If the patient is spitting, place a surgical mask over his or her mouth.

Make sure to have adequate help to restrain a patient safely. When subduing any disturbed patient, use the minimum force necessary. Refer to the *Medical, Legal, and Ethical Issues* chapter and to your EMT-I textbook for further review of the use of restraints.

> **Transition Tip**
>
> Patients with suicidal thoughts, especially those who have made a threat or unsuccessful attempt at suicide, may not be thinking clearly and may behave in very unpredictable ways. Some recognize that if they get into the ambulance or enter the hospital, they will not have the opportunity to complete their threat or gesture, so they may make one last effort to kill themselves. Suicidal/homicidal patients will not hesitate to hurt you or your partner. Be very careful how you assess the situation, making certain that you, your team, and the patient remain safe.

Special Populations

Pediatric Patients

In general, children experience behavioral crises as often as adults do, but the child's situation is usually managed by parents or caregivers. If you are called to help with a child experiencing a behavioral crisis, it is imperative to listen to the caregiver and follow his or her lead on how to best approach the child. Aggressive behavior in children, especially when it seems to be a pattern, may be a symptom of an underlying medical or psychological condition. As a precaution against them hurting themselves or others, children in this situation need a thorough evaluation from a mental health professional.

One specific behavioral problem that is common among teenagers is suicide. Although adults sometimes tend to view a teenager's problems as minor, these problems often appear insurmountable to the affected youth. It is important to never discount a teenager's comments about suicide as being "just an attempt to get attention."

> **Transition Tip**
>
> Suicidal thoughts and actions have no age limits. The youngest reported patient to commit suicide was 6 years old. As such, it is important to take all comments and actions as serious, no matter what the patient's age.

The same risk factors that lead to suicide attempts in adults are often also found in teenagers. Such issues may include termination of a relationship, drug or alcohol problems, a history of disciplinary problems, an unstable home life, social pressures, and peer approval. Another risk factor to consider is that children of parents who commit suicide are more likely to attempt suicide themselves.

Elderly Patients

As the population ages, AEMTs are likely to see more elderly patients with behavioral or psychiatric problems, including depression, dementia, and delirium **FIGURE 17-3**. These mental changes can affect your ability to thoroughly assess and treat an ill or injured geriatric patient. Understanding the causes of altered behavior in geriatric patients will help you administer effective patient care.

Depression is one of the more common mental status problems that you will see in older patients. This condition has a number of potential causes, including dementia, reaction to major illness such as cancer, medications, changes in the endocrine system such as menopause, and imbalance in brain chemicals.

Dementia is another source of abnormal behavior in the elderly. The most common cause in older adults is primary progressive dementia, also known as Alzheimer dementia.

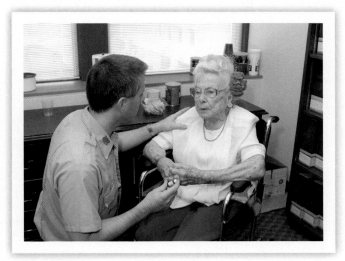

FIGURE 17-3 Understanding the causes of altered behavior in geriatric patients will help you administer effective patient care.

It is estimated that 12.5% of the population older than 65 years and a much higher percentage of the population older than 85 years has Alzheimer dementia. Currently, there is no cure for Alzheimer dementia, but medications are available that can slow the progress of the disease. During the progression of Alzheimer disease, patients may develop openly hostile behavior, kicking, yelling, pinching, and hitting you, your partner, or the patient's caregiver.

Other causes of altered behavior include medical conditions such as diabetic emergencies, heat- and cold-related illnesses, poisoning and overdose, strokes and transient ischemic attacks, and infection. Although the underlying mechanism is not understood, urinary tract infection and constipation can also alter an older person's behavior.

Transition Tip

The medicolegal issues associated with responses to a behavioral crisis put added emphasis on the need for thorough and specific documentation. Record detailed, objective findings that support the conclusion of abnormal behavior (eg, withdrawn, will not talk, crying uncontrollably) and quote the patient's own words when appropriate (eg, "Life isn't worth living anymore," "The voices are telling me to kill people."). Avoid judgmental statements, because they create the impression that you based your care on personal bias rather than the patient's needs.

PREP KIT

Ready for Review

- When the patient's reactions to events interfere with activities of daily living such as bathing, dressing, and eating, the situation is referred to as a behavioral crisis. When the patient becomes a threat to self or to others, it is referred to as a psychiatric emergency.
- An illness with psychological or behavioral symptoms that may result in impaired functioning is a psychiatric disorder. Such a disorder may be the result of the emergency situation, use of mind-altering substances, social and situational stress, psychiatric diseases such as schizophrenia, physical illnesses such as diabetes, or biologic disturbances such as electrolyte imbalances.
- According to the National Institute of Mental Health, at one time or another, one in five Americans has some type of psychiatric disorder.
- Psychotic episodes occur for many reasons. The use of mind-altering substances is one of the most common causes, in which case the experience may be limited to the duration of the substance within the body. Other causes include intense stress, delusional disorders, and more commonly, schizophrenia. Some psychotic episodes last for brief periods; others last for a lifetime.

- To the person experiencing a psychotic episode, the line between reality and fantasy is blurred.
- As an AEMT, you are not responsible for diagnosing the underlying cause of a behavioral crisis or psychiatric emergency; instead, your priorities are to diffuse and control the situation and to safely transport the patient to the hospital.
- The threat of suicide requires immediate intervention. Depression is the most significant risk factor for suicide.
- Patients experiencing delirium are generally not dangerous, but if they exhibit agitated behavior they may strike out irrationally.
- A mentally unstable patient may resist your attempts to provide care. In such situations, you should request that law enforcement personnel handle the patient.
- One of the most important factors to consider in psychiatric emergencies is your own personal safety.
- Aggressive behavior in children, especially when it seems to be a pattern, may be a symptom of a more significant underlying medical or psychological condition.
- As the population ages, AEMTs are likely to see more elderly patients with behavioral or psychiatric problems, including depression, dementia, and delirium.

Case Study

You are dispatched to a disturbance at a medical halfway house on the outskirts of the city. The dispatcher informs you that a 37-year-old man is threatening suicide and appears to be violent toward staff members. You arrive on scene and await the arrival of the police to secure the scene. After the scene has been secured, you are directed by police into the halfway house, where the patient is sitting in the back room. He appears generally agitated and confrontational with police. You attempt to establish a rapport with the patient by asking some general questions. The patient tells you that he has a history of bipolar disorder and that he has been feeling increasingly depressed over the past several days. He reports that he is running out of options and feels that he can no longer deal with the challenges of life. Upon further questioning, you learn the patient has been admitted to the hospital in the past for multiple suicide attempts. The patient says he does not really want to die, but is not sure what to do. He agrees to be cooperative with you and agrees to be transported to a facility for evaluation and treatment. At your request, the police search the patient for weapons before packaging. The patient is transported to the local hospital without incident.

1. On the basis of the information provided by the dispatcher in this scenario, this patient had the potential to be violent. Discuss some of the techniques used for assessing and managing potentially violent patients.

2. What is the difference between a behavioral crisis and a psychiatric emergency?

3. Define psychosis, and discuss the general guidelines to follow when treating a patient with psychosis.

4. A disorder in which there is no known physiologic reason for the abnormal functioning of an organ or organ system is known as a(n):
   A. agitated delirium.
   B. organic brain syndrome.
   C. functional disorder.
   D. psychiatric disorder.

5. Define and discuss the causes of organic brain syndrome.

CHAPTER 18

Gynecologic Emergencies

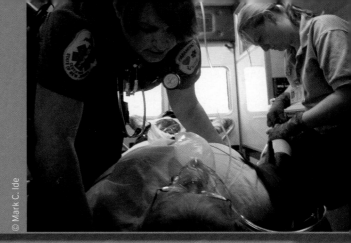

© Mark C. Ide

National EMS Education Standards

Anatomy and Physiology

Integrates complex knowledge of the anatomy and physiology of the airway, respiratory, and circulatory systems to the practice of EMS.

Medicine

Applies fundamental knowledge to provide basic and selected advanced emergency care and transportation based on assessment findings for an acutely ill patient.

Review

One of the primary functions of the female reproductive system is childbirth, making women susceptible to a number of gynecologic problems that do not occur in men. Components of the female reproductive system include the ovaries, fallopian tubes, uterus, and vagina.

What's New

Your EMT-I course focused mainly on obstetrics, pregnancy, and delivery of a newborn. The new standards, however, discuss gynecologic emergencies including sexually transmitted diseases, pelvic inflammatory disease, and vaginal bleeding. Treatment principles for victims of sexual assault are discussed as well. Obstetric emergencies are covered separately in the *Special Populations* chapter of this text.

Introduction

Occasionally, women in their childbearing years, girls, and older women will have major gynecologic problems requiring urgent medical care. The problems include excessive bleeding and soft-tissue injuries to the external genitalia. Some gynecologic conditions can be life threatening without prompt intervention. This chapter provides a brief review of the anatomy and physiology of the female reproductive system and examines complications involving this system, including vaginal bleeding and pelvic inflammatory disease. Principles of managing a woman who has been the victim of sexual assault are also discussed.

Anatomy and Physiology of the Reproductive System: A Review

The ovaries are the primary female reproductive organ **FIGURE 18-1**. They are almond-shaped bodies that lie on either side of the pelvic cavity. The two functions of the ovaries are to produce ova (mature oocytes) and the hormones estrogen and progesterone.

The vagina is the outermost cavity of a woman's reproductive system and forms the lower part of the birth canal. It is about 8 to 12 cm long, beginning at the cervix (the neck of the uterus) and ending as an external opening of

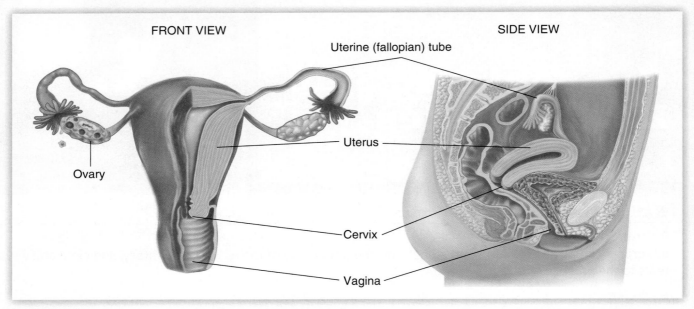

FIGURE 18-1 Front and side views of the female reproductive system.

the body. The uterus, or womb, is the muscular organ where the fetus grows. Essentially, the vagina completes the passageway from the uterus to the outside world for the delivering infant.

The fallopian tubes, or uterine tubes, are tubes or ducts that extend from the uterus and terminate near the ovary on each side. Their purpose is to carry a mature egg, or ovum, from the ovary to the uterus and spermatozoa from the uterus toward the ovary.

Even if the ovum is not fertilized in the fallopian tube, it continues to travel into the uterus. If fertilization has not occurred within about 14 days of ovulation, however, the lining of the uterus begins to separate and menstruation occurs. The menstrual flow consists of blood from the separated lining of the uterus and lasts approximately 1 week. The process of ovulation and menstruation is controlled by female hormones primarily produced in the ovaries. The initial onset of menstruation, known as menarche, occurs during puberty. Menopause is the cessation of menstruation and ovarian function. It generally occurs between the ages of 45 and 55 years.

The external female genitalia consist of the vaginal opening just posterior to the urethral opening **FIGURE 18-2**. The labia majora and labia minora are folds of tissue that surround the urethral and vaginal openings. At the anterior end of the labia is the clitoris, and at the posterior end is the anus. The perineum is the area of skin between the vagina and the anus. The labia are extremely vascular. Because of their location, however, they are usually injured only in cases of sexual assault or abuse.

Pathophysiology of Specific Gynecologic Conditions

Gynecologic emergencies that might be encountered include those associated with sexually transmitted diseases, traumatic injuries, vaginal bleeding, and sexual assault.

Pelvic Inflammatory Disease

Pelvic inflammatory disease (PID) is caused by an acute or chronic infection in the organs of the female pelvic cavity. Its onset is typically acute, within approximately 1 week of the menstrual period. Initial access by the infecting organism is through the vagina, where it ascends to other organs through the cervix, uterus, fallopian tubes, ovaries, uterine and ovarian support structures, and the liver. The chief symptoms of PID are pelvic pain and fever.

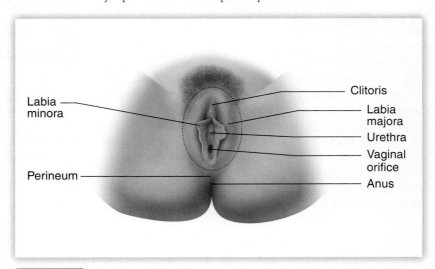

FIGURE 18-2 The external genitalia of the female reproductive system.

Complications that may accompany PID include sepsis, abscess formation, generalized peritonitis, and infertility. Scarring may cause tubal infertility and increase the risk of ectopic pregnancy.

> *Pelvic inflammatory disease (PID)* An infection of the fallopian tubes and the surrounding tissues of the pelvis.

Transition Tip

PID is the most common gynecologic reason why women call for EMS assistance.

The most common presenting sign of PID is generalized lower abdominal pain. Other signs and symptoms include abnormal and often foul-smelling vaginal discharge, increased pain with intercourse, fever, general malaise, and nausea and vomiting.

A patient with PID will complain of abdominal pain. The pain generally starts during or immediately after normal menstruation, so inquiring about the date of the patient's last menstrual period is an important component of the patient's history. Other symptoms may include vaginal discharge, fever and chills, and pain or burning on urination. Patients often walk doubled over and guard the abdomen, and gait tends to be shuffling to avoid excessive movement of the abdominal muscles. Patients often appear ill. Care includes placing the patient in a position of comfort and providing transport to an appropriate facility.

Sexually Transmitted Diseases

Sexually transmitted diseases can lead to more serious conditions. For example, untreated gonorrhea and chlamydia often progress to PID.

Chlamydia is caused by the bacterium *Chlamydia trachomatis*. This infection is a common sexually transmitted disease affecting an estimated 2.8 million Americans each year. Although the symptoms of chlamydia are usually mild or absent, some women may have symptoms including lower abdominal pain, low back pain, nausea, fever, pain during intercourse, and bleeding between menstrual periods. Chlamydial infection of the cervix can spread to the rectum, leading to rectal pain, discharge, or bleeding. If left untreated, the disease may progress to PID. In rare cases, chlamydia causes arthritis that may be accompanied by skin lesions and inflammation of the eye and urethra.

> *Chlamydia* A sexually transmitted disease caused by the bacterium *Chlamydia trachomatis*.

Bacterial vaginosis is one of the most common conditions to afflict women. In this infection, normal bacteria in the vagina are replaced by an overgrowth of other bacterial forms. Symptoms may include itching, burning, or pain and may be accompanied by a "fishy," foul-smelling discharge. If left untreated, bacterial vaginosis can lead to premature birth or low birth weight in the case of pregnancy, make the patient more susceptible to serious infections, and result in PID.

> *Bacterial vaginosis* An overgrowth of bacteria in the vagina, characterized by itching, burning, or pain, and possibly a "fishy" foul-smelling discharge.

Gonorrhea is caused by *Neisseria gonorrhoeae*, a bacterium that can grow and multiply rapidly in the warm, moist areas of the reproductive tract, including the cervix, uterus, and fallopian tubes in women, and in the urethra in both women and men. The bacterium can also grow in the mouth, throat, eyes, and anus. Symptoms are generally more severe in men than in women and appear approximately 2 to 10 days after exposure. Women may be asymptomatic for months until the infection has spread to other parts of the reproductive system. When symptoms do appear in women, they generally manifest as painful urination with associated burning or itching, yellowish or bloody vaginal discharge, usually with a foul odor, and bleeding associated with vaginal intercourse.

> *Gonorrhea* A sexually transmitted disease caused by the bacterium *Neisseria gonorrhoeae*.

More severe infections indicate that the condition has progressed to PID; such patients present with cramping and abdominal pain, nausea and vomiting, and bleeding between periods. Signs and symptoms of rectal infections generally include anal discharge and itching, and occasional painful bowel movements with fecal blood spotting.

Infection of the throat (for which oral sex is the introducing factor) usually results in mild symptoms, including pain or difficulty in swallowing, sore throat, swollen lymph glands, and fever. Headache and nasal congestion may also be present. If the infection is not treated, the bacterium may enter the bloodstream and spread to other parts of the body, including the brain.

Transition Tip

Many sexually transmitted diseases are not only spread through sexual activity, but can also be transmitted by contact with blood. Examples of these diseases include syphilis, many types of hepatitis, and human immunodeficiency virus (HIV).

Vaginal Bleeding

Because menstrual bleeding is a monthly occurrence in most females, vaginal bleeding resulting from other causes may initially be overlooked. Some possible causes of vaginal bleeding include abnormal menstruation, vaginal trauma, ectopic pregnancy, spontaneous abortion (miscarriage), cervical polyps, and cancer. Trauma to the internal female genitalia from any cause other than vaginal penetration is rare because these organs are located deep within the pelvis. Injuries to the vagina and external genitalia are extremely painful and very serious because of the large quantity of nerves and blood vessels in the area. In contrast, internal bleeding from polyps or cancer, while very serious, may be relatively painless.

Ectopic pregnancy and spontaneous abortion are two conditions that can cause vaginal bleeding in women who do not appear to be pregnant and may not even realize that they are pregnant. These two potentially life-threatening conditions are covered in the *Special Populations* chapter.

Patient Assessment of Gynecologic Emergencies

Women are vulnerable to many of the same conditions that cause abdominal pain in men—for example, ulcers and appendicitis. In addition, there are also numerous gynecologic causes of abdominal pain. An old medical axiom states, "Anyone who neglects to consider a gynecologic cause in a woman of childbearing age who complains of abdominal pain will miss the diagnosis at least 50% of the time." For some patients, missing such a diagnosis can be fatal.

Scene Size-up

Gynecologic emergencies can be very messy, sometimes involving large amounts of blood and body fluids contaminated with organisms that cause communicable diseases. As such, it is essential to follow standard precautions and use the appropriate personal protective equipment when treating these patients.

When you are assessing the scene, identify where and in which position the patient is found **FIGURE 18-3**. Document the condition of the patient's residence. This information

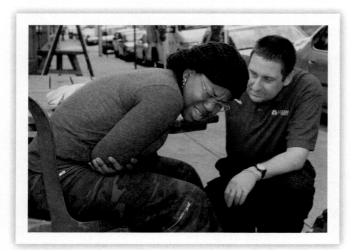

FIGURE 18-3 Note the position of the patient.

will contribute to your assessment of the patient's overall health and the safety of the scene. In the case of a crime scene, you may also be required to testify in court regarding the conditions found upon your arrival.

If any type of assault is suspected, request police assistance. In cases of sexual assault, it is important to have a female AEMT provide patient care if at all possible, so consider calling for one early if you and your partner are both male.

Primary Assessment

As you approach the patient, form a general impression of her condition. Determine responsiveness using the AVPU scale and perform a rapid scan. Assess the ABCs; identifying and treating life threats takes precedence over all other assessment and treatment measures.

If the patient is unresponsive, immediately assess for a pulse while determining if the patient is breathing or has agonal respirations. If there is no pulse, immediately begin CPR. Palpate the pulse to determine its rate, quality, and rhythm. Evaluate skin color, temperature, and moisture to identify any circulatory compromise. If the patient has experienced significant blood loss as a result of vaginal bleeding, she may be hypovolemic without demonstrating obvious signs of shock. If the patient has a weak or rapid pulse or pale, cool, or diaphoretic skin, assume she is in shock and place the patient in a supine position with the legs elevated. Cover the patient for warmth, and provide transport to the emergency department.

Most gynecologic emergencies are not life threatening. Nevertheless, if bleeding is present (either internal or external) or if the patient shows signs of shock, rapid transport is essential. If life threats are present, transport the patient immediately, while performing the remainder of the assessment en route to the hospital.

History Taking

Inquire about the patient's chief complaint, realizing that some of the questions may be extremely personal. Be sensitive to the patient's feelings and ensure that her privacy and dignity are protected. Gynecologic emergencies can be highly embarrassing, and many patients may be extremely uncomfortable discussing their sexual history in front of strangers or family members. An adolescent may want to keep her sexual history from her parents, so it may be necessary to isolate the patient before taking the history.

Obtain a SAMPLE history beginning with current symptoms. Make note of any allergies the patient has and any medications she is taking. Ask about the use of birth control pills or other birth control devices and any medical conditions. Specifically ask the date of the last "normal" menstrual period. Inquire about the possibility of sexually transmitted diseases or pregnancy. Determine when the patient last ate or drank, and which events led to her calling for EMS assistance. Use her mechanism of injury (MOI) or nature of illness (NOI), chief complaint, and answers to questions as the basis for further questioning. For example, if the patient is sexually active, ask her about birth control and any symptoms of possible pregnancy. If she has vaginal bleeding, determine how many pads she is using per hour. This information can help in estimating the amount of blood loss.

Secondary Assessment

Physical examination of a gynecologic patient should be limited and professional. Protect the patient's privacy at all times. Few people are comfortable with having their body exposed to a crowd of family, neighbors, EMS providers, police officers, or fire fighters. Limit the personnel present to those required to perform necessary tasks. Show the patient you respect her by being an advocate for her modesty.

Focus the physical examination on the MOI/NOI and the patient's chief complaint. If significant vaginal bleeding is present, visualize the bleeding and use external pads to control the bleeding, keeping in mind that hypoperfusion (shock) is possible. Ask if there is pain associated with the vaginal bleeding or discharge. Never insert anything into the vagina to control bleeding, including a tampon.

Fever, nausea, and vomiting are common with many medical conditions but should be considered especially significant with gynecologic emergencies. Any report of syncope on the part of the patient, especially if she complains of vaginal bleeding, is considered significant. In such a case, assume that the patient is in shock and treat her accordingly.

Assess the patient's vital signs, including heart rate, rhythm, and quality; respiratory rate, rhythm, and quality; skin color, temperature, and condition; and blood pressure. Determine the presence of tachycardia and hypotension, which could indicate hemorrhage. Use the appropriate monitoring devices, such as a pulse oximeter and noninvasive blood pressure monitor, to track the patient's condition.

Reassessment

Repeat the primary assessment and reassess vital signs every 5 minutes if the patient is unstable and every 15 minutes if she is stable. Determine whether the patient's condition is improving as a result of the interventions administered. Identify and treat any changes in the patient's condition. For example, if the patient appears to be losing consciousness, position her in the supine position, and perform a reassessment. Finally, pay specific attention to the needs of the patient, and accommodate her desire for conversation or silence. Continually offer reassurance.

▌Sexual Assault

Unfortunately, sexual assault is an all too common occurrence. Although most victims are women, men and children can also be targets. Often, there is little you can do beyond providing compassion and transportation to the emergency department. In some cases, the patients will have sustained multiple-system trauma and will also need treatment for shock.

AEMTs called to treat a victim of sexual assault face many complex issues, ranging from obvious medical ones to serious psychological and legal issues. You may be the first person the victim has contact with after the encounter, and how the situation is managed from first contact throughout treatment and transport may have lasting effects for both the patient and you. Professionalism, tact, kindness, and sensitivity are of paramount importance.

Do not examine the genitalia of a victim of sexual assault unless obvious bleeding requires you to apply a dressing. Discourage the patient from washing, douching, urinating, or defecating until after a physician has completed an examination; this will help to preserve any evidence of a crime. If oral penetration has occurred, discourage the patient from eating, drinking, brushing the teeth, or using mouthwash until he or she has been examined. Treat all other injuries according to appropriate procedures and protocols for your EMS system.

> ### Transition Tip
>
> A female victim of rape or sexual assault by a male may experience negative feelings toward men. As such, whenever possible, it is best if the patient is cared for by a female AEMT.

The job of the police is to solve the crime, arrest the perpetrator, and see justice served. Your job, as the AEMT, is to deal with the medical aspects of the case and to act as an advocate for the patient. In this capacity, it is important for you to focus on several key issues.

> ### Transition Tip
>
> Rape is a legal diagnosis, not a medical diagnosis. The medical team can establish only whether sexual intercourse occurred. A court must decide whether intercourse was inflicted forcibly on the victim, against her will.

The most important interventions for sexual assault patients are typically comfort, reassurance, and transport to a facility that has employees who are certified to perform the proper physical examination. Making the patient feel comfortable and safe may help to reassure her. Sometimes just the presence of a female AEMT can be emotionally helpful. Do not insist that the patient talk to you, but rather simply offer the opportunity. Listen carefully and nonjudgmentally. Common reactions may range from anxiety to withdrawal and silence. Denial, anger, and fear are normal behavior patterns. Maintain a professional attitude, and be aware of your own prejudices. **TABLE 18-1** lists the treatment principles to use when dealing with a victim of sexual assault.

> ## Transition Tip
>
> Sexual assault can occur in many settings, with either a stranger or someone well known to the victim. The assault can happen by force or by making the victim vulnerable to the sexual act. The use of drugs to facilitate sexual assault (eg, rape) is by no means a new tactic used by criminals. Indeed, alcohol is a common element at many rape scenes. However, the drugs of choice for commission of a crime of rape are "club drugs," such as ketamine, 3,4-methylenedioxymeth-amphetamine (ecstasy), gamma-hydroxybutyric acid (GHB), and flunitrazepam (Rohypnol). Club drugs (also called "date rape drugs") are used to lower the victim's inhibitions, thereby making the person more vulnerable and inducing amnesia. They are most commonly placed into the victim's drink, where they quickly dissolve and are generally tasteless.

Special Populations

Menarche

The onset of menstruation (menarche) can be an emotionally and physically disturbing event for a child. It is not uncommon for this event to be preceded by cramping pain that can be misinterpreted by a girl who is experiencing menstruation for the first time.

Approach the patient (and her parents) in the most professional manner possible. Empathize with their concerns, and provide transport to the hospital to help allay the concerns of the parents and to help determine whether some other condition is causing or contributing to the situation. Whenever possible, a female AEMT or family member should accompany the patient.

> ## Transition Tip
>
> Gynecologic emergencies can occur at any age.

Menopause

As women age, they reach a time when their menstrual cycles cease—a process called menopause. During this transitional period, the ovaries stop producing eggs and decrease their production of hormones (estrogen and progesterone). Menopause normally occurs between the ages of 45 and 55. For some women menopause is a relief, whereas for others it is a time of disappointment.

The process of menopause is a complicated one. Menstrual periods may become irregular and vary in severity and frequency as menopause approaches. It is not uncommon for women at this stage to continue to have sporadic periods for several months to a year as the transition progresses. The entire process of menopause can take as long as 5 years.

Table 18-1
Treatment Principles for Sexual Assault

In addition to the usual treatment principles that apply to all patients, follow these special steps with patients who have been sexually assaulted:

1. You must document the patient's history, assessment, treatment, and response to treatment in detail because you may have to appear in court as long as 2 or 3 years later. Do not speculate. Record only the facts.

2. Complete the SAMPLE history objectively.

3. Follow any crime scene policy established by your system to protect the scene and any potential evidence for police, particularly that for evidence collection. If the patient will tolerate being wrapped in a sterile burn sheet, this may help investigators to find any hair, fluid, or fiber from the alleged offender.

4. Do not examine the genitalia unless there is major bleeding. If an object has been inserted into the vagina or rectum, do not attempt to remove it.

5. To reduce the patient's anxiety, make sure the AEMT is the same gender as the patient, whenever possible.

6. Discourage the patient from bathing, voiding, or cleaning any wounds until the hospital staff has completed an assessment. Handle the patient's clothes as little as possible, placing articles and any other evidence in paper bags. If the patient insists on urinating, ask the patient to do so in a sterile urine container (if available). Also, deposit the toilet paper in a paper bag. Seal and mark the bag for the police. This can be critical evidence.

Menopause can result in various physical and emotional symptoms. Symptoms, which tend to vary in their severity from woman to woman, may include the following:

- Hot flashes
- Insomnia (difficulty sleeping)
- Night sweats
- Pounding heart
- Mood swings
- Irritability
- Depression

It is important to remember and to remind patients that during this time it is still possible to become pregnant. Women who have discontinued use of birth control because they believed they could not become pregnant may ignore or misinterpret signs of pregnancy when they do occur. Treat patients with compassion and reassurance. Provide transport to the hospital for evaluation by a physician to determine whether pregnancy or something else (such as a tumor or cyst) is causing the problem.

Emergency Care of Gynecologic Emergencies

When you are caring for any patient with a gynecologic emergency, be sure to take standard precautions. As with every patient, the ABCs come first. Intravenous access may be obtained but is typically not necessary unless the patient is demonstrating signs of shock or has excessive vaginal bleeding **FIGURE 18-4**. Ensure maintenance of the airway, give oxygen, take and document vital signs, and treat for shock while arranging for prompt transport. It is more important to provide treatment for shock and transport the patient to the hospital than to determine the actual cause of bleeding. Most women will use sanitary pads to control external bleeding before you arrive. If so, document the number of pads used prior to your arrival, and continue to add pads as necessary. If the woman has a tampon in place, leave it alone, but do not have the patient insert a tampon not already in place. Under no circumstances should you pack dressings inside the vagina.

The external genitalia have a rich nerve supply, making injuries to this area very painful. Treat any external lacerations, abrasions, and tears with moist, sterile compresses, using local pressure to control bleeding and a diaper-type bandage to hold the dressings in place. Leave any foreign bodies in place after stabilizing them with bandages. Continue to assess the patient while transporting to the emergency department. Contusions and other blunt trauma require careful in-hospital evaluation.

Notify staff at the receiving hospital of all relevant information, including any possibility of pregnancy or assault, so that a proper response can be prepared. Carefully document the patient's condition, chief complaint, pertinent information about the scene, and all interventions, especially in cases of sexual assault.

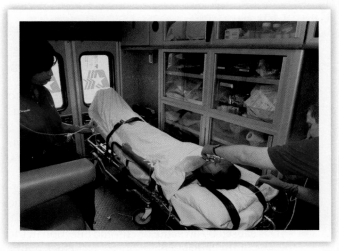

FIGURE 18-4 A patient with vaginal bleeding should be kept lying down. If shock is present, transport in the Trendelenburg position.

Transition Tip

Endometriosis is a painful, chronic gynecologic disorder affecting 6.3 million women in the United States alone. It occurs when the endometrial tissue that lines the uterus, grows outside the uterus—on the ovaries, fallopian tubes, ligaments that support the uterus, and other areas in the pelvis. This tissue responds to the menstrual cycle in the same way that the tissue of the uterine lining does, breaking down and shedding each month. However, while normal menstrual blood flows from the uterus through the vagina and outside the body, the blood and tissue shed from endometrial growths have no way of leaving the body. This results in internal bleeding, inflammation, and the formation of scar tissue. Treatment for endometriosis consists of pain medication, hormone therapy, and if necessary, surgery to remove the uterus (hysterectomy).

Ready for Review

- Occasionally you will be called for a patient experiencing a gynecologic emergency unrelated to pregnancy. The problem may include excessive bleeding, soft-tissue injuries, or infection.
- When a girl reaches puberty (approximately 11 to 16 years of age), she begins to ovulate and experience menstruation.
- Women continue to experience the cycle of ovulation and menstruation until they reach menopause (approximately age 50).
- The causes of gynecologic emergencies vary, ranging from sexually transmitted diseases to traumatic injuries.
- PID is caused by an acute or chronic infection in the organs of the female pelvic cavity. The chief symptoms of PID are pelvic pain and fever, and it typically occurs within 1 week of the menstrual period.
- Sexually transmitted diseases can lead to more serious conditions, such as PID.
- Because menstrual bleeding is a monthly occurrence in most females, vaginal bleeding that is the result of other causes may be initially overlooked. Possible causes of vaginal bleeding include abnormal menstruation, vaginal trauma, ectopic pregnancy, spontaneous abortion (miscarriage), cervical polyps, and even cancer.
- When dealing with patients who have gynecologic problems, it is essential to maintain the patient's privacy as much as possible.
- AEMTs called on to treat a victim of sexual assault face many complex issues, ranging from obvious medical ones to serious psychological and legal issues.
- Most patients experiencing a gynecologic emergency will be treated in the same manner regardless of the cause. Bleeding should be controlled, and the patient's ABCs should be monitored closely. Watch for developing signs of shock, and treat appropriately. Provide transport to the closest appropriate facility.
- The care you provide to a victim of sexual assault may have lasting effects for the patient. Professionalism, tact, kindness, and sensitivity are of paramount importance.

Case Study

You are dispatched to the local college campus for a 20-year-old female with abdominal pain. When you arrive at the scene, you are directed through a dormitory by campus security to the patient's room. Upon entering the room, you seen the patient lying on her left side in bed with her knees pulled up to her chest. She tells you that she has had abdominal pain with a fever for the past several hours that has gotten progressively worse. The patient seems reluctant to offer information. She denies any significant past medical history, medications, or allergies, but is not offering much information about her present illness. Her roommate informs you that the patient is embarrassed about her symptoms as she tries to encourage the patient to talk. After some convincing, the patient tells you that in addition to her abdominal pain, she has had a foul-smelling vaginal discharge for the past few days, a fever today, and a burning sensation when she urinates. She says she knows that she is not pregnant because she finished her menstrual cycle a few days ago. The patient is sexually active with multiple partners and does not always use condoms. Even though the patient is embarrassed, she agrees to be transported and evaluated at the local emergency department.

1. Discuss the process of PID and the signs and symptoms commonly associated with it.

2. Gonorrhea is a sexually transmitted disease that can progress to PID. Discuss the process of a gonorrhea infection and the presenting symptoms commonly seen with this disease.

3. In addition to gonorrhea, chlamydia is another possible cause of PID. Discuss how chlamydia infections affect patients.

4. Discuss the causes of vaginal bleeding.

5. As women age, they go through a process called menopause. Discuss this condition and the symptoms typically experienced by women during this process.

CHAPTER 19

Trauma

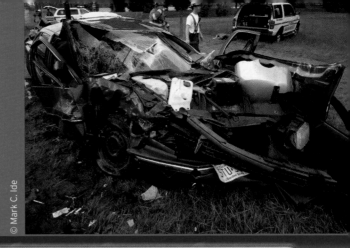

© Mark C. Ide

National EMS Education Standards

Pharmacology
Applies to complex knowledge of the medications that an AEMT may assist/administer to a patient during an emergency.

Trauma
Applies fundamental knowledge to provide basic and selected advanced emergency care and transportation based on assessment findings for an acutely injured patient.

Review

Traumatic emergencies occur as a result of physical forces applied to the body. The kinematics of trauma involve a process of surveying the scene to determine which types of forces and motion are involved in a traumatic event and to predict which injuries might result from those forces. Proper treatment of traumatic injuries involves appropriate assessment, rapid intervention, and management of life threats. It is essential to differentiate between patients requiring rapid transport to definitive care and those for whom on-scene stabilization and treatment are appropriate.

What's New

One of the primary additions to the *National EMS Education Standards* relative to trauma is the pathophysiology of specific traumatic events. A thorough understanding of mechanisms of injury (MOIs) (ie, how injuries occur) will allow you to better anticipate injuries, especially hidden injuries that may occur with certain traumatic events. This chapter discusses specific types of traumatic injuries and their impact on body systems. Transport destinations and trauma center classifications are also discussed.

Introduction

According to the National Institutes of Health (NIH), traumatic injuries are the leading cause of death in the United States among people younger than age 40. Proper prehospital evaluation and care can do much to minimize suffering, long-term disability, and death from trauma.

Different MOIs produce many types of injuries—some significant, others not. Examples of significant MOIs include falls from heights of greater than 10 feet without loss of consciousness, falls from heights of less than 10 feet with loss of consciousness, high speed motor vehicle and motorcycle crashes, car versus pedestrian (or bicycle or motorcycle)

collisions, gunshot wounds, and stabbings. Whether one or more body systems are involved, you should always maintain a high index of suspicion for serious unseen injuries in trauma cases.

Transition Tip

Traumatic injuries can be classified into two categories: blunt trauma and penetrating trauma. Blast injuries can result in both blunt and penetrating injuries.

Energy and Trauma

Traumatic injury occurs when the body's tissues are exposed to energy levels beyond their tolerance. The MOI is the way in which traumatic injuries occur; it describes the forces (or energy transmission) acting on the body that cause injury. Two concepts of energy are typically associated with injury (not including thermal energy, which causes burns): potential energy and kinetic energy. In considering the effects of energy on the human body, it is important to remember that energy can be neither created nor destroyed. It can only be converted or transformed.

> **Transition Tip**
>
> *Potential energy* is the product of mass (weight), force of gravity, and height.
> *Kinetic energy* is the energy of a moving object. Kinetic energy is expressed as follows:
>
> $$\text{Kinetic energy} = \frac{\text{mass}}{2} \times \text{velocity}^2$$
>
> or
>
> $$KE = \frac{m}{2} \times V^2$$

Kinetic energy The energy of a moving object.
Potential energy The product of mass, gravity, and height, which is converted into kinetic energy and results in injury, such as from a fall.

Multisystem Trauma

Multisystem trauma is a term that describes multiple traumatic injuries involving more than one body system, such as head and spinal trauma, chest and abdominal trauma, or chest and multiple extremity trauma. Patients with multisystem trauma experience a high level of morbidity and mortality; therefore, they require teams of physicians to treat their injuries. These teams may include specialists such as orthopaedic surgeons, neurosurgeons, and thoracic surgeons. As an AEMT, it is your job to ensure scene safety and immediately determine the need for additional personnel or equipment, evaluate the kinematics of the MOI, and identify and appropriately manage life threats. When a patient has sustained this type of injury, the on-scene time should be limited to 10 minutes or less whenever possible.

Multisystem trauma Trauma that affects more than one body system.

> **Transition Tip**
>
> Numeric scoring of trauma patients to determine the severity of their injury is common practice in the health care profession. When the various scoring systems were created, it was thought that the implementation of the scoring system would assist in rapidly identifying the severity of the patient's injuries. Several trauma scoring systems are employed. The one most commonly used for patients with head trauma is the *Revised Trauma Score (RTS)* because it is heavily weighted to compensate for major head injury without multisystem injury or major physiologic changes. The RTS is a physiological scoring system that is also used to assess the severity of a trauma patient's injuries. Objective data used to calculate the RTS include the Glasgow Coma Scale (GCS) score **FIGURE 19-1**, systolic blood pressure (SBP), and respiratory rate (RR). In addition to its utility in assessing injury severity, the RTS has demonstrated reliability in predicting survival in patients with severe injuries. The highest RTS a patient can receive is 12; the lowest is 0. The RTS is calculated as follows:
>
> | GCS | SBP | RR | Value |
> | --- | --- | --- | --- |
> | 13 to 15 | > 89 mm Hg | 10 to 29 breaths/min | 4 |
> | 9 to 12 | 76 to 89 mm Hg | > 29 breaths/min | 3 |
> | 6 to 8 | 50 to 75 mm Hg | 6 to 9 breaths/min | 2 |
> | 4 to 5 | 1 to 49 mm Hg | 1 to 5 breaths/min | 1 |
> | 3 | 0 | 0 | 0 |

Revised Trauma Score (RTS) A scoring system used for patients with head trauma.

Begin by assessing and managing the airway, including ventilatory support and high-flow oxygen, while maintaining cervical spine stabilization. Ensure that basic shock therapy, such as controlling hemorrhages and stopping arterial bleeding, is completed. If the patient is bleeding profusely, the hemorrhage must be controlled to ensure sufficient perfusion of organs and tissues. Keep in mind that the patient has sustained multisystem trauma and be aware that the order in which you usually provide treatment and care may need to be adjusted depending on the needs of the patient.

Once threats to the ABCs are corrected, place the patient on a long backboard and transport immediately. During transport, obtain a SAMPLE history and complete a secondary assessment. For critically injured patients, consider ALS intercept and/or air medical transportation. Regardless of

GLASGOW COMA SCALE

Eye Opening

Spontaneous	4
To Voice	3
To Pain	2
None	1

Verbal Response

Oriented	5
Confused	4
Inappropriate Words	3
Incomprehensible Words	2
None	1

Motor Response

Obeys Command	6
Localizes Pain	5
Withdraws (pain)	4
Flexion (pain)	3
Extension (pain)	2
None	1

Glasgow Coma Score Maximum Total	**15**

FIGURE 19-1 The Glasgow Coma Scale is one method of evaluating level of consciousness. The lower the score, the more severe the extent of the brain injury.

the mode of transport, ensure that the patient is transported to an appropriate facility and that the facility is notified of the impending arrival as soon as possible.

Bleeding Control

External Hemorrhaging

The principles of bleeding control have not changed, but recent studies have demonstrated that using pressure points and direct pressure to control severe external hemorrhage is ineffective. If allowed by local protocol and policy, you should apply a tourniquet to control severe bleeding from an extremity, without attempting pressure point control. If a tourniquet is deemed necessary, it should be applied quickly and not be released until a physician is present. Appropriate methods to control external bleeding include the following:

- Direct, even pressure and elevation
- Pressure dressings and/or splints
- Tourniquets for severe bleeding or if either of the other two methods is initially ineffective in controlling bleeding.

It will often be useful to combine these methods. In case of heavier bleeding or major wounds, it is important to continue to apply multiple dressings, without removing existing ones, until the bleeding stops. Do not hesitate to place a tourniquet proximal to an area of bleeding in an extremity if it is not easily controlled with direct pressure or splinting.

Tourniquets

Tourniquets are especially useful for a patient with substantial bleeding from an extremity injury below the axilla or groin. Although a triangular bandage and stick, as you may have learned in a previous EMS course, can still be used as a tourniquet, several new prefabricated tourniquets are now on the market. Follow the steps in **SKILL DRILL 19-1** to apply a commercial tourniquet:

1. Follow standard precautions.

2. Hold direct pressure over the bleeding site.

3. Place the tourniquet around the extremity above the bleeding site and, preferably in the proximal arm or leg just distal to the axilla or groin (**Step 1**).

4. Click the buckle into place and pull the strap tight.

5. Turn the tightening dial clockwise until pulses are no longer palpable distal to the tourniquet or until bleeding has been controlled (**Step 2**).

6. Write "TK" (for "tourniquet") and the exact time (hour and minute) that you applied the tourniquet on a piece of adhesive tape or write directly on the patient's forehead. Use the phrase "time applied." Securely fasten the tape to the patient's forehead. Notify hospital personnel on your arrival that your patient has a tourniquet in place. Record this same information on the ambulance run report form.

7. If instructed by medical control to remove the tourniquet, push the release button and pull the strap back. Be aware that bleeding may rapidly return upon tourniquet release and that you should be prepared to reapply the tourniquet immediately if necessary.

8. As an alternative, you can use a blood pressure cuff as an effective tourniquet. Position the cuff on the upper arm or thigh, and inflate it enough to stop the bleeding—typically to between 200 and 250 mm Hg. Leave the cuff inflated. Continuously monitor the gauge to make sure that the pressure is not gradually dropping. You may have to clamp the tube leading from the cuff to the inflating bulb to prevent loss of pressure or periodically add additional pressure.

Whenever you apply a tourniquet, make sure you observe the following precautions:

- Do not apply a tourniquet directly over a wound, a fracture, or any joint. Keep it near the groin or axilla whenever possible.

SKILL DRILL 19-1

Applying a Commercial Tourniquet

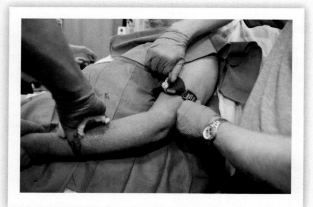

1 Hold pressure over the bleeding site and place the tourniquet above the injury.

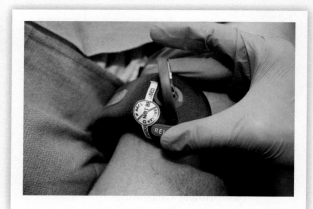

2 Click the buckle into place, pull the strap tight, and turn the tightening dial clockwise until pulses are no longer palpable distal to the tourniquet or until bleeding has been controlled.

- Make sure the tourniquet is tightened securely.
- Never use wire, rope, a belt, or any other narrow material as a tourniquet. It could cut into the skin.
- Use wide padding under the tourniquet if possible. This material will protect the tissues and help with arterial compression.
- Never cover a tourniquet with a bandage. Leave it open and in full view.
- Do not loosen the tourniquet after you have applied it. Hospital personnel will loosen it once they are prepared to manage the bleeding.

Transition Tip

If the use of a tourniquet is not possible because the bleeding is too far proximal, apply direct pressure and maintain it until you arrive at the hospital.

Internal Hemorrhaging

Internal bleeding comprises any bleeding in a cavity or space inside the body. Injury or damage to internal organs commonly results in extensive internal bleeding, which can lead to hypovolemic shock before the extent of blood loss is noticed. A person with a bleeding stomach ulcer may lose a large amount of blood very quickly, for example, as will a person who has a lacerated liver or a ruptured spleen.

Despite the significant effects produced by the blood loss, the patient may not have any outward signs of bleeding.

Internal bleeding is not always caused by trauma. Some of the more common causes of nontraumatic internal bleeding include bleeding ulcers, bleeding from the colon, ruptured ectopic pregnancy, and aneurysms.

The most common symptom of internal bleeding is pain. Abdominal tenderness, guarding, rigidity, pain, bruising, and distention are frequently noted, but are not always present in these situations. In older patients, dizziness, faintness, or weakness may be the first sign of nontraumatic internal bleeding. Ulcers or other gastrointestinal problems may cause vomiting of blood or bloody diarrhea or urine.

Bleeding into the chest may cause dyspnea in addition to tachycardia and hypotension. A bruise is also called a *contusion*, or *ecchymosis*. A *hematoma*—a mass of blood in the soft tissues beneath the skin—indicates bleeding into soft tissues and may be the result of a minor or a severe injury. Bruising or ecchymosis may not be present initially, and the only sign of severe pelvic or abdominal trauma may be redness, skin abrasions, or pain.

Contusion A bruise from an injury that causes bleeding beneath the skin without breaking the skin.
Ecchymosis Bruising or discoloration associated with bleeding within or under the skin.
Hematoma A mass of blood in the soft tissues beneath the skin.

Hemostatic agents promote hemostasis; in other words, they stop bleeding. Products such as Celox, HemCon, and QuikClot are now used in some areas, including the military, to stop profuse bleeding **FIGURE 19-2**.

These agents may take the form of granules that can be poured into a wound or contained in a dressing. They absorb the water component of blood, thereby concentrating the clotting factors, activating platelets, and enhancing the coagulation cascade. Unfortunately, some of these agents have an exothermic effect that can actually result in a burn to the surrounding tissue. Follow local protocols regarding the use of these agents.

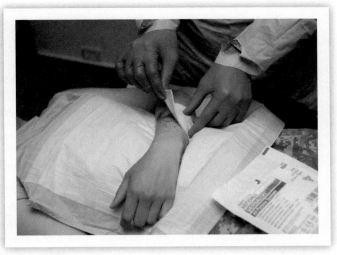

FIGURE 19-2 Hemostatic agents are being used in some areas to stop profuse bleeding.

Bleeding, however slight, from any body opening is serious. It usually indicates internal bleeding that is not easy to see or control. Bright red bleeding from the mouth or rectum or blood in the urine (hematuria) may suggest serious internal injury or disease. Nonmenstrual vaginal bleeding is always significant.

Other signs and symptoms of internal bleeding in both trauma and medical patients include the following:

- Hematemesis: vomiting blood. It may be bright red or dark red, or, if the blood has been partially digested, it may look like coffee-grounds vomitus.
- Melena: a black, foul-smelling, tarry stool that contains digested blood.
- Hemoptysis: bright red blood that is coughed up by the patient.
- Pain, tenderness, bruising, guarding, or swelling. These signs and symptoms may mean that a closed fracture is bleeding.
- Broken ribs, bruises over the lower part of the chest, or a rigid, distended abdomen. These signs and symptoms may indicate a lacerated spleen or liver. Patients with an injury to either organ may have referred pain in the right shoulder (liver) or left shoulder (spleen). You should suspect internal abdominal bleeding in a patient with unexplained shoulder pain.

The first sign of hypovolemic shock (hypoperfusion) is a change in mental status, such as anxiety, restlessness, or combativeness. In nontrauma patients, weakness, faintness, and dizziness on standing are also early signs. Changes in skin color or pallor are often seen in both trauma and medical patients. Later signs of hypoperfusion suggesting internal bleeding include the following:

- Tachycardia
- Weakness, fainting, or dizziness at rest
- Thirst
- Nausea and vomiting
- Cold, moist (clammy) skin

- Shallow, rapid breathing
- Dull eyes
- Slightly dilated pupils that are slow to respond to light
- Capillary refill of more than 2 seconds in infants and children
- Weak, rapid (thready) pulse
- Decreasing blood pressure
- Altered level of consciousness

Patients with these signs and symptoms are at risk; some may be in danger. Even if their bleeding stops, it could begin again at any moment. Given this risk, prompt transport is necessary.

TABLE 19-1 lists various MOIs and associated indicators of internal bleeding.

Controlling internal bleeding or bleeding from major organs usually requires surgery or other procedures that must be performed at the hospital. Keep the patient still and quiet. If spinal injury is not suspected, place the patient in the shock position, with feet elevated. Provide high-flow oxygen and maintain body temperature. You can usually control internal bleeding into the extremities quite well in the field simply by splinting the extremity; an air splint is usually the most effective option. You should never use a tourniquet to control the bleeding from closed, internal, soft-tissue injuries.

Transition Tip

Although it is included in the *National EMS Education Standards*, use of a pneumatic antishock garment (PASG) has been eliminated from the scope of practice in some states, even for use as a splinting device. Instead, the use of a pelvic stabilization device is recommended. As always, follow local protocols.

Table 19-1
The Mechanism of Injury: Indicators of Internal Bleeding

Mechanism of Injury	Potential Internal Bleeding Sources
Fall from a ladder striking the head	Head injury or hematoma
Fall from a ladder striking the extremities	Possible fractures; consider chest injury
Child struck by a car	Head trauma, chest and abdominal injuries, leg fractures
Fall on an outstretched arm	Possible broken bone or joint injury
Child thrown or falls from a height	Children often have a head-first impact, causing head injury
Unrestrained driver in head-on collision	Head and neck, chest, abdomen injuries; knees, femur, hip, and pelvis injuries
Unrestrained front-seat passenger; side-impact collision with intrusion into vehicle	Broken humerus; broken ribs exposing the chest wall (possible flail chest); pelvis and acetabulum injuries; laceration of the liver
Unrestrained driver crushed against steering column	Chest and abdominal injuries; ruptured spleen; neck trauma
Road bike or mountain bike (over the handlebars)	Fractured clavicle; road rash; head trauma if no helmet
Abrupt motorcycle stop causing rider to catapult over the handlebars	Fractured femurs; head and neck injuries
Diving into the shallow end of a swimming pool	Head and neck injuries
Assault or fight	Punching or kicking injury to chest, abdomen, and face
Blast or explosion	Injury from direct strike with debris; indirect and pressure wave in enclosed space. External injuries depend on the anatomic area of the body injured. Internally, air-containing hollow organs such as the middle ear and lungs are the most susceptible to pressure wave injury

Blast Injuries

Although most commonly associated with military conflict, blast injuries are considered significant MOIs. In addition to occurring on the battlefield, these injuries are seen in mines, shipyards, and chemical plants, and increasingly, in association with terrorist activities. Injuries from explosions may involve four different mechanisms FIGURE 19-3.

- **Primary blast injuries.** These injuries are caused entirely by the blast itself, with damage to the body attributable to the pressure wave generated by the explosion. When the victim is close to the blast, the blast wave causes disruption of major blood vessels and rupture of major organs. Hollow organs are the most susceptible to the pressure wave.
- **Secondary blast injuries.** These injuries result from being struck by flying debris, such as shrapnel from the explosive device, or glass or splinters set in motion by the explosion. Objects are propelled by the force of the blast and strike the victim, causing

injury. These objects can travel great distances and at tremendous speeds, up to 3,000 mph for conventional military explosives.

- **Tertiary blast injuries.** These injuries occur when the patient is hurled against a stationary object by the force of the explosion. A "blast wind" may also cause the patient's body to be hurled or thrown, causing further injury. When the body impacts the ground, the physical displacement of the body is referred to as ground shock. In some cases, wind injuries can be so strong as to amputate limbs.
- **Miscellaneous blast injuries.** Other injuries caused by a blast may include burns from hot gases or fires started by the blast, respiratory injury from inhaling toxic gases, and crush injury from the collapse of buildings, among others.

Most patients who survive an explosion have some combination of the four types of injuries mentioned. The discussion here is confined to primary blast injuries, which are the most easily overlooked variety.

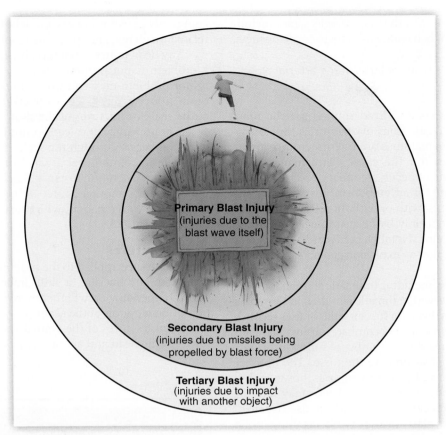

Primary Blast Injury (injuries due to the blast wave itself)

Secondary Blast Injury (injuries due to missiles being propelled by blast force)

Tertiary Blast Injury (injuries due to impact with another object)

FIGURE 19-3 The mechanisms of blast injuries.

Tissues at Risk

Organs that contain air, such as the middle ear, lung, and gastrointestinal tract, are most susceptible to pressure changes. The junction between tissues of different densities, and exposed areas such as head and neck tissues, are prone to injury as well.

The ear is most sensitive to blast injuries. The *tympanic membrane* detects minor changes in pressure and will rupture at pressures of 5 to 7 pounds per square inch above atmospheric pressure. Thus the tympanic membranes are a sensitive indicator whose condition can help you determine the possible presence of other blast injuries. The patient may complain of ringing in the ears, pain in the ears, or some loss of hearing, and blood may be visible in the ear canal. Dislocation of structural components of the ear, such as the ossicles forming the inner ear, may also occur. Permanent hearing loss is possible as a result of a blast injury.

Tympanic membrane The eardrum; a thin, semitransparent membrane in the middle ear that transmits sound vibrations to the internal ear by means of auditory ossicles.

Pulmonary blast injuries are defined as pulmonary trauma (contusions and hemorrhage) that results from short-range exposure to the detonation of explosives. When the explosion occurs in an open space, the patient's side that was toward the explosion is usually injured, but the injury can be bilateral when the victim is located in a confined space at the time of the blast. The patient may complain of tightness or pain in the chest and may cough up blood (hemoptysis) and have tachypnea or other signs of respiratory distress.

Pulmonary blast injury Pulmonary trauma resulting from short-range exposure to the detonation of explosives.

When air is present in the thorax, subcutaneous emphysema (crackling under the skin) can be detected over the chest by palpation. Administer oxygen to any patient with a suspected lung injury resulting from a blast. However, avoid giving oxygen under positive pressure (that is, by demand valve), because such treatment may increase damage to the lung.

One of the most concerning pulmonary blast injuries is *arterial air embolism*, in which air enters the pulmonary vasculature during alveolar disruption. Even small air bubbles can enter a coronary artery and cause myocardial injury. Air embolisms within the cerebrovascular system can produce a variety of other neurologic signs, including changes in vision, behavior, and state of consciousness.

> *Arterial air embolism* Air bubbles in the arterial blood vessels.

Neurologic injuries and head trauma are the most common causes of death from blast injuries. Subarachnoid and subdural hematomas are often seen in patients with primary injuries from this cause. Permanent or transient neurologic deficits occur secondary to concussion, intracerebral bleeding, or air embolism. Instant but transient unresponsiveness, with or without retrograde amnesia, may be caused not only by head trauma, but also by cardiovascular problems. Notably, bradycardia and hypotension are common after an explosion generates an intense pressure wave.

Extremity injuries, including traumatic amputations, are also common. Patients with traumatic amputation caused by the postblast wind are likely to sustain fatal injuries secondary to the blast. In present-day combat, improvements to body armor have increased the number of survivors of blast injuries from shrapnel wounds to the torso. The number of severe orthopaedic and extremity injuries, however, has increased. In addition, whereas body armor may limit or prevent shrapnel from entering the body, it also "catches" more energy from the blast wave, possibly resulting in the victim being thrown backward, which increases the potential for spine and spinal cord injury.

> ### Transition Tip
>
> With partial amputations, make sure to immobilize the part with bulky dressings and a splint to prevent further injury. Do not sever any partial amputations; this may complicate their later reattachment. A partial amputation involving an open fracture is described as a serious injury.

Injuries to the Head, Face, Neck, and Spine

Head Injuries

A head injury is a traumatic insult to the head that may result in injury to soft tissue, bony structures, and the brain. When head injuries are fatal, the cause is either associated brain injury or airway obstruction. In addition to the head injury, and depending on the MOI, it is important to suspect that the patient may have sustained additional trauma such as cervical spine injuries, pelvic injuries, and chest injuries.

Motor vehicle crashes are the MOI most commonly associated with head injuries. Head injuries also occur commonly in victims of assault, falls by the elderly, sports-related incidents, and incidents involving children.

Any head injury is potentially serious. Indeed, if such a problem is not properly treated, what appears to be a minor problem may end up becoming a life-threatening brain injury **TABLE 19-2**. Conversely, severe lacerations of the scalp or fractures of the skull may occur with little or no brain injury and lead to minimal or no long-term consequences. Although the scalp is highly vascular, it is relatively uncommon for a patient to lose enough blood from a scalp laceration to cause shock. As such, it is essential to rule out another source of bleeding or shock when confronted with a patient with a scalp laceration exhibiting signs of shock.

Skull Fractures

Significant force applied to the head may cause a skull fracture. Like any fracture, a skull fracture may be open or closed, depending on whether there is an overlying laceration or penetration of the scalp.

Open fractures of the cranial vault result from severe forces to the head and are often associated with trauma to

---

Table 19-2
General Signs and Symptoms of a Head Injury

Following a head injury, any patient who exhibits one or more of the following signs or symptoms has potentially sustained a very serious underlying brain injury:

- Lacerations, contusions, or hematomas to the scalp
- Soft area or depression of the scalp on palpation
- Visible fractures or deformities of the skull
- Decreased mentation
- Irregular breathing pattern
- Widening pulse pressure
- Slow heart rate
- Ecchymosis about the eyes (raccoon eyes) or behind the ear over the mastoid process (Battle sign)
- Clear or blood-tinged cerebrospinal fluid (CSF) leakage from a scalp wound, nose, or ear
- Failure of the pupils to respond to light
- Unequal pupil size
- Loss of sensation or motor function
- A period of unconsciousness
- Amnesia
- Seizures
- Numbness or tingling in the extremities
- Irregular respirations
- Dizziness
- Visual complaints
- Combative or other abnormal behavior
- Nausea or vomiting
- Posturing (decorticate or decerebrate)
- Unsteady gait

multiple body systems **FIGURE 19-4**. Brain tissue may be exposed to the environment, which significantly increases the risk of a bacterial infection (such as bacterial meningitis). Open cranial vault fractures have an exceedingly high mortality rate. Skull fractures are further classified as linear, depressed, or basilar **TABLE 19-3**.

> ## Transition Tip
>
> The diagnosis of a skull fracture is usually made in the hospital with a computed tomography (CT) scan. Maintain a high index of suspicion that a fracture is present if the patient's head appears deformed or if there is a visible crack in the skull within a scalp laceration or in the presence of raccoon eyes or Battle sign.

Linear skull fracture A type of fracture that accounts for 80% of skull fractures; also referred to as a nondisplaced skull fracture. These fractures commonly occur in the temporal-parietal region of the skull and are not associated with deformities to the skull.

Depressed skull fracture A fracture that results from high-energy direct trauma to the head with a blunt object; patients present with neurologic signs (such as loss of consciousness).

Basilar skull fracture A fracture that typically occurs following diffuse impact to the head (such as in a fall or motor vehicle crash); it generally results from extension of a linear fracture to the base of the skull and can be difficult to diagnose with a radiograph (X-ray).

Traumatic Brain Injuries

The National Head Injury Foundation defines a *traumatic brain injury (TBI)* as "a traumatic insult to the brain capable of producing physical, intellectual, emotional, social, and vocational changes." TBIs are the most serious of all head injuries. They are classified into two broad categories: *primary (direct) injury* and *secondary (indirect) injury*. Primary brain injury is injury to the brain and its associated structures that results instantaneously from an impact to the head. Secondary brain injury refers to a multitude of processes that increase the severity of a primary brain injury and, therefore, negatively impact outcome.

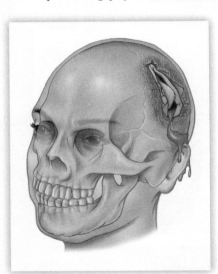

FIGURE 19-4 An open skull fracture.

Traumatic brain injury (TBI) A traumatic insult to the brain capable of producing physical, intellectual, emotional, social, and vocational changes.
Primary (direct) injury An injury to the brain and its associated structures that is a direct result of impact to the head.
Secondary (indirect) injury The "aftereffects" of the primary injury. It includes abnormal processes such as cerebral edema, increased intracranial pressure, cerebral ischemia and hypoxia, and infection; onset of these symptoms is often delayed following the primary brain injury.

Hypoxia and hypotension are the two most common causes of secondary injuries, ultimately resulting from cerebral edema, intracranial hemorrhage, increased intracranial pressure (ICP), cerebral ischemia, and infection. According to the Brain Trauma Foundation, hypoxia or hypotension significantly increases the risk of death and disability in a patient with a head injury. As such, it is important to monitor and address these conditions when they are identified. Secondary brain injury can occur anywhere from a few minutes to several days following the initial head injury.

The brain can be injured directly by a penetrating object, such as a bullet, knife, or other sharp object. More frequently, however, such injuries occur indirectly, as a result of external forces exerted on the skull. The most common cause of brain injury is a motor vehicle crash. When the brain strikes the front of the skull and then slams into the rear of the skull, a *coup-contrecoup brain injury* can occur. The same type of injury may occur on opposite sides of the brain in a lateral collision. In response, the injured brain starts to swell, initially because of cerebral vasodilation. An increase in cerebral water then contributes to further brain swelling. However, cerebral edema (swelling of the brain) may not develop until several hours following the initial injury.

Coup-contrecoup brain injury A brain injury that occurs when force is applied to the head and energy transmission through brain tissue causes injury on the opposite side of original impact.

Cerebral edema is aggravated by low oxygen levels in the blood and improved by high oxygen levels. In fact, the brain consumes more oxygen than any other organ in the body. For this reason, it is essential to ensure that the patient has a patent airway and that adequate ventilations and high-flow oxygen are provided to any patient with a head injury. This is especially true if the patient is unresponsive: Do not wait for cyanosis or other obvious signs of hypoxia to develop.

It is not uncommon for the patient with a head injury to experience a convulsion or seizure. This condition is

Table 19-3
Skull Fractures

Type		
Linear skull fractures **FIGURE 19-5**	Also called nondisplaced skull fractures. CT scan is used to diagnose a linear skull fracture because many patients do not show any physical signs such as deformity.	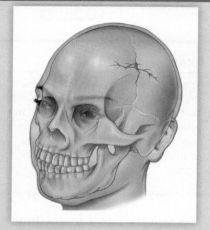 **FIGURE 19-5** A linear skull fracture.
Depressed skull fractures **FIGURE 19-6**	Result from high-energy direct trauma to the head with a blunt object. Patients present with neurologic signs (such as loss of consciousness).	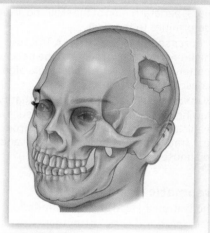 **FIGURE 19-6** A depressed skull fracture.
Basilar skull fractures **FIGURE 19-7**	Also associated with high-energy trauma, but usually occur following diffuse impact to the head (eg, falls, motor vehicle crashes). Result from extension of a linear fracture to the base of the skull and can be difficult to diagnose. Signs and symptoms include CSF drainage from the ears, raccoon eyes, and Battle sign.	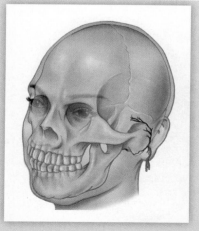 **FIGURE 19-7** A basilar skull fracture.

the result of excessive excitability of the brain, caused by direct injury or the accumulation of fluid within the brain (edema). Be prepared to manage seizures in all patients who have had a head injury because the brain may have sustained an injury as well.

Intracranial Pressure

For adults, the skull is a rigid, unyielding globe that allows little, if any, expansion of intracranial contents. It also provides a hard and somewhat irregular surface against which brain tissue and its blood vessels can be injured when the head sustains trauma.

Accumulation of blood within the skull or swelling of the brain can rapidly lead to an increase in *intracranial pressure (ICP)*, the pressure within the cranial vault. Increased ICP squeezes the brain against the skull.

> **Intracranial pressure (ICP)** The pressure within the cranial vault.

Closely monitor the patient for signs of increased ICP. The precise signs and symptoms will depend on the amount of pressure inside the skull and the extent of brainstem involvement. **TABLE 19-4** lists the levels of ICP and the corresponding signs and symptoms. More ominous signs include decorticate (flexor) posturing characterized by flexion of the arms and extension of the legs, and decerebrate (extensor) posturing characterized by extension of the arms and legs **FIGURE 19-8**.

If the patient's head injuries are significant enough to cause a TBI, the patient may begin to exhibit the signs of Cushing triad: increased blood pressure (hypertension), decreased heart rate (bradycardia), and irregular respirations such as Cheyne-Stokes respirations, central neurogenic hyperventilation, and Biot respirations (irregular rate, pattern, and depth of breathing). Cushing triad is also referred to as a herniation syndrome in which the ICP becomes so great that it forces the brainstem and the midbrain through the foramen magnum (the hole at the base of the skull); if allowed to continue, herniation is uniformly fatal. If the patient exhibits these signs, hyperventilation of the patient via positive-pressure ventilations may be indicated. Follow local protocols and medical direction in regard to hyperventilation in the presence of herniation.

Intracranial Hemorrhage The closed box of the skull has no extra room for an accumulation of blood, so bleeding inside the skull also increases the ICP. Bleeding can occur between the skull and dura mater, beneath the dura mater but outside the brain, or within the tissue of the brain itself.

> **Transition Tip**
>
> It is important to determine if a trauma patient is taking anticoagulants (blood thinners) such as Coumadin (warfarin) or aspirin, because these medications may result in increased bleeding. This information is especially important for patients with head trauma, where even a minor hematoma can become rapidly fatal.

Epidural Hematoma An *epidural hematoma* is an accumulation of blood between the skull and the dura mater

Table 19-4 Levels of Intracranial Pressure	
Mild elevation	<ul><li>Increased blood pressure; decreased pulse rate</li><li>Pupils still reactive</li><li>Cheyne-Stokes respirations (respirations that are fast and then become slow, with intervening periods of apnea)</li><li>Patient initially attempts to localize and remove painful stimuli; this effort is followed by withdrawal and extension</li><li>Effects are reversible with prompt treatment</li></ul>
Moderate elevation (indicates that the middle brainstem is involved)	<ul><li>Widened pulse pressure and bradycardia</li><li>Pupils are sluggish or nonreactive</li><li>Central neurogenic hyperventilation (deep, rapid respirations)</li><li>Decerebrate posturing</li><li>Survival is possible but often with permanent neurologic deficit</li></ul>
Marked elevation (indicates that the lower portion of the brainstem or medulla is involved)	<ul><li>Unilateral fixed and dilated pupil</li><li>Ataxic respirations (characterized by irregular rate, pattern, and volume of breathing with intermittent periods of apnea) or absent respirations</li><li>Flaccid response to painful stimuli</li><li>Irregular pulse rate</li><li>Diminished blood pressure</li><li>Most patients do not survive this level of intracranial pressure elevation</li></ul>

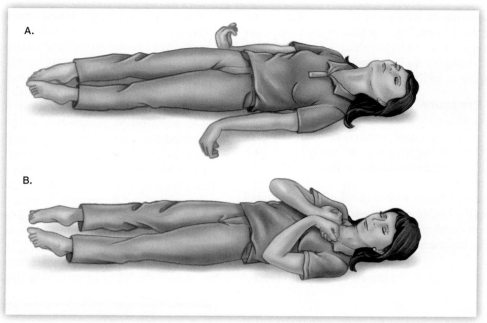

FIGURE 19-8 Posturing indicates significant intracranial pressure. **A.** Decerebrate (extensor) posturing. **B.** Decorticate (flexor) posturing.

FIGURE 19-9. An epidural hematoma is nearly always the result of a blow to the head that produces a linear fracture of the thin temporal bone. The middle meningeal artery runs along a groove in that bone; therefore, it is vulnerable when the temporal bone is fractured. Arterial bleeding into the epidural space will result in rapidly progressing symptoms.

> *Epidural hematoma* An accumulation of blood between the skull and the dura mater.

Often, the patient loses consciousness immediately following the injury; this is often followed by a brief period of consciousness (lucid interval), after which the patient lapses back into unresponsiveness. Meanwhile, as the ICP increases, the pupil on the side of the hematoma becomes fixed and dilated. Without surgery to evacuate the hematoma, death will follow rapidly.

Subdural Hematoma A *subdural hematoma* is an accumulation of blood beneath the dura mater but outside the brain **FIGURE 19-10**. It usually occurs after falls or injuries involving strong deceleration forces. Subdural hematomas are more common than epidural hematomas and may or may not be associated with a skull fracture. Bleeding within the subdural space typically results from rupture of the veins that bridge the cerebral cortex and dura.

> *Subdural hematoma* An accumulation of blood beneath the dura mater but outside the brain.

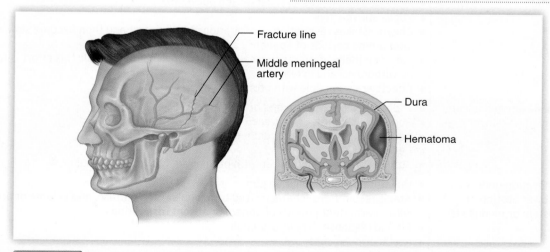

Fracture line

Middle meningeal artery

Dura

Hematoma

FIGURE 19-9 An epidural hematoma is usually the result of a blow to the head that produces a linear fracture of the temporal bone and damages the middle meningeal artery. Blood accumulates between the dura mater and the skull.

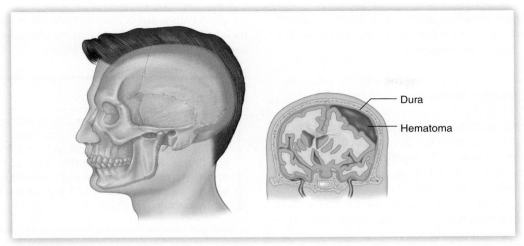

FIGURE 19-10 In a subdural hematoma, venous bleeding occurs beneath the dura mater but outside the brain.

A subdural hematoma is associated with venous bleeding, so this type of hematoma, along with signs of increased ICP, typically develops more gradually than an epidural hematoma. The patient with a subdural hematoma often experiences a fluctuating level of consciousness or slurred speech.

Transition Tip

When you are assessing potential fall injuries, take the following factors into account:
- The height of the fall
- The type of surface struck
- The part of the body that hit first, followed by the path of energy displacement

---

Intracerebral Hematoma An *intracerebral hematoma* involves bleeding within the brain tissue itself **FIGURE 19-11**. This type of injury can occur following a penetrating injury to the head or because of rapid deceleration forces.

> *Intracerebral hematoma* Bleeding within the brain tissue (parenchyma) itself; also referred to as an intraparenchymal hematoma.

Many small, deep intracerebral hemorrhages are associated with other brain injuries. The progression of increased ICP depends on several factors, including the presence of other brain injuries, the region of the brain involved (the frontal and temporal lobes are the most commonly affected locations), and the size of the hemorrhage. Once symptoms appear, the patient's condition often deteriorates quickly. Intracerebral hematomas have a high mortality rate, even if the hematoma is surgically evacuated.

Subarachnoid Hemorrhage In a *subarachnoid hemorrhage*, bleeding occurs into the subarachnoid space, where the CSF circulates. This condition results in bloody CSF and

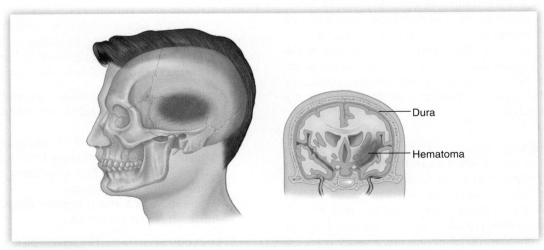

FIGURE 19-11 An intracerebral hematoma involves bleeding within the brain tissue itself.

signs of meningeal irritation (such as neck rigidity and head-ache). Common causes of a subarachnoid hematoma include trauma or rupture of an aneurysm.

> *Subarachnoid hemorrhage* Bleeding into the subarach-noid space, where the cerebrospinal fluid circulates.

The patient with a subarachnoid hematoma often reports a sudden, severe headache. As bleeding into the subarachnoid space increases, the patient experiences signs and symptoms of increased ICP: decreased level of consciousness, changes in the pupils, vomiting, and seizures.

A sudden, severe subarachnoid hematoma usually results in death. People who survive such events often have permanent neurologic impairment.

Concussion

A blow to the head or face may cause concussion of the brain. Concussions are also known as mild TBIs. There is no universal agreement on the exact definition of a concussion, but in general it is considered to be a closed injury with a temporary loss or alteration in the brain's abilities to function without demonstrable physical damage to the brain. For example, a person who "sees stars" after being struck in the head has sustained a concussion that affects the occipital portion of the brain. A concussion may result in unresponsiveness and even the inability to breathe for short periods of time; however, approximately 90% of patients who sustain a concussion do not experience a loss of consciousness.

A patient with a concussion may be confused or have amnesia (loss of memory). Occasionally, the patient can remember everything except the events leading up to the injury; this situation is called retrograde amnesia. Inability to remember events after the injury is called anterograde (posttraumatic) amnesia.

Usually, a concussion lasts only a short period of time. In fact, it has often resolved by the time EMS providers arrive. Nevertheless, it is important to ask about symptoms of concussion, including dizziness, weakness, or visual changes in any patient who has sustained an injury to the head. Additional signs and symptoms of a concussion include nausea or vomiting, ringing in the ears (tinnitus), slurred speech, and inability to focus. Dependent on the severity of the concussion, you may also notice lack of coordination, delay of motor functions, inappropriate emotional responses, or periods of disorientation. Patients may also complain of a temporary headache.

Contusion

Like any other soft tissue in the body, the brain can sustain a contusion, or bruise, when it hits the skull. A contusion is far more serious than a concussion because it involves physical injury to the brain tissue, which may sustain long-lasting and even permanent damage from the event. As with contusions that occur elsewhere in the body, bleeding and swelling from injured blood vessels are associated with a brain contusion. Injury of brain tissue or bleeding inside

the skull causes an increase of pressure within the skull. A patient who has sustained a brain contusion may exhibit any or all of the signs of brain injury.

> ### Transition Tip
>
> Patients with symptoms consistent with concussion may also have a more serious underlying brain injury. A CT scan is necessary to differentiate between these conditions. Always assume that a patient with signs or symptoms of concussion has a more serious injury until proven otherwise by a CT scan at the hospital or by evaluation by a physician.

Other Brain Injuries

Certain medical conditions, such as blood clots or hemorrhages, can also cause brain injuries that produce significant bleeding or swelling. Problems with blood vessels themselves, high blood pressure, or any number of other conditions may cause spontaneous bleeding into the brain, affecting the patient's level of consciousness. Signs and symptoms of nontraumatic injuries are often the same as those of TBIs, except that there is no obvious history of MOI or external evidence of any trauma.

If the respiratory control center of the brain is injured, the rate or depth of breathing may be ineffective. Ventilation may also be limited by chest injuries or, if the spinal cord is injured, by paralysis of some or all of the muscles of respiration. Give high-flow oxygen to any patient with suspected head injury, particularly any patient who is having trouble breathing. This treatment reduces the risk of hypoxia and possible cerebral edema. An injured brain is even less tolerant of hypoxia than a healthy brain, and studies have shown that supplemental oxygen can reduce brain damage. To be effective, however, oxygen must be started as soon as possible.

Emergency Care of Head Injuries

Emergency care for a patient with a head injury has not changed under the new standards. Regardless of the type of head injury, treat the patient according to three general principles that are designed to protect and maintain the critical functions of the central nervous system:

1. Establish an adequate airway. If necessary, begin and maintain ventilation, and always provide high-flow supplemental oxygen.
2. Control bleeding, and provide adequate circulation to maintain cerebral perfusion. Begin cardiopulmonary resuscitation (CPR), if necessary. Be sure to follow standard precautions.
3. Assess and continuously monitor the patient's baseline level of consciousness.

As you continue to treat the patient, do not apply pressure to an open or depressed skull injury. Assess and treat other injuries, dress and bandage open wounds as indicated in the treatment of soft-tissue injuries, anticipate and manage vomiting to prevent aspiration, and be prepared to manage convulsions and changes in the patient's condition. Assume the presence of spinal injury, if appropriate, and transport the patient promptly and with extreme care to the closest appropriate facility.

Eye Injuries

In a normal, uninjured eye, the entire circle of the iris is visible; the pupils are round and usually equal in size, and react equally when exposed to light; and both eyes move together in the same direction when following a moving finger. After injury, however, pupil reaction or shape and eye movement may be disturbed. Any of these conditions should cause you to suspect an injury of the globe of the eye or its associated tissues. Keep in mind, however, that abnormal pupil reactions are often a sign of brain injury rather than eye injury.

Treatment starts with a thorough examination to determine the extent and nature of any damage. Always perform an examination following standard precautions. Look for specific abnormalities or conditions that may suggest the nature of the injury. For burns to the eye, cover both eyes with a sterile dressing moistened with sterile saline as well as with eye shields, if available. Transport the patient promptly. If the patient is wearing contact lenses and has a chemical substance in the eye, remove contact lenses to allow the chemical to drain from the eye. Otherwise, never attempt to remove a contact lens from an eye that has been—or may have been—injured, because manipulating the lens can aggravate the problem.

Lacerations require very careful repair to restore appearance and function. If part of the eyeball is exposed, gently apply a moist, sterile dressing to prevent drying. Never exert pressure on or manipulate the injured eye (globe) in any way. Cover the injured eye with a protective metal eye shield, cup, or sterile dressing.

Foreign Objects

Foreign objects can enter the eye and cause significant damage. Even a very small foreign object, such as a grain of sand lying on the surface of the conjunctiva, may produce severe irritation FIGURE 19-12 . The conjunctiva becomes inflamed and red—a condition known as *conjunctivitis*—almost immediately, and the eye begins to produce tears in an attempt to flush out the object. Irritation of the cornea or conjunctiva causes intense pain. The patient may have difficulty keeping the eyelids open, because the irritation is further aggravated by bright light.

Conjunctivitis Inflammation of the conjunctiva.

If a small foreign object is lying on the surface of the patient's eye, use a normal saline solution to gently irrigate the eye. This treatment will frequently flush away loose,

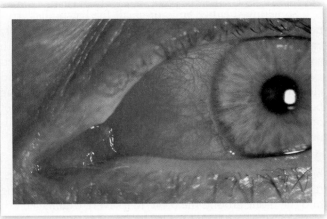

Courtesy of John T. Halgren, MD, University of Nebraska Medical Center

FIGURE 19-12 Conjunctivitis is often associated with the presence of a foreign object in the eye.

small particles. Using a small bulb syringe or a nasal airway or cannula, direct the saline into the affected eye. Always flush from the nose side of the eye toward the outside to avoid flushing material into the other eye FIGURE 19-13 .

Gentle irrigation usually will not wash out foreign bodies that are stuck to the cornea or lying under the upper eyelid. To examine the undersurface of the upper eyelid, pull the lid upward and forward. If you spot a foreign object on the surface of the eyelid, you may be able to remove it with a moist, sterile, cotton-tipped applicator. Conversely, you should never attempt to remove a foreign body that is stuck to the cornea.

Foreign bodies ranging in size from a pencil to a sliver of metal may be impaled in the eye. These objects must be removed by a physician. Emergency care in such cases involves stabilizing the object and preparing the patient for transport to definitive care. Cover the eye with a moist, sterile dressing, and then surround the object with a doughnut-shaped collar made from roller gauze or a small gauze pack.

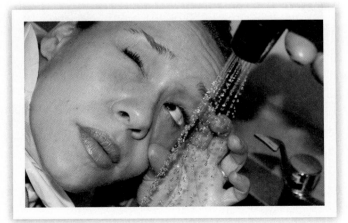

Courtesy of AAOS

FIGURE 19-13 A gently running faucet can be used to irrigate an eye effectively.

Sometimes, either large or small foreign bodies, particularly small metal fragments, may become completely embedded within the eye itself. Bandage both eyes with soft bulky dressings to prevent further injury to the affected eye. The bandage should be loose enough to hold the eyelid closed but not cause pressure on the eye itself. Bandaging both eyes prevents sympathetic motion (the movement of one eye causing both eyes to move), which may cause additional damage to the injured eye.

Blunt Trauma

Blunt trauma can cause a number of serious eye injuries, ranging from the ordinary black eye, resulting from bleeding into the tissue around the orbit, to a severely damaged eye globe. You may see an injury called hyphema, or bleeding into the anterior chamber of the eye, that obscures part or all of the iris FIGURE 19-14 . This injury is often associated with blunt trauma and may seriously impair vision. Twenty-five percent of hyphemas are globe injuries, a serious injury to the eye. Cover the eye to protect it from further injury and provide transportation to the hospital for further medical evaluation.

Blunt trauma can also cause a fracture of the orbit, particularly of the bones that form its floor and support the globe; such an injury is called a *blowout fracture*. The fragments of fractured bone can entrap some of the muscles that control eye movement, leading to double vision FIGURE 19-15 .

> *Blowout fracture* A fracture of the orbit or of the bones that support the floor of the orbit.

Any patient who reports pain, double vision, or impaired vision following blunt injury to the eye should be placed on a stretcher and transported promptly to the emergency department. Protect the eye from further injury

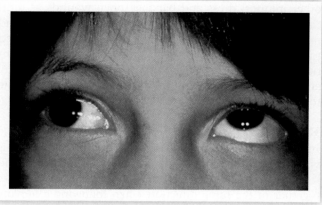

Courtesy of AAOS

FIGURE 19-15   A patient with a blowout fracture may not move his or her eyes together because of muscle entrapment. As a consequence, the patient sees double images of any object.

with a metal shield; cover the other eye to minimize movement on the injured side.

Another possible result of blunt eye injury is retinal detachment—a problem often seen in sports, especially boxing. This condition is painless but produces flashing lights, specks, or "floaters" in the field of vision and a cloud or shade over the patient's vision. Because the retina is separated from the nourishing choroid, this injury requires prompt medical attention to preserve vision in the eye. Transport the patient to a facility capable of handling such emergencies, such as a Level I trauma center or eye specialty center.

Abnormalities in the appearance or function of the eyes often occur following a closed head injury. Any of the following eye findings should alert you to the possibility of a head injury:

- One pupil larger than the other FIGURE 19-16
- The eyes not moving together or pointing in different directions

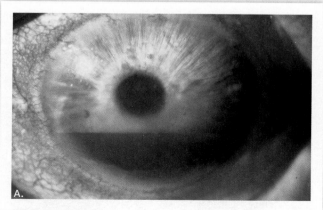

Courtesy of AAOS

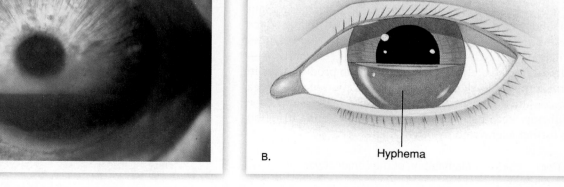

FIGURE 19-14   A. A hyphema, characterized by bleeding into the anterior chamber of the eye, is common following blunt trauma to the eye. This condition may seriously impair vision and should be considered a sight-threatening emergency. B. Illustration of hyphema.

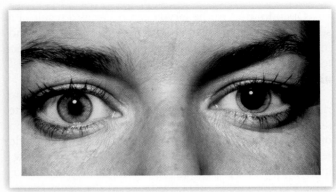

Courtesy of AAOS

FIGURE 19-16 Variation in pupil size may indicate a head injury.

- Failure of the eyes to follow the movement of your finger as instructed
- Bleeding under the conjunctiva, which obscures the sclera (white portion) of the eye
- Protrusion or bulging of one eye

Record any of these observations, along with the time they are made. For an unresponsive patient, keep the eyelids closed, because drying of the ocular tissue can cause permanent injury and may result in blindness. Cover the lids with moist gauze; alternatively, if necessary, hold them closed with clear tape. Normal tears will then keep the tissues moist.

Facial Fractures

Fractures of the facial bones typically result from blunt impact, such as when a patient's head collides with a steering wheel or windshield in an automobile crash or is hit by a baseball bat or pipe in an assault. Assume that any patient who sustained a direct blow to the mouth or nose has a facial fracture. Other clues to the possibility of fracture include bleeding in the mouth, inability to swallow or talk, absent or loose teeth, and loose or movable bone fragments. Patients may also report that "it doesn't feel right" when they close their jaw, signaling an irregularity of bite.

Facial fractures alone are not acute emergencies unless serious bleeding is present; however, they are an indication of significant blunt force trauma applied to that region of the body. Serious bleeding from a facial fracture can be life threatening. In addition to risks associated with external hemorrhage, there is the danger of blood clots lodging in the upper airway and causing an obstruction. Fractures around the face and mouth can also produce deformity and loose bone fragments. Plastic surgeons can repair this kind of damage if the injuries are treated within 7 to 10 days of the injury.

Swelling associated with facial fractures can be extreme within the first 24 hours after injury, and may result in airway obstruction. If you notice swelling during assessment or at any time while the patient is in your care, check for airway obstruction and be prepared to assist with ventilations.

Dental Injuries

Dental injuries can be traumatic to a patient—affecting everything from eating to smiling. Keep this point in mind when providing care.

If a tooth is violently displaced out of its socket, apply direct pressure to stop the bleeding. Suction as necessary, keeping in mind that blood and cracked or loose teeth can obstruct the airway.

When dealing with an avulsed tooth, handle it by its crown and not by the root. When transporting the patient, transport the tooth, placing it in either cold milk or sterile saline. Your agency may also use commercially available kits for this purpose; if so, you should ensure that you are familiar with how the kit is used before you encounter a patient with dental trauma. Notify the receiving facility about the avulsed tooth because reimplantation is recommended within 20 minutes to 1 hour after the trauma.

Be sure to remove and save loose teeth or bone fragments from the mouth, because it is often possible to reimplant them **FIGURE 19-17**. Remove any loose dentures or dental bridges to protect against airway obstruction.

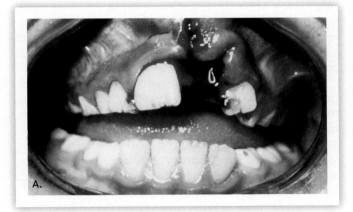

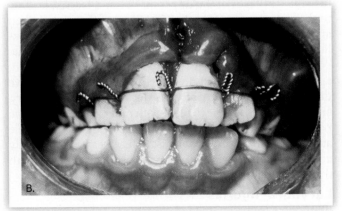

Courtesy of AAOS

FIGURE 19-17 **A.** Save any lost teeth or bone fragments following an injury to the mouth. **B.** Even with traumatic loss of a tooth, the possibility of successful reimplantation is very good.

Injuries to the Neck

Any crushing injury of the upper part of the neck is likely to involve the larynx or trachea. Examples include a collision with a steering wheel, an attempted suicide by hanging, or an off-road biker striking a clothesline or a fixed wire strung across a property line. Once the cartilages forming the upper airway and larynx are fractured, they do not spring back to their normal positions. As a consequence, this type of fracture can lead to loss of voice, difficulty swallowing, severe and sometimes fatal airway obstruction, and leakage of air into the soft tissues of the neck. The presence of air in the soft tissue produces a characteristic crackling sensation called *subcutaneous emphysema*. If you feel this sensation when palpating the neck, maintain the airway as best you can and provide immediate transport.

> *Subcutaneous emphysema* A characteristic crackling sensation felt on palpation of the skin, caused by the presence of air in soft tissues.

As a result of swelling or bleeding into underlying tissues, complete airway obstruction can develop very rapidly in patients with blunt neck injuries. Because it may be very difficult to manage the airway in patients with these injuries, request ALS support early. An incident involving injury to the throat may have also caused a cervical spine injury, requiring spinal stabilization. Always assume a patient with a head or neck injury has cervical spine injury, until proven otherwise.

Penetrating injuries to the neck can cause profuse bleeding from laceration of the great vessels in the neck—that is, the carotid arteries or the jugular veins. When the patient bleeds out, the process is known as exsanguination. Injuries to the great vessels may also allow air to enter the circulatory system, resulting in pulmonary embolism. In addition, the airway, esophagus, and even spinal cord can be damaged by a penetrating injury.

A crushing injury to the upper part of the neck may fracture the cartilages of the upper airway and larynx, leading to the leakage of air into the soft tissue of the neck. When air is trapped in subcutaneous tissue, it produces a crackling sound called crepitation or subcutaneous emphysema.

To manage bleeding of the carotid artery or jugular vein, apply single-digit direct pressure. Apply a sterile occlusive dressing to ensure that air does not enter a vein or artery, and secure the dressing in place with roller gauze around the patient's shoulder (rather than the neck) to avoid possible airway and circulatory problems. If this does not adequately control bleeding, maintain continuous direct pressure with the use of a finger en route to the hospital.

Laryngeal Injuries

Blunt force trauma to the neck can crush the larynx against the cervical spine, resulting in soft-tissue injury, fractures, and/or separation of the fascia that connects the thyroid and cricoid cartilage. These strangulation injuries can also be found in either intentional or unintentional hangings.

Open injuries to the larynx can occur as a result of a stabbing or penetration by a similar object. Penetrating and impaled objects should not be removed unless they interfere with airway maintenance or CPR. Stabilize all impaled objects, providing they are not obstructing the airway.

Significant injuries to the larynx pose an immediate risk of airway compromise because of disruption of the normal passage of air, soft-tissue swelling, or aspiration of blood. Signs and symptoms of larynx injuries include respiratory distress, hoarseness, pain, difficulty swallowing (dysphagia), cyanosis, pale skin, sputum in the wound, subcutaneous emphysema, bruising on the neck, hematoma, or bleeding.

To manage a laryngeal injury, provide oxygenation and ventilation. Apply cervical immobilization but avoid the use of rigid collars, because they may cause further damage to the soft tissues.

Spinal Injuries

The cervical, thoracic, and lumbar portions of the spine can be injured in a variety of ways. Compression injuries can occur as a result of a fall, regardless of whether the patient landed on his or her feet, coccyx, or top of the head. Motor vehicle crashes or other types of trauma can overextend, flex, or rotate the spine. Any one of these unnatural motions, as well as excessive lateral bending, can result in fractures with or without neurologic deficit.

When the spine is pulled along its length, it is called distraction and can cause injuries. For example, hangings often result in fracture of the vertebrae in the upper portion of the cervical spine.

Subluxation of the spine occurs when the vertebrae are no longer aligned. This type of injury pattern may be noted with a hyperextension mechanism or caused by a fracture or a dislocation as well as sports injuries with lateral impact. Common findings include pain and tenderness on palpation of the region. Less frequently you may feel or observe a deformity of the spine, sometimes referred to as a "step-off," where the spinous process may be palpable on physical examination. Regardless of its cause, subluxation is a dangerous injury that can evolve into a debilitating spinal cord injury. If you suspect a subluxation, you should take extra precautions when stabilizing the spine, both manually and with adjuncts.

Emergency medical care of a patient with a possible spinal injury includes maintaining the patient's airway while manually keeping the spine in the proper position, assessing respirations, and providing supplemental oxygen.

▌Injuries to the Chest

Given the location of the heart, lungs, and great blood vessels within the chest cavity, potentially serious injuries may occur with damage to this area of the body. Any injury that interferes with the body's mechanics of normal breathing and circulation must be treated without delay to minimize or prevent permanent damage to tissues that depend on a continuous supply of oxygen.

Blood from lacerations of thoracic organs or major blood vessels can collect in the chest cavity, compressing the lungs or heart. A similar problem may also occur when air collects in the chest and prevents the lungs from expanding. Your ability to act quickly to care for patients with these injuries can make the difference between a successful outcome and death.

Pneumothorax

As was discussed in the *Respiratory Emergencies* chapter, a pneumothorax is the accumulation of air in the pleural space (commonly called a collapsed lung). While this condition can occur spontaneously, a traumatic pneumothorax develops when air enters through a hole in the chest wall or the surface of the lung as the patient attempts to breathe, causing the lung on that side to collapse **FIGURE 19-18**. As a result, any blood that passes through the collapsed portion of the lung is not oxygenated, and hypoxia can develop.

If the lung is collapsed more than 30% to 40%, diminished breath sounds may be evident on that side of the chest. Absent breath sounds are a significant finding in chest trauma and may indicate the development of a tension pneumothorax (discussed later in this section). Depending on the size of the hole and the rate at which air fills the cavity, the lung may collapse in a few seconds or a few hours. If there is a hole in the chest wall, you can actually hear a sucking sound as the patient inhales and the sound of rushing air as he or she exhales. For this reason, an open or penetrating wound to the chest wall is often called an *open pneumothorax* or a sucking chest wound **FIGURE 19-19**.

> *Open pneumothorax* An open or penetrating chest wall wound through which air passes during inspiration and expiration, creating a sucking sound; also referred to as a sucking chest wound.

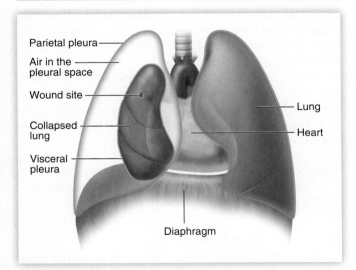

FIGURE 19-18 Pneumothorax occurs when air leaks into the space between the pleural surfaces from an opening in the chest wall or the surface of the lung. The lung collapses as air fills the pleural space.

Parietal pleura
Air in the pleural space
Wound site
Collapsed lung
Visceral pleura
Lung
Heart
Diaphragm

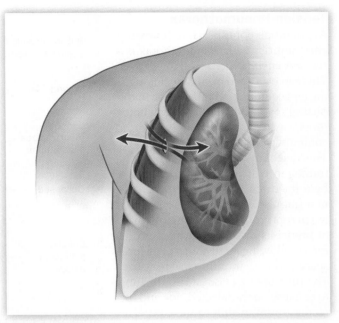

FIGURE 19-19 With a sucking chest wound, air passes from the outside into the pleural space and back out with each breath, creating a sucking sound.

As an AEMT, you should be familiar with treatment of a pneumothorax. For an additional review of this condition, refer to your EMT-I textbook.

Simple Pneumothorax

Any pneumothorax that does not result in major changes in the patient's physiology is referred to as a *simple pneumothorax*. This type of injury is commonly the result of blunt trauma that causes fractured ribs. It is often difficult to diagnose because the lung has to collapse a significant amount before decreased breath sounds are noted.

Patients with a simple pneumothorax may present with tachypnea and tachycardia as a result of hypoxia. As their condition progresses, respiratory distress increases and breath sounds may be decreased or absent on the affected side. Chest wall movement decreases as pressure increases, and hyperresonance can be detected with percussion. The patient may also experience dyspnea, chest pain that is referred to the shoulder or arm on the affected side, and pleuritic chest pain. The patient may also present with subcutaneous emphysema, signs of hypovolemia, or cardiac dysrhythmias.

Immediately cover any open wounds with an occlusive dressing. This is part of the primary assessment. Maintain the ABCs. Use positive-pressure ventilation sparingly because excessive pressure may result in a tension pneumothorax. Call for paramedic backup for treatment of potential cardiac dysrhythmias.

> *Simple pneumothorax* Any pneumothorax that is free from significant physiologic changes and does not cause drastic changes in the vital signs of the patient.

Tension Pneumothorax

A potential complication following chest injuries with pneumothorax is a *tension pneumothorax* **FIGURE 19-20**. This can occur when significant ongoing air accumulation takes place in the pleural space. With a tension pneumothorax, a defect in the airway allows for communication with the pleural space. This defect may be the result of blunt trauma in which a lung is penetrated by a fractured rib, a sudden increase in intrapulmonary pressure culminating in rupture of pulmonary structures, or bronchial disruption from shearing forces, allowing air to enter the pleural space and raise intrathoracic pressure. The pressure increase causes the lung to collapse on the affected side and the mediastinum to shift to the contralateral side. The lung collapse leads to right-to-left intrapulmonary shunting and hypoxia. A reduction in cardiac output occurs as the increased intrathoracic pressure causes compression of the heart and vena cava, reducing preload by decreasing venous return of the heart.

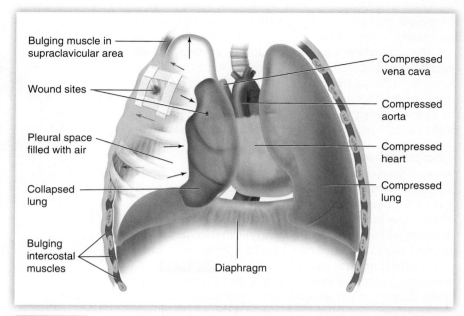

FIGURE 19-20 A tension pneumothorax can develop if a penetrating chest wound is bandaged tightly and air from a damaged lung cannot escape. The air then accumulates in the pleural space, eventually causing compression of the heart and great vessels with resultant circulatory collapse.

Assessment findings in a patient experiencing a pneumothorax that is developing tension include the following:

- Unilaterally decreased or absent breath sounds
- Unequal chest size
- Dyspnea
- Tachypnea
- Respiratory distress
- Extreme anxiety
- Cyanosis
- Bulging of the intercostal muscles
- Tachycardia
- Hypotension
- Narrowed pulse pressure
- Subcutaneous emphysema
- Jugular venous distention
- Tracheal deviation (very late sign)
- Hyperresonance

Tension pneumothorax An accumulation of air or gas in the pleural cavity that progressively increases pressure in the chest, compressing the heart and great vessels and leading eventually to circulatory collapse.

It should be noted that tracheal deviation is a serious late sign and should not be used as the determining factor for initiating invasive treatment.

Maintain the ABCs. Inspect the chest and cover any open wounds with an occlusive or nonporous dressing. If signs of developing tension are present, lift one corner of the dressing to allow air to escape. In the event of a closed tension pneumothorax, call early for paramedic backup to perform a needle chest decompression and for treatment of possible dysrhythmias.

Hemothorax

A *hemothorax* occurs when the potential space between the parietal and visceral pleura is violated and blood begins to accumulate within this space **FIGURE 19-21**. Suspect a hemothorax if a patient has signs and symptoms of shock or decreased breath sounds on the affected side—an indication that the lung is being compressed by the blood. The presence of both air and blood in the pleural space is known as a *hemopneumothorax*. Findings and management are the same as those for a hemothorax.

Manage the ABCs. Provide oxygen and positive-pressure ventilation as needed. If hypovolemia is present, give a fluid bolus, using caution not to increase blood pressure past the point of maintaining perfusion and further increasing bleeding. Provide rapid transport.

Hemothorax A collection of blood in the pleural cavity.
Hemopneumothorax The accumulation of blood and air in the pleural space of the chest.

Cardiac Tamponade

Cardiac tamponade (pericardial tamponade) occurs more commonly in the presence of penetrating chest trauma, although it may also occur in blunt trauma. In cardiac tamponade, blood or other fluid collects in the pericardium,

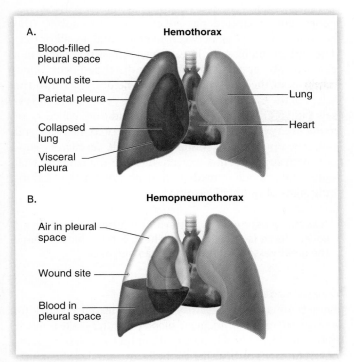

FIGURE 19-21 **A.** A hemothorax is a collection of blood in the pleural space produced by bleeding within the chest. **B.** When both blood and air are present, the condition is called a hemopneumothorax.

the fibrous sac surrounding the heart **FIGURE 19-22**. Accumulation of fluid over minutes to hours leads to increases in intrapericardial pressure. This pressure compresses the heart and decreases cardiac output. It also hampers venous return. Ultimately, as blood accumulates within the pericardial sac, it compresses the heart until it can no longer function and circulatory collapse results.

> *Cardiac tamponade (pericardial tamponade)* Compression of the heart as a result of buildup of blood or other fluid in the pericardial sac, leading to decreased cardiac output.

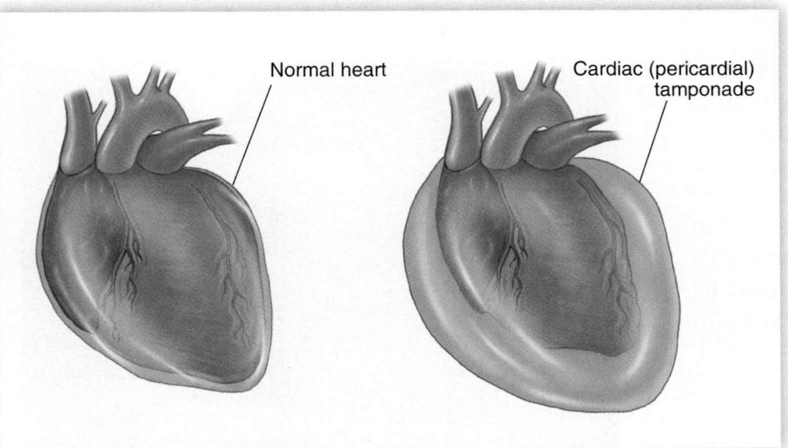

FIGURE 19-22 Cardiac (pericardial) tamponade is a potentially fatal condition in which fluid builds up within the pericardial sac, causing compression of the heart's chambers and dramatically impairing its ability to pump blood to the body.

Signs and symptoms of cardiac tamponade include tachycardia with a weak pulse, respiratory distress, soft, faint heart tones, often called muffled heart sounds, low blood pressure, narrowed pulse pressure, increased diastolic pressure, and jugular vein distention. The patient may also present with pulsus paradoxus or cyanosis in the face, neck, and upper extremities. The Beck triad—composed of narrowing pulse pressure, neck vein distention, and muffled heart tones—makes up the classic signs for diagnosing a cardiac tamponade. However, these signs occur in the advanced stage.

Assess and manage the ABCs, providing oxygen and positive-pressure ventilation as needed. Obtain IV access as a medication route and provide fluid therapy only if the patient becomes hypotensive. Provide rapid transport and call for paramedic backup for treatment of dysrhythmias.

Rib Fractures

A fractured rib that penetrates into the pleural space may lacerate the surface of the lung, causing a pneumothorax, tension pneumothorax, hemothorax, or hemopneumothorax. One sign of this development can be a crackly feeling to the skin in the area (called crepitus or subcutaneous emphysema), which indicates that air is escaping from a lacerated lung and leaking into the chest wall. Be sure to relay this finding to hospital personnel.

Management of rib fractures focuses on decreasing movement, thereby decreasing pain, which allows for better depth of respirations. Allowing the patient to hold a pillow against the affected area can be effective. Note that in young children, the rib cage is very flexible and does not provide the same level of protection as in the adult. This flexibility can allow any significant injury or compression of the rib cage to be masked as the ribs give way to the pressure and do not fracture. Understand, however, that the organs that underlie the rib cage have been exposed to a significant force and are likely injured.

Flail Chest

It is possible for ribs to fracture in more than one place. If several ribs are fractured in two or more places or if the sternum is fractured along with several ribs, a segment of chest wall may become detached from the rest of the thoracic cage **FIGURE 19-23**. This condition is known as flail chest. In what is called paradoxical motion, the detached portion of the chest wall moves in the opposite direction of normal. It moves in instead of out during inhalation, and out instead of in during exhalation. This effect occurs because of the negative pressure that builds up in the thorax. Breathing with a flail chest can be painful and ineffective, rapidly leading to hypoxemia. A flail segment interferes with the body's normal mechanics of ventilation and must be addressed quickly.

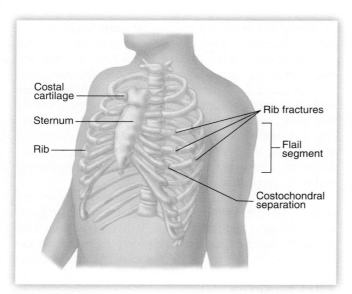

FIGURE 19-23 When several adjacent ribs are fractured in two or more places, a flail chest results. A flail segment shows paradoxical motion when the patient breathes.

Treatment of a patient with a flail chest should focus on maintaining a patent airway, providing respiratory support as necessary, giving supplemental oxygen, and performing ongoing assessments for possible pneumothorax or other respiratory complications. Treatment may also include positive-pressure ventilation with a bag-mask device.

Transition Tip

Stabilizing a flail segment is a controversial issue. Current guidelines suggest that providing positive-pressure ventilation provides internal stabilization and increases oxygenation and ventilation for management of a pulmonary contusion. However, some recent studies have shown that patients may benefit from early operative stabilization with plates and screws to decrease the incidence of further acute complications.

In addition to fracturing ribs, any severe blunt trauma to the chest can injure or bruise the lungs. The pulmonary alveoli may become filled with blood, and fluid can accumulate in the injured area, leaving the patient hypoxic. Severe pulmonary contusion usually develops within a period of hours and should always be suspected in patients with a flail chest. Provide respiratory support and supplemental oxygen to ensure adequate ventilation if you suspect a pulmonary contusion.

Traumatic Asphyxia

Sometimes a patient will experience a sudden, severe compression of the chest, which produces a rapid increase in pressure within the chest. This condition may occur in an unrestrained driver who hits a steering wheel or in a pedestrian or ejected passenger of an automobile who becomes compressed between a vehicle and a wall or tree. The sudden increase in intrathoracic pressure results in a characteristic appearance including distended neck veins, cyanosis in the face and neck, and hemorrhage into the sclera of the eye, signaling the bursting of small blood vessels **FIGURE 19-24**. Findings in this condition, called *traumatic asphyxia*, suggest underlying injury to the heart and possibly a pulmonary contusion. Provide ventilatory support with supplemental oxygen, monitor the patient's vital signs, and provide immediate transport of a patient exhibiting signs of traumatic asphyxia.

> *Traumatic asphyxia* A pattern of injuries seen after a severe force is applied to the chest, forcing blood from the great vessels back into the head and neck.

Myocardial Contusion

Blunt trauma to the chest may injure the heart itself, making it unable to maintain adequate blood pressure. There is much debate in the medical literature about how to assess *myocardial contusion*, or bruising of the heart muscle. Maintain a high index of suspicion for serious injury with blunt chest trauma. Clinical signs will vary based on the area of injury—affected areas include vessels, the myocardium, or the conduction system. Associated injuries include one to three rib fractures and/or a sternal fracture. The patient may also present with retrosternal chest pain. The patient may or may not show external signs, such as bruising. Often the pulse rate is irregular, but life-threatening rhythms such as ventricular tachycardia and ventricular fibrillation are uncommon. The patient may experience a new cardiac murmur.

When you are treating a patient for a myocardial contusion, stay alert for signs of heart failure and beware of administering too much fluid if these signs appear. Assess for jugular vein distention and pulmonary edema. Call for paramedic backup early, and monitor carefully for rapid

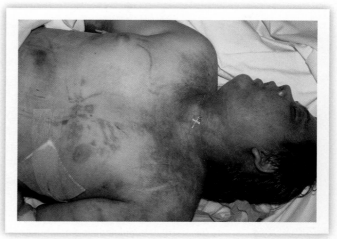

© Chuck Stewart, MD.
FIGURE 19-24 Traumatic asphyxia.

deterioration if the patient presents with tachycardia or an irregular pulse.

> *Myocardial contusion* A bruise of the heart muscle.

Commotio Cordis

Commotio cordis is a blunt chest injury caused by a sudden, direct blow to the chest (over the heart) that occurs only during the critical portion of a person's heartbeat. The result may be immediate cardiac arrest. This phenomenon has been documented to have occurred after patients were struck with softballs, baseballs, bats, snowballs, fists, and even kicks during kickboxing. The blow to the chest typically occurs at speeds in the range of 35 to 40 mph. This blunt force causes a lethal abnormal heart rhythm called ventricular fibrillation, which responds positively to early defibrillation if provided within the first 2 minutes after the injury. Commotio cordis is more commonly associated with sports-related injuries, although you should maintain a high index of suspicion for this condition in all cases in which the person is unresponsive after a blow to the chest.

> *Commotio cordis* A blunt chest injury caused by a sudden, direct blow to the chest that occurs during the critical portion of a person's heartbeat.

Penetrating Wounds of the Great Vessels

The chest contains several large blood vessels: the superior vena cava, the inferior vena cava, the pulmonary arteries, four main pulmonary veins, and the aorta, with its major branches that distribute blood throughout the body. The abdominal aorta and inferior vena cava travel through the abdomen, and the carotid arteries and external jugular veins are located in the neck. Wounds to any of these vessels may be accompanied by massive hemothorax, hypovolemic shock, cardiac tamponade, and enlarging hematomas. Frequently, blood loss is not obvious because it remains within the chest cavity. Hematomas may cause compression of any structure, including the vena cava, trachea, esophagus, great vessels, or heart. Here, particularly, immediate transport to the hospital is critical—a few minutes can mean the difference between life and death.

■ Injuries to the Abdomen

Hollow and Solid Organs

The abdomen contains both hollow and solid organs, any of which may be damaged by trauma. *Hollow organs*, including the stomach, intestines, ureters, and bladder, are structures through which materials pass FIGURE 19-25 . Most of these organs contain food in the process of being digested, urine being passed to the bladder for release, or bile. When ruptured or lacerated, the abdominal organs may spill their acidic contents into the *peritoneal cavity*, setting off an intense inflammatory response (*peritonitis*) that may cause

significant damage to the entire peritoneum and eventually lead to a potentially fatal infection.

> *Hollow organs* Structures through which materials pass, such as the stomach, small intestines, large intestines, ureters, and bladder.
> *Peritoneal cavity* The abdominal cavity.
> *Peritonitis* Inflammation of the peritoneum.

The small intestine is composed of the duodenum, jejunum, and ileum. The large intestine consists of the cecum, colon, and rectum. The intestinal blood supply comes from the mesentery, a fold of tissue that contains a web of vessels, both arteries and veins, as well as nerves and lymphatic tissues. The mesentery connects the small intestine to the posterior abdominal wall. Both blunt and penetrating abdominal injuries can affect this vasculature, resulting in significant bleeding into the peritoneal cavity. A common sign of internal abdominal bleeding is rigidity, with an almost board-like feeling to the abdomen being noted. Occasionally you will find periumbilical bruising or ecchymosis, referred to as the Cullen sign.

Solid organs include the liver, spleen, pancreas, and kidneys FIGURE 19-26 . If injured, these organs can cause significant and rapid blood loss that can be difficult to identify because the patient often does not experience significant pain. Conversely, the organs can slowly ooze blood into the peritoneal cavity, increasing the chance for toxicity to develop, and causing pain to increase slowly over time. Blood in the peritoneal cavity irritates tissue and fills any voids or spaces, making it difficult to determine the exact source of the bleeding.

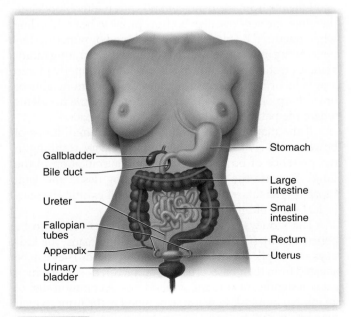

FIGURE 19-25 The hollow organs in the abdominal cavity are structures through which materials pass.

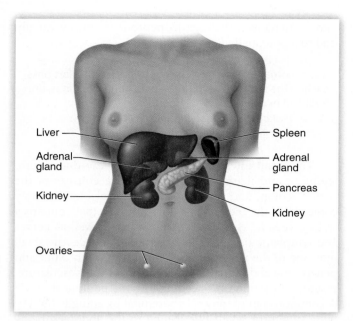

FIGURE 19-26 The solid organs are solid masses of tissue that do much of the chemical work in the body and receive a large, rich supply of blood.

> *Solid organs* Solid masses of tissue in which much of the chemical work of the body takes place (eg, the liver, spleen, pancreas, and kidneys).

The liver—the largest organ in the abdomen—is very vascular. If it is injured, the subsequent blood loss can contribute to hypoperfusion. The liver is often injured by a fractured lower right rib or with penetrating trauma, such as a knife wound.

Like the liver, the pancreas and spleen filter blood and, therefore, are very vascular. Both are prone to heavy bleeding when fractured by blunt force or lacerated or punctured by penetrating injury. The spleen is often injured during motor vehicle crashes, especially in the case of improperly placed seat belts or from the steering wheel, falls from heights or onto sharp objects, and bicycle and motorcycle accidents where the patient hits the handlebars on impact.

If the diaphragm is penetrated or ruptured, loops of bowel are likely to invade the thoracic cavity, resulting in the presence of bowel sounds during auscultation of the lungs. Because the bowel displaces lung tissue and vital capacity, patients with this condition will exhibit dyspnea or feel short of breath.

The kidneys in the retroperitoneal space can also be penetrated by trauma. Like other filtering organs, the kidneys are supplied with large quantities of blood. They can be sheared from their base, crushed, or fractured—all of which cause a significant amount of blood loss. A common sign of an injured kidney is hematuria, or blood in the urine, which may be difficult to detect in the prehospital environment.

Closed Abdominal Injuries

Closed abdominal injuries are those in which blunt force trauma, involving some type of impact to the body, results in injury to the abdomen without breaking the skin. Compression injuries are typically caused by a poorly placed lap belt or when a person is run or rolled over by vehicles or objects. Deceleration injuries commonly occur when a person or the vehicle in which he or she is traveling strikes a large immovable mass such as a larger vehicle, a bridge abutment, or the ground.

In the abdomen, pain can often be deceiving because it is frequently diffuse in nature and may be referred from the site of injury to another location in the body. Most injured organs irritate the surrounding tissues. This commonly predictable radiation pattern can help you determine the source of the pain and possibly the site of the injury. *Kehr sign* is the presence of acute pain in the tip of the shoulder resulting from the presence of blood or other irritants in the peritoneal cavity when a person is lying down and the legs are elevated. Kehr sign in the left shoulder is a classic sign of a ruptured spleen.

> *Kehr sign* Left shoulder pain caused by blood in the peritoneal cavity.

A complaint described as a tearing pain from the abdomen posteriorly often indicates a dissecting abdominal aneurysm. Pain following the angle from the lateral hip to the midline of the groin can be the result of damage to the kidneys or the ureters. Pain primarily located in the right lower quadrant can indicate an inflamed or ruptured appendix. Pain from the gallbladder caused by direct injury or inflammation can be found just under the margin of the ribs on the right side or between the shoulder blades.

> ### Transition Tip
>
> Although pain is the most common symptom of abdominal injury, other significant injuries may mask the pain at first, or the patient may be unresponsive or have altered consciousness, such as after a head injury or a drug or alcohol overdose. Be mindful that the patient may have suffered internal abdominal injury if the MOI is significant.

Determining the location of the pain or referred pain can be more difficult when the patient has voluntary or involuntary guarding. In guarding, the patient consciously or unintentionally stiffens the muscles of the surface of the abdomen. Most often it is the rectus abdominis muscles (that run from the pubis to the xiphoid process) that are held tight, and that tightness can be mistaken for abdominal rigidity. This stiffening is a natural response to abdominal pain; the body is attempting to splint the area to prevent unnecessary movement and to avoid further pain.

Closed abdominal injuries may initially appear as abrasions to the surface of the skin depending on the MOI. In some circumstances, depending on how deep in the abdomen the injury occurs, it may take several minutes to hours for the contusion or hematoma to become visible on the surface. As such, you should not rule out injury based solely on the absence of these findings. For example, when worn properly, a seat belt lies below the anterior superior iliac spines of the pelvis and against the hip joints. If the belt is positioned too high, it can squeeze abdominal organs or great vessels against the spine when the car suddenly decelerates or stops **FIGURE 19-27** .

In later stages of pregnancy, the gravid uterus displaces the bladder anteriorly. This anatomic change renders the normally protected bladder more susceptible to injuries from impacts and the seat belt in motor vehicle crashes. Pregnant patients who adjust the lap belt portion for comfort as opposed to functionality may sustain additional injuries.

Open Abdominal Injuries

In open abdominal injuries, also known as penetrating injuries, a foreign object enters the abdomen and opens the peritoneal cavity to the outside **FIGURE 19-28** . Stab wounds and gunshot wounds are examples of penetrating trauma.

Laceration of the abdomen may cause the intestines to protrude (*eviscerate*). Refer to your EMT-I textbook for a review of abdominal eviscerations. If the injury causes the abdominal contents to spill or leak into the peritoneal cavity, pain and irritation often follow.

Eviscerate To displace organs outside the body.

When a patient has sustained a penetrating injury from a gunshot, it is important to attempt to determine the velocity of the object that penetrated the abdominal wall so as to predict the amount of damage to tissue that has occurred. Three levels of velocities relative to traumatic injuries are distinguished, all of which have the capacity to cause internal damage not apparent during the physical examination:

- **Low-velocity injuries** may be caused by handheld or hand-powered objects such as knives and other edged weapons.
- **Medium-velocity penetrating wounds** may be caused by smaller caliber handguns and shotguns. They create entrance and exit wounds in addition to tissue damage caused by cavitation.
- **High-velocity injuries** may be caused by larger weapons such as high-powered rifles and the higher-powered handguns. They create entrance and exit wounds in addition to tissue damage caused by cavitation.

Tachycardia combined with trauma to the abdomen is a sign of significant abdominal injury indicating compensated hemorrhagic shock. Later signs of progressing shock include decreased blood pressure and pale, cool, moist skin, or changes in the patient's mental status. In some cases, the abdomen may become distended and rigid from the

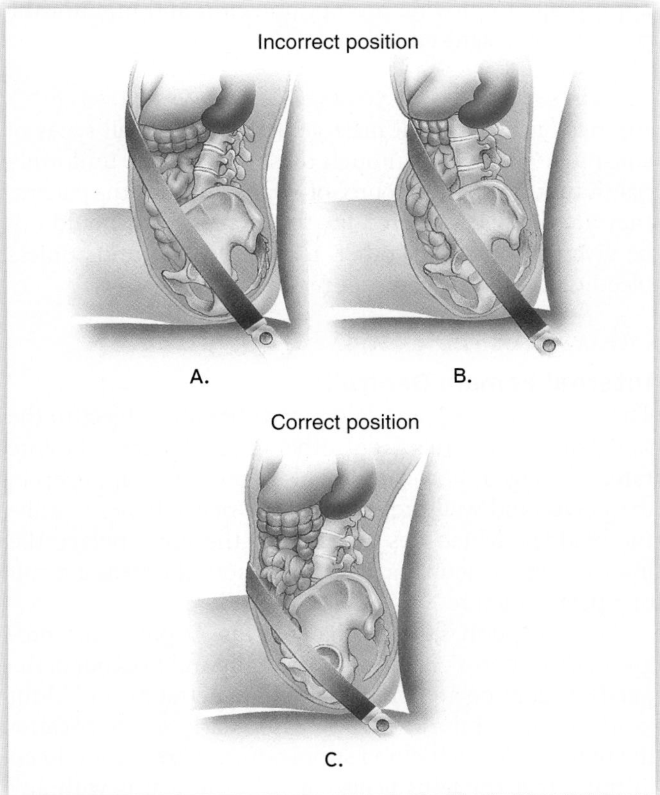

FIGURE 19-27 A. and B. Improper positioning of seat belts. C. The proper position for a seat belt is below the anterior superior iliac spines of the pelvis and against the hip joints.

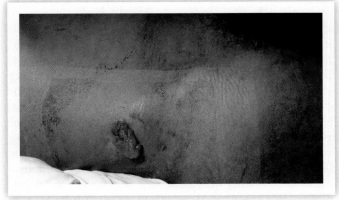

© M. English, MD/Custom Medical Stock Photo

FIGURE 19-28 Because it is difficult to know how deep a penetrating injury is, assume organ damage and transport the patient with an open abdominal injury promptly.

accumulation of blood and fluid, and the patient may feel nauseated and vomit.

Emergency care of abdominal injuries has not changed in the new standards and includes the following measures:

- Monitor ABCs and manage life threats.
- Control external bleeding.
- Stabilize any impaled objects.
- Apply a moist abdominal dressing and cover eviscerations.
- Treat for shock.
- Provide rapid transport to an appropriate facility.

Injuries to the Genitourinary System

Injuries of the Kidney

Injuries of the kidney are not unusual, but rarely occur in isolation because the kidneys lie in a well-protected area of the body. A penetrating wound that reaches the kidneys almost always involves other organs; the same is true with blunt injuries. A blow forceful enough to cause significant kidney damage often results in damage to other intra-abdominal organs. Less significant injuries to the kidneys may result from a direct blow or even from a tackle in football.

Suspect kidney damage if the patient has a history or physical evidence of any of the following:

- An abrasion, laceration, or contusion in the flank
- A penetrating wound in the region of the lower rib cage (the flank) or the upper abdomen
- Fractures on either side of the lower rib cage or of the lower thoracic or upper lumbar vertebrae
- A hematoma in the flank region

When caring for a patient with possible injury of a kidney, treat the patient for shock and associated injuries in the appropriate manner. Provide prompt transport to the hospital, monitoring the patient's vital signs carefully en route.

Injuries to the Urinary Bladder

Injury to the bladder, either blunt or penetrating, may result in rupture of this organ. When this happens, urine spills into the surrounding tissues, and any urine that passes through the urethra is likely to be bloody. Blunt injuries to the lower abdomen or pelvis often cause rupture of the urinary bladder, particularly when the bladder is full and distended. Sharp, bony fragments from a fracture of the pelvis often perforate the urinary bladder **FIGURE 19-29**. Penetrating wounds of the lower abdomen or the perineum (the pelvic floor and associated structures that occupy the pelvic outlet) can directly involve the bladder. In the male, sudden deceleration from a motor vehicle or motorcycle crash can literally shear the bladder from the urethra. In the female, during the last trimester of pregnancy, the bladder is displaced by the uterus, rendering it more susceptible to injury.

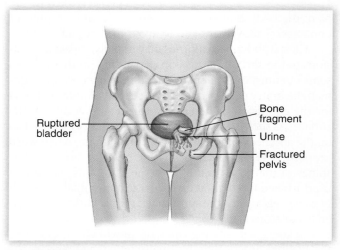

FIGURE 19-29 Fracture of the pelvis can result in laceration of the bladder by the bony fragments. Urine then leaks into the pelvis.

Suspect injury to the urinary bladder if there is blood at the urethral opening or physical signs of trauma on the lower abdomen, pelvis, or perineum. Blood at the tip of the penis or a stain on the patient's underwear may be noted as well. The presence of associated injuries or of shock will dictate the urgency of transport. In most instances, it is appropriate to provide prompt transport and monitor the patient's vital signs en route.

Injuries of the External Male Genitalia

Injuries of the external male genitalia include all types of soft-tissue wounds. Although these injuries are uniformly painful and generally a source of great concern to the patient, they are rarely considered life threatening and should not be given priority over other, more severe wounds unless bleeding cannot be controlled.

Injuries of the Female Genitalia

Internal Female Genitalia

The uterus, ovaries, and fallopian tubes are subject to the same kinds of injuries as any other internal organ. They are rarely damaged, however, because they are small, deep in the pelvis, and well protected by the pelvic bones. Unlike the bladder, which lies adjacent to the bony pelvis, the internal female genitalia are usually not injured as a result of a pelvic fracture.

An exception is the pregnant uterus. As pregnancy progresses, the uterus enlarges substantially and rises out of the pelvis, becoming vulnerable to both penetrating and blunt injuries. These injuries can be particularly severe because the uterus has a rich blood supply during pregnancy. Keep in mind that the fetus is also at risk just as it is with any injury that puts the mother's health in jeopardy. Expect to see the signs and symptoms of shock when these patients experience abdominal injuries.

Provide high-flow oxygen, carefully place the patient on her left side so that the uterus will not lie on the vena cava, and provide prompt transport to an appropriate facility. If the patient is secured to a backboard, tilt the entire board to the left.

External Female Genitalia

The external female genitalia include the vulva, the clitoris, and the major and minor labia (lips) at the entrance of the vagina. Injuries of the external female genitalia can include all types of soft-tissue injuries.

In any case of trauma involving a female patient, it is important to attempt to determine the possibility of pregnancy. Ask the patient for the date of her last known menstrual period or ask whether she has been sexually active. The assumption is that all women of childbearing age are possibly pregnant. This information is medically relevant because certain medications and tests are harmful to the fetus; additional blood loss in the gravid uterus is also a possibility.

In cases of external bleeding and trauma to the external female genitalia, a sterile absorbent sanitary napkin or pad may be applied to the labia. Do not insert instruments, gloved fingers, or a tampon into the vagina, because this can cause further damage.

■ Musculoskeletal Injuries

Musculoskeletal system injuries are often easily identified because of associated pain, swelling, and deformity. Although these injuries are rarely fatal, they frequently result in short- or long-term disability. Providing prompt assessment and treatment may help reduce disability for patients. Despite the sometimes dramatic appearance of these injuries, it is important not to focus solely on a musculoskeletal injury without first determining that no life-threatening injuries exist. Never forget the primary assessment!

Mechanism of Injury

In a healthy person, significant force is generally required to cause fractures and dislocations. This force may be applied to the limb in any of the following ways **FIGURE 19-30**:

- Direct blows (example: the patient's kneecap fractures on impact with the ground)
- Indirect forces (example: a person falls and lands on an outstretched hand resulting in a humerus fracture)
- Twisting forces (a skier becomes caught and falls, applying a twisting force to the tibia)
- High-energy injury (tibial fracture secondary to crush injury)

Types of Musculoskeletal Injuries

A *fracture* is a broken bone. More precisely, it is a break in the continuity of the bone, often occurring as a result of an external force **FIGURE 19-31**. Fractures are classified as either closed or open and are described based on whether

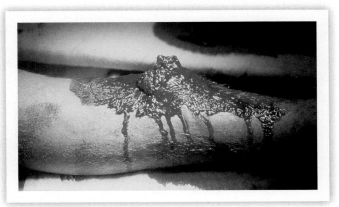

Courtesy of AAOS

FIGURE 19-31 A fracture can occur anywhere on the surface of a bone and may or may not break the skin.

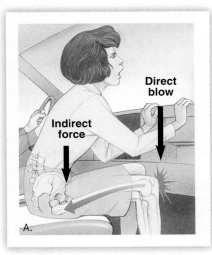

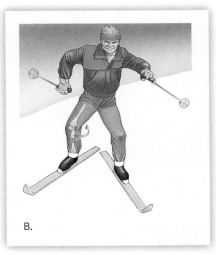

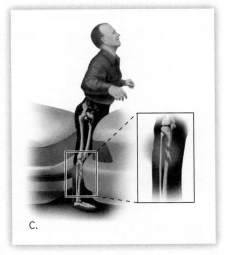

FIGURE 19-30 Significant force is required to cause fractures or dislocations. **A.** Direct blows and indirect forces. **B.** Twisting forces. **C.** High-energy injuries.

the bone is moved from its normal position. A nondisplaced fracture (also known as a hairline fracture) is a simple crack of the bone that may be difficult to distinguish from a sprain or simple contusion. X-ray examinations are required for hospital personnel to diagnose a nondisplaced fracture. A displaced fracture produces actual deformity, or distortion, of the limb by shortening, rotating, or angulating it. Aside from pain, many signs and symptoms of a fracture are possible **TABLE 19-5**.

> *Fracture* A break in the continuity of a bone.

Medical personnel often use special terms to describe particular types of fractures **FIGURE 19-32**.

Transition Tip

The new *National EMS Education Standards* use the term "fracture" instead of "painful swollen deformity"; this term means a broken bone.

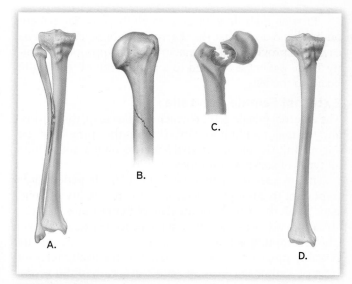

FIGURE 19-32 Special terms to describe fractures. **A.** Greenstick fracture. **B.** Oblique fracture. **C.** Pathologic fracture. **D.** Incomplete fracture.

A *dislocation* is a disruption of a joint in which the bone ends are no longer in contact. The supporting ligaments are often torn, usually completely, allowing the bone ends to

Table 19-5 Signs and Symptoms of Fractures	
Deformity	The limb may appear to be shortened, rotated, or angulated at a point where there is no joint.
Tenderness	Point tenderness may be apparent on palpation in the zone of injury.
Guarding	An inability to use the extremity is the patient's way of immobilizing it to minimize pain.
Swelling	Generalized swelling from fluid buildup may occur several hours after an injury.
Bruising	Within hours or days, blue, purple, and black bruises will appear, followed by yellows and greens as the injured area begins to heal.
Crepitus	A grating or grinding sensation can be felt and sometimes even heard when fractured bone ends rub together.
False motion	Also called free movement, this is motion at a point in the limb where there is no joint.
Exposed fragments	Bone ends may protrude through the skin or be visible within the wound.
Locked joint	A joint that is locked into position is difficult and painful to move.

separate completely from each other **FIGURE 19-33**. A dislocated joint sometimes will spontaneously reduce, or return to its normal position, before your assessment. In this situation, you will be able to confirm the dislocation only by taking a patient history. Often, however, injury to the supporting ligaments and capsule is so severe that the joint surfaces remain completely separated from each other. A dislocation that does not spontaneously reduce is a serious problem. The ends of the bone can become locked in a displaced position, making any attempt to move the joint very difficult and very painful. Commonly dislocated joints include the fingers, shoulder, elbow, and knee. The signs and symptoms of a dislocated joint are similar to those noted with a fracture.

> *Dislocation* Disruption of a joint in which ligaments are damaged and the bone ends become completely displaced.

A *subluxation* is similar to a dislocation except the disruption of the joints is not complete. In other words, a subluxation is an incomplete dislocation of a joint. A fracture-dislocation is a combination injury at the joint in which the joint is dislocated and there is a fracture of the end of one or more of the bones.

> *Subluxation* A partial or incomplete dislocation of a joint.

A *sprain* occurs when a joint is twisted or stretched beyond its normal range of motion. As a result, the supporting capsule and ligaments are stretched or torn. A sprain, particulary a significant sprain, can be considered to be similar to a partial dislocation or subluxation. After the injury, the joint surfaces generally fall back into alignment, so the joint does not remain displaced. Sprains can range from mild to severe, depending on the amount of damage

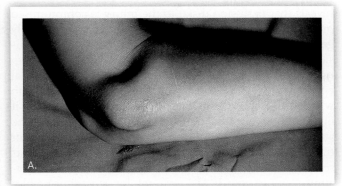

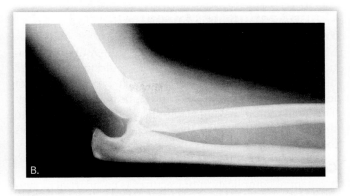

Courtesy of AAOS

FIGURE 19-33 A dislocation is a disruption of a joint in which the bone ends are no longer in contact with each other. **A.** The clinical appearance of an elbow dislocation. **B.** X-ray of the same elbow.

done to the supporting ligaments. The most severe sprains involve actual tearing of the ligament and may allow joint dislocation. Mild sprains are caused by ligament stretching rather than tearing. The joints most vulnerable to this type of injury are the knees, shoulders, and ankles **FIGURE 19-34**.

> *Sprain* A joint injury involving damage to supporting ligaments, and sometimes partial or temporary dislocation of bone ends.

A *strain*, or muscle pull, is a stretching or tearing of the muscle, causing pain, swelling, and bruising of the soft tissues in the area. It occurs because of an abnormal contraction. Strains may range from minute separation to complete rupture. Unlike with a sprain, no ligament or joint damage typically occurs with a strain.

> *Strain* Stretching or tearing of a muscle; also called a muscle pull.

An amputation is an injury in which an extremity is completely severed from the body. Such an injury can potentially damage every aspect of the musculoskeletal system—from bone to ligament to muscle.

Injury to bones and joints is often associated with injury to the surrounding soft tissues, especially to the adjacent nerves and blood vessels. The entire area affected is known as the zone of injury. Depending on the amount of kinetic energy the tissues absorb from forces acting on the body, this zone may extend to a distant point. For this reason, you should not focus on a patient's obvious injury without first completing a rapid scan to check for associated injuries, which may be even more serious. This is especially true when assessing damage from high-energy trauma or gunshots.

> **Transition Tip**
>
> The most common life-threatening musculoskeletal injuries are multiple fractures, open fractures with arterial bleeding, pelvic fractures, bilateral femur fractures, and limb amputations.

A significant MOI is not necessary to fracture a bone in an elderly person. Even a slight force can easily fracture a bone that is weakened by a tumor or osteoporosis, a generalized bone disease common among postmenopausal women. In geriatric patients with osteoporosis, minor falls, simple twisting injuries, or even a muscle contraction can cause a fracture, most often of the wrist, spine, or hip. You should suspect the presence of a fracture in any older patient who has sustained even a mild injury.

> **Transition Tip**
>
> Because it is impossible to differentiate between strains, sprains, dislocations, and fractures in the field, treatment for all of these conditions is the same—primarily splinting the injured extremity.

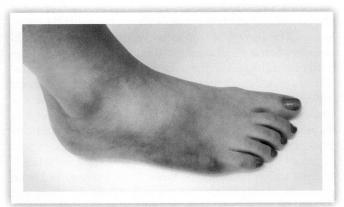

© Sean Gladwell/Dreamstime.com

FIGURE 19-34 Sprains most often occur in the knee or ankle and are characterized by swelling, bruising, point tenderness, pain, and joint instability.

Complications of Musculoskeletal Injuries

Musculoskeletal injuries can lead to numerous complications—not just those involving the musculoskeletal system, but also systemic changes or illness. It is essential to not focus all of your attention on the musculoskeletal injury. The likelihood of having a complication is often related to the magnitude of the force that caused the injury, the injury's location, and the patient's overall health.

Compartment Syndrome

A potential complication of fractures is compartment syndrome. Within a limb, groups of muscles are surrounded by an inelastic membrane called fascia that confines the muscles to an enclosed space, or compartment. This compartment can accommodate only a limited amount of swelling. When bleeding or swelling occurs within a compartment as the result of a fracture or severe soft-tissue injury, the pressure within it rises. Pressure that is too high may impair circulation and lead to pain, sensory changes, and progressive muscle death. This condition, known as compartment syndrome, is one of the most devastating consequences of a musculoskeletal injury. The longer this situation persists, the greater the chance for tissue necrosis.

Be on the alert for compartment syndrome, which most commonly occurs with a fractured tibia or forearm of children and is often overlooked, especially in patients with an altered level of consciousness. Compartment syndrome typically develops within 6 to 12 hours after injury, usually as a result of excessive bleeding, a severely crushed extremity, or the rapid return of blood to an ischemic limb. It is characterized by pain that is out of proportion to the injury, pain on passive stretch of muscles within the compartment, pallor, decreased sensation, and decreased power (ranging from decreased strength and movement of the limb to complete paralysis). A common scenario in which you might encounter compartment syndrome is that of a child who breaks his or her forearm, goes to the emergency room, and has it treated in a cast. The cast can further restrict the capacity of the limb to tolerate swelling. Hours after the child is discharged, compartment syndrome can develop in the limb, triggering the parents to call EMS. Do not mistake these scenarios for routine post-injury pain or be comforted at all that the child was already treated for the injury in the hospital.

Splinting Extremity Injuries

As a general rule, you should splint an orthopaedic injury in the position in which it was found, provided that distal perfusion is intact. In some cases, an injured extremity may be so severely angulated that gentle longitudinal traction may be required to splint the injury effectively, even if distal perfusion is adequate.

Always assess pulses, motor function, and sensation (PMS) before and after application of a splint. If assessment reveals that perfusion distal to the injury is compromised or absent (ie, pallor, absent distal pulses, cold skin), apply gentle longitudinal traction to realign the limb until perfusion is restored. The goal is *not* to return the extremity to its normal anatomic position, but rather to restore distal circulation. In many cases, gentle realignment of the limb will be sufficient to restore adequate perfusion; however, if one attempt (your local protocol may dictate more than one attempt) at realignment is unsuccessful, you should splint the injury in the position found, transport the patient as soon as possible, and notify the receiving facility of the situation. Refer to your EMT-I textbook for general principles and specific steps for applying splints.

■ Environmental Emergencies

Submersion Incidents

Drowning is the process of experiencing respiratory impairment from submersion/immersion in liquid. Some agencies may still use the term "near drowning" to refer to a patient who survives at least temporarily (24 hours) after suffocation in water.

Drowning is often the last stage in a cycle of events caused by panic in the water. It can happen to anyone submerged in water for even a short period of time. Small children can drown in only a few inches of water if left unattended.

> **Transition Tip**
>
> Nothing has changed in the *National EMS Education Standards* regarding hot and cold emergencies or the ways in which they are assessed or managed. As such, they are not discussed in this text. For a review of these types of emergencies, refer to your EMT-I textbook.

Inhaling very small amounts of either fresh water or salt water can severely irritate the larynx, sending the muscles of the larynx and the vocal cords into spasm, called laryngospasm. The average person experiences this effect to a mild degree when a small amount of liquid is inhaled and the patient coughs and seems to be choking for a few seconds. This is the body's attempt at self-preservation; laryngospasm prevents more water from entering the lungs. In severe cases such as water submersion, however, the patient's lungs cannot be ventilated because significant laryngospasm is present. Instead, progressive hypoxia occurs until the patient becomes unresponsive. At this point, the spasm relaxes, making rescue breathing possible. If not yet removed from the water, however, the patient may inhale deeply at this point, and more water may enter the lungs. In 85% to 90% of drowning cases, significant amounts of water enter the lungs of the victim.

Some submersion incidents may be complicated by spinal fractures and spinal cord injuries. Assume that spinal injury exists with the following situations:

- The submersion resulted from a diving mishap or fall from a significant height.
- The patient is unresponsive and no information is available to rule out the possibility of a mechanism causing neck injury.
- The patient is conscious but complains of weakness, paralysis, or numbness in the arms or legs.

Diving Emergencies

Most serious water-related injuries are associated with dives, with or without scuba gear. Some of these problems are related to the nature of the dive; others result from panic.

Medical problems relating to scuba diving techniques and equipment are becoming increasingly common. These problems are separated into three phases of the dive: descent, bottom, and ascent.

Descent problems are usually caused by the sudden increase in pressure on the body as the person moves deeper into the water. Some body cavities cannot adjust to the increased external pressure of the water; the result is severe pain. The areas most commonly affected are the lungs, sinus cavities, middle ear, teeth, and the area of the face surrounded by the diving mask. Usually, the pain caused by these "squeeze problems" forces the diver to return to the surface to equalize pressures, and the problem resolves on its own. A diver who continues to complain of pain, particularly in the ear, after returning to the surface should be transported to the hospital.

A person with a perforated tympanic membrane (ruptured eardrum) may develop a special problem while diving. If cold water enters the middle ear through a ruptured eardrum, the diver may lose his or her balance and orientation, then shoot to the surface and run into ascent problems.

Problems related to the bottom of the dive are rarely seen and usually result from faulty connections in the diving gear. They include inadequate mixing of oxygen and carbon dioxide in the air that the diver breathes, and accidental feeding of poisonous carbon monoxide into the breathing apparatus. Both of these situations can cause drowning, or if recognized by the diver, result in rapid ascent, requiring emergency resuscitation and transport of the patient.

Most serious injuries associated with diving are related to ascending from the bottom and are referred to as ascent problems. These conditions usually require aggressive resuscitation. Two particularly dangerous medical emergencies are air embolism and decompression sickness (also called "the bends").

Air Embolism

The most dangerous, and most commonly encountered emergency in scuba diving is air embolism, a condition involving bubbles of air in the blood vessels. Air embolism may occur on a dive as shallow as 6 feet. This problem starts when the diver holds his or her breath during a rapid ascent. The air pressure in the lungs remains at a high level, while the external pressure on the chest decreases. As a result, the air inside the lungs expands rapidly, causing the alveoli in the lungs to rupture. The air released from this rupture can cause the following injuries:

- Air may enter the pleural space and compress the lungs (a pneumothorax).
- Air may enter the mediastinum (the space within the thorax that contains the heart and great vessels), causing a condition called pneumomediastinum.
- Air may enter the bloodstream and create bubbles of air in the vessels called air emboli.

Both pneumothorax and pneumomediastinum result in pain and severe dyspnea. An air embolus will act as a plug in the circulatory system, preventing the normal flow of blood and oxygen to a specific part of the body. The brain and spinal cord are the organs most severely affected by air embolism because they require a constant supply of oxygen.

The following conditions are potential signs and symptoms of air embolism:

- Blotching (mottling of the skin)
- Froth (often pink or bloody) at the nose and mouth
- Severe pain in the muscles, joints, or abdomen
- Dyspnea or chest pain
- Dizziness, nausea, and vomiting
- Dysphasia (difficulty speaking)
- Cough
- Cyanosis
- Difficulty with vision
- Paralysis or coma
- Irregular pulse and even cardiac arrest

Decompression Sickness

Decompression sickness, commonly called the bends, occurs when bubbles of gas—especially nitrogen—obstruct the blood vessels. This condition results from too rapid an ascent from a dive, too long of a dive at too deep a depth, or repeated dives on the same day without observing the proper time intervals between dives. During the dive, nitrogen that is being breathed dissolves in the blood and tissues because it is under pressure. When the diver ascends, the external pressure is decreased, and the dissolved nitrogen then forms small bubbles within those tissues. These bubbles can lead to problems similar to those noted with air embolism (blockage of tiny blood vessels, depriving parts of the body of their normal blood supply), but severe pain in certain tissues or spaces in the body is the most common problem. The most striking symptom is abdominal and joint pain so severe that the patient literally doubles up, or "bends."

Dive tables and computers are available to show the proper rate of ascent from a dive, including the number and length of pauses that a diver should make on the way up. Even divers who stay within these limits can experience the bends, however.

Decompression sickness can occur from driving a car up a mountain or flying in an unpressurized airplane that climbs too rapidly to a great height, though the risk of this outcome diminishes after 24 to 48 hours. The problem is exactly the same as with the ascent from a deep dive: a sudden decrease of external pressure on the body and release of dissolved nitrogen from the blood that forms bubbles of nitrogen gas within the blood vessels.

It may be difficult to distinguish between air embolism and decompression sickness. As a general rule, air embolism occurs immediately on return to the surface, whereas the symptoms of decompression sickness may not appear for several hours. The emergency treatment is the same for both conditions: basic life support (BLS) followed by recompression in a hyperbaric chamber, a chamber or a small room that is pressurized to more than atmospheric pressure **FIGURE 19-35**. Recompression treatment allows the bubbles of gas to dissolve into the blood and equalizes the pressures inside and outside the lungs. Once these pressures are equalized, gradual decompression can be accomplished under controlled conditions to prevent the bubbles from reforming.

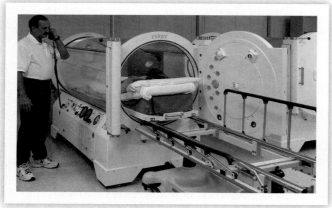

Courtesy of Perry Baromedical Corporation

FIGURE 19-35 A hyperbaric chamber, usually a small room, is pressurized to more than atmospheric pressure and used in the treatment of decompression sickness and air embolism.

Emergency Care for Drowning or Diving Emergencies

If spinal injury is not suspected, turn the patient quickly to the left side to allow substances to drain from the upper airway. Note that water will not drain from the lungs. If evidence of upper airway obstruction by foreign matter is visible, remove the obstruction manually or, if available, by suction. If necessary, use chest compressions, followed by assisted ventilations. Administer oxygen if this intervention was not provided as part of the primary assessment, either by mask for patients who are breathing spontaneously or via a bag-mask device for those requiring assisted ventilation.

Make sure that the patient is kept warm, especially after cold-water immersion. Provide blankets and protection from the environment as needed. When treating conscious patients who are suspected of having air embolism or decompression sickness, follow these accepted treatment steps:

1. Remove the patient from the water. Try to keep the patient calm.
2. Administer oxygen.
3. Place the patient in a left lateral recumbent position with the head down.
4. Provide prompt transport to the nearest recompression facility for treatment.

Injury from decompression sickness is usually reversible with proper treatment. Unfortunately, if the bubbles block critical blood vessels that supply the brain or spinal cord, permanent central nervous system injury may result. Therefore, the key in emergency management of these serious ascent problems is to recognize that an emergency exists, administer oxygen, and provide rapid transport.

Bites and Envenomations

While you may be familiar with bites and stings in general, the new *National EMS Education Standards* include information regarding specific bites and envenomations.

Spider Bites

Spiders are numerous and widespread in the United States. Many species of spiders bite, but only two—the female black widow spider and the brown recluse spider—are able to deliver serious, even life-threatening bites. When caring for a patient who has had some type of bite, be alert to the (unlikely) possibility that the spider may still be in the area. Remember that your safety is of paramount importance.

The female black widow spider (*Latrodectus*) is fairly large, measuring approximately 2 inches long with its legs extended. It is usually black and has a distinctive, bright red-orange marking in the shape of an hourglass on its abdomen **FIGURE 19-36**. The female black widow spider is larger and more toxic than the male. Black widow spiders are found in every state except Alaska. They prefer dry, dim places around buildings, in woodpiles, and among debris.

Most black widow spider bites cause localized pain and agonizing muscle spasms. In some cases, a bite on the abdomen causes muscle spasms so severe that the patient may be thought to have an acute abdominal condition, possibly peritonitis. The main danger with this type of bite, however, is that the black widow's venom is poisonous to nerve tissues (neurotoxic).

Other systemic symptoms of a black widow spider bite include dizziness, sweating, nausea, vomiting, and rashes. Tightness in the chest and difficulty breathing develop within 24 hours, as do severe cramps, with board-like rigidity of the abdominal muscles. Generally, these signs and symptoms subside over 48 hours.

If necessary, a physician can administer a specific antivenin, a serum containing antibodies that counteract the venom. Because of a high incidence of side effects, use of this treatment is reserved for very severe bites, for the aged or very feeble, and for children younger than 5 years. In children, these bites can be fatal. The severe muscle spasms are usually treated in the hospital with IV benzodiazepines such as diazepam (Valium) or lorazepam (Ativan).

The brown recluse spider (*Loxosceles*) is dull brown and, at 1 inch, smaller than the black widow **FIGURE 19-37**. The short-haired body has a violin-shaped mark, brown to yellow in color, on its back. Although the brown recluse

spider lives mostly in the southern and central parts of the country, it may be found throughout the continental United States. The spider takes its name from the fact that it tends to live in dark areas—in corners of old, unused buildings, under rocks, and in woodpiles. In cooler areas, it moves indoors to closets, drawers, cellars, and clothing.

In contrast to the venom of the black widow spider, the venom of the brown recluse spider is not neurotoxic but cytotoxic; that is, it causes severe local tissue damage. Typically, the bite is not painful at first but becomes so within hours. The area becomes swollen and tender, developing a pale, mottled, cyanotic center and possibly a small blister. Over the next several days, a scab of dead skin, fat, and debris forms and digs down into the skin, producing a large ulcer that may not heal unless treated promptly **FIGURE 19-38**. Transport patients with such symptoms as soon as possible.

In general, emergency treatment for spider bites consists of BLS care for the patient in respiratory distress. Much more often, the patient will require only relief from pain. If time permits, apply an ice pack to the bite area and clean the wound with soap and water. Transport the patient to the emergency department as soon as possible for treatment of both pain and muscle rigidity. If possible, bring the spider to the hospital for positive identification.

Hymenoptera Stings

The Hymenoptera family of insects includes bees, wasps, hornets, yellow jackets, and ants. Collectively, these insects kill more people each year than any other venomous animal, including snakes. Death from a Hymenoptera sting is usually the result of anaphylaxis.

Identification of a bee sting is not difficult. There is almost always an immediate local reaction consisting of pain (sometimes extreme), redness, swelling, and itching at the site. Honeybees sting once, usually leaving the barbed stinger and venom sac attached to the skin. Wasps, hornets, yellow jackets, and fire ants can sting repeatedly.

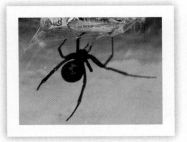

© Crystal Kirk/ShutterStock, Inc.

FIGURE 19-36 Black widow spiders are distinguished by their glossy black color and bright red-orange hourglass marking on the abdomen.

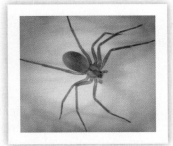

Courtesy of Kenneth Cramer, Monmouth College

FIGURE 19-37 Brown recluse spiders are dull brown and have a dark violin-shaped mark on the back.

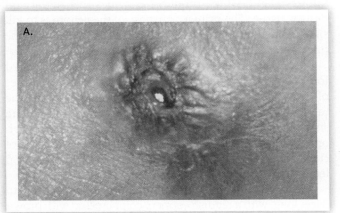

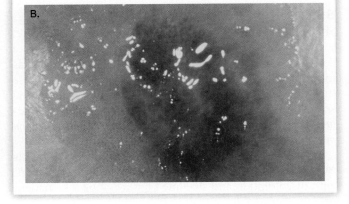

Courtesy of the Department of Entomology, University of Nebraska – Lincoln

FIGURE 19-38 Brown recluse spider bites. **A.** Early stage. **B.** Late stage.

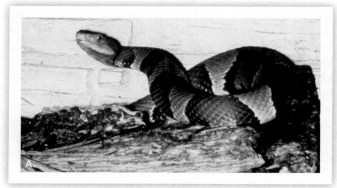

Courtesy of Ray Rauch/U.S. Fish & Wildlife Service

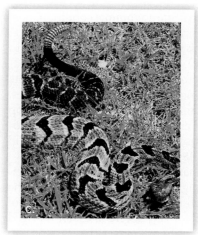

Amee Cross/ShutterStock, Inc.

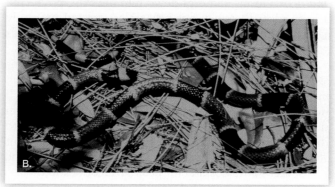

Courtesy of Luther C. Goldman/U.S. Fish & Wildlife Service

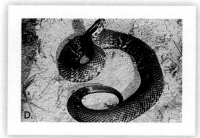

© SuperStock/Alamy Images

FIGURE 19-39 **A.** Copperhead. **B.** Coral snake. **C.** Rattlesnake. **D.** Cottonmouth.

Treatment of a Hymenoptera sting focuses primarily on pain relief and minimization of the risk of infection. Determine whether the stinger and venom sac are still attached to the skin. If so, remove them. This is best done by using a firm-edged item such as a credit card to scrape the stinger and sac off the skin.

If anaphylaxis develops, be prepared to assist the patient in administering an EpiPen auto-injector, if available. Also be prepared to support the airway and breathing should the patient experience significant respiratory compromise.

Snake Bites

Snake bite fatalities in the United States are extremely rare, with only about 15 deaths occurring each year in the entire country. Of the approximately 115 different species of snakes found in the United States, only 19 are venomous. These include the copperhead (*Agkistrodon contortrix*); the coral snakes (*Micrurus* and *Micruroides*); the rattlesnake (*Crotalus*); and the cottonmouth, or water moccasin (*Agkistrodon piscivorus*) **FIGURE 19-39**.

The classic appearance of the poisonous snake bite is two small puncture wounds, usually about ½-inch apart, with discoloration and swelling **FIGURE 19-40**. The patient usually reports pain surrounding the bite.

Rattlesnakes, copperheads, and cottonmouths are all pit vipers, with triangular-shaped, flat heads **FIGURE 19-41**. They take their name from the small pits located just behind each nostril and in front of each eye. The pit is a heat-sensing organ that allows the snake to strike accurately at any warm target, especially in the dark, when it cannot see through its vertical, slit-like pupils.

Pit viper fangs are actually special hollow teeth that act much like hypodermic needles. They are connected to a sac containing a reservoir of venom, which in turn is attached to a poison gland. The gland itself is a specially adapted salivary gland, which produces enzymes that digest and destroy tissue. The primary purpose of the venom is to kill small animals and to start the digestive process prior to the prey being eaten.

In the United States, the most commonly encountered form of pit viper is the rattlesnake. Several different species of rattlesnake can be identified by the rattle on the tail. The rattle is actually numerous layers of dried skin that were shed but failed to fall off, coming to rest against a small knob on the end of the tail. Rattlesnakes have many patterns of color, often with a diamond pattern. They can grow to 6 feet or more in length.

Copperheads are smaller than rattlesnakes, usually 2 to 3 feet long, with a reddish coppery color crossed with brown or red bands. These snakes typically inhabit woodpiles and abandoned dwellings, often close to areas of habitation. Although they account for most of the venomous snake bites

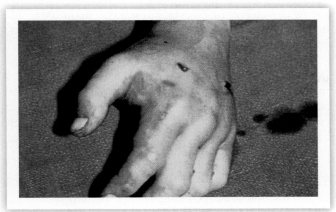

Courtesy of AAOS

FIGURE 19-40 A snake bite wound from a poisonous snake has characteristic markings: two small puncture wounds about ½ inch apart, discoloration, and swelling.

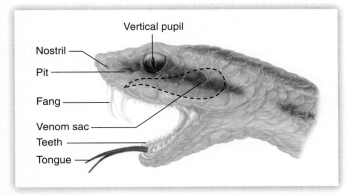

FIGURE 19-41 Pit vipers have small, heat-sensing organs (pits) located in front of their eyes that allow them to strike at warm targets, even in the dark.

in the eastern United States, copperhead bites are almost never fatal. The venom can destroy extremities, however.

Cottonmouths grow to about 4 feet in length. Also called water moccasins, these snakes are olive or brown, with black cross-bands and a yellow undersurface. These water snakes demonstrate a particularly aggressive pattern of behavior. Although fatalities from these snake bites are rare, tissue destruction from the venom may be severe.

Signs and symptoms of envenomation by a pit viper include severe burning pain at the injury site, followed by swelling and a bluish discoloration (ecchymosis) in light-skinned persons that signals bleeding under the skin. These signs are evident within 5 to 10 minutes after the bite has occurred and spread over the next 36 hours. In addition to destroying tissues locally, the venom of the pit viper can interfere with the body's clotting mechanism and cause bleeding at various distant sites. This toxin affects the entire nervous system. Other systemic signs may include weakness, nausea, vomiting, sweating, seizures, fainting, vision problems, changes in level of consciousness, and shock.

The coral snake is a small reptile characterized by a series of bright red, yellow, and black bands completely encircling the body. Many harmless snakes have similar coloring, but only the coral snake has red and yellow bands next to one another, as this helpful rhyme suggests: "Red on yellow will kill a fellow; red on black, venom will lack."

Because of its small mouth and teeth and limited jaw expansion, the coral snake usually bites its victims on a small part of the body, such as a finger or toe.

Coral snake venom is a powerful toxin that causes paralysis of the nervous system. Within a few hours of being bitten, a patient will exhibit bizarre behavior, followed by progressive paralysis of eye movements and respiration. Often, there are limited or no localized signs other than bite marks.

Successful treatment, either emergency or long-term, depends on positive identification of the snake and support of respiration. Antivenin is available, but most hospitals do not stock it. Therefore, you should notify the hospital of the need for it as soon as possible.

To treat snake bites:

1. Immediately quiet and reassure the patient.
2. Flush the area of the bite with 1 to 2 quarts of warm, soapy water to wash away any poison left on the surface of the skin. Do not apply ice to the region.
3. If the patient is hypotensive, a constricting band may be applied 4 to 6 inches above the bite site if called for by local protocols.
4. If the bite occurred on an arm or leg, splint the extremity to minimize movement and the spread of venom at the site, and place the extremity below the level of the heart. If the patient was bitten on the trunk, keep him or her supine.
5. Monitor the patient's vital signs and mark the skin with a pen over the area that is swollen, proximal to the swelling, to note whether swelling is spreading.
6. Keep the patient warm. To prevent shock, place the patient in a position dictated by local protocol for shock patients.
7. Do not give the patient anything by mouth.
8. Administer supplemental oxygen as needed.
9. Transport the patient promptly to the emergency department, giving advance notice that the patient has been bitten by a snake and identifying the type of snake if possible. If the snake has been killed, as is often the case, be sure to bring it with you in a secure container so that physicians can identify it and administer the proper antivenin. Note, however, that as a reflex, a snake can bite for up to one hour after death.

Scorpion Stings

Scorpions are eight-legged arachnids from the biologic group Arachnida that possess a venom gland and a stinger at the end of their tail. Scorpions live in warm climates around the world, including Mexico, India, Africa, South America, and the Caribbean. In the United States, they are primarily found in the Southwest—namely, Arizona, New Mexico, and California. Of course, anyone can have one of these animals as a pet.

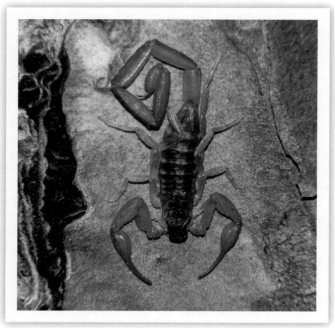

© David Desoer/ShutterStock, Inc.

FIGURE 19-42 A bark scorpion is the only type of scorpion that is commonly associated with death in the United States.

All of the many species of scorpions can deliver a painful sting. Nevertheless, only the bark scorpion is commonly associated with deaths in the United States **FIGURE 19-42**.

A scorpion sting causes immediate pain at the site, followed by numbness or tingling. The pain is usually exacerbated by pressure to the wound. Eventually, the peripheral area surrounding the wound becomes hypersensitive to touch and temperature changes.

The sting of the bark scorpion can cause dramatic neuromuscular signs and symptoms, including uncontrolled roving movements of the eyes, blurred vision, drooling, difficulty swallowing, slurred speech, severe agitation, nausea, vomiting, muscle twitching or spasms, and seizures.

Emergency care for a scorpion bite includes administration of BLS care as necessary, ALS assistance for pain management, and immediate transport of the patient for possible antivenin. If allowed by local protocol, apply a constricting band just above the wound site, tight enough to reduce lymph flow and subsequent spread of venom, but not tight enough to occlude the pulse.

Tick Bites

Only a fraction of an inch long, ticks, especially deer ticks, can easily be mistaken for a freckle, especially given that their bite is not painful **FIGURE 19-43**. The danger with a tick bite is not from the bite itself, but rather from the infecting organisms that the tick carries. Ticks commonly carry pathogens for two infectious diseases—Rocky Mountain spotted fever and Lyme disease. Both are spread through the tick's saliva, which is injected into the skin when the tick attaches itself.

Rocky Mountain spotted fever, which is not limited to the Rocky Mountains, occurs within 7 to 10 days after a bite by an infected tick. Its symptoms include nausea, vomiting, headache, weakness, paralysis, and possibly cardiorespiratory collapse.

Lyme disease is spread by an infected deer tick, which is very small and must be attached for more than 24 hours to infect the host. Originating in Lyme, Connecticut, Lyme disease has now been reported in 35 states. It occurs most frequently in the Northeast, the Great Lake states, and the Pacific Northwest, with New York reporting the largest number of cases. The first symptom, a rash that may spread to several parts of the body, begins about 3 days after the bite of an infected tick. The rash may eventually resemble a target bull's-eye pattern in one-third of patients **FIGURE 19-44**.

Lyme disease can cause a wide variety of symptoms in almost every body system. One of the most common symptoms is painful swelling of joints, so that this infection is

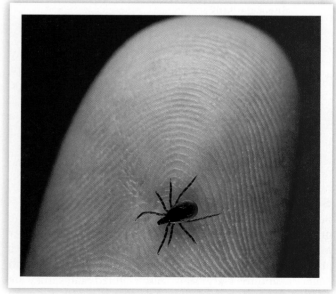

© Scott Camazine/Photo Researchers, Inc.

FIGURE 19-43 Deer ticks may be extremely small, resembling a freckle.

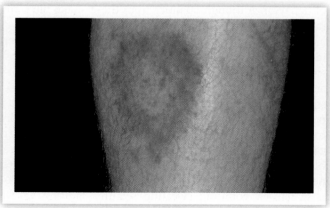

© E.M. Singletary, MD. Used with permission.

FIGURE 19-44 The rash associated with Lyme disease has a characteristic bull's-eye pattern.

often confused with rheumatoid arthritis. If left untreated, Lyme disease may result in permanent disability. However, if it is recognized and treated promptly with antibiotics, the patient often recovers completely.

Electricity-Related Injuries

Personal safety is of particular importance when you are called to the scene of an emergency involving electricity. Obviously, you can be fatally injured by coming in contact with power lines. But you can also be fatally injured by touching a patient who is still in contact with a live power line or any other electrical source. For this reason, you should never attempt to remove someone from an electrical source unless you are specially trained to do so. Likewise, you should never move a downed power line unless you have the special training and equipment necessary. Before even approaching someone who may still be in contact with a power line or electrical appliance, make certain that the power is turned off. Always assume that any downed power line is live.

A burn injury appears where the electricity enters (an entrance wound) and exits (an exit wound) the body. The entrance wound may be quite small, but the exit wound can be extensive and deep FIGURE 19-45. Always look for both entrance and exit wounds.

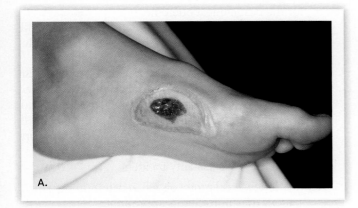

A.

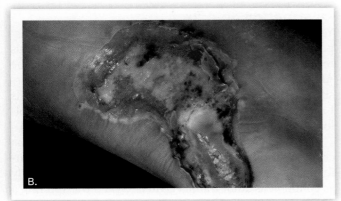

B.

© Chuck Stewart, MD.

FIGURE 19-45 Electrical burns, like gunshot wounds, have entrance and exit wounds. **A.** An entrance wound is often quite small. **B.** The exit wound can be extensive and deep.

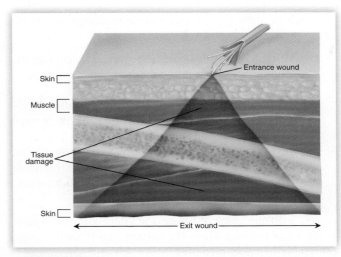

FIGURE 19-46 External signs of an electrical burn may be deceiving. The entrance wound may be a small burn, whereas the damage to deeper tissue may be massive.

Two specific dangers are associated with electrical burns. First, there may be a large amount of deep-tissue injury. Electrical burns are always more severe than the external signs indicate. The patient may have only a small burn to the skin, yet may have massive damage to the deeper tissues, organs, and the nervous system FIGURE 19-46.

Second, the patient may go into cardiac or respiratory arrest from the electric current's disruption of the body's systems. In fact, the two most common causes of death from electrical injury are asphyxia and cardiac arrest. Electrical current can cross the chest and cause cardiac arrest or dysrhythmias.

If indicated, begin CPR on the patient and apply the automated external defibrillator (AED). Although CPR may need to be quite prolonged in patients with electrical burns, it has a high success rate if started promptly. If neither CPR nor defibrillation is indicated, administer supplemental oxygen, and monitor the patient closely for respiratory and cardiac arrest. Treat the soft-tissue injuries by placing dry, sterile dressings on all burn wounds and splinting suspected fractures. Provide prompt transport; all electrical burns are potentially severe injuries that require further treatment in the hospital.

Lightning

Lightning is the third most common cause of death from isolated environmental phenomena. The cardiovascular and nervous systems are most commonly injured during a lightning strike; therefore, respiratory or cardiac arrest is the most common cause of lightning-related deaths. The tissue damage caused by lightning is different from that caused by other electrical-related injuries (ie, high-power line injuries) because the tissue damage pathway usually goes over the skin, rather than through it. During assessment, look for both the entrance and exit wounds. The exit wound will not necessarily appear on the same side of the body. Because the duration of a lightning strike is short, skin burns are usually superficial; full-thickness (third-degree) burns are rare.

Lightning injuries are categorized as being mild, moderate, or severe:

- **Mild:** loss of consciousness, amnesia, confusion, tingling, and other nonspecific signs and symptoms. Burns, if present, are typically superficial.
- **Moderate:** seizures, respiratory arrest, cardiac standstill (asystole) that spontaneously resolves, and superficial burns.
- **Severe:** cardiopulmonary arrest. Because of the delay in resuscitation, often the result of the lightning strike's occurrence in a remote location, many of these patients do not survive.

As with any scene response, the safety of you and your partner has priority. Move the patient to a place of safety, preferably in a sheltered area.

When a person is struck by lightning, the event causes massive direct current shock, with the patient experiencing massive muscle spasms (tetany) that can result in fractures of long bones and spinal vertebrae. Therefore, you should manually stabilize the patient's head in a neutral in-line position and open the airway with the jaw-thrust maneuver. If the patient is in respiratory arrest with a pulse, begin immediate bag-mask device ventilations with 100% oxygen. If the patient is in cardiac arrest, attach an AED as soon as possible and provide immediate defibrillation if indicated. If severe bleeding is present, control it immediately.

Provide full spinal stabilization and transport the patient to the closest appropriate facility. If CPR or ventilations are not required, address other injuries (ie, splint fractures, dress and bandage burns) and provide continuous monitoring while en route to the hospital.

Management: Transport and Destination

Caring for victims of traumatic injuries requires a solid understanding of the US trauma system as well as a good working knowledge of available local resources, including methods of rapid transport and locations of trauma centers and specialized facilities in the area.

Scene Time

Because survival of critically injured trauma patients is time dependent, on-scene time should be limited to the minimum amount necessary to correct life-threatening injuries and package the patient. Optimally, on-scene time for critically injured patients should be less than 10 minutes—the "platinum 10." The following criteria will help you identify a critically injured patient:

- Significant MOI
- Decreased level of consciousness
- Any threats to airway, breathing, or circulation

Patients who present with these criteria or who are very young or old or have chronic illnesses should be considered to be at high risk, requiring rapid treatment and transport.

Type of Transport

Modes of transport ultimately come in one of two categories: ground or air. While ground-transportation EMS units are generally staffed by traditional EMTs and paramedics, air medical units are typically staffed by critical care nurses and paramedics.

The Association of Air Medical Services (AAMS) and MedEvac Foundation International identify the following criteria as indicative of the appropriate use of emergency air medical services for trauma patients:

- There is an extended period required to access or extricate a remote (eg, injured hiker, snowmobiler, or boater) or trapped patient (eg, in a crashed car), which depletes the time window to get the patient to the trauma center by ground.
- The distance to the trauma center is greater than 20 to 25 miles.
- The patient needs medical care and stabilization at the ALS level, and there is no ALS-level ground ambulance service available within a reasonable time frame.
- Traffic conditions or hospital availability make it unlikely that the patient will get to a trauma center via ground ambulance within the ideal time frame for the best clinical outcome.
- The incident involves multiple patients who will overwhelm resources at the trauma center(s) reachable by ground within the ideal time frame.
- EMS systems require bringing a patient to the nearest hospital for initial evaluation and stabilization, rather than bypassing those facilities and going directly to a trauma center. This step may delay the time until definitive surgical care and necessitate air transport to mitigate the impact of that delay.
- There is a mass-casualty incident.

Always follow local protocols when determining which type of patient transportation is appropriate.

Destination Selection

You will often be summoned to accident scenes to transport critically ill trauma patients to definitive care. For this reason, it is important for you to be familiar with how the American College of Surgeons' Committee on Trauma classifies trauma care. Trauma centers are classified into Levels I through IV, with Level I having the most resources, followed by Levels II, III, and IV, respectively **TABLE 19-6**.

Trauma centers are categorized as either adult trauma centers or pediatric trauma centers, but do not necessarily qualify as both. Pediatric trauma centers are not nearly as common as adult trauma centers. When transporting a pediatric trauma patient, be certain to transport the patient to a pediatric trauma center if one is available within a reasonable distance.

Table 19-6
Key Elements for Trauma Centers

Level	Definition	Key Elements
Level I	A comprehensive regional resource that is a tertiary care facility; capable of providing total care for every aspect of injury—from prevention through rehabilitation	1. 24-hour in-house coverage by general surgeons 2. Availability of care in specialties such as orthopaedic surgery, neurosurgery, anesthesiology, emergency medicine, radiology, internal medicine, and critical care 3. Should also include cardiac, hand, pediatric, and microvascular surgery and hemodialysis 4. Provides leadership in prevention, public education, and continuing education of trauma team members 5. Committed to continued improvement through a comprehensive quality assessment program and organized research to help direct new innovations in trauma care
Level II	Able to initiate definitive care for all injured patients	1. 24-hour immediate coverage by general surgeons 2. Availability of orthopaedic surgery, neurosurgery, anesthesiology, emergency medicine, radiology, and critical care 3. Tertiary care needs such as cardiac surgery, hemodialysis, and microvascular surgery may be referred to a Level I trauma center 4. Committed to trauma prevention and continuing education of trauma team members 5. Provides continued improvement in trauma care through a comprehensive quality assessment program
Level III	Ability to provide prompt assessment, resuscitation, and stabilization of injured patients and emergency operations	1. 24-hour immediate coverage by emergency medicine physicians and prompt availability of general surgeons and anesthesiologists 2. Program dedicated to continued improvement in trauma care through a comprehensive quality assessment program 3. Has developed transfer agreements for patients requiring more comprehensive care at a Level I or Level II trauma center 4. Committed to continuing education of nursing and allied health personnel or the trauma team 5. Must be involved with prevention and have an active outreach program for its referring communities
Level IV	Ability to provide advanced trauma life support (ATLS) before transfer of patients to a higher level trauma center	1. Include basic emergency department facilities to implement ATLS protocols and 24-hour laboratory coverage 2. Transfer to higher level trauma centers follows the guidelines outlined in formal transfer agreements 3. Committed to continued improvement of these trauma care activities through a formal quality assessment program 4. Involved in prevention, outreach, and education within its community

Table 19-7
American College of Surgeons Criteria for a Level I Patient

- Confirmed blood pressure of less than 90 mm Hg at any time in adults, and age-specific hypotension in children
- Respiratory compromise, obstruction, and/or intubation
- Receiving blood to maintain vital signs
- Emergency physician's discretion
- Glasgow Coma Scale score of less than or equal to 8 with mechanism attributed to trauma
- Gunshot wound to the abdomen, neck, or chest

Table 19-8
American College of Surgeons Recommendations for a Level II Patient

Patient characteristic/ condition indicators	1. Glasgow Coma Scale score of less than 14 when associated with trauma 2. Respiratory rate of fewer than 10 or more than 29 breaths/min (fewer than 20 breaths/min in an infant younger than 1 year of age) when associated with trauma 3. Penetrating wounds (other than gunshot wounds) to the head, neck, torso, and extremities proximal to the elbow and knee 4. Flail chest 5. Combination of trauma with burns 6. Two or more proximal long-bone fractures 7. Pelvic fractures 8. Limb paralysis and/or spinal cord injury 9. Amputation proximal to the wrist and/or ankle

Mechanism of injury indicators	1. High-speed vehicle crash
	  ▪ Initial speed of greater than 40 mph
	  ▪ Major vehicle deformity
	  ▪ Intrusion into the passenger compartment
	2. Ejection from the vehicle
	3. Death in same passenger compartment
	4. Extrication time of greater than 20 minutes
	5. Falls of greater than 20 feet or significant falls in children or elderly
	6. Vehicle rollover
	7. Car-versus-pedestrian or car-versus-bicycle impact of greater than 5 mph
	8. All-terrain vehicle (ATV) or motorcycle crash of greater than 20 mph or separation of rider from ATV or motorcycle
	
	Pediatric indicators include:
	9. Falls of greater than 10 feet without loss of consciousness
	10. Falls of less than 10 feet with loss of consciousness
	11. Medium- to high-speed vehicle crash (greater than 25 mph)

Consider Level II classification with the following preexisting conditions	12. Age younger than 5 years or older than 55 years 13. Cardiac disease, respiratory disease 14. Type 1 diabetes mellitus, cirrhosis of the liver, morbid obesity 15. Pregnancy 16. Immunosuppressed patients 17. Patients with a bleeding disorder or on anticoagulants

The American College of Surgeons' Committee on Trauma has developed criteria for Level I trauma patient classification **TABLE 19-7**. When one or more of the criteria listed are present in the trauma patient, he or she is classified as a Level I trauma patient. Although the American College of Surgeons' Committee on Trauma does not cite required criteria for a Level II patient, it has provided recommendations for such patients, which are listed in **TABLE 19-8**.

Transition Tip

Because traumatic injuries are as varied as the mechanisms that cause them, it is almost impossible to prepare for every possible situation that you may face as an AEMT. In all situations, you must remain calm, complete an organized assessment, correct life-threatening injuries, and do no harm. Never hesitate to request ALS assistance or medical control for guidance. Follow your local protocols.

PREP KIT

Ready for Review

- Multisystem trauma is a term that describes multiple traumatic injuries involving more than one body system.
- Two concepts of energy are typically associated with injury: potential energy and kinetic energy.
- Recent studies have brought into question the effectiveness of using pressure points to control severe external hemorrhage. If allowed by local protocol and policy, you should use a tourniquet without attempting pressure point control.
- The most common symptom of internal bleeding is pain. Significant internal bleeding will generally cause swelling in the area of bleeding. Intra-abdominal bleeding will often cause pain and distention. Bruising is a sign of internal bleeding.
- Injuries from explosions occur from primary blast injuries, secondary blast injuries, tertiary blast injuries, and miscellaneous blast injuries.
- Head injuries commonly occur in victims of motor vehicle crashes, assault, falls by the elderly, sports-related incidents, and incidents involving children.
- A skull fracture may be open or closed, depending on whether an overlying laceration or penetration of the scalp is present.
- TBIs are the most serious of all head injuries. Concussions are known as mild TBIs.
- Accumulation of blood within the skull or swelling of the brain can rapidly lead to an increase in ICP.
- The face and neck are particularly vulnerable to injury because of their relatively unprotected positions on the body.
- Proper emergency care of eye injuries will minimize pain and may very well help prevent permanent loss of vision.
- Blunt trauma to the chest may injure the heart itself, making it unable to maintain adequate blood pressure.
- The chest contains several large blood vessels; injury to any of these vessels can result in massive, rapidly fatal hemorrhage.
- Hollow organs include the stomach, intestines, ureters, and bladder; they are structures through which materials pass. Solid organs include the liver, spleen, pancreas, and kidneys.
- Closed abdominal injuries are those in which blunt force trauma—that is, some type of impact to the body—results in injury to the abdomen without breaking the skin.
- Open abdominal injuries, also known as penetrating injuries, are those in which a foreign object enters the abdomen and opens the peritoneal cavity to the outside.
- Injuries of the kidney are not unusual, but rarely occur in isolation because the kidneys lie in a well-protected area of the body.
- Injury to the bladder, either blunt or penetrating, may result in rupture of this organ.
- Injuries to the male external genitalia are rarely considered life threatening.
- The internal female genitalia are rarely damaged because they are small, deep in the pelvis, and well protected by the pelvic bones. An exception is the pregnant uterus, which is highly vulnerable to injury.
- Because the external female genitalia have a rich nerve supply, injuries in this area are very painful.
- Musculoskeletal injuries are among the most common reasons why patients seek medical attention.
- Drowning is the process of experiencing respiratory impairment from submersion or immersion in liquid.
- Injuries associated with scuba diving may be immediately apparent or may show up hours later. Patients with air embolism or decompression sickness may have pain, paralysis, or altered mental status. Be prepared to transport such patients to a recompression facility with a hyperbaric chamber.
- Poisonous spiders include the black widow spider and the brown recluse spider.
- Poisonous snakes include pit vipers and coral snakes.
- The Hymenoptera family of insects includes bees, wasps, hornets, yellow jackets, and ants. Collectively, these insects kill more people each year than any other venomous animal.
- Caring for victims of traumatic injuries requires a solid understanding of the US trauma system as well as a good working knowledge of available local resources, including methods of rapid transport and locations of trauma centers and specialized facilities in the area.
- Modes of transport ultimately come in one of two categories: ground or air.

Case Study

You are dispatched to a local industrial site for a 42-year-old man with a "traumatic injury." The dispatcher informs you that the patient was using a table saw to cut large pieces of wood and apparently slipped, causing injury to the right upper extremity.

When you arrive on scene, you are immediately greeted by employees who direct you to the patient's location. As you approach the patient, you notice what appear to be large quantities of blood on the floor and sprayed on the walls. Bystanders applied a dressing to the injury before your arrival; however, you can clearly see that blood is soaking through the bulky dressings. The patient appears agitated and in pain. Your partner puts an additional dressing over the wound while you talk to the patient.

The patient tells you that his hands were wet with sweat and slipped while guiding a section of wood through the saw. His hand pushed back the guard and his arm struck the saw. Bystanders reported hearing a scream come from the patient's workstation and seeing blood sprayed on the wall.

The dressings your partner applied are now soaked through with blood. Concerns for being able to control bleeding lead you to the decision to apply a tourniquet to the right upper extremity and rapidly transport the patient to the trauma center.

1. What are the appropriate methods to control external bleeding?

2. What are the precautions to consider when applying a tourniquet?

3. Given the MOI for this patient, a partial amputation is likely. Explain the treatment for a partial amputation.

4. If this patient is experiencing a partial amputation involving an open fracture, which of the following classifications would best describe the injury based on the musculoskeletal injury grading system?
   A. Moderate injury
   B. Serious injury
   C. Severe, life-threatening injury (survival is probable)
   D. Critical injury (survival is uncertain)

5. Which of the following is not considered a later sign of hypoperfusion associated with internal bleeding?
   A. Tachycardia
   B. Decreased thirst
   C. Dull eyes
   D. Shallow, rapid breathing

CHAPTER 20

Special Patient Populations

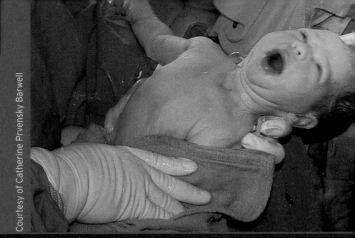

Courtesy of Catherine Prvensky Barwell

National EMS Education Standards

Anatomy and Physiology

Applies complex knowledge of the anatomy and function of all human systems to the practice of EMS.

Pathophysiology

Applies complex knowledge of the pathophysiology of respiration and perfusion to patient assessment and management.

Special Patient Populations

Applies a fundamental knowledge of growth, development, and aging and assessment findings to provide basic and selected advanced emergency care and transportation for a patient with special needs.

Review

Obstetrics and pediatrics were covered in detail during your EMT-I training. The majority of that training has not changed. Complications, such as prolapsed umbilical cord, breech presentation, arm or leg presentation, still require rapid transport to the hospital. Pediatric assessment and emergency care have also remained the same, with each age group having anatomic and psychosocial differences.

What's New

While delivery of a newborn is not a new skill to the AEMT, information regarding certain complications of pregnancy and delivery has been added to the *National EMS Education Standards*. In addition, some changes have been made to the standards regarding neonatal resuscitation. Pediatric emergencies have not changed significantly, although some additional steps related to assessment of a child are included. Emergency care relevant to geriatric patients has been added to the new standards, as has the topic of patients with special challenges.

▌Introduction

Special populations refers to the pediatric and geriatric populations as well as to obstetrics/newborns cases and those patients with special needs. The members of these populations have unique characteristics and pose some challenges to the AEMT regarding emergency care.

▌Obstetric Emergencies

Although childbirth may seem like an emergency, it is actually a normal, routine part of life. Sometimes, however, complications may occur, whether during the pregnancy itself, during labor and delivery, or after delivery.

Complications of Pregnancy

Most births are uneventful and require little or no medical intervention beyond basic interventions, such as suctioning, drying, and warming the baby; others, however, may be life threatening to both the woman and baby. The most common of these conditions are discussed.

Hypertension

Hypertension is a major cause of mortality and morbidity in the pregnant woman. In some women, hypertension is the result of a condition called *preeclampsia*, or pregnancy-induced hypertension. Preeclampsia is defined as an increase in blood pressure after the 20th week of gestation. It is accompanied by a protein release in the urine and often by edema, particularly in the upper body. The protein in the urine will not typically be detected by EMS personnel and edema can be normal for a pregnant woman. The most important feature of preeclampsia for the AEMT to recognize is hypertension. Preeclampsia is characterized by the following signs and symptoms:

- Headache
- Swelling in the hands, face, and feet
- Anxiety
- Nausea/vomiting

In severe preeclampsia, you may also find:

- Pulmonary edema/shortness of breath
- Confusion or other altered level of consciousness
- Visual disturbances, such as blurry vision or scotomata (seeing spots)
- Upper abdominal pain
- Myoclonus (hyperactive reflexes)

> *Preeclampsia* A condition of late pregnancy that involves headache, visual changes, and swelling of the hands and feet; also called pregnancy-induced hypertension.

Another pregnancy-related condition, *eclampsia*, is characterized by a seizure in a pregnant woman who has preeclampsia and no other cause for the seizure. The treatment of a woman with preeclampsia is mostly supportive. Ensure the ABCs and try to keep the patient calm. The patient should be kept in a position of comfort and monitored closely. At a minimum, she should receive supplemental oxygen to prevent fetal distress and an intravenous (IV) line of an isotonic crystalloid solution at a keep-vein-open rate for medication administration if it becomes necessary.

> *Eclampsia* Seizures (convulsions) resulting from severe hypertension in a pregnant woman.

Gestational Diabetes

Pregnancy increases the demand for carbohydrates. Because the insulin molecule is too large to pass through the placental barrier, several hormones are used to compensate for the increased carbohydrate requirement. Women who are predisposed to a diabetic state may develop chemical diabetes during pregnancy, but return to a normal carbohydrate metabolism postpartum. This condition is called gestational diabetes. Usually, gestational diabetes spontaneously resolves following delivery. If you encounter a woman who is pregnant with an altered or decreased mental status, you should suspect diabetes and check her blood glucose level. If hypoglycemia is present, administer 25 g of dextrose 50% IV. This medication should be given slowly through a large IV line. If hyperglycemia or diabetic ketoacidosis (DKA) is present, crystalloid fluid boluses may be necessary to treat the associated dehydration. Several fluid boluses may be required because DKA is commonly associated with severe hypovolemia, possibly even shock. Monitor blood pressure carefully when administering fluid to a pregnant patient.

Refer to the *Endocrine and Hematologic Emergencies* chapter for additional information on diabetes.

Bleeding

Bleeding during pregnancy is an alarming sign that something is wrong. Aside from traumatic injury, the primary reasons for bleeding during pregnancy are ectopic pregnancy, spontaneous abortion, and abruptio placenta and placenta previa.

Ectopic Pregnancy An *ectopic pregnancy* is the implantation and growth of the embryo outside of the uterus, such as in a fallopian tube **FIGURE 20-1**, on the ovary, in the abdominal cavity or peritoneum, or in the cervix. The most common place to find an ectopic pregnancy is in the fallopian tube. If implantation occurs in a fallopian tube, the tube will rupture as the fetus begins to grow, resulting in internal hemorrhage. The woman usually feels lower abdominal pain and cramping and usually, but not always, has vaginal bleeding. For this reason, you should always consider the possibility of an ectopic pregnancy in women who have missed a menstrual cycle and complain of sudden stabbing, usually unilateral, pain in the lower abdomen. This is probably the most life-threatening emergency for the pregnant woman during the first trimester. A history of pelvic inflammatory disease, tubal ligation

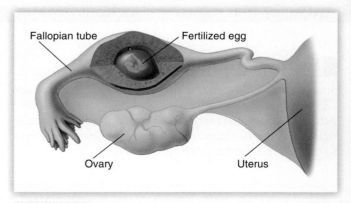

FIGURE 20-1 In an ectopic pregnancy, a fertilized egg implants somewhere other than in the uterus. Here it is implanted in one of the fallopian tubes.

surgery, and previous ectopic pregnancies are risk factors that should heighten your suspicion for a possible ectopic pregnancy. The treatment of the patient with a suspected ectopic pregnancy is focused on supporting the ABCs. She should receive high-flow oxygen, at least one large-bore (14- or 16-gauge) IV line of an isotonic crystalloid, and rapid transport to a hospital that can provide immediate surgery. If she is already in shock, she should receive 20-mL/kg fluid boluses to maintain perfusion and receive airway management as indicated.

> *Ectopic pregnancy* A pregnancy that develops outside the uterus, typically in a fallopian tube.

Transition Tip

Pregnant women face an increased chance of domestic violence and abuse. Abuse is one of the more common causes of complications in pregnancy that may harm the woman or the unborn child (fetus). Some studies have indicated that 15% to 25% of pregnant women are victims of physical or sexual abuse. Abuse during pregnancy increases the chance of miscarriage, premature delivery, and low birth weight, and puts the woman at risk from bleeding, infection, and uterine rupture.

Spontaneous Abortion The most common cause of vaginal bleeding during the first and second trimesters of pregnancy is spontaneous abortion or miscarriage. The term abortion does not imply any cause and simply means that the fetus is released from the uterus before 20 weeks of gestation. It may be an elective procedure (induced) if the woman decides to terminate the pregnancy, or it can be a spontaneous abortion, without any known cause, or it could be induced by trauma, medications, or other medical causes.

There is no specific treatment that you must provide to the patient with a suspected abortion. The patient should receive high-flow oxygen, a large-bore IV line of isotonic crystalloid (ie, normal saline or lactated Ringer's) in the event fluid boluses are required for severe bleeding and shock, and transport to an appropriate hospital. Support the patient emotionally, without giving false hope, and try to keep her calm.

Transition Tip

In the event of heavy bleeding, only administer enough fluid to maintain radial pulses. Increasing the blood pressure will also increase bleeding.

Abruptio Placenta *Abruptio placenta* is the premature separation of the placenta from the wall of the uterus prior to delivery of the fetus **FIGURE 20-2** . Depending on the location of the bleeding compared with the position of the placenta, hemorrhaging may be internal or external. Abruptio placenta most commonly occurs during the third trimester of pregnancy. A patient with abruptio placenta typically presents with severe abdominal pain commonly described as a tearing sensation and dark venous blood from the vagina.

> *Abruptio placenta* A premature separation of the placenta from the wall of the uterus.

Due to the blood loss, the patient is at risk for developing hypovolemic shock.

Emergency care includes providing emotional support for the patient, administering high-flow oxygen and IV therapy, and providing immediate transport to an appropriate facility.

Placenta Previa In *placenta previa*, the placenta implants in an abnormal location on the uterine wall, covering the cervix **FIGURE 20-3** . This condition usually causes no problems until the pregnancy is near term and the fetus starts to descend into the birth canal. This bleeding is usually external through the vagina and is typically bright red. The bleeding is usually painless. The patient may show signs of shock depending on how much blood is lost.

> *Placenta previa* A condition in which the placenta develops over and covers the cervix.

Placenta previa is a true emergency requiring immediate transport to an appropriate facility. As with abruptio placenta, emergency care involves administering high-flow oxygen and treating the patient for shock.

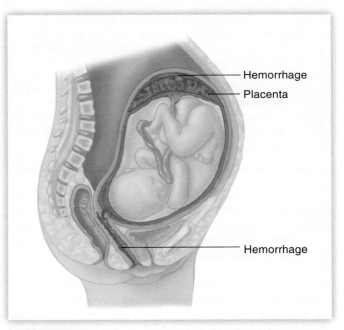

FIGURE 20-2 In abruptio placenta, the placenta separates prematurely from the wall of the uterus.

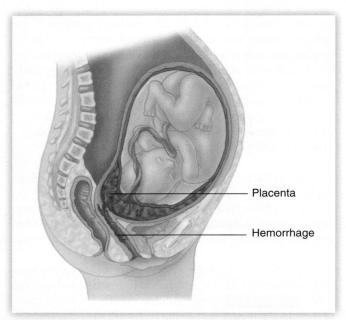

FIGURE 20-3 In placenta previa, the placenta develops over and covers the cervix.

Transition Tip

Regardless of the cause, a pregnant patient who is bleeding from the vagina will likely be emotional and very concerned about her infant. Your professional approach in communicating with the patient will be crucial in calming her emotions. Decreasing the patient's anxiety will directly affect how she and the fetus respond during an emergency. Any bleeding from the vagina in a pregnant woman is a serious sign that should be treated promptly at an appropriate facility. If the mother shows signs of shock, position her on her left side and administer high-flow oxygen. Place a sterile pad or sanitary napkin over the vagina, and replace it as often as necessary. Never insert anything into the vagina. Save blood-soaked pads so that hospital personnel can estimate how much blood has been lost. Also save any tissue that may be passed from the vagina.

Trauma and Pregnancy

On some occasions, a trauma call involves a pregnant woman. In these situations, keep in mind that you have two patients to care for—the woman and the unborn fetus. Any trauma to the expectant mother has a direct effect on the condition of her fetus. Pregnant women may be victims of many types of trauma, including assaults, motor vehicle crashes, shootings, and, unfortunately, domestic abuse.

Pregnant women are also at an increased risk of falls. This risk is heightened during pregnancy because hormonal changes loosen up the joints in the musculoskeletal system,

and the weight of the uterus and displacement of abdominal organs can change the patient's center of gravity, causing her to lose her balance. Treatment of a pregnant trauma patient in the field is as follows:

- **Maintain an open airway.** A pregnant patient has an increased risk of vomiting and aspiration compared with patients who are not pregnant. Be prepared. Keep your suction unit ready.
- **Administer high-flow oxygen.** Provide 100% supplemental oxygen via a nonrebreathing mask if the patient is responsive.
- **Ensure adequate ventilation.** Assess lung sounds and provide or assist ventilation with a bag-mask device and 100% oxygen. Because the uterus of a pregnant woman presses up against the diaphragm, ventilation will be more difficult than in a women who is not pregnant.
- **Assess circulation.** Control external bleeding with direct pressure or tourniquets as appropriate. Suspect internal bleeding and shock based on the mechanism of injury (MOI). Keep the patient warm and provide spinal immobilization if indicated.
- **Provide IV fluids.** Start one or two IV lines of normal saline using large-bore catheters and macrodrip sets.
- **Transport considerations.** During the third trimester of pregnancy, transport the woman on her left side (to anticipate vomiting and to avoid hypotensive syndrome) maintaining appropriate spinal precautions.

Complications of Delivery

Unruptured Amniotic Sac

Usually, the amniotic sac will break or rupture at the beginning of labor. The sac may also rupture during contractions. If the amniotic sac has not ruptured by the time the newborn emerges from the vagina, it will appear as a fluid-filled sac (like a water balloon). This situation is serious because the sac will suffocate the newborn if it is not removed. You may need to puncture the sac as the newborn's head is crowning (not before) by pulling it away from the newborn and tearing it with your fingers or a clamp, away from the newborn's face. Amniotic fluid will gush out. Push the sac away from the newborn's face and clear the newborn's mouth and nose immediately, using the bulb syringe and gauze sponge.

Meconium Staining

If the amniotic fluid is green or brown instead of clear or has a foul odor, suspect *meconium staining*, which can cause a depressed newborn and airway obstruction. If an infection has resulted from meconium aspiration prior to birth, the newborn may respond only to prolonged resuscitation or may not respond at all. Call for paramedic backup early if there is any indication of meconium staining or fetal distress, and be sure to notify the hospital. Aggressive suctioning of the newborn's mouth and oropharynx before delivery of the body may prevent meconium aspiration and respiratory distress.

Meconium staining The occurrence of a dark green material in the amniotic fluid that can cause lung disease in the newborn.

Umbilical Cord Around the Neck

The cord wrapped around the neck is called a nuchal cord. It is usually easy to remove from around the newborn's neck by slipping the cord gently over the head or shoulder. A nuchal cord that is tightly wound around the neck, however, could cause the newborn to asphyxiate. In this situation, you must cut the cord immediately. Start by placing two clamps 2 inches apart on the cord and cut between the clamps. Once you have cut the cord, unwrap it from around the neck very carefully because it is fragile and easily torn.

Breech Delivery

Occasionally during delivery the buttocks or both feet come out first. This is called a breech presentation. The newborn who presents breech is at greater risk for delivery trauma. If the newborn's buttocks have already passed through the vagina, delivery is underway and you must prepare to assist. Call for paramedic backup and contact medical control for guidance if time permits. Preparations for a breech delivery are the same as those for a vertex delivery. Position the patient, unwrap the emergency delivery kit, and place yourself and your partner as you would for a normal delivery. Allow the legs and buttocks to deliver spontaneously, supporting them to prevent rapid expulsion. The head is usually face down and should be allowed to deliver spontaneously. However, you must ensure that the newborn's airway is open by pushing the walls of the vagina away from the mouth and nose of the newborn. This is a true emergency and requires rapid transport.

Uterine Rupture

If the uterus ruptures, it will happen during labor. The patient usually complains of severe abdominal pain, and the abdomen may be rigid from peritonitis. Physical examination will show signs of shock—sweating, tachycardia, and falling blood pressure. Significant vaginal bleeding may or may not be obvious.

Postpartum Hemorrhage

The average blood loss during the third stage of labor is normally about 150 mL. When blood loss exceeds 500 mL during the first 24 hours after giving birth, it is considered postpartum hemorrhage (bleeding after birth). To manage postpartum hemorrhage in the field, perform the following:

- Continue uterine massage.
- Place the newborn(s) at the mother's breast(s).
- Notify the hospital of the mother's status and your estimated time of arrival (ETA).
- Transport without delay.
- Start another large-bore IV line with normal saline wide open.

- Do not attempt an internal vaginal examination.
- Do not attempt to pack the vagina with dressings.
- Manage external bleeding with firm pressure. It may be necessary to open the labia and place packs at the bleeding site if bleeding is not coming from the vagina but is external to it.

Pulmonary Embolism

One of the most common causes of maternal death during childbirth or in the postpartum period is pulmonary embolism. A pulmonary embolism is a clot that travels through the bloodstream and ultimately becomes lodged in the pulmonary circulation, obstructing blood flow to the lungs. It is a serious and potentially life-threatening complication of pregnancy.

Should a pregnant woman experience sudden dyspnea, tachycardia, or hypotension in the postpartum state, you should suspect pulmonary embolism. The patient may complain of sudden sharp chest pain or abdominal pain or may experience syncope. Physical examination may reveal nothing unusual except for an increased pulse rate, tachypnea, and hypotension—signs that may be mistaken for shock. Management of a postpartum embolism is the same as management of pulmonary embolism occurring in nonpregnant women. In the prehospital environment, this should include supplemental oxygen and rapid transport to the hospital.

Transition Tip

Suspect a pulmonary embolism in any patient who has recently delivered a child with sudden onset of difficulty breathing or altered mental status. Provide high-flow oxygen and immediate transport to the hospital. Be prepared to provide resuscitation as needed.

Stillborn Babies

On rare occasions, the happiness of childbirth is overshadowed by despair when the newborn is dead (stillborn). Good prenatal care most often identifies a stillborn child well before delivery, but in the absence of such care, it may be totally unexpected. Do not attempt to resuscitate an obviously dead newborn (ie, signs of putrification are evident). When a newborn is dead, prepare yourself for dealing with the emotions of the parents as the trauma sets in. Educating yourself about the cultural and ethnic heritage of patients you may encounter in the area where you work will help you prepare for this situation.

Neonatal Assessment and Resuscitation

While you should be familiar with neonatal resuscitation efforts, there are changes. As always, follow your local protocols.

- **A-B-C sequence.** Research has shown that neonatal cardiac arrest is most likely asphyxial in nature. As such, the A-B-C sequence of resuscitation is suggested, with a 3:1 compression-to-ventilation ratio except when the cause of arrest is clearly cardiac in nature.
- **Assessment of heart rate, respiratory rate, and oxygenation.** Once supplemental oxygen has been delivered through either assisted ventilations or blow-by oxygen, begin a simultaneous evaluation of three clinical characteristics: heart rate, respiratory rate, and the state of oxygenation (as determined by pulse oximetry). Research has shown that assessment of the skin color of a newborn is subjective and that oxyhemoglobin saturation is best monitored by a pulse oximeter applied to the neonate's upper right extremity (wrist or palm).
- **Supplemental oxygen.** For full-term neonates, research has shown it is best to begin resuscitation using room air rather than with 100% supplemental oxygen. Term neonates are born with oxyhemoglobin saturation of less than 60%, and hyperoxia (excess oxygen) can actually be toxic, especially in a premature newborn.
- **Suctioning.** Research has shown that there is no benefit to airway suctioning of a newborn, even in the presence of meconium staining, and that there is a documented risk associated with suctioning. As such, the new standard states that immediate suctioning after birth should be reserved for neonates who require positive-pressure ventilation.
- **Compression-to-ventilation ratio.** The recommended ratio of compressions to ventilations during neonatal resuscitation remains 3:1, which was determined to be critical for the majority of newborns suffering from asphyxial arrest. If the cause of arrest is thought to be cardiac in nature, however, rescuers should deliver a compression-to-ventilation ratio of 15:2.
- **Delayed cord clamping.** There is increased evidence that delaying clamping of the umbilical cord for at least 1 minute is beneficial in neonates not requiring resuscitation. There is no benefit or detriment to delaying clamping in neonates requiring resuscitation. Follow your local protocols.

Pediatric Emergencies

Even as a seasoned EMS provider, you may experience a certain level of discomfort when responding to and caring for a pediatric patient in distress. Pediatric patients differ in how they respond physiologically and emotionally to a stressful event. In most situations, caring for an infant or child means you must care for the parents or caregivers as well **FIGURE 20-4**. As such, it is imperative to remain calm and professional, and to effectively communicate with the patient and caregivers regarding your plan of care.

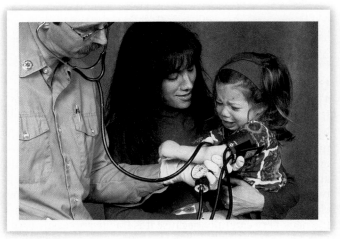

FIGURE 20-4 Treating a sick or injured child can be extremely challenging. A calm, professional demeanor is of utmost importance as you care for both the child and the parents.

> ### Transition Tip
>
> With the exception of the pediatric assessment triangle (PAT) described later in this chapter, pediatric assessment and emergency care have not changed with the *National EMS Education Standards*. As such, the topic of pediatric emergencies is limited in this chapter to pathophysiology and epidemiology of certain conditions, and an overview of patient assessment. Certain information specific to pediatric patients, such as communication techniques, age-specific assessment techniques, and life-span development, was discussed throughout this text, as were specific medical and traumatic conditions that a child may endure. For an additional review of pediatrics, including anatomy, refer to your EMT-I textbook.

Pathophysiology of Pediatric Conditions Based on Body Systems

The Respiratory System

Proportionally, tidal volume in children is similar to that in adolescents and adults; however, their metabolic oxygen demand is doubled. According to a report by the Institute of Medicine in 2007, respiratory illnesses are among the top 10 reasons for emergency department visits in children younger than 17 years in the United States. Asthma is the most common cause of respiratory emergency in children. Other causes include bronchiolitis and pneumonia, both of which are discussed in the *Infectious Diseases* chapter. Foreign bodies, infection, and trauma can also cause respiratory emergencies.

Failure to recognize and treat declining respiratory status will lead to certain death. A pediatric patient in respiratory distress still has the compensatory mechanisms and the ability to exchange oxygen and carbon dioxide. During respiratory distress, the pediatric patient is working harder to breathe and will eventually go into respiratory failure if left untreated. Respiratory failure occurs when the pediatric patient has exhausted all compensatory mechanisms and waste products begin to collect. If this condition is not treated, a total shutdown of the respiratory system will occur—that is, respiratory arrest. Respiratory arrest is the leading cause of cardiopulmonary arrest in the pediatric population.

Transition Tip

Children, especially those younger than 5 years, can (and do) obstruct their airway with any object that they can fit into their mouths: hot dogs, balloons, grapes, toys, or coins. In cases of trauma, a child's teeth may become dislodged and block the airway. Blood, vomitus, or other secretions can also cause mild or severe airway obstruction. In addition, some medical conditions can cause an obstruction of the airway, such as with croup, epiglottitis, and bacterial tracheitis.

Cardiovascular System

It is important to know the normal pulse ranges when evaluating children **TABLE 20-1**. The pediatric cardiovascular system is similar to that of an adult. Even though pediatric patients have a larger proportional amount of circulating blood volume than adults, they are more dependent on the actual cardiac output of the heart (amount of blood being pumped out of the heart in 1 minute). Suspect shock when an infant or child presents with tachycardia. Bradycardia, however, usually indicates severe hypoxia and must be managed aggressively. Remember that hypotension, when it occurs in a child, is an ominous sign and often indicates impending cardiopulmonary arrest. Assessment of capillary refill in children younger than 6 years is a valuable indicator of tissue perfusion.

Table 20-1 Pediatric Pulse Rates	
Age	**Pulse Rate (beats/min)**
Neonate: 0 to 1 month	100 to 180
Infant: 1 month to 1 year	100 to 160
Toddler: 1 to 3 years	90 to 150
Preschool-age: 3 to 6 years	80 to 140
School-age: 6 to 12 years	70 to 120
Adolescent: 12 to 18 years	60 to 100
Adult: Older than 18 years	60 to 100

The Nervous System

The nervous system continually develops throughout childhood. The brain and spinal cord are not well protected by the developing skull and spinal vertebrae. Therefore brain injuries in young children, when they occur, are frequently more devastating than those in adults. Bruising and damage to the brain may be the result of head momentum such as is seen with shaken baby syndrome. The pediatric brain also requires twice the cerebral blood flow as an adult's brain, making even minor injuries significant. Spinal cord injuries are less common in pediatric patients.

The Gastrointestinal System

The abdominal musculature in the child is immature and offers less protection to solid, vascular organs such as the spleen and liver, both of which are proportionally larger and more vascular in children. In addition, the abdominal organs are nearer to one another. For these reasons, pediatric patients are at higher risk for splenic and hepatic injuries than adults. Multiple organ injuries are more common.

The Musculoskeletal System

Bones in children are softer and more porous until adolescence. A child's softer bones make incomplete fractures more likely in this population. Treat any sprain as though a fracture exists, and immobilize the injury accordingly.

Injury to the epiphyseal plate (growth plate) of the bone during its development may result in abnormalities in normal bone growth and development.

The Integumentary System

The thermoregulatory system in children is immature. In addition, children have thinner skin and a lack of subcutaneous fat, making the pediatric population more prone to hypothermic events. Infants younger than 6 months lack the ability to shiver in response to a cold stimulus and, therefore, cannot generate heat. Newborns and infants younger than 1 month are the most susceptible to hypothermia. Nevertheless, newborns should not be overwarmed, as this practice can worsen neurologic outcomes.

Infants and young children should be kept warm during a transport or when exposed for assessment of an injury. Because the head in infants and young children is larger in proportion to the rest of the body, as much as 50% of the body's total heat can be lost when the child's head is exposed to the environment. As such, the head should be covered with a hat or blanket. Without recognition and treatment of a hypothermic event, the pediatric patient may progress to an unconscious state and lapse into convulsive seizure activity.

Pediatric Patient Assessment

On the way to a scene involving a pediatric patient, you should prepare to interact with the family, have pediatric equipment available, and prepare to perform an age-appropriate physical assessment. To form a general impression of a pediatric patient, the PAT is used. To perform a physical assessment of a pediatric patient, a hands-on assessment of the ABCs is done. Otherwise, the assessment of the pediatric patient is the same as it is for an adult.

Pediatric Assessment Triangle

The *pediatric assessment triangle (PAT)* is a structured assessment tool that allows you to rapidly form a general impression of the pediatric patient's condition without touching him or her. It provides a first-glance assessment to identify the general category of the pediatric patient's physiologic problem and to establish urgency for treatment and/or transport. The PAT is a 15- to 30-second visual assessment of the pediatric patient.

> *Pediatric assessment triangle (PAT)* A structured assessment tool that allows the health care provider to rapidly form a general impression of an infant or child without touching him or her; it consists of assessing appearance, work of breathing, and circulation to the skin.

The PAT is a valuable tool in the field when confronted with conditions that may have a variety of etiologies, such as respiratory distress or failure, cardiovascular shock leading to cardiopulmonary failure or arrest, isolated head injury, ingestion of a toxic substance, and neurologic injuries—or even as an approach to assessment of a stable pediatric patient. The PAT **FIGURE 20-5** consists of three elements: appearance (muscle tone and mental status), *work of breathing*, and circulation to the skin. The only equipment required for the PAT are your own eyes and ears; no stethoscope, blood pressure cuff, cardiac monitor, or pulse oximeter is required.

> *Work of breathing* An indicator of oxygenation and ventilation; it reflects the patient's attempt to compensate for hypoxia.

Appearance

Evaluating the pediatric patient's appearance involves noting the level of consciousness or interactiveness and muscle tone—signs that will provide you with information about the adequacy of the pediatric patient's cerebral perfusion (mentation) and overall function of the central nervous system.

Much of the information regarding the pediatric patient's level of consciousness can be obtained by using the PAT. In addition, you can evaluate the pediatric patient's level of consciousness by using the AVPU scale, modified as necessary for the pediatric patient's age **TABLE 20-2**, as well as the pediatric Glasgow Coma Scale **TABLE 20-3**.

An infant or child with a normal level of consciousness will act appropriately for his or her age, exhibiting good muscle tone and maintaining good eye contact. An abnormal level of consciousness is characterized by inappropriate behavior or interactiveness for the child's age, poor muscle tone, or poor eye contact with the caregiver or with you **FIGURE 20-6**.

A helpful mnemonic called TICLS (or tickles) can also help you determine whether the pediatric patient is sick or not sick. TICLS stands for Tone, Interactiveness, Consolability, Look or gaze, and Speech or cry **TABLE 20-4**.

Work of Breathing

A child's breathing becomes more labored as the body attempts to compensate for abnormalities in oxygenation and ventilation. Increased work of breathing often manifests as tachypnea, abnormal airway noise (grunting, stridor, or wheezing), retractions of the intercostal muscles or sternum **FIGURE 20-7**, or the way the pediatric patient positions himself or herself.

Circulation to Skin

Skin color, temperature, and condition are all important signs of tissue perfusion. When cardiac output falls, blood vessels constrict to redirect blood from areas of lesser need (such as the skin) to areas of greater need (such as the brain, heart, and kidneys). This effect results in

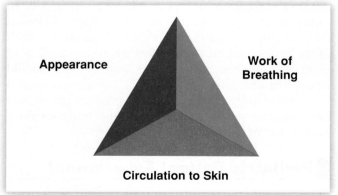

Used with permission of the American Academy of Pediatrics, Pediatric Education for Preshospital Professionals, © American Academy of Pediatrics, 2000.

FIGURE 20-5 The three components of the pediatric assessment triangle (PAT) are appearance, work of breathing, and circulation to the skin.

Table 20-2 The Pediatric AVPU Scale	
Alert	Normal interactiveness for age
Verbal	Appropriate: Responds to name Inappropriate: Nonspecific or confused
Painful	Appropriate: Withdraws from pain Inappropriate: Sound or movement without purpose or localization of pain
Unresponsive	No response to any stimulus

Table 20-3
Pediatric Glasgow Coma Scale (GCS)

Activity	Score	Infant	Score	Child
Eye opening	4 3 2 1	Open spontaneously Open to speech or sound Open to painful stimuli No response	4 3 2 1	Open spontaneously Open to speech Open to painful stimuli No response
Verbal	5 4 3 2 1	Coos, babbles Irritable cry Cries to pain Moans to pain No response	5 4 3 2 1	Oriented conversation Confused conversation Cries Inappropriate words Moans Incomprehensible words/sounds No response
Motor	6 5 4 3 2 1	Normal spontaneous movement Localizes pain Withdraws to pain Abnormal flexion (decorticate) Abnormal extension (decerebrate) No response (flaccid)	6 5 4 3 2 1	Obeys verbal commands Localizes pain Withdraws to pain Abnormal flexion (decorticate) Abnormal extension (decerebrate) No response (flaccid)

Table 20-4
Characteristics of Appearance: The TICLS Mnemonic

Characteristic	Features to Look For
Tone	Is the child moving or resisting examination vigorously? Does the child have good muscle tone? Or is the child limp, listless, or flaccid?
Interactiveness	How alert is the child? How readily does a person, object, or sound distract the child or draw the child's attention? Will the child reach for, grasp, and play with a toy or exam instrument, such as a penlight or tongue blade? Or is the child uninterested in playing or interacting with the caregiver or AEMT?
Consolability	Can the child be consoled or comforted by the caregiver or by the AEMT? Or is the child's crying or agitation unrelieved by gentle reassurance?
Look or gaze	Does the child fix his or her gaze on a face, or is there a "nobody home," glassy-eyed stare?
Speech or cry	Is the child's cry strong and spontaneous or weak or high pitched? Is the content of speech age appropriate or confused and garbled?

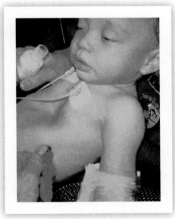

Courtesy of Health Resources and Services Administration, Maternal and Child Health Bureau, Emergency Medical Services for Children Program.

FIGURE 20-6 A limp child who is unable to maintain eye contact may be critically ill or injured.

pallor or cyanosis and coolness of extremities. Likewise, clammy skin is a sign of shock.

Pallor of skin and mucous membranes may be seen in compensated shock; this pale color may also be a sign of anemia or hypoxia. Mottling is caused by constriction of peripheral blood vessels and is another sign of poor perfusion **FIGURE 20-8**.

Cyanosis of the skin and mucous membranes reflects a decreased level of oxygen in the blood. It is a late sign of respiratory failure or shock; absence of discoloration, however, does not rule out these conditions. Never wait for the development of cyanosis before you start administering oxygen!

Stay or Go

On the basis of the findings related to the PAT, you should decide whether the child is stable or whether the child requires urgent care. If a pediatric patient is unstable, assess ABCs, treat any life threats, and provide immediate transport to an appropriate facility. If the patient is stable, you have time to continue with the remainder of the patient assessment process.

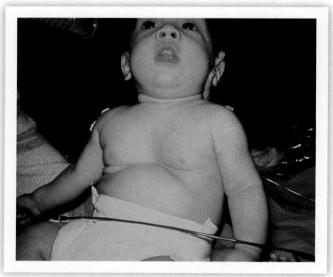

Courtesy of Health Resources and Services Administration, Maternal and Child Health Bureau, Emergency Medical Services for Children Program.

FIGURE 20-7 Retractions of the intercostal muscles or sternum indicate increased work of breathing.

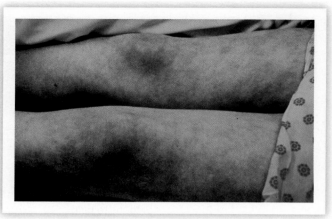

Courtesy of Health Resources and Services Administration, Maternal and Child Health Bureau, Emergency Medical Services for Children Program.

FIGURE 20-8 Mottling of the skin indicates poor perfusion and is the result of constriction of peripheral blood vessels.

Hands-on ABCs

Now that you have completed the PAT, the *National EMS Education Standards* call for a hands-on assessment of a pediatric patient. Assess and treat any life threats by following the ABCDE pathway:

- **A**irway
- **B**reathing
- **C**irculation
- **D**isability
- **E**xposure

Disability refers to assessment of the patient's level of consciousness, pupillary response, symmetric movement of extremities (assessing neurologic motor function), and pain level.

Exposure of the pediatric patient is necessary for completing the hands-on ABCs. The PAT requires removal of part of the pediatric patient's clothing to allow for careful observation of the face, chest wall, and skin. Completing the components requires further exposure, as needed, to fully evaluate physiologic functions, anatomic abnormalities, and unsuspected injuries or rashes. Be careful to avoid heat loss, especially in infants, by covering the patient as soon as possible.

Transition Tip

The approach to, and process of, pediatric assessment and physical examinations depends on the patient's age. Refer to your EMT-I textbook for a review of assessment for specific age groups.

Transition Tip

The intentional injury of a child, whether physical or emotional, unfortunately is not rare in our society. More than 2 million cases of child abuse are reported to child protection agencies in the United States annually. Many of these children suffer life-threatening injuries, and some die. If suspected child abuse is not reported, the child is likely to be abused again and again, perhaps suffering permanent injuries or even dying. As a health care provider, you are a mandated reporter of any suspected child abuse. An easy way to remember assessment points for the pediatric population is the mnemonic CHILD ABUSE, shown in **TABLE 20-5**. For an additional review of pediatric abuse, refer to your EMT-I textbook.

Table 20-5 Mnemonic for Assessing Possible Child Abuse	
C	Consistency of the injury with the child's developmental age
H	History inconsistent with injury
I	Inappropriate parental concerns
L	Lack of supervision
D	Delay in seeking care
A	Affect
B	Bruises of varying ages
U	Unusual injury patterns
S	Suspicious circumstances
E	Environmental clues

Geriatric Emergencies

The process of aging is gradual and starts much earlier than most people realize. A decline in the systems of the human body starts as early as the late 20s and progresses slowly throughout life.

Geriatric patients present as a special problem because the classic presentation of disease is often altered by the presence of chronic conditions and the physiology of aging. In addition, geriatric patients may be taking multiple medications that can interact and have toxic effects.

Providing effective treatment for this growing population of patients requires that you understand the issues related to aging and that you modify your assessment and treatment approach.

Transition Tip

It takes time and patience to interact with an elderly person, which can sometimes be frustrating. Have patience and treat the patient with respect. Make every attempt to avoid "ageism," which is a stereotyping of elderly people that often leads to discrimination. Common stereotypes include assuming that the patient has dementia, is hard of hearing, has a sedentary lifestyle, or is immobile.

General Considerations

The changing physiology of geriatric patients can predispose this population to a host of problems not seen in youth. A simple rib fracture in a 30- or 40-year-old patient may be inconsequential; by comparison, the same injury in a geriatric patient who is 80 or 90 years old can result in pneumonia and even death. A hip fracture from a low-mechanism fall is common in elderly people due to bones weakened by osteoporosis or infection, and may have dire consequences. Sedentary behavior while healing can predispose the patient to pneumonia and blood clots that may interfere with healing and can even cause death. Many patients who experience hip fractures never return to their preinjury levels of activity. In fact, research has shown that the risk of death within one year after a hip fracture ranges from 25% to 30% in the elderly population. All of these factors make assessment and treatment decisions more complex and patient complaints potentially more serious when you are dealing with elderly patients.

Common Complaints

The most frequently occurring conditions in older persons are hypertension, respiratory diseases, arthritis, and heart disease. Leading causes of death in the geriatric population include heart disease, cancer, stroke, chronic obstructive pulmonary disease and other respiratory illnesses, diabetes, and trauma **TABLE 20-6**.

Table 20-6
Common Conditions and Leading Causes of Death in Geriatric Patients

Common Conditions

- Hypertension (48%)
- Diagnosed arthritis (47%)
- Heart disease (32%)
- Cancer (20%)
- Diabetes (16%)
- Sinusitis (14%)

Leading Causes of Death

- Heart disease
- Cancer
- Stroke
- Chronic obstructive pulmonary disease
- Pneumonia and influenza
- Diabetes
- Trauma

Source: Sahyoun RN, Lentzner H, Hoyert D, Robinson KN. *Trends in Causes of Death Among the Elderly.* Hyattsville, MD: National Center of Health Statistics; March 2001. Aging Trends Series No. 1.

Special Considerations in Assessing a Geriatric Medical Patient

Assessing an elderly patient can often be challenging because of communication issues, hearing and vision deficits, altered consciousness and mentation, complicated medical histories, and the effects of medication **TABLE 20-7**. Previous injury or illnesses, although not associated with the current problem, may also alter assessment findings. For example, medications may mask changes in vital signs, and a previous stroke may have changed a patient's baseline level of consciousness and neurologic status.

Investigation of the Chief Complaint

Start the assessment by investigating the chief complaint or history of the present illness. Find and account for all medications. If a patient lives alone, look for evidence of medical information such as a list of medications and medical conditions that may have been put in a specific place (on the refrigerator or "Vial of Life") to provide a medication history for caregivers or EMS personnel.

Determining the chief complaint can be extremely difficult at times. As an AEMT, you will have to play the role of detective many times to determine the actual complaint. The more facts and information that you can obtain from the patient and bystanders or caregivers, the more informed your treatment decision will be.

Table 20-7
Geriatric Patient Assessment Guidelines

- When entering the home, take note of issues that would make it environmentally unsafe.

- Introduce yourself, show respect, and use patience to gain an older patient's confidence.

- Assessment of an elderly patient can be complicated by a combination of multiple medical and traumatic conditions, age-related changes in level of consciousness, and hearing and vision impairments.

- Airway, breathing, circulation, and vital signs are changed by the normal process of aging.

- Many older patients use multiple medications. Be aware of the possibility of overdose, underdose, or interactions if a new medication was recently added to this regimen.

- An older person's body does not have the flexibility or reserves of a younger person's body when facing illness or injury.

- Elderly persons are more readily affected by poor nutrition and dehydration.

- Older people cannot thermoregulate easily and tend to be cold.

- The memory and cognition of an older person may be impaired because of the process of aging, or such changes may be an acute sign. If possible, ask family members or neighbors whether the patient's current mentation is new.

- The skin of an older adult may be fragile and can tear easily. Consider patient movement options that are safe and appropriate.

Transition Tip

When you are assessing a geriatric patient, it is important to determine your patient's baseline mental status early. Is an acute change in level of consciousness the reason why you were called or has an altered level of consciousness been present for some time? Use family members, if available, to establish baseline mental status.

Vital Signs

Vital signs may be different in elderly people because of the physiologic changes that come with aging, chronic disease, and the effects of medications. Although the heart rate should be in the normal adult range, this rate may be altered by medications such as beta-blockers. Such medications keep the heart rate low and prevent the tachycardia that might be typically seen in dehydration or shock. Weaker and irregular pulses are also common in elderly patients. The pulse may be irregular secondary to atrial fibrillation. Circulatory compromise may make it difficult to feel a radial pulse on an older patient, so other pulse points may need to be considered.

Blood pressure tends to be higher in elderly people. An elderly patient who has a blood pressure in a normal adult range could actually be hypotensive. Hypertension, in contrast, could signal impending stroke. Try to determine whether the patient has missed taking medications for hypertension, or any medications for that matter. It is not uncommon for the elderly to stop taking medications or to miss doses due to forgetfulness or financial constraints causing them to have lapses between refills.

The respiratory rate in an older patient should be in the same range as in a younger adult, but remember that chest rise is often compromised by increased chest wall stiffness. Auscultate breath sounds to listen for rales associated with pulmonary edema, rhonchi or rales associated with pneumonia, or wheezes associated with asthma.

Transition Tip

Careful interpretation of pulse oximetry data is necessary in older adults, because the pulse oximetry device requires adequate perfusion to get an accurate reading. Older adults may have poor circulation, vasoconstriction, hypotension, hypothermia, lack of red blood cells, or carbon monoxide poisoning that could result in an inaccurate reading. An alternative approach such as adhesive temporal probes, if available and approved by the local protocol, might help confirm accuracy of the data.

The GEMS Diamond

When you are called to care for older patients, it is important to remember certain key concepts. The GEMS diamond **FIGURE 20-9** was designed to assist the prehospital professional in the assessment and treatment of older patients. It is not intended to be a format for the approach to geriatric patients, nor is it intended to replace the ABCs of care. Instead, it serves as an acronym for the issues to be considered when assessing older patients.

The "G" of the GEMS diamond stands for "geriatric." When responding to an emergency involving an older patient, consider that older patients are different from younger patients and may present atypically.

The "E" of the GEMS diamond stands for an environmental assessment. Assessment of the environment can provide clues to the patient's condition and the cause of the emergency. Is the home too hot or too cold? Is the home well-kept and secure? Is there a strange odor present?

G Geriatric Patients

- Present atypically
- Deserve respect
- Experience normal changes with age

E Environmental Assessment

- Check for hazardous conditions that may be present (eg, poor wiring, rotted floors, unventilated gas heaters, broken window glass, clutter that prevents adequate egress).
- Are smoke detectors present and working?
- Is the home too hot or too cold?
- Is there an odor of feces or urine in the home? Is bedding soiled or urine-soaked?
- Is food present in the home? Is it adequate and unspoiled?
- Are liquor bottles present? If so, are they lying empty?
- If the patient has a disability, are appropriate assistive devices (eg, ramps, rails, wheelchairs, or walkers) present?
- Does the patient have access to a telephone?
- Are medications out of date or unmarked, or are prescriptions for the same or similar medications from many physicians? Are any of the medications prescribed to other people?
- If living with others, is the patient confined to one part of the home?
- If the patient is residing in a nursing facility, does the care appear to be adequate to meet the patient's needs?

M Medical Assessment

- Older patients tend to have a variety of medical problems, making assessment more complex. Keep this in mind in all cases—both trauma and medical. A trauma patient may have an underlying medical condition that could have caused or may be exacerbated by the injury.
- Obtaining a medical history is important in older patients, regardless of the chief complaint.
- Primary assessment
- Reassessment

S Social Assessment

- Assess activities of daily living (eating, dressing, bathing, toileting).
- Are these activities being provided for the patient? If so, by whom?
- Are there delays in obtaining food, medication, or other necessary items? The patient may complain of this, or the environment may suggest this.
- If in an institutional setting, is the patient able to feed himself or herself? If not, is food still sitting on the food tray? Has the patient been lying in his or her own urine or feces for prolonged periods?
- Does the patient have a social network? Does the patient have a mechanism to interact socially with others on a daily basis?

FIGURE 20-9 The GEMS diamond provides a concise way to remember the most important issues related to older patients.

Are there risk factors suggesting carbon monoxide poisoning? Are hazardous conditions present? Preventive care is also very important for a geriatric patient, who may not carefully study the environment or may not realize where risks exist.

The "M" of the GEMS diamond stands for medical assessment. Older patients tend to have a variety of medical problems that lead them to take numerous prescription, over-the-counter (OTC) products, and herbal medications. Obtaining a thorough medical history is very important in older patients.

The "S" stands for social assessment. Older people may have less of a social network because of the deaths of spouses, family members, and friends. They may also need assistance with activities of daily living, such as dressing and eating. Numerous social agencies are readily available to help geriatric patients, but many people are unaware of such services.

The GEMS diamond provides a concise way to remember the important issues for older patients. Using this concept can help you make appropriate referrals and, as a result, help older patients maintain their quality of life.

Changes in the Body

As was discussed in the *Life Span Development* chapter, the body goes through certain changes as it ages. **TABLE 20-8** reviews these changes.

Pathophysiology of the Respiratory System: A Review

Age-related changes in the respiratory system can predispose an older adult to respiratory illness. In this population, even a minor lung infection can become a life-threatening event.

The alveoli in an older person's lung tissue can become enlarged and the elasticity decreases, making it more difficult to expel used air. This change in lung tissue quality is comparable to a balloon that has been expanded and then deflated. The balloon loses some of its ability to contract to its original state after inflation. This lack of elasticity results in a decreased ability to exchange oxygen and carbon dioxide. The body's chemoreceptors, which monitor the changes in oxygen and carbon dioxide levels in the blood, slow with age. This change can present as lower pulse oximetry readings, even in healthy people.

Pneumonia

Although tobacco abuse seems to be decreasing among elderly people, chronic lower respiratory disease, influenza, and pneumonia remain among the top five causes of geriatric deaths. In fact, one of the most common causes of death in older patients is infection with *Pneumococcus* bacteria.

Pulmonary Embolism

Another condition that can cause respiratory distress in the elderly is a pulmonary embolism, a condition in which a

Table 20-8
Effects of Aging

System	Effects of Aging
Respiratory system	■ Weakened airway musculature, often resulting in decreased breathing capacity and increased difficulty breathing. ■ Loss of elastic recoil in the chest wall, resulting in air trapping and an increase in the amount of air left in the lungs at the end of an exhalation. ■ Loss of mechanisms that protect the upper airway, including decreased cough and gag reflexes, resulting in a decreased ability to clear secretions. ■ Decrease in the number of cilia that line the bronchial tree, lessening a person's ability to cough and, therefore, increasing the chances of infection. ■ Enlarged alveoli and decreased elasticity, making it harder to expel used air.
Cardiovascular system	■ Overall decrease in the efficiency of the cardiovascular system. ■ Hypertrophy (enlargement) of the heart with age, probably in response to the chronically increased afterload imposed by stiffened blood vessels. ■ Gradual decrease in cardiac output, mostly as a result of a decreasing stroke volume. ■ Arteriosclerosis—stiffening of blood vessel walls—is common, contributing to systolic hypertension, which places an extra burden on the heart. ■ Widening pulse pressure, decreased coronary artery perfusion, and changes in cardiac ejection efficiency resulting from overproduction of abnormal collagen and decreased quantities of elastin, leading to vascular stiffening.
Nervous system	■ Decline in mental function, which results in slower processing of sensory stimuli and language, and longer retrieval times for short- and long-term memory. ■ Decreased size and weight (10% to 20% of the younger adult averages) of the brain, which increases the space in the cranium and, therefore, raises the risk for head injuries. Head injuries with a minimal mechanism are commonly missed in the elderly population until it is too late. ■ Slowed motor and sensory neural networks caused by a 5% to 50% loss of neurons responsible for transmission of impulses. ■ Diminished senses of taste and smell. ■ Visual changes as early as age 40 years, with as many as 50% of patients older than 65 years having vision problems.
Gastrointestinal system	■ Reduction in the volume of saliva, resulting in dryness of the mouth. ■ Dental loss resulting from disease of the teeth and gums. ■ Decreased sense of taste, which may lead to poor nutrition. ■ Reduced gastric secretions. ■ Changes in gastric motility, leading to slower gastric emptying and increased risk of aspiration. ■ Decreased absorption of nutrients from food. ■ Decreased blood flow to the liver. ■ Decline in the activity of the enzyme systems involved with the detoxification of drugs. ■ Poor muscle tone of the smooth muscle sphincter between the esophagus and stomach. ■ Slowing peristalsis (motion that moves feces through the colon), leading to constipation. ■ Weakened rectal sphincter, resulting in fecal incontinence (lack of bowel control). ■ Shrinking of the liver, which is responsible for removing toxins and breaking down drugs in the body.
Genitourinary system	■ Reduction in renal function, renal blood flow (by as much as 50%), and tubule degeneration. ■ Decreased bladder capacity. ■ Decline in sphincter muscle control. ■ Decline in voiding senses with increase in nocturnal voiding. ■ Benign prostatic hypertrophy (enlarged prostate) in men.

Table 20-8
Effects of Aging (*continued*)

System	Effects of Aging
Endocrine system	• Decreased metabolism of thyroxine, a thyroid hormone that has an effect on metabolism in the body. • Decreased conversion of thyroxine to triiodothyronine leading to a slower heart rate, fatigue, drier skin and hair, cold intolerance, and weight gain. • Increased secretion of antidiuretic hormones, causing fluid imbalance. • Increases in the levels of norepinephrine, possibly having a harmful effect on the cardiovascular system. • Reduction in pancreatic beta cell secretion, leading to hyperglycemia.
Immune system	• Decreased effectiveness of systemic and cellular immune responses at fighting infection.

venous clot suddenly blocks an artery. In the elderly, this potentially life-threatening condition is often confused with a cardiac, lung, or musculoskeletal problem.

> **Transition Tip**
>
> Specific respiratory conditions, including pneumonia and pulmonary embolism, are discussed in detail in the *Respiratory Emergencies* chapter.

Pathophysiology of the Cardiovascular System: A Review

Geriatric patients are at risk for atherosclerosis, an accumulation of fatty material in the arteries, increasing the likelihood of myocardial infarction (heart attack) and stroke. Atherosclerotic disease typically begins in the teenage years and affects more than 60% of people older than 65 years. The presence of arteriosclerosis—a disease that causes the arteries to thicken, harden, and calcify—makes stroke, heart disease, hypertension, and bowel infarction more likely.

Older people are also at an increased risk for aneurysm—an abnormal, blood-filled dilation of the wall of a blood vessel. Severe blood loss can occur if an aneurysm ruptures.

Rupture of an *abdominal aortic aneurysm (AAA)* is one of the most rapidly fatal conditions. With an AAA, the walls of the aorta weaken and blood begins to leak into the layers of the vessel, causing the aorta to bulge like a bubble on a tire. If enough blood is lost into the vessel wall itself, shock occurs. If the wall bursts, fatal blood loss typically results.

> *Abdominal aortic aneurysm (AAA)* A condition in which the walls of the aorta in the abdomen weaken and blood leaks into the layers of the vessel, causing it to bulge.

> **Transition Tip**
>
> Some changes in cardiovascular performance do not result from aging, but rather reflect deconditioning because of a sedentary lifestyle. Many people tend to limit physical activity and exercise as they grow older, whether as the result of a medical condition or for psychosocial reasons. The phrase, "Use it or lose it," applies just as much to the cardiac muscle as to the biceps muscle.

Heart Attack (Myocardial Infarction)

Chest pain is a common complaint of the elderly and can often indicate heart-related issues such as myocardial infarction. It is important to remember that the classic symptoms of a heart attack or myocardial infarction are often not present in geriatric patients. As many as one third of older patients experience "silent" heart attacks in which the usual chest pain is not present. This presentation is particularly common in women and people with diabetes. Do not assume your patient is not having a myocardial infarction simply because the classic, pressure-type, substernal chest pain is not reported.

With older people, treat associated symptoms such as dyspnea; epigastric and abdominal pain; nausea and vomiting; weakness, dizziness, light-headedness, and syncope; fatigue; and confusion as seriously as if the patient had chest pain. Other signs and symptoms that can indicate a cardiovascular problem in elderly persons include issues with circulation; diaphoresis (profound sweating); pale, cyanotic (blue) mottled skin; adventitious (outside of normal) or decreased breath sounds; and increased peripheral edema (swelling).

It is important to obtain as much information as possible from the patient. Even if the patient has an altered mental status or is having a hard time communicating, elicit as much information as possible. No one can describe subjective symptoms such as pain or shortness of breath as well as the patient.

As in all prehospital emergencies, health care providers must prioritize the ABCs. Use the appropriate oxygen delivery device and airway adjunct consistent with the patient's condition. Remember to reassess the patient often.

TABLE 20-9 lists signs and symptoms commonly noted in geriatric patients experiencing a myocardial infarction.

Congestive Heart Failure

Signs and symptoms of heart failure differ depending on the extent to which the right or left side of the heart is not functioning correctly. In heart failure, the heart is not able to maintain cardiac output sufficient to meet the needs of the body because it is no longer able to pump effectively. Hypertension may be seen early on, but as the muscle becomes more fatigued and cardiac output is decreased, the patient may experience hypotension. Acute exacerbations of heart failure are often related to poor diet, medication noncompliance, onset of dysrhythmias such as atrial fibrillation, or acute myocardial infarction.

> **Transition Tip**
>
> Specific cardiovascular conditions, including myocardial infarction, heart failure, and aneurysm, are discussed in detail in the *Cardiovascular Emergencies* chapter.

Pathophysiology of the Nervous System: A Review

Dementia

Dementia is the slow onset of progressive disorientation, shortened attention span, and loss of cognitive function. It is a chronic, generally irreversible condition that causes a progressive loss of cognitive abilities, psychomotor skills, and social skills. Dementia develops slowly over a period of years rather than a few days and is the result of many neurologic diseases. Alzheimer disease, cerebrovascular accidents, and genetic factors, for example, may all cause dementia.

> *Dementia* The slow onset of progressive disorientation, shortened attention span, and loss of cognitive function.

When assessing the patient with dementia, you may note delusions, hallucinations, or aggressive behavior. The patient might exhibit loss of cognitive function. Determine whether this is an acute finding or whether it evolved as a progressive condition over a period of time. Patients with dementia may have short- and long-term memory problems and a decreased attention span, or be unable to perform their daily routines. They may show a decreased ability to communicate and appear confused. Determine the reason you were called, and establish a baseline of the person's cognitive function. Never assume that dementia is chronic. In the absence of a specific history of dementia, assume any signs represent new findings and treat appropriately.

Other aspects of dementia can also complicate your ability to assess and manage the patient. Sometimes patients are not only confused but also angry. They will generally have poor memory and impaired judgment, and may be unable to vocalize symptoms or areas of pain, or follow commands. In addition, these patients often exhibit disorganized thoughts, inattention, memory loss, disorientation, hallucinations, delusions, and a reduced level of consciousness.

Table 20-9 Common Signs and Symptoms of Myocardial Infarction in an Older Patient	
Signs/ Symptoms	**Potential Causes**
Dyspnea	Dyspnea, the feeling of shortness of breath or difficulty in breathing, is a common complaint in older people and is commonly associated with an MI. It is often combined with other symptoms, such as nausea, weakness, and sweating. In older persons, chest pain is often not present, but dyspnea on exertion is noted.
Generalized weakness	Generalized weakness (malaise) can be caused by many things. However, you should suspect an MI in a patient with a sudden onset of weakness. Weakness is often associated with sweating.
Syncope/ confusion/ altered mental status	Syncope can have many causes, and in older people, none of these causes should be presumed to be minor. Syncope often has a cardiac cause. Altered mental status is usually a signal of poor blood supply to the brain, often from a cardiac arrhythmia and MI.

Abbreviation: MI indicates myocardial infarction.

> **Transition Tip**
>
> Be alert when dealing with any patient exhibiting an altered mental status, even if it is normal for that patient. Some patients with dementia, Alzheimer disease, or other illnesses can become extremely violent, posing a danger to family as well as rescuers.

Patients with dementia may express anxiety over movement out of their current environment. They may not understand the need to go to the hospital and often express anxiety and fear of treatment. Their level of tolerance to changes in routine may be very low. Exercise extreme patience with these patients.

Delirium

Delirium is a sudden change in mental status, consciousness, or cognitive processes. It is marked by the inability to focus, think logically, and maintain attention. Delirium affects 15% to 50% of hospitalized people aged 70 years or older.

> *Delirium* A more or less sudden change in mental status marked by the inability to focus, think logically, and maintain attention.

Delirium is commonly an acute condition indicating some type of new health problem. It is usually the result of a reversible physical ailment, such as tumors or fever, but it can also derive from metabolic causes. Acute anxiety may be present, but memory remains intact. Any time a patient has a sudden change in mental status, thoroughly evaluate the history, including an assessment of possible risk factors and current medications, looking for potential clues as to the underlying pathophysiology.

Other important things to look for in the history are intoxication or withdrawal from alcohol; withdrawal from sedatives; medical conditions such as urinary tract infections, bowel obstructions, dehydration, fever, cardiovascular disease, and hyperglycemia or hypoglycemia; psychiatric disorders such as depression; malnutrition/vitamin deficiencies; and environmental emergencies.

Assess the patient for the three specific conditions that can be managed at the prehospital level:

- Hypoxia
- Hypovolemia
- Hypoglycemia

Any of these three conditions, if unrecognized or untreated, can be rapidly fatal. With these conditions, delirium has a rapid onset—described in terms of minutes, hours, or days—and is usually curable if identified early. Geriatric patients will respond to oxygen for hypoxia, placement in the shock position for hypovolemia, and glucose for hypoglycemia.

During physical examination, you may see changes in circulation, response of the pupils, or response to motor tests, or you may find adventitious breath sounds. A low blood pressure can indicate hypovolemia. Dilated pupils could suggest hypoxia or drug use; wheezing, rales, and rhonchi are the result of disease processes that impair breathing and oxygenation.

Treatment for patients with delirium is mostly supportive. Monitor vital signs, including breath sounds. Use airway adjuncts if the patient is unable to maintain his or her airway and obtain IV access to use as a fluid resuscitation route if needed.

> **Transition Tip**
>
> Sundown syndrome (or Sundowning) is a term that describes the onset of confusion and agitation that generally affects people with dementia or cognitive impairment and usually strikes around sunset. Although this condition is generally associated with dementia, people without dementia sometimes develop delirious and agitated behavior in a hospital or similar setting as a reaction to pain, medical procedures, infection, or simply a change in environment. The patient with sundown syndrome will usually act perfectly normal after leaving the hospital environment.

Syncope

Always assume that a syncopal episode in an older patient is a life-threatening problem until proven otherwise. Syncope (fainting) is often caused by an interruption of blood flow to the brain. It has many causes—some serious, some not. In any event, an older person who has a period of unconsciousness should be examined to determine the cause of the syncope. **TABLE 20-10** lists some of the causes of syncope in geriatric patients.

Table 20-10
Possible Causes of Syncope in Geriatric Patients

Cause	Mechanism
Cardiac arrhythmias/ myocardial infarction	The heart is beating too fast or too slow, the cardiac output drops, and blood flow to the brain is interrupted. A myocardial infarction can also cause syncope.
Vascular and volume changes	Medication interaction can cause venous pooling and vasodilation, widening of a blood vessel, resulting in a drop in blood pressure and inadequate blood flow to the brain. Another cause of syncope can be a decrease in blood volume because of hidden bleeding from a condition such as a leaking aortic aneurysm.
Neurologic	A transient ischemic attack, or a small stroke, can sometimes cause syncope.

Stroke

Stroke (cerebrovascular accident, or CVA) is a leading cause of death in the elderly. The likelihood of having a stroke becomes greater as a person gets older. Both preventable and nonpreventable causes of stroke have been identified. Preventable risk factors include smoking, obesity, and a sedentary lifestyle. Less preventable causes are high cholesterol and hypertension. Uncontrollable factors include cardiac disease and atrial fibrillation.

> ### Transition Tip
>
> Specific neurologic conditions, including syncope and stroke, are discussed in detail in the *Neurologic Emergencies* chapter.

Neuropathy

Neuropathy is a disorder of the nerves of the peripheral nervous system in which function and structure of the peripheral motor, sensory, and autonomic neurons are impaired. Symptoms depend on the types of nerves affected and where they are located:

- **Motor nerves.** Impairment causes muscle weakness, cramps, spasms, loss of balance, and loss of coordination.
- **Sensory nerves.** Impairment causes tingling, numbness, itching, and pain; burning, freezing, or extreme sensitivity to touch.
- **Autonomic nerves.** Impairment affects involuntary functions that could include changes in blood pressure and heart rate, constipation, and bladder and sexual dysfunction.

> **Neuropathy** A group of conditions in which the nerves leaving the spinal cord are damaged, resulting in distortion of signals to or from the brain.

Neuropathies are treated with medication and other therapies not available in the prehospital setting. Emergency care should focus on making the patient as comfortable as possible and transporting him or her for further evaluation and care.

Pathophysiology of the Gastrointestinal System: A Review

Specific gastrointestinal problems that are more common in older patients include bleeding in the upper and lower gastrointestinal tract and nausea, vomiting, and diarrhea.

Gastrointestinal Bleeding

Upper gastrointestinal bleeding occurs in the esophagus, stomach, or duodenum. These bleeding episodes are sometimes seen in people who are long-term users of nonsteroidal anti-inflammatory drugs (NSAIDs) such as celecoxib (Celebrex), ibuprofen, and naproxen or people who are long-term alcohol users. Irritation of the lining of the stomach or ulcers can cause forceful vomiting that tears the esophagus. Hepatitis and cancer can also contribute to bleeding problems. Gastrointestinal bleeding is usually noted by the vomiting of blood or coffee ground–like vomitus.

Lower gastrointestinal bleeding occurs in the colon or rectum. This condition is usually not as critical a threat as upper gastrointestinal bleeding unless the patient presents with tachycardia and hypotension. Bleeding that travels through the lower digestive tract usually manifests as melena (black, tarry stools), whereas red blood usually means a local source of bleeding, such as hemorrhoids. Melena, not pain, is the most common presenting symptom of GI bleeding. Treat the patient for shock. Manage the ABCs and use appropriate oxygen therapy and adjuncts as needed. Severe lower gastrointestinal tract bleeding requires immediate transportation to the nearest emergency department.

Nausea, Vomiting, and Diarrhea

The complaint of nausea, vomiting, and diarrhea needs to be investigated to determine the underlying cause. These complaints may be attributed to conditions inside or outside the gastrointestinal tract. Nausea may be an older person's complaint during a cardiac episode. During your assessment of the patient who reports having nausea, vomiting, or diarrhea, remember to ask the color associated with the vomiting and/or diarrhea. Bloody emesis or diarrhea is a clinically significant finding and may indicate serious gastrointestinal bleeding.

Pathophysiology of the Renal System: A Review

Although the kidneys of an elderly person may be capable of dealing with day-to-day demands, they may not be able to meet unusual challenges, such as those imposed by illness. For that reason, acute illness in elderly patients is often accompanied by derangements in fluid and electrolyte balance. Aging kidneys, for example, respond sluggishly to sodium deficiency. An elderly patient may lose a great deal of sodium before the kidneys halt urinary sodium excretion—a problem that is exacerbated by the markedly decreased thirst mechanism in elderly people. The net result may be rapid development of severe dehydration.

Bowel and bladder continence require anatomically correct gastrointestinal and genitourinary tracts, functioning and intact sphincters, and properly working cognitive and physical functions. Urinary incontinence (involuntary loss of urine) can have significant social and emotional impact, but relatively few people admit to the problem and even fewer seek treatment for it.

As people age, the capacity of the bladder decreases. As a consequence, an older person may find it difficult to postpone voiding or may have involuntary bladder contractions. An increase in nocturnal voiding is common.

Incontinence can lead to skin irritation, skin breakdown, and urinary tract infections.

Two major types of incontinence are distinguished: stress and urge. Stress incontinence occurs during activities such as coughing, laughing, sneezing, lifting, and exercise. Urge incontinence is triggered by hot or cold fluids, running water, and even thinking about going to the bathroom. Treatment of incontinence consists of medications, physical therapy, and, in some cases, surgery.

Older patients may also complain of urinary retention or difficulty urinating. They may have difficulty voiding or absence of voiding as a result of many medical causes. In men, enlargement of the prostate can place pressure on the urethra, making voiding difficult. Bladder and urinary tract infections can also cause inflammation. In severe cases of urinary retention, patients may have acute or chronic renal failure.

> ### Transition Tip
>
> Refer back to the *Gastrointestinal and Urologic Emergencies* chapter for additional information on specific gastrointestinal or renal diseases, including pathophysiology, assessment, and emergency care.

Pathophysiology of the Endocrine System: A Review

Hyperosmolar hyperglycemic state (HHS) is a complication of type 2 diabetes that is sometimes seen in elderly people. Unlike in DKA, which occurs in conjunction with type 1 diabetes, the resulting high blood glucose level does not cause ketosis. Instead, it leads to osmotic diuresis and a shift of fluid to the intravascular space that results in dehydration. The signs and symptoms of HHS and DKA often overlap, however. Associated signs and symptoms include hyperglycemia, polydipsia (thirst), polyuria (urination), and polyphagia (hunger), as well as dizziness, confusion, altered mental status, and possibly seizures.

On assessment, you may see changes in circulation such as warm, flushed skin; poor skin turgor; pale, dry oral mucosa; and a furrowed tongue. The patient may also present with signs and symptoms of hypotension and shock, including tachycardia. The blood glucose level will be greater than 500 mg/dL in DKA; by comparison, in HHS, this value is greater than 300 mg/dL. Another assessment difference is that DKA will present with Kussmaul respirations (deep and labored), whereas HHS does not. Rehydration through fluid boluses is the prehospital treatment of choice along with supportive care for either condition.

Pathophysiology of the Musculoskeletal System: A Review

The stooped posture of older people comes from atrophy of the supporting structures of the body. Two of every three older patients will show some degree of *kyphosis* (also called humpback or hunchback). Lost height in older adults generally results from compression in the spinal column, first in the disks and then from the process of *osteoporosis*, which results in compression fractures of the vertebral bodies.

> *Kyphosis* A forward curling of the back caused by an abnormal increase in the curvature of the spine.
> *Osteoporosis* A generalized bone disease in which a reduction in the amount of bone mass leads to compression fractures after minimal trauma; this disease can occur in both men and women, although it is more prevalent in postmenopausal women.

Osteoporosis, a condition that affects both men and women, is characterized by a decrease in bone mass leading to reduction in bone strength and greater susceptibility to fracture. The extent of bone loss that a person undergoes is influenced by numerous factors, including genetics, smoking, level of activity, diet, alcohol consumption, hormonal factors, and body weight. The most rapid loss of bone occurs in women during the years following menopause. In fact, many postmenopausal women use hormone replacement therapy as a means to reduce the loss of bone. Calcium and vitamin D supplements and other medications are available to improve bone strength. Older people should be encouraged to remain active and perform low-impact exercises to maintain bone and muscle strength.

Osteoarthritis is a progressive disease of the joints that destroys cartilage, promotes the formation of bone spurs in joints, and leads to joint stiffness. This type of arthritis is thought to result from wear and tear and, in some cases, repetitive trauma to the joints. It affects 35% to 45% of people older than 65 years. Typically, osteoarthritis affects several joints of the body—most commonly those in the hands, knees, hips, and spine. Patients complain of pain and stiffness on rising and pain that gets worse with exertion. The end result is often substantial disability and disfigurement. Patients are typically treated with anti-inflammatory medications and physical therapy to improve range of motion.

Pathophysiology of the Integumentary System: A Review

Collagen is a protein that is the chief component of connective tissue and bones, and elastin is a protein that helps to make the skin pliable. Reproduction of these proteins slows as the body ages, bringing on a thinner and less robust appearance in older people. The layer of fat under the skin also becomes thinner because of the redistribution of fluids and proteins. As the elasticity of the skin declines, bruising becomes more common, because the skin can tear more easily. In addition, exocrine (sweat) glands do not respond as readily to heat because of atrophy and because of remodeling of the tissues of the dermal layer of the skin.

A common problem that affects the skin of the elderly is pressure ulcers, sometimes referred to as bedsores or *decubitis ulcers*. Pressure ulcers form when a patient remains lying or sitting in the same position for a long time. The pressure from the weight of the body cuts off the blood flow to the area of skin; in turn, because of the lack of blood flow to the skin, a sore develops. Such sores can develop in as little as 45 minutes. Decubitis ulcers can be painful and cause complications such as bleeding, sepsis, and a type of bone infection called osteomyelitis.

> **Decubitis ulcers** Sores caused by the pressure of skin against a surface for long periods; they can range from a pink discoloration of the skin to a deep wound that may invade into bone or organs. Also known as bedsores.

To help prevent these ulcers, take special care to pad voids in a patient who may be on a backboard for an extended period of time. Special pads are available to prevent the development of ulcers during transport.

Toxicologic Emergencies

Several pathophysiologic changes cause elderly people to be more susceptible to toxicity than their younger-adult counterparts. These changes include decreased kidney function, altered gastrointestinal absorption, and decreased vascular flow in the liver, which in turn alters metabolism and excretion. These metabolic issues can also make it difficult for physicians to find the appropriate dosage for new medications. For the most part, dosages for older people need to be reduced compared with those for younger patients.

The elderly account for one fourth of all prescribed medications and one third of OTC medications sold in the United States. Typical OTC medicines used by elderly people include aspirin, antacids, cough syrups, and decongestants. Many people believe OTC medications cannot be dangerous; these medications, however, can have negative effects when mixed with each other and/or with herbal substances, alcohol, and prescription medications.

Many older people take a variety of drugs. Polypharmacy refers to the use of multiple medications by one patient. Many patients have more than one physician and may not remember which medications each doctor prescribed or may not want to tell one doctor about seeing another. Patients may also take OTC medications, including herbal remedies, or medications prescribed for a family member or friend. Any of these actions may have adverse or cumulative effects.

Although almost any drug can produce toxic effects in an older person, certain drugs and classes of drugs are implicated more often than others. Typically, toxic effects present with psychiatric symptoms (such as hallucinations, paranoia, delusions, agitation, and psychosis) and cognitive impairment (such as delirium, confusion, disorientation, amnesia, stupor, and coma).

Trauma and Geriatric Patients

Trauma is one of the top 10 causes of death among elderly people. Falls are the leading cause of trauma-related disability in older patients. The incidence of falls increases with increasing age. Although most falls do not produce serious injury, in 2006 more than 20,800 patients died of fall-related injuries, with 17,700 of these occurring in patients aged 65 years and older.

Motor vehicle trauma is the second leading cause of trauma death in the geriatric population. An older patient is five times more likely than a younger patient to be fatally injured in a car crash, even though excessive speed is rarely a causative factor in the older age group. Pedestrian accidents and burns are also common mechanisms of injury in older patients, resulting in death, serious injury, or disability.

Elder Abuse and Neglect

Reports and complaints of abuse, neglect, and other related problems among the nation's older population are on the rise. Elder abuse is defined as any action by an older person's family member, caregiver, or other associated person that takes advantage of the older person's person, property, or emotional state. It is sometimes called parent battering.

The exact extent of elder abuse is not known for several reasons, including the following:

- Elder abuse is a problem that has been largely hidden from society.
- The definitions of abuse and neglect among the geriatric population vary.
- Victims of elder abuse are often hesitant to report the problem to law enforcement agencies or human and social welfare personnel.

An older adult who is being abused by his or her relative or caregiver may feel ashamed or guilty. The abused person may feel shame, anger, or guilt (or all three) for being in an abusive situation. If the caregiver/abuser is a family member, the abused person may fear retribution or anger from other family members for reporting the abuse to an outside agency.

The physical and emotional signs of abuse, such as rape, spouse beating, and nutritional deprivation, are often overlooked or not accurately identified in the elderly population. Older women, in particular, are not likely to report incidents of sexual assault to law enforcement agencies. Patients with sensory deficits, dementia, and other forms of altered mental status, such as drug-induced depression, may not be able to report abuse.

Elder abuse occurs most often in women older than 75 years. The abused person is often frail and has multiple chronic medical conditions including dementia. He or she may sleepwalk, have an impaired sleep cycle, and periodically shout at others. Such a person may also be incontinent and, in general, is dependent on others for activities of daily living.

Abusers of older people have often been victims of child abuse themselves, and the abuse that is inflicted on the older person may be in retaliation. Most of these abusers are not trained in the particular care that older people require and have little relief time from the constant care demands of their own family, children, and spouse. Their lives are now complicated by the constant, demanding needs of the older person they have to care for.

The abuser may also have marked fatigue, be unemployed with financial difficulties, and abuse one or more substances. With a careful eye, you can recognize the clues to these stressful situations and help guide the family toward programs in their community that are geared to helping the whole family. Programs such as adult day care, Meals on Wheels, and many local individualized programs help to decrease the stress put on the family and lower the risk of abuse.

Abuse is not restricted to the home, however. Environments such as nursing, convalescent, and continuing care centers are also sites where older people may sustain physical, psychological, financial, or pharmacologic harm. Often, care providers in these environments consider older people to be management problems or categorize them as obstinate and undesirable patients.

Patient Assessment of Elder Abuse

While you are assessing the patient, try to obtain an explanation of what happened. As with abuse in any age group, suspect abuse when answers to questions about what caused the injury are concealed or avoided, or when you are given unbelievable answers. Information that may be important in assessing possible abuse includes the following:

- Repeated visits to the emergency department or clinic
- A history of being accident prone
- Repeated or multiple soft-tissue injuries
- Unbelievable or vague explanations of injuries
- Psychosomatic complaints
- Chronic pain without medical explanation
- Self-destructive behavior
- Eating and sleep disorders
- Depression or a lack of energy
- Substance and/or sexual abuse history

Like any other abused patients, elderly victims of abuse may be so afraid of retribution that they make false statements. A geriatric patient who is being abused by family members may lie about the origin of abuse for fear of being thrown out of the home. In other cases of elder abuse, sensory deprivation or dementia may hinder adequate explanation.

Repeated abuse can lead to a high risk of death. A preventive measure for reducing additional maltreatment of the patient is identification of the abuse by emergency medical

Table 20-11 Categories of Elder Abuse	
Physical	- Assault - Neglect - Dietary - Poor maintenance of home - Poor personal hygiene
Psychological	- Benign neglect - Verbal - Treating the person as an infant - Deprivation of sensory stimulation
Financial	- Theft of valuables - Embezzlement

providers **TABLE 20-11**. This step may allow for referral and protective services of human services, social services, and public safety agencies.

Signs of Physical Abuse

Signs of abuse may be quite obvious or very subtle. Inflicted bruises are usually found on the buttocks and lower back, genitals and inner thighs, cheeks or earlobes, neck, upper lip, and inside the mouth. Pressure bruises caused by the human hand may be identified by oval grab marks, pinch marks, or handprints. Human bites are typically inflicted on the upper extremities and can cause lacerations and infection. You should inspect the patient's ears for indications of twisting, pulling, or pinching and evidence of frequent blows to the outer ears. Multiple bruises in various states of healing are common in abused patients.

Burns are a widely encountered form of abuse. If you see burns—especially cigarette burns or physical marks that indicate that certain parts of the patient's body have been scalded systematically—suspect abuse. The damage from burns is often caused by contact with cigarettes, matches, heated metal, forced immersion in hot liquids, chemicals, and electrical power sources.

It may be difficult to detect a failure to thrive in an older patient who has been abused. Observe the patient's weight and try to determine whether the patient appears undernourished or has been unable to gain weight in the current environment. Does the patient have a ravenous appetite? Has medication been withheld? Is money being withheld, so that the patient cannot buy food or medicine? Check for signs of neglect, such as evidence of a lack of hygiene, poor dental hygiene, poor temperature regulation, or lack of reasonable amenities in the home **FIGURE 20-10**.

Regard injuries to the genitals or rectum with no reported trauma as evidence of sexual abuse in any patient. Geriatric patients with altered mental status may never be able to report sexual abuse. In addition, many women do not report cases of sexual abuse because of shame and the pressure to forget.

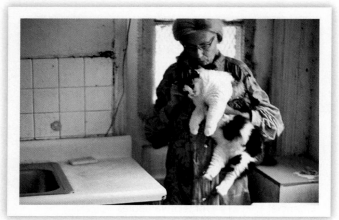

© Jeff Greenberg/PhotoEdit, Inc.

FIGURE 20-10 Check for signs of neglect, such as evidence of a lack of hygiene, poor dental hygiene, poor temperature regulation, or lack of reasonable amenities in the home.

▌Patients With Special Challenges

As medicine and medical technology continue to improve, the number of people both adults and children—with chronic diseases and injuries who are living at home or in other environments outside of a hospital setting continues to grow. As such, it is important to become familiar with the special needs created by patients with chronic diseases and conditions.

Examples of patients with special needs include the following groups:

- Children who were born prematurely, with associated respiratory problems
- Infants or small children with congenital heart disease
- Patients with neurologic disease (occasionally caused by hypoxemia at the time of birth, as with cerebral palsy)
- Patients with congenital or acquired diseases resulting in altered body function that requires medical assistance for breathing, eating, urination, or bowel function
- Patients with sensory deficits such as hearing or visual impairments
- Geriatric patients with chronic diseases requiring visitation from a home health care service

You may be called on to treat a patient who is dependent on mechanical ventilators, IV pumps, or other devices to live. Assess and care for all patients with special needs the same way you care for other patients. Specifically, assessment and treatment of the ABCs remains the priority. Do not allow yourself to be distracted by the noise and mechanics of the medical equipment—your focus needs to remain on the patient whom the medical equipment may be assisting. If the emergency is the result of medical equipment failure, use the equipment on the ambulance. In some cases, the patient will have a "go bag," which contains a collection of spare equipment and supplies for such situations.

Developmental Disability

A *developmental disability* is caused by insufficient cognitive development of the brain, resulting in a person's inability to learn and socially adapt at a normal developmental rate. A developmental disability may be caused by genetic factors, congenital infections, complications during the labor and delivery process, malnutrition, or environmental factors. Prenatal drug or alcohol use, as in fetal alcohol syndrome, may also cause developmental disability, as can traumatic brain injury and poisons (eg, lead or other toxins).

> *Developmental disability* Insufficient development of the brain, resulting in some level of dysfunction or impairment.

A person with slight impairment may appear slow to understand or have a limited vocabulary. Such patients will often behave immaturely in comparison to their peers. Severely disabled persons may not have the ability to care for themselves, communicate, understand, or respond to their surroundings.

Speaking to patients and family members will give you a good idea of how well a patient can understand and how the patient will interact with you. Family or friends may also be able to supply additional medical information regarding the patient.

Because patients with disabilities may have difficulty adjusting to change or a break in routine, an emergency call that generates an invasion by a roomful of strangers can be overwhelming. The patient may become more difficult to interact with as his or her anxiety level increases. Make every effort to respect the patient's wishes and concerns. Patience is key. Take as much time as necessary to explain in a calming, understandable way the treatment the patient is about to receive.

Patients with developmental disabilities are susceptible to the same disease processes as other patients, including diabetes, heart attack, and respiratory difficulties. Assess and treat the patient according to the chief complaint, ensuring that emergency care and transport are accomplished with as little stress as possible.

Autism

Autism is a pervasive developmental disorder characterized by impairment of social interaction. Other characteristics can include severe behavioral problems, repetitive motor activities, and impairment in verbal and nonverbal skills. The spectrum of disability is wide, which explains why the name of the disorder has evolved from autism to autism spectrum disorder (ASD). Some children with ASD will grow up to be independent, whereas others will be unable to care for themselves.

> *Autism* A pervasive developmental disorder characterized by impairment of social interaction.

On the more severe end of the spectrum, patients with autism fail to use or understand nonverbal means of communicating messages. They frequently have difficulty making eye-to-eye contact and resist encouragement to do so. They have extreme difficulty with complex tasks that require many steps and do best with simple, one-step directions ("Please roll up your sleeve."). Patients with autism tend to get lost in long conversations and have trouble answering open-ended questions (eg, "What sorts of things do you enjoy doing?"). They tend to talk in robotic or monotone speech patterns, sometimes repeat phrases over and over, and may make up their own words. Many patients with autism confuse pronouns and will say "you" when they really mean "I," as in "You are going to the hospital," when they really mean, "I am going to the hospital." A small percentage of patients with autism do not speak at all, but instead rely on pulling parents and caregivers around by the hand to get their needs met.

There is no simple explanation as to why autism develops in children. According to the Centers for Disease Control and Prevention, approximately 1 in every 150 American children is diagnosed with autism. Autism affects males four times more often than females. It is typically diagnosed by 3 years of age. The parents or caregivers often report unique repetitive movement (hand-flapping, twirling objects), fascination with limited objects or subjects, or odd or eccentric behaviors. Today children with ASD receive special instruction and care in school-based settings. It is likely that some older adults with autism have never been diagnosed and have never received assistance.

Patients with autism generally do not have other medical disorders and will have medical needs similar to their peers without autism. When you are caring for a patient with autism, rely on parents or caregivers for information and keep them involved in the treatment of the patient.

Down Syndrome

Down syndrome is produced by a genetic chromosomal defect that can occur during fetal development, resulting in mild to severe mental retardation **FIGURE 20-11**. The normal human somatic cell contains 23 chromosomes. Down syndrome, which is also known as trisomy 21, occurs when chromosome 21 fails to separate, so that the ovum contains 24 chromosomes. When the ovum is fertilized by a normal sperm with 23 chromosomes, a triplication ("trisomy") of chromosome 21 occurs.

> *Down syndrome* A genetic chromosomal defect that occurs during fetal development and that results in mental retardation as well as certain physical characteristics, such as a round head with a flat occiput and slanted, wide-set eyes.

Increased maternal age during pregnancy and a family history of Down syndrome are known risk factors for this condition. A variety of abnormalities are associated with the condition, including a round head with a flat occiput;

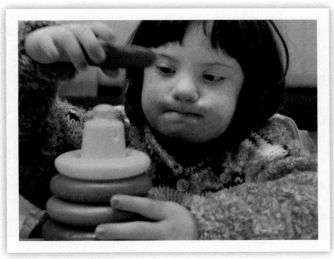
© PhotoCreate/ShutterStock, Inc.
FIGURE 20-11 A child with Down syndrome.

an enlarged, protruding tongue; slanted, wide-set eyes and folded skin on either side of the nose, covering the inner corners of the eye; short, wide hands; a small face and features; congenital heart defects; thyroid problems; and hearing and vision problems. Persons with Down syndrome do not usually have all of these signs, but a diagnosis is able to be made rapidly at birth because a combination of signs can be seen. Depending on their level of mental disability, persons with Down syndrome may lead more independent lives through employment, voting, and getting involved in the community.

Patients with Down syndrome are at increased risk for medical complications, including those that affect the cardiovascular, sensory, endocrine, orthopaedic, dental, gastrointestinal, and neurologic development. As many as 40% of these patients may have underlying heart conditions and hearing or vision problems. Two thirds of children born with Down syndrome have congenital heart disease.

Persons with Down syndrome often have large tongues and small oral and nasal cavities. They may also have misalignment of teeth and other dental anomalies. The enlarged tongue and dental anomalies can lead to speech abnormalities as well. In an emergency situation, if airway management is necessary, mask ventilation can be challenging. In the case of airway obstruction, a jaw-thrust maneuver may be all that is needed to clear the airway. In an unconscious patient, either the jaw-thrust maneuver or a nasopharyngeal airway may be necessary.

Many persons with Down syndrome also have epilepsy. In such cases, the person typically has tonic–clonic seizures, and patient management is the same as with other patients with seizures.

Patient Interaction

It is normal to feel somewhat uncomfortable when initiating contact with a developmentally disabled patient. The best plan of action is to treat the patient as you would any other patient. Approach the patient in a calm, friendly manner, watching for signs of increased anxiety or fear. You are a stranger, most likely approaching with a group of people. The patient may not understand your uniform or realize that you and your crew are there to help. It may be helpful to have the other members of your team hold back slightly until you can establish a rapport with the patient. You can then slowly introduce the team members and explain what they are going to do.

Move slowly but deliberately, explaining beforehand what you plan to do. Watch carefully for signs of fear or reluctance from the patient. Make sure you are at eye level with the patient. If the patient is sitting, kneel or sit down beside the patient. This is important in communicating with all patients, of course, but it is even more important in making the patient with special challenges comfortable.

Do your best to soothe the patient's anxiety and discomfort as you work through your assessment and provide treatment. By initially establishing trust and communication, you will have a much better chance for a successful outcome.

Patients who previously experienced head and traumatic brain injuries may be difficult to assess and treat. These patients may face a complex array of challenges related to their injury. In such cases, family and friends may need to assist you in obtaining a complete medical history from the patient. Interaction with a patient with brain injury needs to be tailored to the person's specific abilities. Take the time to speak with the patient and family to establish what is considered normal behavior for the patient; for example, determine whether the patient has cognitive, sensory, communication, motor, behavioral, or psychological deficits.

When you are caring for a patient with a previous brain injury, talk in a calm, soothing tone, and watch the patient closely for signs of anxiety or aggression. In some cases, the patient may need to be specially positioned or restrained to ensure your safety and the safety of the patient. Do not expect the patient to walk to the ambulance or stretcher. Above all, treat the patient with respect. Use his or her name, explain procedures, and continue to reassure the patient throughout the process.

▐ Sensory Disabilities

Visual impairments may result from many different causes, including congenital defect, disease, injury, and degeneration of the eye, optic nerve, or nerve pathway (eg, with aging). The degree of blindness may range from partial to total. Some patients lose peripheral or central vision; others can merely distinguish light from dark or discern general shapes.

Hearing impairment may range from a slight hearing loss to total deafness. Some patients may have difficulty with pitch, volume, and speaking distinctly. Some hearing-impaired people learn to speak even though they have never heard sounds. Others may have heard speech and learned to speak, but have since lost some or all of their hearing, leading them to speak too loudly. Parkinson disease or other disease processes may cause patients to slur words, speak very slowly, or speak in a monotone.

The two most common forms of hearing loss are known as sensorineural deafness and conductive hearing loss. *Sensorineural deafness*, or nerve damage, is the type of hearing loss most frequently encountered in the field. Sensorineural deafness occurs from a lesion or damage to the inner ear. Elderly persons will often have some degree of sensorineural hearing loss because of advanced age. In contrast, conductive hearing loss is caused by a faulty transmission of sound waves, which can occur when a person has an accumulation of wax within the ear canal or a perforated eardrum.

> *Sensorineural deafness* A permanent lack of hearing caused by a lesion or damage of the inner ear.

Communication with a patient who is hearing impaired can be challenging at best without hearing aids. A piece of paper and a writing utensil may prove helpful until the hearing aid(s) can be located.

Emergency care of patients with visual or hearing impairments is the same regardless of the cause. Specific steps to take during the assessment and treatment of patients with sensory disabilities have been discussed in other areas of this text. In general, make patients feel as comfortable as possible; use any special aids they have to minimize their disability, and treat them with respect.

▐ Physical Disabilities

Cerebral Palsy

Cerebral palsy is a term for a group of disorders characterized by poorly controlled body movement `FIGURE 20-12`. This disorder is a result of damage to the developing fetal brain while in utero, traumatic brain injury at birth or early during childhood, or a postpartum infection such as meningitis. Patients with cerebral palsy can have symptoms that range from mild to severe, involving poor posture and uncontrolled, spastic movements of the limb.

> *Cerebral palsy* A group of disorders characterized by poorly controlled body movement.

This disorder is also associated with other conditions such as visual and hearing impairments, difficulty communicating, epilepsy (seizures), and mental retardation. A significant majority (75%) of patients with cerebral palsy possess some varying degrees of developmental delay, but others have a normal intelligence level and are able to live independently with minimal support.

Patients with cerebral palsy may have an unsteady gait (ataxia) and may require the assistance of a wheelchair or walker. This type of equipment should be transported with the patient, providing it can be secured properly in the ambulance. One in every four patients with cerebral palsy may also have a seizure disorder.

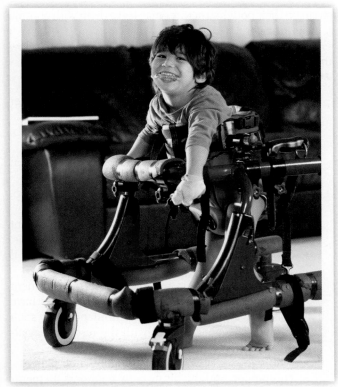

© Jaren Jal Wicklund/ShutterStock, Inc.

FIGURE 20-12 A child with cerebral palsy.

As with all patients, assessing the ABCs is of the utmost importance. The airway status of a patient with cerebral palsy should be observed closely because the patient may have increased secretion production and difficulty swallowing (dysphagia), requiring aggressive suctioning to clear.

When caring for a patient with cerebral palsy, note the following:

- Never assume that a patient with cerebral palsy is mentally disabled. Although 75% of affected persons do have some developmental disability, many have a normal IQ or only slight mental impairment.
- Limbs are often underdeveloped and prone to injury (eg, from a fall from a wheelchair).
- Patients who have the ability to walk may have an ataxic or unsteady gait, causing them to be more prone to falls.
- If a pediatric patient has a specially made pillow or chair, he or she may prefer to use it during transport. Remember to pad the patient to ensure his or her comfort, and never force a patient's extremities into any position.
- Whenever possible, take the person's walker or wheelchair along during transport so the patient can use it at the hospital and on the return trip home.
- Approximately 25% of patients with cerebral palsy also have seizures. Be prepared to provide care for a seizure if one occurs, and be prepared to provide suctioning as well.

Spina Bifida

Spina bifida is a birth defect caused by incomplete closure of the spinal column, which results in an exposed spinal cord and undeveloped vertebrae **FIGURE 20-13**. Although this opening can be surgically closed, the child is left with spinal damage. To reduce the occurrences of such disabling birth defects, pregnant women are advised to take vitamin B (folic acid). Unfortunately, spina bifida remains one of the most common disabling birth defects in the United States. Most patients with spina bifida also have hydrocephalus ("water on the brain"), which requires the placement of a shunt to drain excessive amounts of cerebrospinal fluid from the brain.

> *Spina bifida* A developmental defect in which a portion of the spinal cord or meninges protrudes outside of the vertebrae and possibly even outside of the body, usually at the lower third of the spine in the lumbar area.

Patients with spina bifida will often have partial or full paralysis of the lower extremities, loss of bowel and bladder control, and an extreme allergy to latex products. A supply of latex-free products should be kept on the ambulance to avoid a severe anaphylactic reaction in patients with spina bifida.

Patients with spina bifida benefit from the same considerations offered when treating any patient with paralysis or difficulty moving. Take special care to use a gentle touch. Ask the patient the best method for movement before initiating transfer to the stretcher.

Paralysis

Paralysis is the inability to voluntarily move one or more body parts. It may be caused by stroke, trauma, or a birth defect. Paralysis does not always entail a loss of sensation. In some cases, the patient will have normal sensation or even hyperesthesia (increased sensitivity), which may cause the patient to interpret touch as pain in the affected area. Paralysis of one side of the face may make communication a challenge.

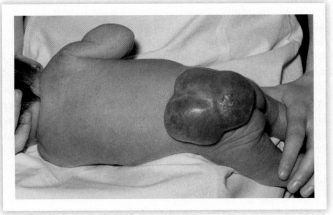

© Biophoto Associates/Photo Researchers, Inc.

FIGURE 20-13 Spina bifida is still one of the most disabling birth defects in the United States.

The diaphragm of some paralyzed patients may not function correctly, requiring the use of a ventilator. Patients may also rely on specialized equipment such as urinary catheters, tracheotomies, colostomies, or feeding tubes, which are discussed later in this chapter. Some patients may have difficulty swallowing, creating the need for suctioning. Each type of spinal cord paralysis requires its own equipment for treatment and may have its own complications.

Bariatric Patients

Obesity is a condition in which a person has an excessive amount of body fat, resulting from an imbalance between calories consumed and calories used. The solution to the obesity problem may sound relatively simple—reestablish the balance and cure the problem. Unfortunately, obesity can be a much more complex situation. The causes of obesity are not fully understood. Oftentimes, this problem may be attributed to a low metabolic rate or genetic predisposition.

> *Obesity* A condition in which a person has an excessive amount of body fat.

The term "obese" is used when someone is 20% to 30% over his or her ideal weight. In severe or morbid obesity, the person is 50 to 100 lb over the ideal weight. Severe obesity afflicts approximately 9 million adult Americans. Obese persons are often ridiculed publicly and sometimes are victims of discrimination. The person's mobility and general quality of life are often negatively affected by his or her size, and the extra weight can cause a myriad of health problems, such as diabetes, hypertension, heart disease, and stroke.

Interaction With Obese Patients

Obese patients may be embarrassed by their condition and fearful of ridicule as a result of past experiences. As with any patient, work hard to put these patients at ease. Establish the patient's chief complaint and then communicate your plan to help. Many severely obese patients have a complex and extensive medical history.

If transport is necessary, plan early for extra help and call for additional assistance if necessary. In particular, send a member of your team to find the easiest and safest exit to use. Remember, everyone's safety is at stake! You do not want to risk dropping the patient or injuring a team member by trying to lift too much weight. Moves, no matter how simple they may seem, become far more complex with an oversized patient. Depending on the size of the patient, you may need specialized equipment and additional manpower for lifting assistance.

Interaction With Morbidly Obese Patients

Morbidly obese patients may overcome mobility difficulties by pulling, rocking, or rolling into a position. The constant strain on their body's structures may leave them with chronic joint injuries or osteoarthritis.

When you are moving a morbidly obese patient, follow these tips:

- Treat the patient with dignity and respect.
- Ask your patient how it is best to move him or her before attempting to do so.
- Avoid trying to lift the patient by only one limb, which would risk injury to overtaxed joints.
- Coordinate and communicate all moves to all team members prior to starting to lift.
- If the move becomes uncontrolled at any point, stop, reposition, and resume.
- Look for pinch or pressure points from equipment because they could cause deep venous thrombosis.
- Very large patients may have difficulty breathing if placed in a supine position.
- Many manufacturers make specialized equipment for morbidly obese patients, and some areas have specially equipped bariatric ambulances for such patients. Become familiar with the resources available in your area.
- Plan egress routes to accommodate large patients, equipment, and the lifting crew members. Remember: Do no harm!
- Notify the receiving facility early to allow special arrangements to be made prior to your arrival to accommodate the patient's needs.

Patients With Medical Technology Assistance

Advances in medicine have resulted in a growing number of patients being treated in their own homes or in other nonhospital settings with devices such as mechanical ventilators, tracheostomy tubes, gastrostomy tubes, and central venous catheters. As a consequence, you may encounter—and need to be able to deal with—a wide variety of medical technologies when responding to an emergency call.

Tracheostomy Tubes

A *tracheostomy tube* is a plastic tube placed in a surgical opening from the anterior part of the neck into the trachea. This tube, which can be either temporary or permanent, passes from the neck directly into the major airways **FIGURE 20-14**.

> *Tracheostomy tube* A plastic tube placed within the tracheostomy site (stoma).

Patients who depend on home automatic ventilators or those who have chronic pulmonary medical conditions may breathe through a tracheostomy tube. Because these tubes bypass the nose and mouth, such devices are foreign to the respiratory tract. The body reacts to the presence of

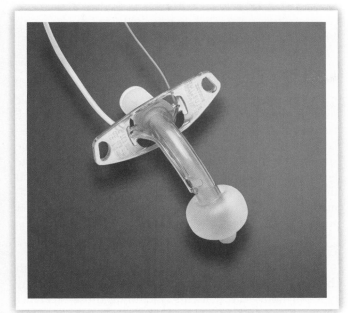

Portex® Blue Line® Ultra Tracheostomy courtesy of Smiths Medical.

FIGURE 20-14 Some patients require a tracheostomy tube to breathe.

this foreign object by building up secretions in or around the tube, such that the tube may become obstructed by mucus plugs or other items. Routine care provided by caregivers includes keeping the stoma clean and dry and suctioning any secretions.

Obstructions of the tracheostomy tube are emergency events that require you to intervene immediately. This type of emergency can be stressful to deal with, so it is imperative to remember the ABCs and airway management.

Other complications include air leaking around the tube, which usually happens with new tracheostomies, and the tube becoming loose or dislodged. Occasionally, the opening around the tube may become infected. Emergency care of a patient with a tracheostomy tube includes maintaining an open airway, suctioning the tube if necessary to clear a mucus plug, maintaining the patient in a position of comfort, administering supplemental oxygen, and providing transport to the hospital.

Refer to your EMT-I textbook to review the Skill Drill on suctioning and cleaning a tracheostomy tube.

Mechanical Ventilators

Patients who are on a mechanical ventilator cannot breathe without assistance. Patients who require these devices may or may not have an underlying respiratory drive as a result of a congenital defect or a chronic lung disease process. Other patients may have a traumatic brain injury, muscular dystrophy, or another disease process that weakens their ability to breathe and requires a permanent tracheostomy and mechanical ventilator.

If the ventilator malfunctions, remove the patient from the ventilator and begin ventilations with a bag-valve device.

To do so, remove the mask from a bag-valve device and attach the bag and valve directly to the tracheostomy tube. Patients with tracheostomies do not breathe through their mouth or nose. As such, a face mask or nasal cannula cannot be used on these patients. Masks designed specifically for patients with tracheostomies cover the tracheostomy hole and have a strap that goes around the neck. These masks are usually available in intensive care units, where many patients have tracheostomies, and may or may not be available in a prehospital setting. If you do not have a tracheostomy mask, you can improvise by placing a face mask over the stoma **FIGURE 20-15**. Even though the mask is shaped to fit the face, you can usually achieve an adequate fit over the patient's neck by adjusting the strap.

Patients on home mechanical ventilators require assisted ventilation throughout transport. Recognize that the patient's caregivers will know how the mechanical ventilator works and will be of great help to you in attaching the bag and valve from a bag-mask device to the tracheostomy tube in preparation for transport. Again, solicit the help of the patient, family, and caregivers.

Apnea Monitors

While caring for infants with special challenges, you may come across an apnea monitor. This device is typically used when an infant is born prematurely, has severe gastroesophageal reflux that causes choking episodes, has a family history of sudden infant death syndrome, or has experienced an apparently life-threatening event such as a period of apnea shortly after birth.

A typical episode of apnea may last for only 15 to 20 seconds and occur during periods of sleep. The apnea monitor is attached with electrodes or a belt wrapped around the infant's chest or stomach. It is designed to sound an alarm if the infant experiences bradycardia or if an episode of apnea occurs. It also stores information related to the infant's cardiorespiratory events. The apnea monitor is typically used for 2 weeks to 2 months after birth to monitor the respiratory

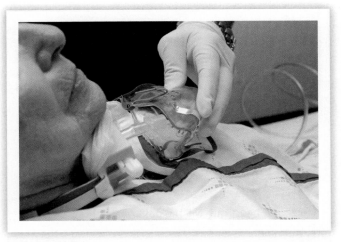

FIGURE 20-15 If you do not have a tracheostomy mask, use a face mask instead.

system, although it has been used in patients from birth to as much as 1 year of age.

If you are called to care for a patient on an apnea monitor, bring the apnea monitor to the receiving hospital with the pediatric patient, if possible, so that it may be evaluated and any stored data may be retrieved for analysis.

Internal Cardiac Pacemakers

An *internal cardiac pacemaker* is a device implanted under the patient's skin to regulate the heart rate in patients with underlying conductive heart conditions. These devices are typically placed on the nondominant side of the patient's chest so that normal activities are not hindered. In patients who are small or extremely thin, the device may be implanted in the abdomen. In some cases, the pacemaker may also include an automated implanted cardioverter defibrillator, which monitors the patient's heart rhythm and is able to slow down or stop accelerated heart rates.

> *Internal cardiac pacemaker* A device implanted under the patient's skin to regulate the heart rate in patients with underlying conductive heart conditions.

When using an automated external defibrillator (AED) in patients with these kinds of pacemakers, avoid placing the defibrillator pads directly over the implanted device. While obtaining the patient's history during the patient assessment process, gather specific information for the benefit of the receiving hospital staff, such as the type of cardiac pacemaker **TABLE 20-12**.

Left Ventricular Assist Devices

A *left ventricular assist device* is a piece of medical equipment that takes over the function of either one or both heart ventricles. These types of devices are used as a bridge to heart transplantation while a donor heart is being located. To date, there is only one approved ventricular assist device designed for persons aged 5 to 16 years.

> *Left ventricular assist device* A piece of medical equipment that takes over the function of either one or both heart ventricles.

If you encounter a patient with such a device, you will primarily provide support measures and basic care while using the caregiver as a resource during the transport. Risk factors associated with the implantation of a left ventricular assist device include excessive bleeding following the surgery, infection, blood clots leading to strokes, and acute heart failure. Although medical equipment failure is rare in these cases, be prepared to provide CPR if necessary. Paramedics should be notified as soon as possible so that other supportive measures may be initiated.

Central Venous Catheters

A *central venous catheter* is a venous access device with the tip of the catheter in the vena cava. It is used for many types of home care patients, including those receiving chemotherapy, long-term antibiotic or pain management, high-concentration glucose solutions, and hemodialysis **FIGURE 20-16**. Central venous catheters are often located in the chest, upper arm, or subclavicular area.

> *Central venous catheter* An intravenous access device used in many types of home care patients, including those receiving chemotherapy, long-term antibiotic or pain management, high-concentration glucose solutions, and hemodialysis.

Problems associated with these devices include the following complications: infiltration, where the catheter dislodges from the vessel; a broken line; infections around the line; obstruction of the line by a blood clot; bleeding around the line or from the tubing attached to the line; and sepsis developing from an infected line. If bleeding occurs, apply direct pressure to the tubing and provide immediate transport to the hospital.

Table 20-12
Questions for Patients With Pacemakers or Automated Implanted Defibrillators
▪ Which type of heart disorder does the patient have?
▪ How long has this device been implanted?
▪ What is the patient's normal baseline rhythm and heart rate?
▪ Is the patient's heart completely dependent on the pacemaker device?
▪ At what heart rate will the defibrillator fire?
▪ How many times has the defibrillator shocked the patient?

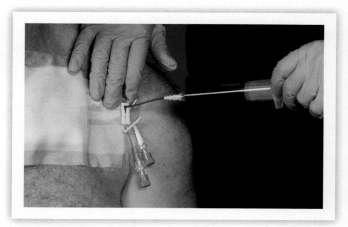

FIGURE 20-16 Patients who require frequent intravenous medications may have a central line in place.

Gastrostomy Tubes

Gastrostomy tubes are sometimes referred to as gastric tubes or G-tubes. They are placed directly into the stomach to provide nutrition for patients who cannot ingest fluids, food, or medication by mouth **FIGURE 20-17**. These tubes may alternately be inserted through the nose or mouth into the stomach (such as a nasogastric or orogastric tube).

> *Gastrostomy tube* A tube that is placed directly through the skin into the stomach to provide nutrition for patients who cannot ingest fluids, food, or medication by mouth. Also referred to as a gastric tube or G-tube.

In some cases, a gastric tube may be placed surgically directly into the stomach and sutured in place; however, it may become dislodged during the patient's normal daily activity. If such a situation arises, assess the patient for signs or symptoms of bleeding into the stomach such as vague abdominal discomfort, nausea, vomiting (especially "coffee grounds" emesis), and bloody emesis.

Patients who have a gastric tube in place may still be at risk of aspiration. Always have suction readily available to clear any materials from the patient's mouth and to prevent airway problems. Patients with gastric tubes who have difficulty breathing should be transported while sitting or lying on the right side with the head elevated 30° to prevent the contents of the stomach from passing into the lungs. Administer supplemental oxygen if the patient has any difficulty breathing.

Patients with diabetes who receive insulin and gastric tube feedings may become hypoglycemic quickly if the gastric tube feedings are discontinued for any reason. Be alert for an altered mental status or a change in the baseline behavior if the patient falls into this group.

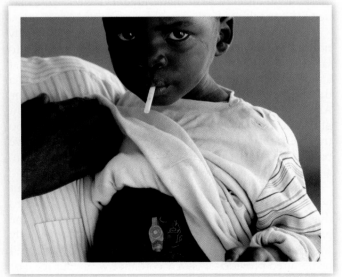

© DELOCHE/age fotostock

FIGURE 20-17 Gastric tubes are placed through the skin into the stomach for children or adults who cannot be fed by mouth.

Shunts

Some patients with chronic neurologic conditions may have shunts, such as a patient with hydrocephalus. A *shunt* is a tube that drains fluid from the brain to another part of the body outside of the brain.

> *Shunt* A tube that drains fluid from the brain to another part of the body outside of the brain, such as the abdomen; it lowers pressure in the brain.

Several different types of shunts are available, such as a ventriculo-peritoneal shunt or a ventriculo-atrial shunt. A ventriculo-peritoneal shunt drains excess fluid from the ventricles of the brain into the peritoneum of the abdomen. A ventriculo-atrial shunt drains excess fluid from the ventricles of the brain into the right atrium of the heart. These devices keep pressure from building up too much in the skull.

If a shunt becomes blocked or infected, changes in mental status and respiratory arrest may occur. Infection of a shunt occurs most frequently within the first 2 months after the insertion. A blocked shunt may also present as a medical emergency. If the shunt is unable to drain properly, intracranial pressure may increase and the patient will experience an altered mental status.

During assessment of a patient with a shunt, you will likely feel a device beneath the skin on the side of the head, behind the ear. This device is a fluid reservoir, and its presence should alert you to the possibility that the patient has an underlying shunt. Should the shunt become dysfunctional, the patient could be predisposed to respiratory arrest.

Signs that a patient is in distress include bulging fontanelles (in infants), headache, projectile vomiting, altered mental status, irritability, high-pitched cry, fever, nausea, difficulty with coordination (walking), blurred vision, seizures, redness along the shunt track, bradycardia, and heart arrhythmias. Emergency medical care includes airway management and artificial ventilation during transport.

Colostomies and Ileostomies

A *colostomy* or *ileostomy* is a surgical procedure that creates an opening between the small or large intestine and the surface of the body, allowing for elimination of waste products. A urostomy is a surgically created opening in the abdominal wall through which urine passes. The special opening is referred to as a stoma. Either urine or feces is expelled through the stoma and collected into a clear external bag or pouch, which is frequently emptied or changed.

> *Colostomy* A surgical procedure that establishes an opening between the colon and the surface of the body.
> *Ileostomy* A surgical procedure that creates an opening between the small intestine and the surface of the body.

If you encounter a patient with a colostomy or ileostomy bag who has been complaining of diarrhea or vomiting, assess the patient for signs and symptoms of dehydration. The area around the stoma is prone to infection, so patients and caregivers must be diligent with daily hygiene. Signs of infection include redness, warm skin around the stoma, and tenderness on palpation over the colostomy or ileostomy site. Contact medical control or follow your local protocols when caring for a patient with a colostomy or ileostomy.

Patient Assessment for Patients With Special Challenges

Interaction with the caregiver of a child or adult with special needs will be an important part of the patient assessment process. Always speak with the caregiver or family members; they have likely become experts on the illness or disability. The parents, caregivers, or home health care staff members are trained to use and troubleshoot problems with medical equipment on a daily basis. Assess the patient's baseline vital signs, note any allergies (eg, to latex), medications, and other pertinent medical history. You must first determine the patient's normal baseline status before an assessment of the current condition can be made. To do so, it is often helpful to ask, "What is different today?"

Home Care

Home care occurs within a patient's home environment. Patients requiring home services encompass people with a wide spectrum of special health care needs, including infants and the elderly, patients with chronic illnesses, and patients with developmental disabilities. For example, such services are commonly needed among patients older than 65 years as a means to keep them at home rather than in a long-term care facility.

Services offered by home care agencies include, but are not limited to, delivering prepared meals, house cleaning, washing laundry, yard maintenance, providing physical therapy, and providing personal hygiene, including bathing and wound care. Oftentimes, EMS is called to a residence when a home care provider has either found the patient injured or recognized a change in the patient's health status. Home care personnel can be an important resource for providing a patient's baseline health status and the history of the present illness or condition as well as health care documentation or medication lists that should be transported with the patient to the hospital.

Hospice Care and Terminally Ill Patients

Unfortunately, not all illnesses can be cured. As health care providers, you and your team may be called on to assist a patient who has a terminal illness. Such a patient may be receiving hospice care either at a hospice facility or at home.

Patients receiving hospice care are terminally ill. They may have diseases such as cancer, heart and lung failure, end-stage Alzheimer disease, or acquired immunodeficiency syndrome (AIDS). As part of the person's enrollment in hospice care, the patient's physician has determined the illness is terminal and has completed a do not resuscitate (DNR) order or given medical orders for the scope of treatment, outlining the care agreed upon by the patient and/or the family. Hospice care provides comfort care (pain medications) during a person's last days. Palliative care, or comfort care, improves the patient's quality of life before the patient dies and allows the patient to be with family and friends during the last days. If called to a facility that provides hospice care or to a home with a patient receiving hospice care, you will need to follow local protocols, the patient's wishes, or legal documents such as a DNR order. All necessary documentation must be brought with the patient to the hospital and noted in the patient care report.

If you are called to the home of a terminally ill patient, the care you give will have a lasting impact on the family. This is a time when compassion, understanding, and sensitivity are most needed. Some homes with patients receiving hospice care may be chaotic. Family members may be having a difficult time coping with the situation, and they may exhibit anger and hostility. Treat everyone with compassion and understanding. Members of your team may be able to separate family members to speak with them privately to defuse intense emotions and restore order.

Some terminally ill patients at home may also receive outpatient care from a hospice or a home health nurse. You may be called to the home because of a delay in the arrival of the regular care provider or for transport so that a physician can address an immediate need, such as mitigation of increasing pain. Because terminally ill patients may use a complex array of pain medications, transdermal patches, or self-administered pain management devices, you may need to consult medical control for guidance.

Even if a DNR order is in place, family members may not understand what to do and they may not be ready to face the death of a loved one. Other legal documents that a terminally ill patient may have include a living will and a durable power of attorney. Though these orders require the AEMTs to withhold life-sustaining treatment in the event of cardiac or respiratory arrest, they do not mean that no treatment should be given; that is, patients should receive pain medication, supplemental oxygen therapy, nutrition, and hydration as needed based on assessment.

Ascertain the family's wishes about having the patient remain in the home or having the patient transported to the hospital. If a family member requests to accompany the patient, he or she should be allowed to do so. If the family wishes the patient to remain at home, this request should be honored provided it is in accordance with your local or state protocol.

Local protocols for handling the death of a patient vary, so be familiar with local or state regulations. Protocols should identify whether the coroner needs to be called, whether a pronouncement of death is required, and, if so, who is responsible for the determination. Make sure you understand your local protocols before you are called to respond to such a circumstance.

Poverty and Homelessness

According to a US Bureau of the Census report published in 2007, 12.5% of the US population lives in poverty. People who live in these circumstances are unable to provide for all of their basic needs such as housing, food, child care, health insurance, and medication. An impoverished person or family may have housing but may go without food or medication to pay for that housing. Disease prevention strategies such as dental care, good nutrition, and exercise are unlikely to be implemented by such persons, increasing the likelihood of disease in people who live in poverty.

It is estimated that nearly 4 million people in the United States are homeless. Of those 4 million, approximately 40% are women and children. The homeless population includes persons with mental illness, victims of domestic violence, persons with addiction disorders, and impoverished families.

Part of your job as an AEMT is to be an advocate for all patients. Your job is to provide emergency medical care and transport patients to the appropriate facility. Remember, all health care facilities *must* provide a medical assessment and required treatment, regardless of the patient's ability to pay under the Emergency Medical Treatment and Active Labor Act (referred to as EMTALA). You can also act as an advocate by becoming familiar with the social services resources within your community so you can refer patients to these lifelines.

Ready for Review

- Complications of pregnancy may include hypertension, bleeding, and diabetes.
- During a trauma call that involves a pregnant woman, you have two patients to consider—the woman and the unborn fetus. Any trauma to the woman will have a direct effect on the condition of her fetus.
- Use the PAT to develop a general impression of the infant or child.
- The aging process is accompanied by changes in physiologic function. The decrease in the functional capacity of various organ systems can affect the way in which the patient responds to illness.
- Assessing an elderly person can be challenging because of communication issues, hearing and vision deficits, alteration in consciousness, complicated medical history, and the effects of multiple medications.
- To obtain an accurate history for a geriatric patient, patience and good communication skills are essential. A slow, deliberate approach to the patient history, with one AEMT asking questions, is generally the best strategy.
- The risk of serious injury or death is higher in elderly patients who experience a traumatic injury than in younger persons in the same situation.
- When you treat a geriatric trauma patient, assess the injuries and carefully look for the cause of the injury. A medical condition such as fainting could actually be the cause of a fall. In such a case, both the injuries from the fall and the medical condition will need to be addressed.
- As medicine and medical technology continue to improve, the number of children and adults living with chronic diseases is increasing. Assess and care for patients with special needs in the same manner as all other patients.
- You may find children and adults living at home who depend on mechanical ventilators, IV pumps, or other medical devices to maintain their lives.
- You and your team may be called on to assist a patient who is terminally ill. Terminally ill patients may be in a hospice facility or at home.

Case Study

It is 10:00 in the morning when you arrive at the scene where a pregnant 16-year-old girl is experiencing vaginal bleeding. The patient tells you she is 32 weeks along in her pregnancy and receives regular prenatal care. Your partner obtains a set of vital signs while you take the patient's history. The patient said she woke up at 8 o'clock this morning with terrible abdominal pain and noticed bright red bleeding from her vagina. She initially thought she was just having some false labor; however, the bleeding and pain continued. She reports that she has needed to change her sanitary napkin multiple times since she woke up. She does

not recall any trauma. The patient says she was going to call her physician, but began to panic and called for EMS assistance. She has no significant past medical history, but she has been diagnosed with pregnancy-induced hypertension. Vital signs are as follows: pulse, 102 beats/min; respirations, 22 breaths/min; and blood pressure, 98/60 mm Hg. The patient appears very upset and tells you she is concerned about her baby.

1. What is the difference between abruptio placenta and placenta previa?

2. What is the treatment for a pregnant patient who is experiencing vaginal bleeding?

3. What is the physiology behind pregnancy that makes pregnant patients more prone to trauma?

4. Which of the following is not typically associated with preeclampsia?
   A. Headache
   B. Seeing spots
   C. Decreased respiratory rate
   D. High blood pressure

5. What is the treatment for a pregnant patient experiencing eclampsia?

CHAPTER 21

EMS Operations

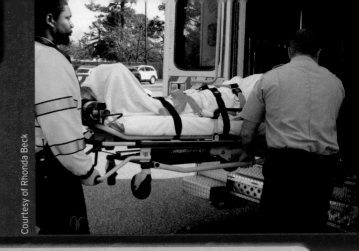

Courtesy of Rhonda Beck

Introduction

EMS operations involves the many aspects of an emergency call that do not constitute direct patient care, yet significantly influence the outcome of direct patient care. Ambulance operations includes the various phases of an emergency call, from pre-dispatch procedures such as daily vehicle inspections; to dispatch, response, and transport; and finally to post-run procedures. Phases of an emergency call are discussed in detail in your EMT-I textbook. This chapter focuses on safety during ambulance operations, vehicle extrication and rescue, mass-casualty incidents, terrorist activities, and disaster management.

Ambulance Operations

Learning how to properly operate your vehicle is just as important as learning how to care for patients when you arrive on the scene. An ambulance involved in a crash delays patient care, at a minimum, and may take the lives of the EMS providers, other motorists, or pedestrians at worst. While it is suggested that you take an Emergency Vehicle Operator's course (EVOC) prior to driving an ambulance, this section provides basic information regarding safe operations of the ground ambulance.

Safe Driving Practices

All proficient and safe drivers of an ambulance know that the first rule of safe driving in an emergency vehicle is that speed does not save lives; good care does. The second rule is that the driver and passengers must wear seat belts and shoulder restraints at all times because they are the most important items of safety equipment on the ambulance. Other important aspects of safe driving practices include learning how your vehicle accelerates, corners, sways, and

Table 21-1
Guidelines for Safe Ambulance Driving

1. Select the shortest and least congested route to the scene at the time of the dispatch.

2. Avoid routes with heavy traffic congestion; know alternative routes to each hospital during rush hours.

3. Avoid one-way streets; they may become clogged. Do not go against the flow of traffic on a one-way street, unless absolutely necessary.

4. Watch carefully for bystanders as you approach the scene. Curiosity seekers rarely move out of the way.

5. Park the ambulance in a safe place once you arrive at the scene. If you park facing into traffic, turn off your headlights so that they do not blind oncoming cars unless they are needed to illuminate the scene. If the vehicle is blocking part of the road, keep your warning lights on to alert oncoming motorists; otherwise, turn them off.

6. Drive within the speed limit while transporting patients, except in the rare extreme emergency.

7. Go with the flow of the traffic.

8. Always drive defensively.

9. Always maintain a safe following distance. Use the "4-second rule": Stay at least 4 seconds behind another vehicle in the same lane.

10. Try to maintain an open space or cushion in the lane next to you as an escape route in case the vehicle in front of you stops suddenly.

11. Use your siren if you turn on the emergency lights, except when you are on a freeway.

12. Always assume that the other drivers do not hear the siren or see your emergency lights.

stops. You must know exactly how your vehicle will respond to steering, braking, and accelerating under various conditions. **TABLE 21-1** lists further guidelines to follow when you are en route to a call.

Safety

You must always be prepared, mentally and physically, for any incident that requires rescue or extrication. The most important part of this preparation is thinking about your safety and the safety of your team. Safety begins with the proper mind-set and the proper protective equipment.

The equipment that you use and the gear that you wear will depend on the situation you expect to encounter, as well as what you observe during your scene size-up. Such protective gear may include turnout gear, helmets, hearing

protection, and a fire extinguisher. However, the importance of wearing blood- and fluid-inpenetrable gloves at all times during patient contact cannot be emphasized enough. If you will be involved with extrication, you should wear a pair of leather gloves over your disposable gloves to protect you from injury when handling ropes, tools, broken glass, hot or cold objects, or sharp metal.

Vehicle Safety Systems

A variety of safety systems are used in modern vehicles. Although many of these devices are useful when the vehicle is in motion, they can become hazards after the vehicle has been involved in a crash.

Shock-absorbing bumpers provide vehicle protection from low-speed impact. Following a front- or rear-end crash, the shock absorbers within these bumpers may be compressed or "loaded." You should avoid standing directly in front of such bumpers, and always approach vehicles from the side, because the shock absorbers can release and injure your knees and legs.

Manufacturers are now mandated to incorporate supplemental restraint systems or air bags into their vehicles. These air bags fill with a nonharmful gas on impact and quickly deflate after the crash. Air bags are located in the steering wheel and the dash in front of the passenger, and they deploy when the vehicle is struck from the front or rear. Additional bags may be present to protect the driver and passengers from side impacts. These bags may be located in the doors or seats. Air bags should normally deploy and deflate before your arrival on the scene. Air bags have, however, inflated while EMS providers were providing patient care, causing injury to the providers. Use caution when working in damaged vehicles in which air bags have not inflated. Generally, you should maintain at least a 5-inch clearance around side-impact air bags that have not deployed, 10 inches around driver air bags that have not deployed, and 20 inches around passenger-side air bags that have not deployed.

You may notice a haze similar to smoke inside vehicles in which air bags have deployed. Manufacturers use cornstarch or talc on the air bags to reduce friction; the substance may cause minor skin irritation. Appropriate protective gear, including eye protection, will reduce the potential for such irritation.

Fundamentals of Extrication

Hazard Control
A variety of hazards may be present at the extrication scene. Law enforcement personnel are responsible for traffic control and direction, maintaining order at the scene, investigating the crash or crime scene, and establishing and maintaining lines so that bystanders are kept at a safe distance and out of the way of rescuers. Fire fighters are responsible for extinguishing any fire, preventing additional

ignition, ensuring that the scene is safe, and washing down any spilled fuel **FIGURE 21-1**. Downed electrical lines are a common hazard at vehicle crash scenes. You should never attempt to move downed electrical lines. If power lines are touching or located in proximity to a vehicle involved in the crash, patients should be instructed to remain in the vehicle until power is removed. In occasional incidents involving significant hazards, there will be an area designated as the *safe zone*. You and the ambulance should remain in that area, outside of the *danger zone (hot zone)*. A danger zone (hot zone) is an area where people can be exposed to sharp metal edges, broken glass, toxic substances, or ignition or explosion of hazardous materials.

> *Safe zone* An area of protection providing safety from the danger zone (hot zone).
>
> *Danger zone (hot zone)* An area where people can be exposed to sharp metal edges, broken glass, toxic substances, lethal rays, or ignition or explosion of hazardous materials.

Sometimes, the scene at a crash or fire is further complicated by the presence of *hazardous materials (HazMat)*. A hazardous material is any substance that is toxic, poisonous, radioactive, flammable, or explosive and can cause injury or death with exposure. In addition to posing a threat to you and others at the immediate scene, hazardous materials may pose a threat to a much larger area and population. Whenever there is a possibility that a hazardous material is involved, you will need to follow a number of additional special procedures.

> *Hazardous materials (HazMat)* Any substance that is toxic, poisonous, radioactive, flammable, or explosive and causes injury or death with exposure.

Bystanders and family members can be hazards themselves. If they are allowed to get too close, they are at risk of injury and may also interfere with the overall management of the incident. For these reasons, the rescue group will set up a danger zone that is off-limits to bystanders. You should help to set up and enforce this zone. If you arrive before the rescue group, you should coordinate crowd control with law enforcement officials.

The vehicle also can be a hazard. An unstable vehicle on its side or roof can be a danger to you. Rescue personnel can stabilize the vehicle with a variety of jacks or cribbing (wooden blocks). Prior to attempting to gain access to a vehicle involved in a crash, you should ensure that the vehicle is in "park" with the parking brake set and the ignition is turned off. The battery should also be disconnected, negative side first, to minimize the possibility of sparks or fire. Other hazards include vehicles with headrests that deploy in the event of a crash and vehicles that are already on fire or are leaking fuel.

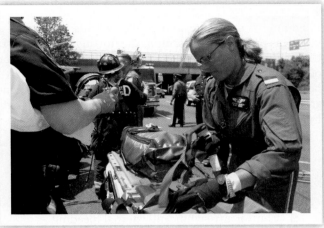

© Mark C. Ide

FIGURE 21-1 Every crash requires cooperation, as each responder has a specific role at the scene. Fire fighters, law enforcement, the rescue team, and EMS personnel all have individual responsibilities.

Do not approach a vehicle that is on fire or leaking fuel without proper turnout gear, and never use flares around these vehicles. The first step in responding to these hazards when dealing with an alternative fuel vehicle is to turn the valve of the fuel cylinder into the "off" position. If you are not properly attired or trained in the management of this vehicle hazard, set up a safety zone and call for qualified personnel.

Alternative Fuel Vehicles

Today, with advances in automotive technology, EMS responders should keep in mind that some vehicles on the road are powered by alternative fuel. Vehicles may be powered by electricity and electricity/gasoline hybrids or fuels such as propane, natural gas, methanol, or hydrogen. Although each type of vehicle has its own unique features, one feature is common throughout—the need for responders to disconnect the battery to prevent further fire or explosion.

Electric and alternative fuel vehicles are usually identified by markings on the vehicle. You should not approach an electric or alternative fuel vehicle without proper turnout gear. Toxic fumes and vapors from electric vehicle batteries can occasionally be carried in smoke or steam.

In more than 40% of today's alternative fuel vehicles, the batteries are not located in the engine compartment but in other areas, such as the trunk or under the seats. Furthermore, there also may be more than one battery present. You must remain vigilant when presented with these alternative types of vehicles and their inherent dangers. For example, hybrid batteries have higher amperes than a traditional vehicle's battery, and these amperes can injure you.

Support Operations

Support operations include lighting the scene, establishing tool and equipment staging areas, and marking helicopter landing zones. Fire and rescue personnel will work together on these functions.

Emergency Care

Providing medical care to a patient who is trapped in a vehicle is principally the same as that for any other patient. Unless there is an immediate threat of fire, explosion, or other danger, once entrance and access to the patient have been provided, you should perform a primary assessment and perform any critical interventions before further extrication begins, as follows:

1. Provide manual stabilization to protect the cervical spine, as needed.
2. Open the airway.
3. Provide high-flow oxygen.
4. Assist or provide for adequate ventilation.
5. Control any significant external bleeding.
6. Treat all critical injuries.

Good communication among team members and clear leadership are essential to safe, efficient provision of proper emergency care. Although your input at the scene is important, one member of your team must be clearly in charge. The team leader's assessment of the patient and the situation will dictate the way in which medical care, packaging, and transport will proceed. Customarily, the senior medical person is responsible for this role. If a team leader has not been identified, this must be decided and agreed on before you arrive at the scene. A lack of identifiable leadership at the scene hinders the rescue effort and patient care. Leaders should be identified as part of a larger incident command system (ICS). They should be medically trained and qualified to judge the priorities of patient care, and they must also be experienced in extrication. For a full review of extrication principles, refer to your EMT-I textbook.

Specialized Rescue Situations

On most calls, you can drive the ambulance to within a short distance of the patient's location and, with either simple or complex access, you can reach and treat the patient. However, in some situations, the patient can be reached only by teams trained in special technical rescues. Specialized skills of these teams include the following:

- Cave rescue
- Confined space rescue
- Cross-field and trail rescue (park rangers)
- Dive rescue
- Lost person search and rescue
- Mine rescue
- Mountain-, rock-, and ice-climbing rescue
- Ski slope and cross-country or trail snow rescue (ski patrol)
- Structural collapse rescue
- Special weapons and tactics (SWAT) rescue
- Technical rope rescue (low- and high-angle rescue)
- Trench rescue
- Water and small-craft rescue
- White-water rescue

National Incident Management System

Although most incidents are handled at the local level, the president directed the Secretary of Homeland Security to implement the *National Incident Management System (NIMS)* in March 2004. Major incidents require the involvement and coordination of multiple jurisdictions, functional agencies, and emergency response disciplines. The NIMS provides a consistent nationwide template to enable federal, state, and local governments, as well as private-sector and nongovernmental organizations, to work together effectively and efficiently. The NIMS is used to prepare for, prevent, respond to, and recover from domestic incidents, regardless of cause, size, or complexity, including acts of catastrophic terrorism and HazMat incidents.

National Incident Management System (NIMS) A Department of Homeland Security system designed to enable federal, state, and local governments and private-sector and nongovernmental organizations to effectively and efficiently prepare for, prevent, respond to, and recover from domestic incidents, regardless of cause, size, or complexity, including acts of catastrophic terrorism.

Two important underlying principles of the NIMS are flexibility and standardization. The organizational structure must be flexible enough to be rapidly adapted for use in any situation. The NIMS provides standardization in terminology, resource classification, personnel training, certification, and more. Another important feature of the NIMS is the concept of interoperability, which refers to the ability of agencies of different types or from different jurisdictions to communicate with each other.

The ICS is one component of the NIMS. The major NIMS components are as follows:

- **Command and management.** The NIMS standardizes incident management for all hazards and across all levels of government. The NIMS standard incident command structures are based on three key constructs: ICS, multiagency coordination systems, and public information systems.
- **Preparedness.** The NIMS establishes measures for all responders to incorporate into their systems to prepare for their response to all incidents at any time.
- **Resource management.** The NIMS sets up mechanisms to describe, inventory, track, and dispatch resources before, during, and after an incident. The NIMS also defines standard procedures to recover equipment used during the incident.
- **Communications and information management.** Effective communications, information management, and sharing are critical aspects of domestic incident management. The NIMS communications and information systems enable the essential functions needed to provide interoperability.

- **Supporting technologies.** The NIMS promotes national standards and interoperability for supporting technologies to successfully implement the NIMS and standard technologies for professions or incidents. It provides structure for the science and technology used in incident management.
- **Ongoing management and maintenance.** The US Department of Homeland Security (DHS) will establish a multijurisdictional, multidisciplinary NIMS Integration Center. This center will provide strategic direction for and oversight of the NIMS, supporting routine maintenance and continuous improvement of the system in the long term.

Incident Command System

It is important for you to be familiar with the terminology and concepts of the ICS. Some agencies refer to the ICS as the incident management system. However, the terminology under NIMS is incident command system. The purpose of the ICS is to ensure responder and public safety, achieving incident management goals, and ensuring the efficient use of resources.

As you know, communication is the building block of good patient care. Common terminology and the use of "clear text" communications (plain English as opposed to 10-codes) help responders from multiple agencies work efficiently together.

Using the ICS gives you a modular organizational structure built on the size and complexity of the incident. The goal of the ICS is to make the best use of your resources to manage the environment around the incident and to treat patients during an emergency. The ICS is designed to control duplication of effort and freelancing, in which individual units or different organizations make independent and often inefficient decisions about the next appropriate action. Follow your local standard operating procedures for establishing the ICS.

One of the organizing principles of the ICS is limiting the span of control of any one person. This principle refers to keeping the supervisor/worker ratio at one supervisor for three to seven workers. A supervisor who has more than seven people reporting to him or her is exceeding an effective span of control and needs to divide tasks and delegate the supervision of some tasks to another person.

Organizational divisions may include sections, branches, divisions, and groups. In some regions, emergency operations centers may exist. The centers are usually operated by the city, state, or federal government. These centers will usually only be activated in a large catastrophic event that may go on for days, involve hundreds of patients, and tax the whole system.

The people who will participate in the many tasks in a mass-casualty incident (MCI) or a disaster should use the ICS. You should find out from your service if one exists, who is in charge, how it is activated, and what your expected role will be.

There are many roles defined in the ICS. The general staff includes command, finance, logistics, operations, and planning. It is important for you to understand the specific duties of each and how they work in coordinating the response. Command functions include the public information officer (PIO), safety officer, and liaison officer.

Communications and Information Management

Communication has historically been the weak point at most major incidents. To minimize the effects of communications problems, it is recommended that communications be integrated. This means that all agencies involved should be able to communicate quickly and effortlessly via radios. Communications allow for accountability throughout the incident, as well as instant communication between recipients. As always, and more so during a large incident, it is important to maintain professionalism on all radio communications, remembering to communicate clearly, concisely, and using clear text (no codes).

Mobilization and Deployment

When an incident has been declared and the need for additional resources has been identified, a request is made for additional resources. Once a request is made, these resources are mobilized and deployed to the scene. It is important to wait until the request is made, to minimize the potential for freelancing.

EMS Response Within the Incident Command System

Preparedness

Preparedness involves the decisions made and basic planning done before an incident occurs. Every area is prone to natural disasters, such as hurricanes, tornadoes, earthquakes, and wildfires. Therefore, preparedness in a given area involves decisions and planning for the most likely natural disasters for the area, among other disasters.

Your EMS agency should have written disaster plans that you are regularly trained to carry out. A copy of the disaster plan should be kept in each EMS vehicle. EMS facilities need to have disaster supplies for at least a 72-hour period for self-sufficiency. Also, your EMS service should have mutual aid agreements with surrounding organizations to help expedite requests for help in an emergency. All groups with mutual aid agreements should practice using the plans frequently. Organizations should share a list of resources so they will know what help can be accessed. Also, your local EMS organizations should develop an assistance program for the families of EMS responders. If EMS responders have concerns about their families during a disaster, their effectiveness on the job could be diminished.

Of course, you should have a personal disaster plan for your family. Families need to be prepared and know what to expect should you be required to be a disaster responder. You also should be up to date on immunizations for influenza, hepatitis A and B, and tetanus.

Scene Size-up

Remember that sizing up a scene starts with dispatch. If dispatch information indicates a possible unsafe scene, you should stay away from the scene or get only close enough to make an assessment without putting yourself in harm's way. When you arrive first on the scene of an MCI, you will make an initial assessment and some preliminary decisions. The size-up will be driven by three basic questions that responders must ask themselves:

- What do I have?
- What do I need to do?
- What resources do I need?

These questions have a symbiotic relationship. The answer from one helps to answer the others, and each answer represents a piece to the puzzle. Work as a team when you answer these questions because overlooking just one safety issue early on can start a chain reaction of problems.

What Do I Have?

Start with scene safety. First, assess the scene for hazards. Warn all other responders about hazardous materials, fuel spills, electrical hazards, or other safety concerns as soon as possible. Confirm the incident location. Estimate the number of casualties. Report immediately to dispatch. An example of such a report would say: "AEMT unit number one arriving on scene, multiple vehicles involved, full road blockage, no apparent hazards at this time, AEMT unit number one is assuming command."

What Do I Need to Do?

You should keep the following priorities in mind:

- Safety
- Incident stabilization
- Provision of care to injured persons
- Preservation of property and the environment

You need to consider these priorities in the order they are given. Safety is paramount. Safety includes your life, your partner's life, and other rescuers' lives. Then, consider the safety of the patient and any bystanders. This will be difficult for anyone dedicated to saving lives, but it is important to put yourself and your partner first—you have the skills, and bystanders usually do not; the situation can be far worse if you do not put yourself first. Often, if a responder is injured, other responders will focus on "their own," removing available resources from the incident.

You may have to initially work to isolate or stabilize the incident before providing care to injured persons—this is another difficult concept for all emergency workers. Remember, you cannot help the injured if the scene is unstable. An unstable scene can lead to an injured AEMT.

What Do I Need?

Decide what resources are needed. You may need more EMS responders, ambulances, or other forms of transportation. If extrication is required, a rescue unit and fire department response may be needed. If hazardous materials are at the scene, get a HazMat team immediately. Many large EMS systems deploy specialized MCI units or mobile emergency room vehicles that are able to treat dozens of patients on the scene.

Establishing Command

Once you have performed a good scene size-up and answered the three basic questions, command should be established by the most senior official, notification to other responders should go out, and necessary resources should be requested. A command system ensures that resources are effectively and efficiently coordinated. Command must be established early, preferably by the first-arriving, most experienced public safety official. These officials may include police, fire, or EMS personnel.

Communications

Communications is often the key problem at an MCI or a disaster. The infrastructure may be damaged, or communications capabilities may be overwhelmed. If possible, use face-to-face communications to limit radio traffic. Some organizations responding to a disaster might not know how to use a radio. If you communicate via radio, do not use codes or signals. Most communications problems should be worked out before a disaster happens by designating channels strictly for command during a disaster. Whatever form of communications equipment is used, it must be reliable, durable, and field-tested. Be sure there are backups in place if the primary communications system does not work. Some regions have mobile self-contained communications centers, whereas others use local radio groups such as ham radio operators to assist with communications. Most important, your plan should include a "Plan B" in case of communications failure.

Medical Incident Command

What has traditionally been referred to as medical incident command is also known as the medical (or EMS) branch of the ICS **FIGURE 21-2**. At incidents that have a significant medical factor, the Incident Commander (IC) should appoint someone as the medical branch director. This person will supervise the primary roles of the medical branch—triage, treatment, and transport of injured people. The medical branch director should help ensure that EMS units responding to the scene are working within the ICS, each medical division or group receives a clear assignment before beginning work at the scene, and personnel remain with their vehicle in the staging area until they are assigned their duties. Depending on the scale of the incident, EMS may be a branch or may fall under the logistics section as a unit.

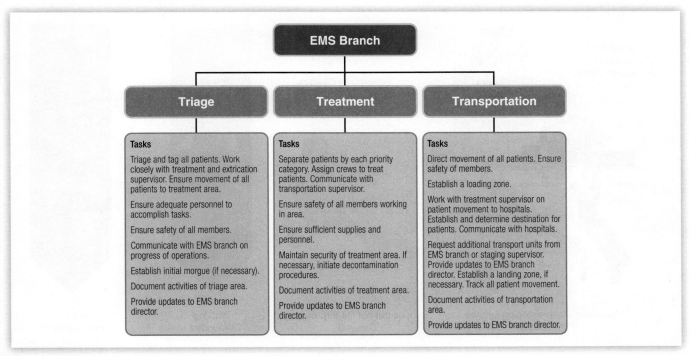

Triage

START Triage

START triage is one of the easiest methods of triage. START stands for Simple Triage And Rapid Treatment. The staff members at Hoag Memorial Hospital, Newport Beach, CA, are responsible for developing this method of triage. It is easily mastered with practice and will give you the ability to rapidly categorize patients at an MCI. START triage uses a limited assessment of the patient's ability to walk, respiratory status, hemodynamic status (pulse), and neurologic status **FIGURE 21-3**.

The first step of the START triage system is performed on arrival at the scene by calling out to patients at the disaster site, "If you can hear my voice and are able to walk …" and then directing patients to an easily identifiable landmark. The injured persons in this group are the walking wounded and are considered minimal (green) priority, or third-priority patients.

The second step in the START process is directed toward nonwalking patients. You move to the first nonambulatory patient and assess the respiratory status. If the patient is not breathing, you should open the airway by using a simple manual maneuver. A patient who still does not begin to breathe is triaged as expectant (black). If the patient begins to breathe, tag him or her as immediate (red) and place in the recovery position and move on to the next patient.

If the patient is breathing, a quick estimation of the respiratory rate should be made. A patient who is breathing faster than 30 breaths/min or slower than 10 breaths/min is triaged as an immediate priority (red). If the patient is breathing from 10 to 29 breaths/min, move to the next step of the assessment.

The next step is to assess the hemodynamic status of the patient by checking for bilateral radial pulses. An absent radial pulse implies the patient is hypotensive and should be triaged as an immediate priority. If a radial pulse is present, go to the next assessment.

The final assessment in START triage is to assess the patient's neurologic status, which simply means to assess the patient's ability to follow simple commands, such as "show me three fingers." This assessment establishes that the patient can understand and follow commands. A patient who is unresponsive or cannot follow simple commands is an immediate priority patient. A patient who complies with a simple command should be triaged in the delayed category.

JumpSTART Triage for Pediatric Patients

Lou Romig, MD, recognized that the START triage system does not take into account the physiologic and developmental differences of pediatric patients. She developed the Jump-START triage system for pediatric patients. JumpSTART is intended for use in children younger than 8 years or who appear to weigh less than 100 lb. As in START, the Jump-START system begins by identifying the walking wounded. Infants or children not developed enough to walk or follow commands (including children with special needs) should be taken as soon as possible to the treatment sector for immediate secondary triage. This action assists in getting

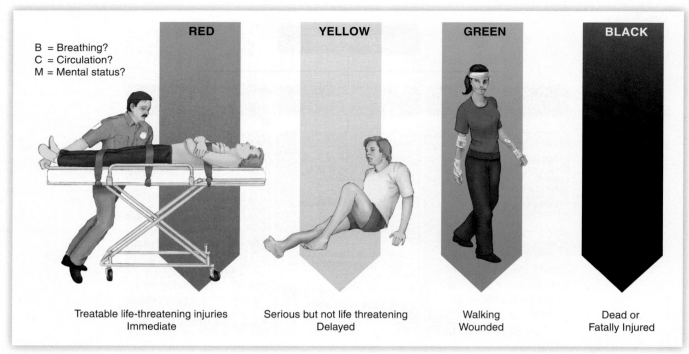

B = Breathing?
C = Circulation?
M = Mental status?

| RED | YELLOW | GREEN | BLACK |

Treatable life-threatening injuries
Immediate

Serious but not life threatening
Delayed

Walking
Wounded

Dead or
Fatally Injured

FIGURE 21-3 Use the START triage system to sort patients into appropriate groups for treatment.

children who cannot take care of their own basic needs into a caregiver's hands. There are several differences within the respiratory status assessment compared with that in START. First, if you find that a pediatric patient is not breathing, immediately check the pulse. If there is no pulse, label the patient as expectant. If the patient is not breathing but has a pulse, open the airway with a manual maneuver. If the patient does not begin to breathe, give five rescue breaths and check respirations again. A child who does not begin to breathe should be labeled expectant. The primary reason for this difference is that the most common cause of cardiac arrest in children is respiratory arrest.

The next step of the JumpSTART process is to assess the approximate rate of respirations. A patient who is breathing fewer than 15 breaths/min or more than 45 breaths/min is tagged as immediate priority, and you move on to the next patient. If the respirations are within the range of 15 to 45 breaths/min, the patient is assessed further.

The next assessment in JumpSTART triage is also the hemodynamic status of the patient. Just like in START, you are simply checking for a distal pulse. This does not need to be the brachial pulse; assess the pulse that you feel the most competent and comfortable checking. If there is an absence of a distal pulse, label the child as an immediate priority and move to the next patient. If the child has a distal pulse, move on to the next assessment.

The final assessment is for neurologic status. Because of the developmental differences in children, their responses will vary. For JumpSTART, a modified AVPU (*Alert* to person, place, and day; responsive to *Verbal* stimuli; responsive to *Pain*; or *Unresponsive*) score is used. A child who is unresponsive or responds to pain by posturing or with incomprehensible sounds or is unable to localize pain is considered an immediate priority and tagged as such. A child who responds to pain by localizing it or withdrawing from it or is alert is considered a delayed priority patient.

Triage Special Considerations

There are a few special situations in triage. Patients who are hysterical and disruptive to rescue efforts may need to be made an immediate priority and transported out of the disaster site, even if they are not seriously injured. Panic breeds panic, and this type of behavior could have a detrimental impact on other patients and on the rescuers.

A rescuer who becomes sick or injured during the rescue effort should be handled as an immediate priority and be transported off the site as soon as possible to avoid negative impact to the morale of remaining rescuers.

HazMat and weapons of mass destruction incidents force the HazMat team to identify patients as contaminated or decontaminated before the regular triage process. Contamination by chemicals or biologic weapons in a treatment area, a hospital, or trauma center could obstruct all systems and organizations coping with the MCI. Bear in mind that some incidents may require multiple triage areas or teams because the victims are located far apart.

Destination Decisions

All patients triaged as immediate (red) or delayed (yellow) should preferably be transported by ground ambulance or air ambulance, if available. In extremely large situations, a bus may transport the walking wounded. If a bus is used for minimal-priority patients, it is strongly suggested that they be transported to a hospital or clinic distant from the MCI or disaster site to avoid overwhelming the local area hospital resources. It is advisable when using a bus to plan for at least one AEMT or paramedic to ride on the bus and to have an ambulance follow the bus. If a minimal-priority patient's condition worsens, the patient could be moved to the ambulance and transported to a closer facility. The AEMT or paramedic can stay with the patients triaged as needing minimal care until their arrival at the designated hospital. Any worsening of a patient's condition must be relayed to the receiving hospital as soon as possible in whatever manner the incident dictates.

Immediate-priority patients should be transported two at a time until all are transported from the site. Then patients in the delayed category can be transported two or three at a time until all are at a hospital. Finally, the slightly injured are transported. Expectant patients who are still alive would receive treatment and transport at this time. Dead victims are handled or transported according to the standing operating procedure for the area.

It is important to remember that during an MCI, local hospitals may have their resources overwhelmed as well. Early notification to receiving facilities will allow for the hospitals to increase staffing and move patients within their facility as required. Typically, EMS agencies will know a hospital's surge capacity, which will tell the agency how many patients of each category the hospital is able to safely handle and care for.

Hazardous Materials

Your training has taught you that rapid response to the scene of a crash can save lives. However, you were also taught that when you arrive at the scene of a possible HazMat incident, it is necessary to step back and assess the situation. This can be very stressful, particularly if you can see a patient. Unfortunately, rushing into such scenes can have catastrophic results for both you and the patient.

Because of the unique aspects of responding to and working at a HazMat incident, the Occupational Safety and Health Administration (OSHA) has issued minimum training requirements for such incidents in its publication "29 CFR 1910.120—Hazardous Waste Operations and Emergency Response Standard" (HAZWOPER); all individuals, including AEMTs, must meet the OSHA requirements before they are permitted to become involved in these situations. In addition, you need to meet training requirements published in "1910.120(q)(6)(i)—First Responder Awareness Level." This text does not include the skills and information needed to meet the training requirements that must be satisfied before individuals are approved to respond to HazMat incidents at the awareness level. Check with your agency for information about specific HazMat awareness-level training.

> **Transition Tip**
>
> A helpful resource for responders responding to a HazMat incident is the US Department of Transportation's (DOT) *Emergency Response Guidebook* (ERG). The ERG, which is available on the Internet, provides guidance on the initial actions to take when responding to HazMat incidents and aids responders in the identification of hazardous materials.

On the basis of the HAZWOPER regulation, first responders at the awareness level should have sufficient training or experience to objectively demonstrate competency in the following areas:

- An understanding of what hazardous substances are and the risks associated with them
- An understanding of the potential outcomes of a HazMat incident
- The ability to recognize the presence of hazardous substances
- The ability to identify the hazardous substances, if possible
- An understanding of the role of the AEMT trained at the HAZWOPER first responder awareness level in the emergency response plan
- The ability to determine the need for additional resources and to notify the communications center

> **Transition Tip**
>
> As an AEMT, you should have a basic understanding of hazardous materials. The *National EMS Education Standards* require that entry-level students be certified in the HAZWOPER standard, 29 CFR 1910.120(q)(6)(i)—First Responder Awareness Level. Most AEMT training programs based on the 1994 NSC provided only a general overview of hazardous materials. If you are not currently certified at the HAZWOPER first responder awareness level, it is recommended that you attend a certification course. Additional information regarding hazardous materials can be found in your EMT-I textbook.

Terrorism Response and Disaster Management

When the 1994 NSC was developed, terrorism was not even a consideration for most people. It was a far-reaching possibility at best. Today, this concern has become a part of life. Although your EMT-I textbook may have discussed terrorism, it is considered new to the *National EMS Education Standards*.

Terrorism is defined by the Federal Code of Regulations as the unlawful use of force and violence against persons or property to intimidate or coerce a government, the civilian population, or any segment thereof, in furtherance of political or social objectives. In recent years, both international terrorists and domestic groups have increased their targeting of civilian populations with acts of terror. The question is not whether terrorists will strike again, but rather when and where they will strike. As a result of the increase in terrorist activity, it is possible that you may be called on to respond to a terrorist event at some point during your career. In that event, you must be prepared for the incident, both mentally and physically.

> *Terrorism* As defined by the Federal Code of Regulations, the unlawful use of force and violence against persons or property to intimidate or coerce a government, the civilian population, or any segment thereof, in furtherance of political or social objectives.

The use of weapons of mass destruction, or weapons of mass casualty, further complicates the management of the terrorist incident and places you in greater danger. Although it is difficult to plan and anticipate a response to many terrorist events, several key principles apply to every response.

No one is quite sure who the first terrorist was, but terrorist forces have been at work since early civilizations. Today, terrorists pose a threat to nations and cultures everywhere, both international and domestic.

Terrorist organizations are generally categorized based on their goals, such as the following:

1. **Violent religious groups/doomsday cults**, which include groups such as Aum Shinrikyo, whose members carried out chemical attacks in Tokyo in 1994 and 1995. Some of these groups may participate in apocalyptic violence.
2. **Extremist political groups**, such as violent separatist groups and those who seek political, religious, economic, and social freedom.
3. **Technology terrorists** who attack a population's technological infrastructure as a means to draw attention to their cause, such as cyber-terrorists.
4. **Single-issue groups**, which include antiabortion groups, animal rights groups, anarchists, racists, and even ecoterrorists who threaten or use violence as a means to protect the environment.

Most terrorist attacks require the coordination of multiple terrorists working together. Nineteen hijackers worked together to commit the worst act of terrorism in US history on September 11, 2001. At least four terrorists worked together to commit the London Subway bombings on July 7, 2005. In a few instances, however, a single terrorist has struck with devastating results. A sole terrorist carried out all of the Atlanta abortion clinic attacks and the 1996 Summer Olympics attack in Atlanta, for example.

Weapons of Mass Destruction

A *weapon of mass destruction (WMD)*, or weapon of mass casualty (WMC), is any agent designed to bring about mass death, casualties, or massive damage to property and infrastructure (bridges, tunnels, airports, and seaports). These instruments of death and destruction include biologic, nuclear, incendiary, chemical, and explosive weapons (B-NICE), also known as chemical, biologic, radiologic, nuclear, and explosive (CBRNE) weapons. B-NICE and CBRNE are helpful mnemonics that may be used to remember the kinds of WMD.

> *Weapon of mass destruction (WMD)* Any agent designed to bring about mass death, casualties, and/or massive damage to property and infrastructure (bridges, tunnels, airports, and seaports); also known as a weapon of mass casualty.

To date, the preferred WMD for terrorists has been explosive devices. Terrorist groups have favored tactics relying on truck bombs or car or pedestrian suicide bombers. Many previous terrorist attempts to use either chemical or biologic weapons to their full capacity have been unsuccessful. Nonetheless, as an AEMT, you should understand the destructive potential of these weapons.

The motives and tactics of the new-age terrorist groups have begun to change. Like the doomsday cults that have carried out attacks in the past, many terrorist groups now advocate apocalyptic, indiscriminate killing. This doctrine of total carnage would make the use of WMDs highly desirable. WMDs are relatively easy to obtain or create and are specifically geared toward killing large numbers of people. Had the proper techniques been used during the 1995 Aum Shinrikyo attack on the Tokyo subway, there might have been tens of thousands of casualties. With the fall of the former Soviet Union, the technology and expertise to produce WMDs may be available to terrorist groups with sufficient funding. Moreover, the technical recipes for making B-NICE weapons can be found readily on the Internet; in fact, they have even been published on terrorist groups' web sites.

Chemical Terrorism/Warfare

Chemical agents are manufactured substances that can have devastating effects on living organisms. They can be produced in liquid, powder, or vapor form depending on the desired route of exposure and dissemination technique. Developed during World War I, these agents have been implicated in thousands of deaths since their introduction on the battlefield and have been used to terrorize civilian populations. These chemical agents consist of the following types:

- Vesicants (blister agents)
- Respiratory agents (choking agents)
- Nerve agents
- Metabolic agents (cyanides)

Biologic Terrorism/Warfare

Biologic agents are organisms that cause disease. They are generally found in nature. For terroristic use, however, they are cultivated, synthesized, and mutated in a laboratory. The weaponization of biologic agents is performed to artificially maximize the target population's exposure to the germ, thereby affecting the greatest number of people and achieving the desired result.

The primary types of biologic agents that you may come into contact with during a biologic event include the following:

- Viruses
- Bacteria
- Toxins

Nuclear/Radiologic Terrorism/Warfare

There have been only two publicly known incidents involving the use of a nuclear device. During World War II, Hiroshima and Nagasaki were devastated when they were targeted with nuclear bombs. The awesome destructive power demonstrated by this attack ended World War II and has served as a deterrent to nuclear war. Since then, however, some nations that have close ties with terrorist groups (known as state-sponsored terrorism) have obtained some degree of nuclear capability.

It is also possible for a terrorist to secure radioactive materials or waste to perpetrate an act of terror. These materials are far easier for a determined terrorist to obtain and require less expertise to use. The difficulties in developing a nuclear weapon are well documented. Radioactive materials, however, such as those in radiologic dispersal devices (RDDs), also known as "dirty bombs," can cause widespread panic and civil disturbances.

AEMT Response to Terrorism

When you are responding to a terrorist event, the basic foundations of patient care remain the same, but the treatment can and will vary. Terrorist events can produce a single casualty, hundreds of casualties, or even thousands of casualties. When you are presented with widespread mass casualties, you must remember to maintain situational awareness. What you may do in one situation may not be appropriate for another situation. In large-scale terrorist events, it is important to use triage and base patient care on the available resources.

Recognizing a Terrorist Event (Indicators)

Most acts of terror are covert, which means that the public safety community generally has no prior knowledge of the time, location, or nature of the attack. This element of surprise makes responding to such an event more complex. You must constantly be aware of your surroundings and understand the possible risks for terrorism associated with certain locations at certain times. For this reason, it is important that you know the current threat level issued by the federal government through the DHS.

The Homeland Security National Terror Advisory System (NTAS) alerts responders to the potential for an attack. This system replaces the color-coded Homeland Security Advisory System (HSAS). On the basis of the current threat level, it is important to take appropriate actions and precautions while continuing to perform your daily duties and respond to calls. The Homeland Security system is used to inform the public safety community of the climate of terrorism (derived from intelligence gathering and the amount of terrorist communication) and to heighten the awareness of the potential for a terrorist attack. It is designed to save lives, including yours.

The DHS has not issued specific recommendations for EMS personnel to follow in response to the alert system. Always follow your local protocols.

Understanding and being aware of the current threat is just the first step in responding safely to calls. Once on duty, you must be able to make appropriate decisions regarding the potential for a terrorist event. In determining the potential for a terrorist attack, make the following observations:

- **Type of location.** Is the location a monument, an infrastructure facility, a government building, or a specific type of location such as a temple? Is there a large gathering? Is there a special event taking place?
- **Type of call.** Is there a report of an explosion or suspicious device nearby? Does the call come into dispatch as someone having unexplained coughing and difficulty breathing? Are there reports of people fleeing the scene?
- **Number of patients.** Are there multiple victims with similar signs and symptoms? This is probably the single most important clue that a terrorist attack or an incident involving a WMD has occurred.
- **Victims' statements.** This is probably the second-best indication of a terrorist or WMD event. Are the victims fleeing the scene giving statements such as "Everyone is passing out," "There was a loud explosion," or "There are a lot of people shaking on the ground"? If so, something is occurring that you do not want to rush into, even if it is determined not to be a terrorist event.

Transition Tip

One of the easiest ways to distinguish between a non-terrorist mass-casualty event and a terrorist event is that the intentional use of a WMD affects multiple persons. These patients will generally exhibit the same signs and symptoms. It is highly unlikely for more than one person to experience a seizure at any given time, for example. It is not uncommon to find multiple patients complaining of difficulty breathing at the scene of a fire, but the same report in the subway at rush hour, when no smell of smoke has been reported, is certainly cause for suspicion. In these situations, you must use good judgment and resist the urge to "rush in and help," especially when the incident involves multiple victims and an unknown cause.

- **Preincident indicators.** Has there been a recent increase in violent political activism? Are you aware of any credible threats made against the location, gathering, or occasion?

Response Actions

Once you suspect that a terrorist event has occurred or a WMD has been used, there are certain actions you must take to ensure that you will be safe and in the proper position to help the community.

Scene Safety Ensure that the scene is safe, remembering to stage your vehicle at a safe distance (usually one to two blocks) from the incident, and wait for law enforcement or HazMat personnel to advise you that the scene has been made secure. If you have any doubts about whether the area is safe, do not enter it. When dealing with a WMD scene, you likely will not be able to enter where the event has occurred—nor do you want to.

The best location for staging is upwind and uphill from the incident. Wait for assistance from those who are trained in assessing and managing WMD scenes. You should expect that a perimeter will be created, usually by law enforcement personnel, in an effort to isolate the scene, prevent further contamination of evidence, and protect rescuers and the public from further danger. Also remember the following rules:

- Failure to park your vehicle at a safe location can place you and your partner in danger. Always identify an escape plan before leaving the vehicle in case the scene becomes unsafe.
- If your vehicle is blocked in by other emergency vehicles or damaged by a secondary device (or event), you will be unable to provide victims with transportation **FIGURE 21-4** or escape yourself.

Responder Safety (Personnel Protection) The best form of protection from a WMD agent is to avoid coming into contact with the agent. The greatest threats facing responders in a WMD attack are contamination and cross-contamination.

Contamination with an agent occurs when you have direct contact with the WMD or are exposed to it. _Cross-contamination_ occurs when you come into contact with a contaminated person who has not yet been decontaminated.

> _Contamination_ The spread of a disease-causing agent through direct contact or exposure to a weapon of mass destruction.
> _Cross-contamination_ The spread of a disease-causing agent as a result of coming into contact with another contaminated person.

Notification Procedures When you suspect a terrorist or WMD event has taken place, notify the dispatcher, providing that communications function properly. Vital information needs to be shared effectively if you are to receive the appropriate assistance. Inform dispatch of the nature of the event, any additional resources that may be required, the estimated number of patients, and the upwind route or optimal route of approach for assisting personnel.

It is important to establish a staging area for other units to converge. Be mindful of access and exit routes when directing units to respond to a location. For example, it is unwise to have units respond to the front entrance of a hotel or apartment building that has experienced an explosion. In addition, note that only responders in the proper protective equipment are equipped to handle the WMD incident.

> ### Transition Tip
>
> During the terrorist attacks on September 11, 2001, communications were severely affected by the collapse of the World Trade Center. The primary communications repeater was situated on top of one of the towers. In addition, excess radio traffic made transmitting and receiving messages extremely difficult. Not only were radio communications affected, but most cellular phones and the majority of radio and television stations were disabled as well. The lesson learned from this event is to have multiple backup systems in place to ensure your ability to communicate with your dispatcher. In the event of a terrorist or WMD event, refrain from using the radio unless you have something important to transmit. If you do transmit, gather your thoughts and speak in as calm a tone as possible, avoiding unnecessary chatter. Remember, while you are transmitting, others may be unable to call for help.

Establishing Command The provider arriving first on the scene must begin to sort out the chaos and define his or her responsibilities under the ICS. As the first person on scene, you may need to establish command until additional personnel arrive. Depending on the circumstances and stage of the operation, you and other AEMTs may function as medical branch directors, triage officers, treatment officers, transportation officers, logistic officers, or other important

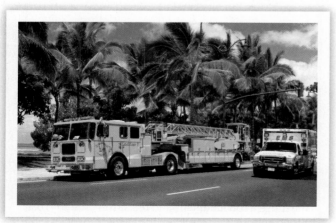

© pbpgalleries/Alamy Images

FIGURE 21-4 Make sure your vehicle is not blocked in by other emergency vehicles.

positions. If the initial ICS is already in place, you should immediately seek out the medical staging officer to receive your assignment.

Secondary Device or Event (Reassessing Scene Safety) Terrorists have been known to plant additional explosives set to explode after the initial bomb. This type of *secondary device* is intended primarily to injure responders and to secure media coverage since the media generally arrive on scene immediately. Secondary devices may include various types of electronic equipment, such as cell phones or pagers, that are detonated when "answered."

> *Secondary device* A type of explosive used by terrorists that is set to explode after the initial bomb goes off.

Do not rely on others to secure your safety. It is every AEMT's responsibility to constantly assess and reassess the scene for safety. It is easy to overlook a suspicious package lying on the floor while you are treating casualties. Stay alert. Something as subtle as a change in the wind direction during a gas attack or an increase in the number of contaminated patients can place you in danger. Never become so involved with the tasks you are performing that you do not maintain appropriate situational awareness and look around to make sure that the scene remains safe.

Chemical Agents

Chemical agents are liquids or gases that are dispersed to kill or injure their intended victims. Modern-day chemicals were first developed during World War I and World War II. During the Cold War, many of these agents were perfected and stockpiled. Whereas the United States has long since renounced the use of chemical weapons, many nations continue to develop and stockpile them. These agents are deadly and pose a serious threat if acquired by terrorists.

Several systems are used to classify chemical weapons. The properties or characteristics of an agent can be described as liquid, gas, or solid material. Persistency and volatility are terms used to describe how long the agent will stay on a surface before it evaporates. Persistent or nonvolatile agents can remain on a surface for long periods, usually longer than 24 hours. By comparison, nonpersistent or volatile agents evaporate relatively quickly when left on a surface in the optimal temperature range. An agent that is described as highly persistent (such as VX, a nerve agent) can remain in the environment for weeks to months, whereas an agent that is highly volatile (such as sarin, also a nerve agent) will turn from liquid to gas (evaporate) within minutes to seconds.

Route of exposure is a term used to describe how the agent most effectively enters the body. Chemical agents can pose either a vapor or contact hazard. Agents with a vapor hazard enter the body through the respiratory tract in the form of vapors. Agents with a contact hazard (or skin hazard) give off very little vapor or no vapors and enter the body through the skin.

> *Route of exposure* Manner by which a toxic substance enters the body.

> ## Transition Tip
>
> Always make sure that patients have been thoroughly decontaminated by trained personnel prior to providing emergency care. Chemical agents are primarily a vapor hazard, and all of the patient's clothing must be removed prior to providing treatment to prevent off-gassing to you. Finally, never perform mouth-to-mouth or mouth-to-mask ventilation on a victim of a chemical agent exposure. The noxious vapors may linger in the patient's airway, and cross-contamination may occur.

Vesicants (Blister Agents)

The primary route of exposure of blister agents, or *vesicants*, is the skin (contact); however, if vesicants are left on the skin or clothing long enough, they produce vapors that can enter the respiratory tract. Vesicants cause burn-like blisters to form on the victim's skin and in the respiratory tract. Vesicant agents include sulfur mustard (H), Lewisite (L), and phosgene oxime (CX) (the symbols H, L, and CX are military designations for these chemicals). Vesicants usually cause the most damage to damp or moist areas of the body, such as the armpits, groin, and respiratory tract. Signs of vesicant exposure on the skin include the following:

- Skin irritation, burning, and reddening
- Immediate, intense skin pain (with L and CX)
- Formation of large blisters
- Gray discoloration of skin (a sign of permanent damage seen with L and CX)
- Swollen and closed or irritated eyes
- Permanent eye injury (including blindness)

If vapors were inhaled, the patient may experience the following signs and symptoms:

- Hoarseness and stridor
- Severe cough
- Hemoptysis (coughing up blood)
- Severe dyspnea

> *Vesicants* Blister agents. Their primary route of entry into the body is through the skin.

Sulfur mustard (H) is a brownish, yellowish oily substance that is generally considered very persistent. When released, it has the distinct smell of garlic or mustard and is quickly absorbed into the skin and mucous membranes. As this agent is absorbed into the skin, it begins an irreversible process of damage to the cells. Absorption through the skin or mucous membranes usually occurs within seconds, and damage to the underlying cells takes place within 1 to 2 minutes.

> *Sulfur mustard (H)* A vesicant; a brownish-yellowish oily substance that is generally considered very persistent. This agent has the distinct smell of garlic or mustard, is quickly absorbed into the skin and mucous membranes, and begins an irreversible process of damaging the cells.

Mustard is considered a mutagen, which means that it mutates, damages, and changes the structures of cells. Eventually, cellular death will occur. On the surface, the patient will generally not produce any signs or symptoms until 4 to 6 hours after exposure (depending on the concentration and amount of exposure) **FIGURE 21-5** .

A person exposed to sulfur mustard will develop a progressive reddening of the affected area, which gradually evolves into large blisters. These blisters are very similar in shape and appearance to those associated with thermal second-degree burns. The fluid within the blisters does not contain any of the agent; however, the skin covering the area is considered to be contaminated until decontamination by trained personnel has been performed.

Mustard also attacks vulnerable cells within the bone marrow and depletes the body's ability to reproduce white blood cells. As with burns, the primary complication associated with vesicant blisters is secondary infection. If the patient survives the initial direct injury from the agent, the depletion of the white blood cells leaves the patient with a decreased resistance to infections.

Although sulfur mustard is regarded as persistent, it releases enough vapors when dispersed to be inhaled. This type of exposure creates upper and lower airway compromise, resulting in damage and swelling of the airways. Such airway compromise makes the patient's condition far more serious.

Lewisite (L) and *phosgene oxime (CX)* produce blister wounds very similar to those caused by mustard. Both are highly volatile and have a rapid onset of symptoms, as opposed to the delayed onset seen with mustard. These agents produce immediate intense pain and discomfort when contact is made. The patient may have a grayish discoloration at the contaminated site. Although tissue damage also occurs with exposure to Lewisite and phosgene oxime, they do not cause the secondary cellular injury associated with mustard.

> *Lewisite (L)* A blistering agent that has a rapid onset of symptoms and produces immediate intense pain and discomfort on contact.
> *Phosgene oxime (CX)* A blistering agent that has a rapid onset of symptoms and produces immediate intense pain and discomfort on contact.

Vesicant Agent Treatment

There are no antidotes for mustard or CX exposure. British anti-Lewisite is the antidote for agent L; however, it is not carried by civilian EMS personnel. When vesicant exposure is suspected, always ensure that the patient has been decontaminated before initiating patient care. The patient may require prompt airway support if any agent has been inhaled, but this should not occur until after decontamination. Transport should be initiated as soon as possible. Generally, burn centers are best equipped to handle the wounds and subsequent infections produced by vesicants. Follow local protocols when deciding the transport destination.

Pulmonary Agents (Choking Agents)

The pulmonary agents are gases that cause immediate harm to persons exposed to them. The primary route of exposure for these agents is the respiratory tract, which makes them an inhalation or vapor hazard. Once inside the lungs, they damage lung tissue, allowing fluid to leak into the lungs. Pulmonary edema develops in the patient, resulting in difficulty breathing because of the inability for air exchange. These agents produce respiratory-related symptoms such as dyspnea, tachypnea, and pulmonary edema. This class of chemical agents consists of chlorine and phosgene.

Chlorine (CL) was the first chemical agent ever used in warfare. It has a distinct odor of bleach and creates a green haze when released as a gas. Initially it produces upper airway irritation and a choking sensation. The patient may later experience the following signs and symptoms:

- Shortness of breath
- Chest tightness
- Hoarseness and stridor as the result of upper airway constriction
- Gasping and coughing

> *Chlorine (CL)* The first chemical agent ever used in warfare. It has a distinct odor of bleach, creates a green haze when released as a gas, and initially produces upper airway irritation and a choking sensation.

With serious exposures, patients may experience pulmonary edema, complete airway constriction, and death.

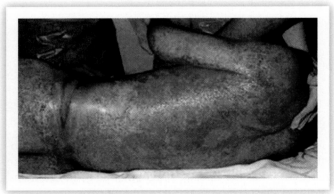

Courtesy of Dr. Saeed Keshavarz/RCCI, Research Center of Chemical Injuries/IRAN

FIGURE 21-5 Skin damage resulting from exposure to sulfur mustard (H).

The fumes from a mixture of household bleach (CL) and ammonia create an acid gas that produces similar effects. Each year, such poisonous mixtures send hundreds of people to the hospital.

The choking agent known as *phosgene* should not be confused with phosgene oxime, the blistering agent (vesicant). Not only has phosgene been produced for chemical warfare, but it is also a product of combustion that might be generated in a fire at a textile factory or house or from metalwork or burning Freon (a liquid chemical used in refrigeration). Given this risk, you may encounter a victim of exposure to this gas during the course of a normal call or at a fire scene.

> *Phosgene* A pulmonary agent that is a product of combustion, and that might be generated in a fire at a textile factory or house, or from metalwork or burning Freon. This very potent agent has a delayed onset of symptoms, usually in the range of hours.

Phosgene is a very potent agent for which the onset of symptoms is delayed following exposure, usually for several hours. Unlike with CL, when phosgene enters the body, it generally does not produce severe irritation that might cause the victim to leave the area or hold his or her breath. In fact, the odor produced by the chemical is similar to that of freshly mowed grass or hay. This results in much more gas entering the body unnoticed.

Initially, a mild exposure to phosgene may produce the following signs and symptoms:

- Nausea
- Chest tightness
- Severe cough
- Dyspnea on exertion

The victim of a severe exposure may present with dyspnea at rest and excessive pulmonary edema. (The patient will actually expel large amounts of fluid from the pulmonary edema in the lungs.) A severe exposure produces such large amounts of fluid in the lungs that the patient may actually become hypovolemic and subsequently hypotensive.

Pulmonary Agent Treatment

The best initial treatment for any patient who has been exposed to a pulmonary agent is removal from the contaminated environment. This extrication should be done by trained personnel who are wearing the proper personal protective equipment. Aggressive management of the ABCs should be initiated, paying particular attention to oxygenation, ventilation, and suctioning if required. Do not allow the patient to be active, because such movement will worsen the condition much more rapidly.

No antidotes are available that can counteract the pulmonary agents. Managing the ABCs, allowing the patient to rest in a position of comfort with the head elevated, and initiating rapid transport are the primary goals for prehospital emergency care.

Nerve Agents

Nerve agents are among the most deadly chemicals developed. Designed to kill large numbers of people with small quantities, nerve agents can cause cardiac arrest within seconds to minutes of exposure. Nerve agents, which were discovered while researchers were trying to develop a superior pesticide, comprise a class of chemicals called organophosphates. Organophosphates are found in household bug sprays, agricultural pesticides, and some industrial chemicals, albeit at far lower strengths than in nerve agents. These chemicals block an essential enzyme in the nervous system, causing the body's organs to become overstimulated and burn out.

> *Nerve agents* A class of chemicals called organophosphates; they function by blocking an essential enzyme in the nervous system, which causes the body's organs to become overstimulated and burn out.

G agents came from the early nerve agents, the G series, which were developed by German scientists (hence the G) in the period between the first two world wars. Three G series agents exist, all of which were designed with the same basic chemical structure but with slight variations to produce different properties. The two characteristics on which these agents vary are lethality and volatility.

> *G agents* Early nerve agents that were developed by German scientists in the period between World War I and World War II. There are three G agents: sarin, soman, and tabun.

The following G agents are listed from high volatility to low volatility:

- *Sarin (GB)*: A highly volatile colorless and odorless liquid, sarin turns from liquid to gas within seconds to minutes at room temperature. It is highly lethal, with an LD_{50} of 1,700 mg/70 kg (about 1 drop, depending on the purity). The LD_{50} is the amount of an agent that will kill 50% of people who are exposed to this level. Sarin is primarily a vapor hazard, with the respiratory tract being its main route of entry into the human body. This agent is especially dangerous in enclosed environments such as office buildings, shopping malls, and subway cars. When it comes into contact with the skin, it is quickly absorbed and evaporates. When sarin is on clothing, it has the effect of off-gassing, which means that the vapors are continuously released over a period of time (like perfume). This effect renders both the victim and the victim's clothing contaminated.

> *Sarin (GB)* A nerve agent that is one of the G agents; a highly volatile, colorless and odorless liquid that turns from liquid to gas within seconds to minutes at room temperature.

- *Soman (GD)*: Twice as persistent as sarin and five times as lethal, soman has a fruity odor as a result of the type of alcohol used in the agent, and it generally has no color. This agent is a contact and an inhalation hazard that can enter the body through skin absorption and through the respiratory tract. A unique additive in soman causes it to bind to the cells that it attacks faster than any other agent. This irreversible binding is called aging, which makes it more difficult to treat patients who have been exposed to soman.

> *Soman (GD)* A nerve agent that is one of the G agents; it has a fruity odor and is both a contact and inhalation hazard—it can enter the body through either skin absorption or the respiratory tract.

- *Tabun (GA)*: Approximately half as lethal as sarin, but 36 times more persistent, under the proper conditions tabun will remain present in the contaminated area for several days. It also has a fruity smell and an appearance similar to sarin. The components used to manufacture this nerve agent are easy to acquire, and the agent is easy to manufacture, which make it unique. Tabun is a contact and an inhalation hazard that can enter the body through skin absorption and through the respiratory tract.

> *Tabun (GA)* A nerve agent that is one of the G agents; it has a fruity smell and is unique because the components used to manufacture the agent are easy to acquire and the agent is easy to manufacture.

- *V agent (VX)*: A clear oily agent that has no odor and looks like baby oil, V agent was developed by the British after World War II. It has chemical properties similar to the G series agents. The difference is that VX is more than 100 times more lethal than sarin and is extremely persistent **FIGURE 21-6**. In fact, VX is so persistent that given the proper conditions, it will remain relatively unchanged for weeks or even months. These properties make VX primarily a contact hazard because it gives off very little vapor. It is easily absorbed into the skin, and the oily residue that remains on the skin's surface is extremely difficult to decontaminate.

> *V agent (VX)* A clear, oily agent that has no odor and looks like baby oil; more than 100 times more lethal than sarin and is extremely persistent.

Nerve agents all produce similar symptoms but have varying routes of entry. They differ slightly in their lethal concentration or dose as well as in their volatility. Some agents are designed to become a gas quickly (nonpersistent or highly volatile), whereas others remain liquid for a period of time (persistent or nonvolatile). Nerve agents have been used successfully in warfare, and to date represent the only type of chemical agent that has been used

successfully in a terrorist act. Once the agent enters the body through skin contact or through the respiratory system, the patient will begin to exhibit a pattern of predictable symptoms.

Like all chemical agents, the severity of the symptoms will depend on the route of exposure and the amount of agent to which the patient was exposed. The resulting symptoms are described using the military mnemonic SLUDGEM and the medical mnemonic DUMBELS **TABLE 21-2**. The medical mnemonic is more useful to you as an AEMT because it lists the more dangerous symptoms associated with exposure to nerve agents.

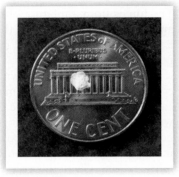
FIGURE 21-6 VX is the most toxic chemical ever created. The dot on the penny demonstrates the amount needed to achieve a lethal dose.

Only a handful of medical conditions are characterized by the bilateral pinpoint constricted pupils (miosis) seen with nerve agent exposure. Conditions such as a cerebrovascular accident, direct light to both eyes, and a drug overdose also can cause bilateral constricted pupils. When this sign is present, you should assess the patient for all of the SLUDGEM/DUMBELS signs and symptoms to determine whether the patient has been exposed to a nerve agent.

Miosis is the most common symptom of nerve agent exposure and can remain for days to weeks. Seizures associated with nerve agent exposure are unlike those noted in patients with a history of seizure. These seizures will

Table 21-2
Symptoms of Persons Exposed to Nerve Agents

Military Mnemonic: SLUDGEM	Medical Mnemonic: DUMBELS
Salivation, **S**weating	**D**iarrhea; **D**iaphoresis (excessive sweating)
Lacrimation (excessive tearing)	**U**rination
Urination	**M**iosis (pinpoint pupils)
Defecation, **D**rooling, **D**iarrhea	**B**radycardia; **B**ronchospasm (spasm of the bronchioles)
Gastric upset and cramps	**E**mesis (vomiting)
Emesis (vomiting)	**L**acrimation (excessive tearing); **L**ethargy (fatigue)
Muscle twitching; **M**iosis (pinpoint pupils)	**S**eizures, **S**alivation, **S**weating

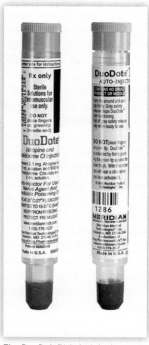

The DuoDote™ Auto-Injector courtesy of Meridian Medical Technologies, Inc., a subsidiary of King Pharmaceuticals, Inc.

FIGURE 21-7 The DuoDote™ Auto-Injector.

continue until the patient dies or until treatment is given with an antidote.

Nerve Agent Treatment

Fatalities from severe nerve agent exposure occur as a result of respiratory complications, which lead to respiratory arrest. Once the patient has been decontaminated, be prepared to treat the patient aggressively. You can greatly increase the patient's chances of survival simply by providing airway and ventilatory support. As with all emergencies, managing the ABCs is the best and most important treatment you can provide. Often in patients exposed to these agents, seizures will begin and not stop. These patients require administration of nerve agent antidote kits in addition to support of the ABCs.

In terms of medical treatment for nerve agent exposure, the most common treatment is the *DuoDote Auto-Injector*, which contains 2.1 mg of atropine and 600 mg of 2-PAM and is delivered as a single dose through one needle **FIGURE 21-7**.

> *DuoDote Auto-Injector* A nerve agent kit containing atropine and 2-PAM chloride (pralidoxime chloride); delivered as a single dose through one needle.

Atropine is used to block the nerve agent from affecting the body. Because the nerve agent may remain in the body for long periods, however, 2-PAM is used to eliminate the agent from the body. Many of the symptoms described in the DUMBELS mnemonic will be reversed with the use of atropine, but multiple doses may need to be administered to achieve these results. If your service carries a nerve agent antidote, refer to local protocols for dose and use information.

In some regions, AEMTs may carry DuoDote kits on the unit and will be called on to administer one or both of the antidotes to themselves, coworkers, or patients.

If your service carries a nerve agent antidote kit, refer to local protocols for dose and use information. **TABLE 21-3** summarizes and compares the nerve agents.

> ### Transition Tip
>
> On March 20, 1995, members of Aum Shinrikyo, a Japanese cult, released sarin (GB) in the Tokyo subway. The first-arriving medical responders were met with chaos as hundreds and then thousands of people fled the subway system. Many of these people were contaminated and showing signs and symptoms of nerve agent exposure. In the end, more than 5,000 people sought medical care for exposure to sarin, and 12 people died. None of the EMS personnel wore protective clothing, and most became cross-contaminated. Remember—you can avoid becoming exposed; do not become a victim.

Metabolic Agents (Cyanides)

Hydrogen cyanide (AC) and cyanogen chloride (CK) are both agents that affect the body's ability to use oxygen. *Cyanide* is a colorless gas that has an odor similar to almonds. The effects of cyanide begin on the cellular level and are

Table 21-3 The Nerve Agents						
Name	**Military Designation**	**Odor**	**Special Features**	**Onset of Symptoms**	**Volatility**	**Route of Exposure**
Tabun	GA	Fruity	Easy to manufacture	Immediate	Low	Contact and vapor hazard
Sarin	GB	None (if pure) or strong	Will off-gas while on victim's clothing	Immediate	High	Primarily respiratory vapor hazard; extremely lethal if skin contact is made
Soman	GD	Fruity	Ages rapidly, making it difficult to treat	Immediate	Moderate	Contact with skin; minimal vapor hazard
V agent	VX	None	Most lethal chemical agent; difficult to decontaminate	Immediate	Very low	Contact with skin; no vapor hazard (unless aerosolized)

very rapidly seen at the organ and system levels. Besides the nerve agents, metabolic agents are the only chemical weapons known to kill within seconds. Unlike nerve agents, however, these deadly gases are commonly found in many industrial settings.

> *Cyanide* An agent that affects the body's ability to use oxygen; a colorless gas that has an odor similar to almonds. The effects of cyanide poisoning begin on the cellular level and are seen very rapidly at the organ system level.

> ## Transition Tip
>
> The basic chemical ingredient in nerve agents is organophosphate, which is widely used, albeit in lesser concentrations, in insecticides. Whereas industrial chemicals do not possess sufficient lethality to be effective WMDs, they are easy to acquire and inexpensive and would have similar effects as the nerve agents. Crop-duster planes could be used to disseminate these chemicals. Be cautious when responding to calls where insecticide equipment is stored and used, such as a farm or supply store that sells these products. The symptoms and medical management of victims of organophosphate insecticide poisoning are identical to those of victims of nerve agents.

Cyanides are produced in massive quantities throughout the United States every year for industrial uses such as gold and silver mining, photography, and plastics processing. They are often present in fires associated with textile and plastic factories. In fact, cyanide is naturally found in the pits of many fruits in very low doses.

The symptoms noted with AC and CK exposure do not differ very much. In low doses, these chemicals are associated with dizziness, light-headedness, headache, and vomiting. Higher doses will produce the following symptoms:

- Shortness of breath and gasping respirations
- Tachypnea
- Flushed skin
- Tachycardia
- Altered mental status
- Seizures
- Coma
- Apnea
- Cardiac arrest

Symptoms associated with the inhalation of a large amount of cyanide will all appear within several minutes. Unless the patient is treated promptly, death is likely.

Cyanide Agent Treatment

Cyanide binds to the body's cells, preventing oxygen from being used. Although several medications can act as antidotes to this agent, most services do not carry them. When cyanide is present in the environment, trained personnel

wearing the proper personal protective equipment must remove the patient from the source of exposure, even if there is no liquid contamination. In addition, all of the patient's clothes must be removed to prevent off-gassing in the ambulance.

Mild effects of cyanide exposure can generally be resolved by simply removing the victim from the source of contamination and administering supplemental oxygen. Severe exposure, however, requires aggressive oxygenation and perhaps ventilation with supplemental oxygen. Always use a bag-mask device or oxygen-powered ventilator device to ventilate a victim of a metabolic agent. The agent can easily be passed from the patient to the rescuer through mouth-to-mouth or mouth-to-mask ventilations. If no antidote is available, initiate transport immediately.

TABLE 21-4 summarizes the chemical agents. The odors of the particular chemicals are provided for informational purposes only. The sense of smell is a poor tool to use to determine whether a chemical agent is present. Many persons are unable to smell these agents, and the odor could originate from another source. This information is useful to you if you receive reports from victims who claimed to smell bleach or garlic, for example. Never enter a potentially hazardous area and "smell" the area to determine whether a chemical agent is present.

▌Biologic Agents

Biologic agents pose many difficult issues when used as WMDs. They can be almost completely undetectable. Also, most of the diseases caused by these agents will be similar to other minor illnesses commonly seen by EMS providers.

Biologic agents are grouped as viruses, bacteria, and neurotoxins and may be spread in various ways. *Dissemination* is the means that a terrorist uses to spread the agent—for example, poisoning the water supply or aerosolizing the agent into the air or ventilation system of a building. A disease vector is an animal that, once infected, spreads disease to another animal. For example, bubonic plague can be spread by infected rats, smallpox by infected persons, and West Nile virus by infected mosquitoes.

> *Dissemination* The means that a terrorist uses to spread a disease—for example, poisoning of the water supply or aerosolizing the agent into the air or ventilation system of a building.

How easily the disease is able to spread from person to person is called communicability. Some diseases, such as infection with the human immunodeficiency virus, are difficult to spread by routine contact so their communicability is considered low. In other instances when communicability is high, such as with smallpox, the person is considered contagious. Typically, routine standard precautions are enough to prevent contamination from contagious biologic organisms.

**Table 21-4
Chemical Agents**

Name	Military Designations	Odor	Lethality	Onset of Symptoms	Volatility	Primary Route of Exposure
Nerve agents	Tabun (GA) Sarin (GB) Soman (GD) VX	Fruity or none	Most lethal chemical agents; can kill within minutes; effects are reversible with antidotes	Immediate	Moderate (GA, GD) Very high (GB) Low (VX)	GA—both vapor and contact hazard GB—vapor hazard GD—both VX—contact hazard
Vesicants	Mustard (H) Lewisite (L) Phosgene oxime (CX)	Garlic (H) Geranium (L)	Causes large blisters to form on victims; may severely damage the upper airway if vapors are inhaled; severe, intense pain and grayish skin discoloration (L and CX)	Delayed (H) Immediate (L, CX)	Very low (H, L) Moderate (CX)	Primarily contact, with some vapor hazard
Pulmonary agents	Chlorine (CL) Phosgene (CG)	Bleach (CL) Cut grass (CG)	Causes irritation choking (CL); severe pulmonary edema (CG)	Immediate (CL) Delayed (CG)	Very high	Vapor hazard
Metabolic agents	Hydrogen cyanide (AC) Cyanogen chloride (CK)	Almonds (AC) Irritating (CK)	Highly lethal chemical gases; can kill within minutes; effects are reversible with antidotes	Immediate	Very high	Vapor hazard

Incubation describes the period of time between when the person is exposed to the agent and when symptoms begin. The incubation period is especially important to understand. Although your patient may not exhibit signs or symptoms, he or she may still be contagious.

> **Incubation** The period of time from when a person is exposed to a disease to when symptoms begin.

AEMTs need to be aware of the circumstances in which they should suspect the use of biologic agents. If the agent is in the form of a powder, such as in the October 2001 American attacks involving anthrax powder mailed in letters, the incident must be handled by HazMat specialists. Patients who have come into direct contact with the agent need to be decontaminated before any contact with EMS personnel occurs or treatment is initiated.

Transition Tip

Because humans are acceptable hosts and vectors for many viruses and bacteria, it is important to use standard precautions at all times. If you fail to use standard precautions, you may not only become a host for a virus, but you may also spread the pathogen to others. Remember, a virus moves from person to person to survive, and many infectious diseases present like common colds.

Viruses

Viruses are germs that require a living host to multiply and survive. A virus is a simple organism that cannot thrive outside of a host (living body). Once in the body, the virus invades healthy cells and replicates itself, thereby spreading through the host. As the virus spreads, so does the disease that it carries. Viruses may move from host to host by direct methods, such as respiratory droplets, or through vectors. A vector is any agent that acts as a carrier or transporter.

> **Viruses** Germs that require a living host to multiply and survive.

Viral agents that may be used during a biologic terrorism incident pose an extraordinary problem for health care providers, especially those in EMS. Although some viral agents have vaccines, there is no treatment for a viral infection other than the limited number of antiviral medications available for some agents. The viruses described in the following section are considered to have the potential to be used by terrorists.

Smallpox

Smallpox is a highly contagious disease. All forms of standard precautions must be used to prevent cross-contamination of this virus to health care providers. By simply wearing examination gloves, a high-efficiency particulate air (HEPA)–filtered respirator, and eye protection, you will greatly reduce your risk of contamination.

Smallpox A highly contagious viral disease; it is most contagious when blisters begin to form.

The last natural case of smallpox in the world was seen in 1977. The illness starts with a high fever, body aches, and headaches, with the patient's temperature usually being in the range of 101°F to 104°F. Later, the rash and blisters that are hallmarks of smallpox become evident.

An easy, quick way to differentiate the smallpox rash from other skin disorders is to observe the size, shape, and location of the lesions. In smallpox, all of the lesions are identical in their development. In other skin disorders, the lesions will be in various stages of healing and development. Smallpox blisters also begin on the face and extremities and eventually move toward the chest and abdomen. The disease is in its most contagious phase when the blisters begin to form **FIGURE 21-8**.

Unprotected contact with these blisters will promote transmission of the disease **TABLE 21-5**. There is a vaccine to prevent smallpox; however, it has been linked to medical complications and in rare cases, death. Should an outbreak occur, the US government has enough vaccine to vaccinate every person in the United States.

Viral Hemorrhagic Fevers

Viral hemorrhagic fevers (VHF) comprise a group of diseases caused by the Ebola, Rift Valley, and yellow fever viruses, among others. This group of viruses causes the blood in the body to seep out from the tissues and blood vessels **FIGURE 21-9**. Initially, the patient will have flulike symptoms, which then progress to more serious symptoms such as internal and external hemorrhaging. VHF outbreaks are not uncommon in Africa and South America, but are extremely rare in the United States. All standard precautions must be taken when treating patients with these illnesses. Mortality rates can range from 5% to 90%, depending on

Table 21-5 Characteristics of Smallpox	
Dissemination	Aerosolized for warfare or terrorist uses
Communicability	High from infected individuals or items (such as blankets used by infected patients); person-to-person transmission possible
Route of entry	Inhalation of coughed droplets or direct skin contact with blisters
Signs and symptoms	Severe fever, malaise, body aches, headaches, small blisters on the skin, bleeding of the skin and mucous membranes; incubation period of 10 to 12 days; duration of the illness, approximately 4 weeks
Medical management	Standard precautions; no specific treatment for smallpox, provide with supportive care (ABCs)

the strain of virus, the victim's age and health condition, and the availability of a modern health care system **TABLE 21-6**.

Viral hemorrhagic fevers (VHF) A group of diseases that include the Ebola, Rift Valley, and yellow fever viruses, among others. They cause the blood in the body to seep out from the tissues and blood vessels.

Bacteria

Unlike viruses, *bacteria* do not require a host to multiply. These organisms are much more complex and larger than viruses, growing up to 100 times larger than the largest virus.

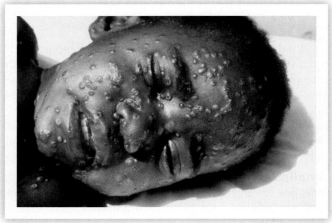

Courtesy of CDC

FIGURE 21-8 In smallpox, all of the lesions are identical in their development. In other skin disorders, the lesions will be in various stages of healing and development.

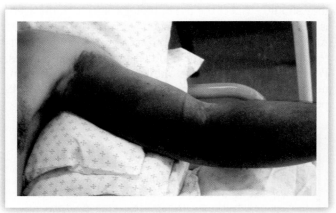

Courtesy of Professor Robert Swanepoel, University of Pretoria

FIGURE 21-9 Viral hemorrhagic fevers cause the blood vessels and tissues to seep blood. The end result is ecchymosis, hemoptysis, and blood in the patient's stool. Notice the severe discoloration in this patient with Crimean-Congo hemorrhagic fever, indicating internal bleeding.

Table 21-6 Characteristics of Viral Hemorrhagic Fevers	
Dissemination	Direct contact with an infected person's body fluids; can also be aerosolized for use in an attack
Communicability	Moderate from person-to-person or contaminated items
Route of entry	Direct contact with an infected person's body fluids
Signs and symptoms	Sudden onset of fever, weakness, muscle pain, headache, and sore throat; all followed by vomiting and, as the virus runs its course, internal and external bleeding
Medical management	Standard precautions; no specific treatment for viral hemorrhagic fever; provide supportive care (ABCs) and treatment for shock and hypotension, if present

Table 21-7 Characteristics of Anthrax	
Dissemination	Aerosol
Communicability	Only in the cutaneous form (rare)
Route of entry	Through inhalation of spores or skin contact with spores or direct contact with skin wound (cutaneous)
Signs and symptoms	Flu-like symptoms, fever, respiratory distress with tachycardia, shock, pulmonary edema, and respiratory failure after 3 to 5 days of flu-like symptoms
Medical management	Pulmonary/inhalation: standard precautions, oxygen, ventilatory support for a patient with pulmonary edema or respiratory failure, and transport Cutaneous: standard precautions, apply dry sterile dressing to prevent accidental contact with wound and fluids

Bacteria contain all the cellular structures of a normal cell and are completely self-sufficient. Most bacterial infections can be fought with antibiotics.

> ***Bacteria*** Microorganisms that reproduce by binary fission. These single-cell creatures reproduce rapidly. Some can form spores (encysted variants) when environmental conditions are harsh.

Most bacterial infections will generally begin with flu-like symptoms, which can make it quite difficult for health care providers to identify whether the cause is a biologic attack or a natural epidemic.

Inhalation and Cutaneous Anthrax *(Bacillus anthracis)* Anthrax is caused by a deadly bacterium that lays dormant in a spore (protective shell). When exposed to the optimal temperature and moisture, this germ is released from the spore. The routes of entry for anthrax bacteria are inhalation, cutaneous, and gastrointestinal (from consuming food that contains spores) **FIGURE 21-10**. The inhalational form, or pulmonary

anthrax, is the most deadly and often presents as a severe cold. Unless treated, pulmonary anthrax is associated with a 90% death rate. Once infected, antibiotics can be used to treat anthrax successfully. A vaccine is also available to prevent anthrax infections **TABLE 21-7**.

> ***Anthrax*** A deadly bacterium (*Bacillus anthracis*) that lays dormant in a spore (protective shell); the germ is released from the spore when exposed to the optimal temperature and moisture. The route of entry into the body may be inhalation, cutaneous, or gastrointestinal (from consuming food that contains spores).

Plague (Bubonic/Pneumonic)

The 14th century plague that ravaged Asia, the Middle East, and finally Europe (the Black Death) killed an estimated 33 to 42 million people. Nearly 500 years later, in the early 19th century, almost 20 million people in India and China died because of plague. The plague's natural vectors are infected rodents and fleas. When a person is bitten by an infected flea or comes into contact with an infected rodent (or the waste of the rodent), the person can contract bubonic plague.

Bubonic plague infects the lymphatic system (a passive circulatory system in the body that bathes the tissues in lymph and works with the immune system). When such infection occurs, the patient's lymph nodes (the area of the lymphatic system where infection-fighting cells are housed) become infected and grow. The glands of the nodes will grow large (up to the size of a tennis ball) and round, forming *buboes* **FIGURE 21-11**. If left untreated, the infection may spread through the body, leading to sepsis and possibly

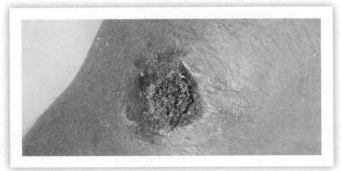

Courtesy of James H. Steele/CDC

FIGURE 21-10 Cutaneous anthrax.

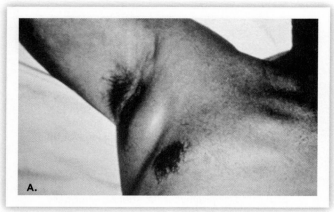

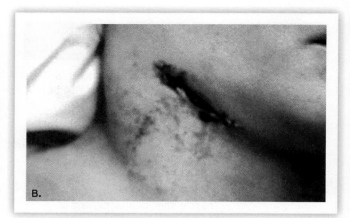

Courtesy of CDC

FIGURE 21-11 **A.** Plague buboe at lymph node under arm. **B.** Plague buboe at lymph node on neck.

death. This form of plague is not contagious and is not likely to be seen in a bioterrorist incident.

> *Bubonic plague* An infection transmitted by infected fleas that is characterized by acute malaise, fever, and the formation of tender, enlarged, inflamed lymph nodes that appear as lesions, called buboes.
>
> *Buboes* Enlarged lymph nodes (up to the size of a tennis ball) that are characteristic of people infected with the bubonic plague.

Pneumonic plague is a lung infection, also known as plague pneumonia, that results from inhalation of plague bacteria. This form of the disease is contagious and has a much higher death rate than the bubonic form **TABLE 21-8**.

> *Pneumonic plague* A lung infection, also known as plague pneumonia, that results from inhalation of plague bacteria.

Table 21-8 Characteristics of Plague	
Dissemination	Aerosol
Communicability	Bubonic: low, only from contact with fluid buboes Pneumonic: high, from person-to-person
Route of entry	Ingestion, inhalation, or cutaneous
Signs and symptoms	Fever, headache, muscle pain and tenderness, pneumonia, shortness of breath, extreme lymph node pain and enlargement (bubonic)
Medical management	Standard precautions, ABCs, provide oxygen, and transport

Neurotoxins

Neurotoxins are the most deadly substances known to humans. The strongest neurotoxin is 15,000 times more lethal than VX and 100,000 times more lethal than sarin. These toxins are produced from plants, marine animals, molds, and bacteria. The route of entry for these toxins is through ingestion, inhalation from aerosols, or injection. Unlike viruses and bacteria, neurotoxins are not contagious and produce a faster onset of symptoms. Although these biologic toxins have immense destructive potential, they have not been used successfully as WMDs.

> *Neurotoxins* Biologic agents that are the most deadly substances known to humans; they include botulinum toxin and ricin.

Botulinum Toxin

The most potent neurotoxin is *botulinum*, which is produced by bacteria. When introduced into the body, this neurotoxin affects the nervous system's ability to function. Voluntary muscle control diminishes as the toxin spreads. Eventually the toxin causes muscle paralysis that begins at the head and face and travels downward throughout the body. The patient's accessory muscles and diaphragm become paralyzed, and the patient goes into respiratory arrest **TABLE 21-9**.

> *Botulinum* A very potent neurotoxin produced by bacteria. When introduced into the body, it affects the nervous system's ability to function and causes botulism.

Ricin

While not as deadly as botulinum, *ricin* is still five times more lethal than VX. This toxin is derived from mash that is left from the castor bean **FIGURE 21-12**. When introduced into the body, ricin causes pulmonary edema and respiratory and circulatory failure leading to death **TABLE 21-10**.

Table 21-9 Characteristics of Botulinum Toxin	
Dissemination	Aerosol or food supply sabotage or injection
Communicability	None
Route of entry	Ingestion, inhalation
Signs and symptoms	Dry mouth, intestinal obstruction, urinary retention, constipation, nausea and vomiting, abnormal pupil dilation, blurred vision, double vision, drooping eyelids, difficulty swallowing, difficulty speaking, and respiratory failure as the result of paralysis
Medical management	ABCs, provide oxygen, and transport; ventilatory support in case of paralysis of the respiratory muscles; vaccine available

Table 21-10 Characteristics of Ricin	
Dissemination	Aerosol or contamination of a food or water supply sabotage
Communicability	None
Route of entry	Inhalation, ingestion, injection
Signs and symptoms	Inhaled: cough, difficulty breathing, chest tightness, nausea, muscle aches, pulmonary edema, and hypoxia Ingested: nausea and vomiting, internal bleeding, and death Injection: no signs except swelling at the injection site and death
Medical management	ABCs, no treatment or vaccine available

> *Ricin* A neurotoxin derived from mash that is left from the castor bean; it causes pulmonary edema and respiratory and circulatory failure, leading to death.

The clinical picture depends on the route of exposure to ricin. This toxin is quite stable and extremely toxic by many routes of exposure, including inhalation. It is likely that 1 to 3 mg of ricin can kill an adult, and the ingestion of just one seed can most likely kill a child.

Although all parts of the castor bean are actually poisonous, it is the seeds that are the most toxic. Castor bean ingestion causes a rapid onset of nausea, vomiting, abdominal cramps, and severe diarrhea, followed by vascular collapse. Death usually occurs on the third day in the absence of appropriate medical intervention.

Ricin is least toxic when ingested by the oral route. This difference probably reflects its poor absorption in the gastrointestinal tract, some digestion in the gut, and possibly some expulsion of the agent as a result of the rapid onset of vomiting. Ingestion causes local hemorrhage and necrosis of the liver, spleen, kidneys, and gastrointestinal tract. Signs and symptoms appear 4 to 8 hours after exposure. Signs and symptoms of ricin ingestion are as follows:

- Fever
- Chills
- Headache
- Muscle aches
- Nausea
- Vomiting
- Diarrhea
- Severe abdominal cramping
- Dehydration
- Gastrointestinal bleeding
- Necrosis of the liver, spleen, kidneys, and gastrointestinal tract

Inhalation of ricin causes nonspecific weakness, cough, fever, hypothermia, and hypotension. Symptoms occur about 4 to 8 hours after inhalation, depending on the inhaled dose. The onset of profuse sweating some hours later signifies the termination of the symptoms. Signs and symptoms of ricin inhalation are as follows:

- Fever
- Chills
- Nausea
- Local irritation of eyes, nose, and throat
- Profuse sweating
- Headache
- Muscle aches
- Nonproductive cough
- Chest pain
- Dyspnea
- Pulmonary edema
- Severe lung inflammation
- Cyanosis
- Seizures
- Respiratory failure

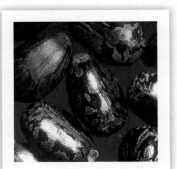

Courtesy of Brian Prechtel/USDA

FIGURE 21-12 These seemingly harmless castor beans contain the key ingredient for ricin, one of the most potent toxins known to humans.

Treatment for ricin exposure is supportive and includes both respiratory support and cardiovascular support as needed. Early intubation and ventilation, combined with treatment of pulmonary edema, are appropriate. Intravenous fluids and electrolyte replacement are useful for treating the dehydration caused by profound vomiting and diarrhea. **TABLE 21-11** summarizes the biologic agents.

Other AEMT Roles During a Biologic Event

Syndromic Surveillance

Syndromic surveillance is the monitoring, usually by local or state health departments, of patients presenting to emergency departments and alternative care facilities, the recording of EMS call volume, and monitoring the use of over-the-counter medications. Surveillance for patients with signs and symptoms that resemble influenza is particularly important when a biologic event is suspected. In such a case, local and state health departments monitor for an unusual influx of patients with these symptoms in hopes of discovering an outbreak early.

The EMS role in syndromic surveillance is a small one, yet is valuable in the overall tracking of a biologic terrorist event or infectious disease outbreak. Quality assurance and dispatch operations need to be aware of an unusual number of calls from patients with "unexplainable flu" coming from a particular region or community.

Points of Distribution (Strategic National Stockpile)

Points of distribution (PODs) are existing facilities that are established for the mass distribution of antibiotics, antidotes, vaccinations, and other medications and supplies in a time of need. These medications may be delivered in large containers known as "push packs" by the Centers for Disease Control and Prevention (CDC) National Pharmaceutical Stockpile. Push packs have a delivery time of 12 hours anywhere in the country and include antibiotics, chemical antidotes, antitoxins, life-support medications, intravenous administration supplies, airway maintenance supplies, and medical/surgical items. In some regions, local and state municipalities have started to stockpile their own supplies to reduce the time delay in providing these items in an MCI.

EMTs, AEMTs, and paramedics may be called on to assist in the delivery of the medications to the public (depending on local emergency management planning). As an AEMT, your role may include triage, treatment of seriously ill patients, and transport of patients to the hospital. Most plans for PODs include at least one ambulance on standby for the transport of seriously ill patients.

▉ Radiologic/Nuclear Devices

What Is Radiation?

Ionizing radiation is energy that is emitted in the form of rays or particles. This energy can be found in radioactive material, such as rocks and metals. Radioactive material is any material that emits radiation. This material is unstable, and it attempts to stabilize itself by changing its structure in a natural process called decay. As the substance decays, it gives off radiation until eventually it reaches a stable state. The process of radioactive decay can take from as little as minutes to billions of years; meanwhile, the substance remains radioactive.

> *Ionizing radiation* Energy that is emitted in the form of rays or particles.

Table 21-11
Biologic Agents

Disease	Transmission Person to Person	Incubation Period	Duration of Illness	Lethality (Approximate Case Fatality Rates)
Inhalation anthrax	No	1 to 6 d	3 to 5 d (usually fatal if untreated)	High
Pneumonic plague	High	2 to 3 d	1 to 6 d (usually fatal)	High unless treated within 12 to 24 h
Smallpox	High	7 to 17 d (average, 12 d)	4 wk	High to moderate
Viral hemorrhagic fevers	Moderate	4 to 21 d	Death between 7 and 16 d	High to moderate, depending on type of fever
Botulinum poisoning	No	1 to 5 d	Death in 24 to 72 h; lasts months if patient does not die	High without respiratory support
Ricin poisoning	No	18 to 24 h	Days; death within 10 to 12 d for ingestion	High

The energy that is emitted from a strong radiologic source consists of *alpha radiation*, *beta radiation*, *gamma (X-ray) radiation*, or *neutron radiation*. Alpha radiation is the least harmful penetrating type of radiation and cannot move through most objects. In fact, a sheet of paper or the body's skin easily stops it. Beta radiation is slightly more penetrating than alpha radiation and requires a layer of clothing to stop it. Gamma rays are far faster and stronger than alpha and beta rays. These rays easily penetrate the human body and require lead or several inches of concrete to stop them. Neutron particles are among the most powerful forms of radiation. They easily penetrate lead and require several feet of concrete to stop them **FIGURE 21-13**.

> *Alpha radiation* Type of energy that is emitted from a strong radiologic source; it is the least harmful penetrating type of radiation and cannot travel fast or through most objects.
>
> *Beta radiation* Type of energy that is emitted from a strong radiologic source; it is slightly more penetrating than alpha radiation and requires a layer of clothing to stop it.
>
> *Gamma (X-ray) radiation* Type of energy that is emitted from a strong radiologic source that is far faster and stronger than alpha and beta rays. Gamma rays easily penetrate through the human body and require either several inches of lead or concrete to prevent penetration.
>
> *Neutron radiation* Type of energy that is emitted from a strong radiologic source; the fastest-moving and most powerful form of radiation. Neutrons easily penetrate through lead and require several feet of concrete to stop them.

Sources of Radiologic Material

There are thousands of radioactive materials found on the earth. These materials are generally used for purposes that benefit humankind, such as radiography, cancer treatment,

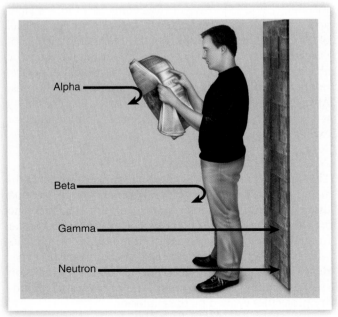

FIGURE 21-13 The penetrating potential of radiation: Alpha radiation, Beta radiation, Gamma radiation, Neutron radiation.

sterilization of supplies, killing germs in food (irradiation), construction work, and other various industrial and scientific uses. Once radiologic material has been used for its purpose, the material remaining is called radiologic waste. Radiologic waste remains radioactive but has no more usefulness. Such waste materials can be found at the following locations:

- Hospitals
- Colleges and universities
- Chemical and industrial sites

Not all radioactive material is tightly guarded, and the waste is often not guarded. This makes use of radioactive material and substances appealing to terrorists.

Radiologic Dispersal Devices (RDD)

A *radiologic dispersal device (RDD)* is any container that is designed to disperse radioactive material. The spread of radiation would generally require the use of a bomb—hence the nickname "*dirty bomb*." A dirty bomb has the potential to injure victims with not only the radioactive material, but also the explosive material used to deliver it. Just the thought of an RDD creates fear in a population, so the ultimate goal of some terrorists—fear—is accomplished. In reality, the destructive capability of a dirty bomb is limited to the explosives that are attached to it. Thus, if the explosive is sufficient to kill 10 persons without radioactive material, it will also kill 10 persons with the radioactive material added. Long-term injuries and illness may be associated with the use of an RDD, yet not much more damage than the bomb by itself would create. In short, the dirty bomb is an ineffective WMD.

> *Radiologic dispersal device (RDD)* Any container that is designed to disperse radioactive material.
>
> *Dirty bomb* Nickname for a bomb that is used as a radiologic dispersal device.

Nuclear Energy

Nuclear energy is artificially made by altering (splitting) radioactive atoms. The result is an immense amount of energy that usually takes the form of heat. Nuclear material is used in medicine, weapons, naval vessels, and power plants. It gives off all forms of radiation, including neutrons (the most deadly type of radiation). When nuclear material is no longer useful, it becomes radioactive waste.

Nuclear Weapons

The destructive energy of a nuclear explosion is unlike any other weapon in the world. That enormous power explains why nuclear weapons are kept only in secure facilities throughout the world. Some nations with ties to terrorists have actively attempted to build nuclear weapons. So far, none of these nations have the ability to deliver a fully capable nuclear weapon such as a missile or bomb. Nuclear weapons also have the formidable deterrent of complete mutual annihilation that argues against their use. Therefore, the likelihood of a nuclear attack is extremely remote.

Unfortunately, however, due to the collapse of the former Soviet Union, the whereabouts of many small nuclear devices is unknown. These suitcase-sized nuclear weapons are called Special Atomic Demolition Munitions (SADM). The SADM, or "suitcase nuke," was designed to destroy individual targets, such as important buildings, bridges, tunnels, and large ships. As of 1998, perhaps as many as 80 of these devices were missing. No other information or updates on the whereabouts of these devices have been made public.

Symptomatology

The effects of radiation exposure vary depending on the amount of radiation a person receives and the route of entry. Radiation can be introduced into the body by all routes of entry as well as through the body (irradiation). A person can inhale radioactive dust from nuclear fallout or from a dirty bomb, or absorb radioactive liquid into the body through the skin. Once in the body, the radiation source irradiates the person from within rather than from an external source (such as x-ray equipment). Common signs of acute radiation sickness are listed in **TABLE 21-12**. Additional injuries will occur with a nuclear blast such as thermal and blast trauma, trauma from flying objects, and eye injuries.

Medical Management

Being exposed to a radiation source does not contaminate a patient or make him or her radioactive. However, when patients have a radioactive source on their body (such as debris from a dirty bomb), they are contaminated and must be initially cared for by a HazMat responder. Once the patient is decontaminated and there is no threat to you as an AEMT, you may begin treatment with the ABCs and treat the patient for any burns or trauma.

Protective Measures

There are no suits or protective gear designed to completely shield AEMTs from radiation. The people who work in high-risk areas wear some protection (lead-lined suits), but this equipment is not typically available to AEMTs. The best ways to protect yourself from the effects of radiation are to use time and distance wisely and to shield yourself using buildings and walls for protection. Do not enter a HazMat area unless you are trained as a HazMat responder and have proper training in the use of self-contained breathing apparatus.

- **Time.** Radiation has a cumulative effect on the body. The less time you are exposed to the source, the milder the effects will be. If you realize that the patient is near a radiation source, leave the area immediately.
- **Distance.** Radiation is limited as to how far it can travel. Depending on the type of radiation, often moving only a few feet away is enough to remove you from immediate danger. Alpha radiation cannot travel more than a few inches, whereas gamma rays can travel hundreds or thousands of meters. Take this factor into account when responding to a nuclear or radiologic incident and make certain that you and other responders are stationed far enough from the incident.
- **Shielding.** As discussed earlier, the path of all radiation can be stopped by a specific object. It will be impossible for you to recognize the type of radiation being emitted or even from which direction it is coming. Therefore, you should always assume that you are dealing with the strongest form of radiation and place concrete shielding (such as buildings or walls) between yourself and the incident. The importance of shielding cannot be overemphasized.

Incendiary and Explosive Devices

Incendiary and explosive devices come in various shapes and sizes. Although you are not tasked with recognizing all of the possible types of explosive devices, including improvised explosive devices (IEDs), it is important for you to be able to identify an object you believe is a potential device, notify the proper authorities, and safely evacuate the area. Always remember that a secondary device is a possibility when you are responding to the scene of an incendiary or explosive device call.

Mechanisms of Injury

The type and severity of wounds sustained from incendiary and explosive devices primarily depend on the patient's distance from the epicenter of the explosion. Patients who are close to the epicenter of the explosion are likely to suffer from all wound-causing agents of the munitions. Patients who are farther away from the epicenter are likely to experience a combination of blast injuries from the explosion and penetrating trauma injuries from primary and secondary projectiles created by the explosion.

Table 21-12 Common Signs of Acute Radiation Sickness	
Low Exposure	**Nausea, Vomiting, Diarrhea**
Moderate exposure	First-degree burns, hair loss, depletion of the immune system (death of white cells), and cancer
Severe exposure	Second- and third-degree burns, cancer, and death

PREP KIT

Ready for Review

- The first rule for safely driving an emergency vehicle is that speed does not save lives—good care does. The second rule is that the driver, AEMTs, and patients must wear seat belts and shoulder restraints at all times.
- The new *National EMS Education Standards* expand upon the vehicle extrication information provided in the past. The most important change is the increased emphasis on safety.
- During extrication operations, the rescue team is responsible for securing and stabilizing vehicles, providing safe entrance and access to patients, extricating patients, and protecting patients during extrication. In contrast, EMS personnel are responsible for assessment, medical care, triage, packaging, and transport of patients in these incidents.
- The NIMS provides a consistent nationwide template to enable federal, state, and local governments, as well as private-sector and nongovernmental organizations, to work together effectively and efficiently. The NIMS is used to prepare for, prevent, respond to, and recover from domestic incidents, regardless of cause, size, or complexity, including acts of catastrophic terrorism and HazMat incidents.
- The purposes of the ICS are threefold: ensuring responder and public safety, achieving incident management goals, and ensuring the efficient use of resources.
- The goal of triage is to do the greatest good for the greatest number. As a consequence, the triage assessment is brief and the patient condition categories are basic.
- The four basic triage categories can be recalled using the mnemonic IDME:
  - Immediate (red)
  - Delayed (yellow)
  - Minimal (green; hold)
  - Expectant (black; likely to die or dead)
- Types of groups that tend to use terrorism include violent religious groups or doomsday cults, extremist political groups, technology terrorists, and single-issue groups.
- A WMD is any agent designed to bring about mass death, casualties, and/or massive damage to property and infrastructure (bridges, tunnels, airports, and seaports). WMDs may include biologic, nuclear, incendiary, chemical, and explosive weapons (B-NICE).
- Terrorists may set secondary devices that are designed to explode after the initial bomb, with the intent to injure responders and attract media coverage. Given this risk, it is essential for AEMTs to constantly assess and reassess the scene for safety.
- The route of exposure is how the agent most effectively enters the body.
- Explosive and incendiary devices come in various shapes and sizes. It is important to be able to identify an object you believe is a potential device and notify the proper authorities, while safely evacuating the area.

Case Study

You are responding to the downtown area for a building explosion. The scene sounds chaotic based on the radio chatter, and you and your partner are not sure what to expect. When you arrive at the scene, you see several EMS units staging and what looks like an established triage area. You are instructed by the EMS Operations Officer to report to the Triage Officer and assist with triaging patients. Near the scene is an area designated for triage; you see several patients lying there on colored tarps. The tarps are colored red, yellow, green, and black. There seem to be only a few patients in the triage area, but you notice more patients being evacuated from the building.

1. What are the major components of the NIMS, and what is the reasoning for inclusion of each component?

2. While driving to this scene, what are some general guidelines to consider?

3. While triaging patients, you notice your partner has sent several patients to the "red" area. Explain the meaning behind the "red" triage category and list some conditions that would fit into this category.

4. You notice that many patients in the triage area are coughing forcefully and appear to be having trouble breathing. You suspect that these patients may have been exposed to some form of pulmonary agent in the explosion. What is the pathophysiology behind pulmonary agents, and what is the basic treatment for this exposure?

5. The IC informs your area that there is a possibility of radiation exposure from the explosion. Describe in detail the three elements to consider when protecting yourself against exposure to radiation.

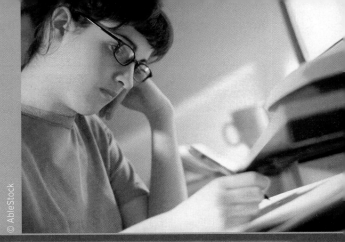

CHAPTER 22

Medical Terminology

National EMS Education Standard

Medical Terminology
Uses foundational anatomic and medical terms and abbreviations in written and oral communication with colleagues and other health care professionals.

Review

Effective communication with members of other health care professions requires the ability to understand medical terms. These terms have been around for many years. You undoubtedly learned the most common terms during your EMT-I course including terms such as hypertension, hypothermia, apnea, tachycardia, and hepatitis. At that time, you most likely learned these terms by simply memorizing their meaning.

What's New

The new *National EMS Education Standards* includes a section on medical terminology. When you understand how medical terms are built, you can enhance your knowledge of medical terms by being able to take terms apart to derive their meanings. This chapter presents the most common terms used in the prehospital arena as well as abbreviations and symbols frequently used during documentation.

Introduction

As an EMS professional, it is important to possess a strong working knowledge of medical terminology. The language of medicine is primarily derived from Greek and Latin. Understanding terminology involves breaking words down into their separate components of prefixes, suffixes, root words, and combining forms. Understanding and using medical terminology are key skills necessary for communicating effectively with other medical personnel.

Root Words

A *root word* is the main part or stem of a word. It conveys the essential meaning of the word. All medical terms contain at least one root word. Sometimes multiple root words have the same meaning. For example, *nephr* and *ren* are both root words for kidneys. A root word frequently indicates a body part. It may be combined with another root word, a prefix, or a suffix. **TABLE 22-1** provides a list of common root words.

> **Root word** The main part or stem of a word.

Transition Tip

The terms listed in this chapter represent only a select few of the most commonly used prefixes, suffixes, and root words. As your career continues, you will add a wealth of terms to your medical vocabulary.

Combining Forms

A *combining form* is created when a root word is combined with a vowel, usually an *o*, but sometimes an *i*. The combining vowel has no meaning on its own, but is used to

> **Combining form** A form created when a root word is combined with a vowel, usually an *o*, but sometimes an *i*.

Table 22-1
Root Words

Root Word	Meaning	Root Word	Meaning
abdomin	abdomen	cyan	blue
acou	hear	cycl	circle or cycle
acr	extremity	cyst	bladder
aden	gland	cyt	cell
adip	fat	derm(at)	skin
alb	white	digit	finger or toe
andr	male	enter	intestines
angi	vessel	erythr	red
ante	anterior, front	esthe	sensation or perception
aort	aorta	febr	fever
append	appendix	foramen	opening
aqua	water	fract	break
arteri	artery	gastr	stomach
arthr	joint	gest	carry, produce, congestion
asthen	weak	glyc(y)	sugar
audi	to hear	gno	know
auto	self, own	gyn(ec)	female
bio	life	hem(at)	blood
blast	germ or cell	hepat(ic)	liver
blephar	eyelid	histo	tissue
bronch	bronchus	humerus	the bone in the upper arm
bucc	cheek	hydr	water
bursa	pouch or sac	hypn	sleep
calcane	calcaneum (heel bone)	hyster	uterus (womb)
callus	hard, thick skin	idi	separate, distinct
carcin	cancer	lact	milk
cardi	heart	later	side
carp	wrist	leuk	white
cent	one hundredth or 100	lingu	tongue
cephal	head	lith	stone, calculus
cerebr	cerebrum	mamm	breast, mammary gland
cervic	neck	melan	black
chol	bile or gall	menses	menstruation
chondr	cartilage	mening	membrane, usually refers to the meninges
cili	eyelid	myel	bone marrow, spinal cord, or myelin
cleid	clavicle	my	muscle
cost	rib	nas	nose
cubitus	elbow	nephr	kidney
cutan	skin		

Table 22-1
Root Words (*continued*)

Root Word	Meaning	Root Word	Meaning
neur	nerve	quadr, quar, quat	four
noct	night	ren	kidney
ocul	eye	retin	inner nerve-containing layer of the eye
olig	little, scanty, or minimal	retro	backward or behind
oophor	ovary	rhin	nose
ophthalm	eye	sangui(n)	blood
or	mouth	scler	hardening, sclera
orchid	testis	sebum	a fatty secretion of the sebaceous glands
ortho	straight	sect	cut
ost(e)	bone	sept	partition, divider; also seven
ot	ear	ser	the clear portion of body fluids, including blood
ov	egg	sinus	cavity, channel, or hollow space
ox	oxygen	somat	body
palp	to examine by touch	spir	breathe
path	disease or abnormal	stasis	slowing or stopping of the normal flow of a fluid, such as blood
ped	child or foot	stature	height
percuss	to tap	stern	sternum (breastbone)
phag	eat	tact	touch
pharyng	throat	tetra	four
phleb	vein	therm	heat
phot	light	thorac	chest
pleur	rib, side	tom	to cut
pneum(at)	breath	toxic	poisonous
pneum(on)	lung, air, gas	trich	hair
pod	foot	ur	urine, urinary tract
proct	anus, rectum	varic	varicose vein
pseudo	false	vas	vessel
psych	mind	viscer	internal organs
ptyal	saliva	xen	stranger, foreign (material)
pulm	lung	xer	dry
pur, py	pus		
pyel	renal pelvis		
pyr	fire		

connect two word elements such as two root words or a root word and a suffix if the suffix begins with a consonant. For example, to combine *gastr* (root word for stomach) and *enter* (root word for intestines), an *o* is necessary.

Example: *gastr/o* (combining form for stomach) + *enter* (root word for intestines) + *-itis* (suffix meaning inflammation) = *gastroenteritis* (inflammation of the stomach and intestines)

Examples of Combining Forms

erythr/ + o = erythr/ red (eg, erythrocyte or red blood cell)

gastr/ + o = gastr/o stomach (eg, gastroenteritis or inflammation of the stomach and intestines)

cardi/ + o = cardi/o heart (eg, cardiomegaly or enlargement of the heart)

arthr/ + o = arthr/o joint (eg, arthritis or inflammation of the joints)

immun/ += o = immune/o immune (eg, immunodeficiency or deficiency of the immune system)

hepat/ + o = hepat/o liver (eg, hepatocyte or liver cell)

Transition Tip

As a rule, a combining form (root word + *o*) is used to link a root to a suffix that begins with a consonant or two root words, even if the second root word begins with a vowel (eg, osteoarthritis).

Prefixes

A *prefix* is a word element that appears at the beginning of a word. Not all medical terms have prefixes. When used, the prefix changes the meaning of the word. For example, *-pnea* is a suffix meaning breathing. Adding different prefixes alters the meaning of the word.

> *Prefix* A word element that appears at the beginning of a word.

a- (without, not) + *-pnea* (breathing) = *apnea* (not breathing)

dys- (difficulty) + *-pnea* (breathing) = *dyspnea* (difficulty breathing)

brady- (slow) + *-pnea* (breathing) = *bradypnea* (slow breathing)

tachy- (fast) + *-pnea* (breathing) = *tachypnea* (rapid breathing)

A prefix is typically used to indicate location, intensity, direction, number, time, position, or negation. By learning to recognize a few of the more commonly used medical prefixes, you can figure out the meaning of terms that may not be immediately familiar. **TABLE 22-2** provides a list of common prefixes.

Suffixes

A *suffix* is a word element that appears at the end of a word. Like a prefix, a suffix changes the meaning of the word. For example, by adding different suffixes to the root word *hem* or *hemat*, meaning blood, different words are created.

> *Suffix* A word element that appears at the end of a word.

Table 22-2
Common Prefixes

Prefix	Meaning	Prefix	Meaning
a	without, lack of	di	twice, double
ab	away from	dia	through, across
ad	to, toward	dys	difficult, painful, abnormal
an	without, lack of	ecto	outside, outward
ana	up, back, again	endo	in, within
ante	before, in front of	epi	upon, on
anti	against, opposed to	eu	easy, good, normal
auto	self	ex	out, out from
bi	two	extra	outside, in addition
brady	slow	hemi	half
circum	around, about	heter	other, different
contra	against, opposite	hom	the same
de	down from, cessation	homeo	same or like

Table 22-2
Common Prefixes (*continued*)

Prefix	Meaning	Prefix	Meaning
hyper	over, excessive	peri	around
hypo	under, deficient	poly	many
infra	inferior to, beneath, below	post	after, behind
inter	between	pre	before
intra	within	pro	before, in front of
iso	same, equal	pseudo	false
macro	large	quadri	four
mal	abnormal or bad	semi	half or partial
medi	middle	sub	under, moderately
mega	large	super	high, excessive, or more than normal
micro	small	supra	above
mono	one	tachy	fast
neo	new	trans	across, through
para	near, beside, beyond	tri	three
per	through	uni	one

hemat (blood) + *-ologist* (specialist) = *hematologist* (physician who specializes in blood disorders)

hemat (blood) + *-ology* (study of) = *hematology* (the study of blood)

hem/o (blood) + *-ptysis* (spitting) = *hemoptysis* (spitting up blood)

hem/o (blood) + *-rrhage* (bursting forth of) = *hemorrhage* (bursting forth of blood)

hemat (blood) + *-emesis* (vomiting) = *hematemesis* (vomiting blood)

hemat (blood) + *-uria* (urine) = *hematuria* (blood in the urine)

In medical terminology, a suffix usually indicates a procedure, condition, disease, or part of speech. **TABLE 22-3** provides a list of common suffixes.

Table 22-3
Common Suffixes

Suffix	Meaning	Suffix	Meaning
-ac	pertaining to	-ary	pertaining to, having the form of, possessing
-al	pertaining to	-asthen	weakness
-algesia	pain	-ation	process of
-algia	pain	-blast	immature cell
-ar	pertaining to	-capnia	carbon dioxide (CO_2)
-arche	beginning	-cardia	heart condition

(continues)

**Table 22-3
Common Suffixes (continued)**

Suffix	Meaning	Suffix	Meaning
-cele	hernia, swelling	-itis	inflammation
-centesis	surgical puncture (usually to remove fluid)	-ization	process of
		-kinesia	movement
-ception	conceiving	-lepsy	seizure
-cide	killing	-lysis	separation, destruction, loosening
-cision	a cutting	-megaly	enlargement of
-crine	secrete	-meter	instrument for measuring
-cyte	cell	-metry	act of measuring
-derma	skin	-ology	science of
-dipsia	thirst	-oma	tumor
-duction	act of leading, bringing, conducting	-opia	vision
-dynia	pain	-opsy	view of
-eal	pertaining to	-orexia	appetite
-ectasis	dilation, expansion	-ory	pertaining to
-ectomy	surgical removal of	-osis	abnormal condition
-edema	swelling	-oxia	oxygen
-ema	state of, condition	-paresis	partial paralysis
-emesis	vomiting	-pathy	disease
-emia	blood condition	-penia	decrease, deficiency
-esis	condition	-pepsia	digestion
-esthesia	feeling	-phagia	eating or swallowing
-gen	forming, producing, causing	-phasia	speech
-globin	protein	-phobia	fear
-gnosis	knowing	-phonia	voice
-graft	transplantation	-phoresis	carrying, transmission
-gram	record, writing	-phoria	feeling (mental state)
-graph	instrument for recording	-plasia	formation, growth
-graphy	process of recording	-plasty	surgical repair
-gravida	pregnant woman	-plegia	paralysis
-ia	condition	-plexy	stroke
-iac	pertaining to	-pnea	breathing
-iatry	medicine, treatment	-ptosis	drooping
-ic	pertaining to	-ptysis	spitting
-ical	pertaining to	-rrhage	abnormal or excessive flow or discharge
-ician	specialist	-rrhaphy	suture of; repair of
-icle	small, minute		
-ile	pertaining to	-rrhea	flow or discharge
-ism	condition	-scope	instrument for examination
-ist	specialist	-scopy	visual examination

Table 22-3
Common Suffixes (*continued*)

Suffix	Meaning	Suffix	Meaning
-sis	a process, action, or condition	-toxic	poison
-spasm	involuntary contraction, twitching	-tripsy	crushing
-stenosis	narrowing, stricture	-trophic	development, nutrition
-stomy	surgical creation of an opening (mouth)	-tropin	stimulate
-taxia	order, coordination	-ula	small, minute
-tension	to stretch	-um	structure, thing
-therapy	treatment	-uria	urine
-thorax	chest	-us	condition, structure
-thymia	mind, emotion	-version	turning
-tic	pertaining to	-y	condition, process
-tomy	incision		

Abbreviations

Abbreviations take the place of words to shorten notes or documentation. When using abbreviations on patient care reports, it is important to use only standard, generally accepted abbreviations to avoid confusion and documentation errors. Never use abbreviations when speaking to a patient. **TABLE 22-4** provides a list of commonly used abbreviations and symbols. This list is intended to help you decipher documents written by other health care professionals.

> *Abbreviations* Letters or symbols that take the place of words and are used to shorten notes or documentation.

Table 22-4
Common Abbreviations and Symbols

Sometimes abbreviations are written with periods (for example, abd. and a.c.), and sometimes different capitalization might be used and might convey a different meaning. Not all possible meanings for the abbreviations in this table are given here. Unless you are certain about the meaning, ask the person who used the abbreviation.

Abbreviation	Meaning	Abbreviation	Meaning
ā	before	AED	automated external defibrillator
ā ā	of each (used in writing prescriptions)	AF	atrial fibrillation
AAA	abdominal aortic aneurysm	AIDS	acquired immunodeficiency syndrome
abd	abdomen	AK	above the knee
ABG	arterial blood gas	AKA	above-the-knee amputation
ac	before meals	A-line	arterial line
ACLS	Advanced Cardiac Life Support	AMA	against medical advice
ACS	acute coronary syndrome	amb	ambulatory
ADL	activity of daily living	AMI	acute myocardial infarction
ad lib	as much as desired	AMS	altered mental status

(*continues*)

Table 22-4
Common Abbreviations and Symbols (*continued*)

Abbreviation	Meaning	Abbreviation	Meaning
ant	anterior	CNS	central nervous system
AO × 4	alert and oriented to person, place, time, and event	c/o	complaining of
A & P	anatomy and physiology	CO	cardiac output, carbon monoxide
AP	anteroposterior, front-to-back, action potential, angina pectoris, anterior pituitary, arterial pressure	CO_2	carbon dioxide
		COLD	chronic obstructive lung disease
		COPD	chronic obstructive pulmonary disease
APC	atrial premature complex, activated protein C, aspirin–phenacetin–caffeine	CP	chest pain, chemically pure, cerebral palsy
Aq	water	CPR	cardiopulmonary resuscitation
ARDS	adult respiratory distress syndrome	CRNA	certified registered nurse anesthetist
ASA	aspirin (acetylsalicylic acid)	CRT	capillary refill time, cathode-ray tube
ASAP	as soon as possible	CSF	cerebrospinal fluid
ASHD	arteriosclerotic or atherosclerotic heart disease	CSM	carotid sinus massage, cerebrospinal meningitis
AV, A-V	atrioventricular, arteriovenous	CVA	cerebrovascular accident
BBB	bundle branch block	CVP	central venous pressure
bid	twice daily	CXR	chest x-ray
BKA	below-the-knee amputation	D & C	dilatation and curettage
BM	bowel movement	D/C	discontinue
BP	blood pressure	diff	differential
BS	blood sugar, breath sounds, bowel sounds, bachelor of science (degree)	dig	digoxin
		DM	diabetes mellitus
BSA	body surface area	DOA	dead on arrival
BVM	bag-valve-mask (ventilation device)	DOE	dyspnea on exertion
bx	biopsy	DON	director of nursing
c̄	with	DOS	dead on scene
°C	degrees Celsius (centigrade)	DPT	diphtheria and tetanus toxoids and pertussis vaccine
Ca	calcium	DSD	dry sterile dressing
CA	cancer, cardiac arrest, chronological age, coronary artery, cold agglutinin	DtaP	diphtheria and tetanus toxoids and acellular pertussis vaccine
CABG	coronary artery bypass graft	DTP	diphtheria and tetanus toxoids and pertussis vaccine
CAD	coronary artery disease		
CBC	complete blood count	DTs	delirium tremens
cc	cubic centimeter	DVT	deep venous thrombosis
CC, C/C	chief complaint	D_5W	dextrose 5% in water
CCU	coronary care unit	Dx	diagnosis
CHF	congestive heart failure	ECG	electrocardiogram
Cl	chloride	ED	emergency department
cm	centimeter	EDC	estimated date of confinement
cm³	cubic centimeter		

Table 22-4
Common Abbreviations and Symbols (*continued*)

Abbreviation	Meaning	Abbreviation	Meaning
EEG	electroencephalogram	H_2O	water
eg	for example	H_2O_2	hydrogen peroxide
EKG	electrocardiogram	H & P	history and physical
ENT	ears, nose, and throat	HPI	history of present illness
ER	emergency room	hr	hour
ET	endotracheal tube, endotracheal	hs	at bedtime
ETA	estimated time of arrival	HTN	hypertension
ETOH	ethyl alcohol	Hx	history
ETT	endotracheal tube	Hz	hertz
°F	degrees Fahrenheit	IABP	intra-aortic balloon pump
FiO_2	fraction of inspired oxygen	IC	intracardiac, inspiratory capacity, irritable colon
FBS	fasting blood sugar		
Fe	iron	ICP	intracranial pressure
FHR	fetal heart rate	ICU	intensive care unit
FHT	fetal heart tones	IM	intramuscular
FHx	family history	I & O	intake and output
fL	femtoliter	IO	intraosseous
fl, fld	fluid	IPPB	intermittent positive-pressure breathing
FSH	follicle-stimulating hormone		
fx	fracture	IUD	intrauterine (contraceptive) device
g	gram	IV	intravenous
GB	gallbladder	JVD	jugular venous distention
GI	gastrointestinal	K^+	potassium
gm	gram	KCl	potassium chloride
gr	grain	kg	kilogram
GSW	gunshot wound	KUB	kidneys, ureters, and bladder
gtt	drop(s)	KVO	keep vein open
GTT	glucose tolerance test	L	liter
GU	genitourinary	LAC	laceration, laparoscopic-assisted colectomy
gyn	gynecology		
h	hour	lb	pound
H, (H)	hypodermic	LE	lower extremity
H/A	headache	LHD	left hand dominant
Hb, Hgb	hemoglobin	LLL	left lower lobe (of the lung)
Hct	hematocrit	LLQ	left lower quadrant (of the abdomen)
Hg	mercury	L/M	liters per minute
H & H	hemoglobin and hematocrit	LMP	last menstrual period
HH	hiatal hernia	LOC	level of consciousness, loss of consciousness
HIV	human immunodeficiency virus		
		lpm	liters per minute

(*continues*)

Table 22-4
Common Abbreviations and Symbols (*continued*)

Abbreviation	Meaning	Abbreviation	Meaning
LPN	licensed practical nurse	NPA	nasopharyngeal airway
LR	lactated Ringer's (solution)	NPO	nil per os (nothing by mouth)
LSD	lysergic acid diethylamide	NS	normal saline
LUL	left upper lobe (of the lung)	NSR	normal sinus rhythm
LUQ	left upper quadrant (of the abdomen)	NTG	nitroglycerin
LVN	licensed vocational nurse	N/V	nausea and vomiting
m	meter	N/V/D	nausea, vomiting, and diarrhea
MAE	moves all extremities	NVD	neck vein distention
MAEW	moves all extremities well	O_2	oxygen
MAP	mean arterial pressure	OB	obstetrics
mcg	microgram	OBS	organic brain syndrome
MCL	midclavicular line, modified chest lead	OD	overdose, right eye, optical density, outside diameter, doctor of optometry
MDI	metered-dose inhaler		
mEq	milliequivalent	OP	outpatient
mg	milligram (mgm is a symbol formerly)	OPA	oropharyngeal airway
MI	myocardial infarction	OR	operating room
MICU	mobile intensive care unit, medical intensive care unit	OS	left eye
		OTC	over-the-counter
min	minute	OU	both eyes
mL	milliliter	oz	ounce
mm	millimeter	p̄	after
mm Hg	millimeters of mercury	pc	after meals
MRI	magnetic resonance imaging	P_{CO_2}	partial pressure of carbon dioxide
MS	morphine sulfate, multiple sclerosis	PDR	*Physician's Desk Reference*
MSO_4	morphine sulfate	PE	pulmonary embolism, physical examination
MVA	motor vehicle accident		
MVC	motor vehicle crash, motor vehicle collision	PEA	pulseless electrical activity
		PEARL, PERL	pupils equal and reactive to light
MVP	mitral valve prolapse	ped, peds	pediatric
Na	sodium	PEEP	positive end-expiratory pressure
NA, N/A	not applicable	PERRL	pupils equal, round, and reactive to light
NaCl	sodium chloride		
NAD	no apparent distress, no appreciable disease	pH	hydrogen ion concentration
		PID	pelvic inflammatory disease
$NaHCO_3$	sodium bicarbonate	PND	paroxysmal nocturnal dyspnea
NC	nasal cannula	po	per os (by mouth)
NG	nasogastric	PO	postoperative, "post op"
NICU	neonatal intensive care unit	P_{O_2}	partial pressure of oxygen
NKA	no known allergies	PRN	pro re nata (as needed)
NKDA	no known drug allergies	psi	pounds per square inch

Table 22-4
Common Abbreviations and Symbols (*continued*)

Abbreviation	Meaning	Abbreviation	Meaning
PSVT	paroxysmal supraventricular tachycardia	S/S	signs and symptoms
pt	patient	stat	immediately
PT	physical therapy	STD	sexually transmitted disease
PTA	prior to admission, plasma thromboplastin antecedent	Sub Q	subcutaneous
PTT	partial thromboplastin time	SVT	supraventricular tachycardia
PVC	premature ventricular complex, polyvinyl chloride	Sym, Sx	symptoms
		tab	tablet
PVD	peripheral vascular disease	TB	tuberculosis
q	every	TBA	to be admitted, to be announced
qd	every day	tbsp	tablespoon
qh	every hour	tech	technician, technologist
qid	four times a day	TIA	transient ischemic attack
qod	every other day	tid	three times a day
RA	rheumatoid arthritis, right atrium	TKO	to keep open
RAD	reactive airway disease, right axis deviation	TPR	temperature, pulse, respiration
		tsp	teaspoon
RBC	red blood cell	Tx	treatment
Rh	Rhesus blood factor, rhodium	U	unit
RHD	rheumatic heart disease, right hand dominant	UA	urinalysis
		UE	upper extremity
RL	Ringer's lactate	URI	upper respiratory infection
RLL	right lower lobe (of the lung)	USP	United States Pharmacopeia
RLQ	right lower quadrant (of the abdomen)	UTI	urinary tract infection
RN	registered nurse	VD	venereal disease
R/O	rule out	vol	volume
ROM	range of motion, rupture of membranes	VS	vital signs
		w/	with
RUL	right upper lobe (of the lung)	WBC	white blood cell
RUQ	right upper quadrant (of the abdomen)	WNL	within normal limits
Rx	prescription	wt	weight
$\bar{s}$	without	yo, y/o	year old
SC	subcutaneous, secretory component	$\bar{x}$	except
SICU	surgical intensive care unit	1°	first, first degree, primary
SIDS	sudden infant death syndrome	2°	second, second degree, secondary
SL	sublingual	↑	increased
SOB	shortness of breath	↓	decreased
SQ	subcutaneous	Ø	no, not, none
ss	half	Ⓡ	right
		Ⓛ	left

(*continues*)

Table 22-4
Common Abbreviations and Symbols (*continued*)

Abbreviation	Meaning	Abbreviation	Meaning
μ	micro	<	less than
α	alpha	?	questionable, possible
β	beta	–	negative
@	at	♀	female
~	approximately	♂	male
×2	times two	Δ	treatment, delta (indicating a difference or change between two values of something)
/	per		
✢, ≠	not equal		
>	greater than		

Defining Medical Words

Defining medical terms is a three-step approach:

1. Identify and define the suffix (the last part of the word).
2. Identify and define the first part of the word. This may be a root word, combining form, or prefix.
3. Identify and define the middle parts of the word (often the root word).

For example, take the term hypoglycemia.

Hypo- (prefix meaning low) + *glyc* (root word meaning sugar) + *-emia* (suffix meaning blood condition).

Hypoglycemia is the medical term meaning low blood sugar.

Take the term gastroenteritis:

1. Define the suffix *-itis*, which means inflammation.
2. Define the beginning of the term—in this case, it is the combining form *gastr/o* meaning stomach.
3. Define the middle part of the word—it this case, it is *enter*, which is the root word for intestines.

Analyzing all the components, you can see that the meaning of the term *gastroenteritis* is inflammation of the stomach and intestines.

Building Medical Words

Three general rules apply when building medical terms:

1. A root word can link directly to a suffix that begins with a vowel.
   Example: gastrectomy [*gastr* is the root word for stomach; *-ectomy* is the suffix meaning surgical removal]
2. A combining form is used to link a root word with a suffix that begins with a consonant.

Example: lymphocyte [*lymph/o* is the combining form for white; *-cyte* is the suffix meaning cell]

3. A combining form is used to link one root word to another root word, even if the second root word begins with a vowel.
   Example: osteoarthritis [*oste/o* is the combining form for bone; *arthr* is the root word for joint; *-itis* is the suffix for inflammation]

Here are some additional examples:

Bradycardia: *brady-* (prefix for slow) + *card* (root word for heart) + *-ia* (suffix for condition) = *bradycardia* (a condition of a slow heart)

Tachycardia: *tachy-* (prefix for rapid) + *card* (root word for heart) + *-ia* (suffix for condition) = *tachycardia* (a condition of a fast heart)

Endocarditis: *endo-* (prefix for within) + *card* (root word for heart) + *-itis* (suffix for inflammation) = *endocarditis* (inflammation within the heart)

Mammography: *mamm/o* (combining form for breast) + *-graphy* (process of recording) = *mammography* (recording of the breast—used to find tumors within the breast)

Arthritis: *arthr* (root word for joint) + *-itis* (suffix for inflammation) = *arthritis* (inflammation of the joints)

Rhinoplasty: *rhin/o* (combining form for nose) + *-plasty* (suffix for surgical repair) = *rhinoplasty* (surgical repair of the nose)

Transition Tip

Before using any abbreviations in your own reports, familiarize yourself with the accepted use of abbreviations in your local jurisdiction or service area.

PREP KIT

Ready for Review

- By learning some of the most common root words, prefixes, and suffixes, and using a medical dictionary, you will gain a good working knowledge of medical terminology.
- An understanding of medical terminology is essential for communicating with patients, other health care professionals, and coworkers.
- A prefix appears at the beginning of a word. It generally describes location and intensity.
- A root word is the main part or stem of a word, which conveys the essential meaning of the word and frequently indicates a body part in medical terminology.
- A suffix is placed at the end of a word to change its meaning. It usually indicates a procedure, condition, disease, or part of speech.
- Learning abbreviations will assist with documentation and decrease the length of your reports.
- Only use standard, accepted, and approved abbreviations when completing patient care reports or other medical documentation.

Case Study

You arrive at the scene of a 42-year-old woman who has been experiencing abd pain for the past hour. The patient tells you that she has been having episodes of abd pain intermittently for the past several weeks. These episodes typically follow meals, particularly consumption of meals including fried foods. The patient denies pregnancy, trauma, or ETOH use. As your partner applies oxygen, you inquire about her past medical history. She tells you that she has a history of HTN, HH, and a recent URI. During the physical exam, you note the patient has tenderness to the RUQ. After performing a physical exam, you load the patient into the unit and transport her to the local hospital.

1. A diagnosis of cholecystitis is likely for this patient. Define cholecystitis based on the root, prefix, and suffix of the word.

2. The patient has a past medical history of HTN, HH, and a URI. What do these abbreviations stand for?

   HTN:

   HH:

   URI:

3. On the basis of the information presented in the scenario, describe the exact location of the patient's pain.

4. Which of the following root words is used when discussing the elbow?
   A. Chondr-
   B. Calcane-
   C. Cubitus
   D. Carp-

5. The suffix "-ectasis" is used to describe:
   A. surgical excision.
   B. dilation and expansion.
   C. surgical drainage.
   D. formation and growth.

APPENDIX A

Drugs Used at the AEMT Level

Specific Medications

A certified AEMT is allowed to administer or help patients self-administer numerous medications. Details about each of these are provided in **TABLE A-1**. As an AEMT, you may administer the following:

- Oxygen
- Oral glucose
- Glucagon
- 50% dextrose ($D_{50}W$)
- Intravenous fluids—D_5W (5% dextrose), normal saline, lactated Ringer's
- Epinephrine (intramuscular or subcutaneous)
- MDI medications—albuterol
- Nebulized medications—albuterol
- Nitroglycerin—spray, tablets, paste
- Nitrous oxide
- Naloxone
- Aspirin
- Others based on local protocols

However, you may administer or help to administer these medications only under the following conditions:

- A licensed physician gives you a direct order to administer a medication and/or the local medical protocols under which you are working permit you to administer the medication. Some local protocols exclude one or more of the medications in the preceding list.
- The local medical protocols under which you are working include standing orders for the use of a medication in defined situations. It is imperative that you do not give or help patients take any other medications under any circumstances.

Table A-1
Drugs, Fluids, and Routes Used at the AEMT Level*

Drugs	
Albuterol (Proventil, Ventolin)	
Class	Sympathomimetic, bronchodilator
Mechanism of action	Beta-2 agonist that stimulates adrenergic receptors of the sympathomimetic nervous system; causes smooth muscle relaxation in the bronchial tree and peripheral vasculature
Indications	Treatment of bronchospasm in patients with reversible obstructive airway disease (COPD/asthma)
Contraindications	Known prior hypersensitivity reactions to albuterol; tachycardia arrhythmias, especially those caused by digitalis; synergistic with other sympathomimetics
Adverse reactions	Often dose-related; include restlessness, tremors, dizziness, palpitations, tachycardia, nervousness, peripheral vasodilation, nausea, vomiting, hyperglycemia, increased blood pressure, and paradoxical bronchospasm

(continues)

Table A-1
Drugs, Fluids, and Routes Used at the AEMT Level* (continued)

Drugs	
Albuterol (Proventil, Ventolin)	
Drug interactions	Tricyclic antidepressants may potentiate vasculature effects. Beta blockers are antagonistic. May potentiate hypokalemia caused by diuretics.
How supplied	Solution for aerosolization: 0.5% (5 mg/mL). MDI: 90 mg/metered spray (17 g canister with 200 inhalations).
Route	Inhalation (nebulizer or MDI)
Dosage and administration	Adult: Administer 2.5 mg. Dilute 0.5 mL of 0.5% solution for inhalation with 2.5 mL normal saline in nebulizer and administer over 5–10 minutes. MDI: 1–2 inhalations (90–180 μg). Five minutes between inhalations. Pediatric: Administer solution of 0.01–0.03 mL (0.05–0.15 mg/kg/dose diluted in 2 mL of 0.9% normal saline). May repeat every 20 minutes three times.
Duration of action	Onset: 5–15 minutes. Peak effect: 30 minutes to 2 hours. Duration: 3–4 hours.
Special considerations	Pregnancy safety: Animal studies suggest the drug may be dangerous to the fetus. Antagonized by beta blockers (eg, propranolol [Inderal], metoprolol [Lopressor]). May precipitate angina pectoris and arrhythmias.
Aspirin	
Class	Platelet inhibitor, anti-inflammatory agent
Mechanism of action	Prostaglandin inhibition
Indications	New-onset chest pain suggestive of acute myocardial infarction
Contraindications	Hypersensitivity; relatively contraindicated in patients with active ulcer disease or asthma
Adverse reactions	Heartburn, GI bleeding, prolonged bleeding, nausea, and vomiting; wheezing in allergic patients
Drug interactions	Use with caution in patients allergic to NSAIDs.
How supplied	81-mg, 160-mg, or 325-mg tablets (chewable and standard)
Route	Oral (chewable tablet[s])
Dosage and administration	160 mg to 325 mg PO (chewed if possible)
Duration of action	Onset: 30–45 minutes. Peak effect: Variable. Duration: Variable.
Special considerations	Pregnancy safety: The drug may pose a risk to the human fetus. Not recommended in pediatric population.
Dextrose 50%	
Class	Carbohydrate, hypertonic solution
Mechanism of action	Rapidly increases serum glucose levels; short-term osmotic diuresis
Indications	Hypoglycemia, altered level of consciousness, coma of unknown etiology, seizure of unknown etiology, status epilepticus
Contraindications	Intracranial hemorrhage
Adverse reactions	Extravasation leads to tissue necrosis; warmth, pain, burning, thrombophlebitis, rhabdomyolysis (muscle breakdown), hyperglycemia
Drug interactions	Sodium bicarbonate, warfarin (Coumadin)
How supplied	25-g/50-mL prefilled syringes (500 mg/mL)
Route	IV, IO
Dosage and administration	Adult: 12.5–25 g slow IV; may be repeated as necessary. Pediatric: 0.5–1 g/kg/dose slow IV; may be repeated as necessary.

Table A-1
Drugs, Fluids, and Routes Used at the AEMT Level* (*continued*)

Drugs	
Dextrose 50%	
Duration of action	Onset: Less than 1 minute. Peak effects: Variable. Duration: Variable.
Special considerations	Determine glucose level before administering. Do not administer to patients with known CVA unless hypoglycemia documented.
Epinephrine (Adrenalin)	
Class	Sympathomimetic
Mechanism of action	Direct-acting alpha- and beta-agonist. Alpha: vasoconstriction. Beta-1: Positive inotropic, chronotropic, and dromotropic effects. Beta-2: Bronchial smooth muscle relaxation and dilation of skeletal vasculature.
Indications	Allergic reactions, anaphylaxis, asthma
Contraindications	Hypertension, hypothermia, pulmonary edema, myocardial ischemia, hypovolemic shock
Adverse reactions	Hypertension, tachycardia, arrhythmias, pulmonary edema, anxiety, restlessness, psychomotor agitation, nausea, headache, angina
Drug interactions	Potentiates other sympathomimetics; MAOIs may potentiate effects; beta blockers may blunt effects
How supplied	1:1,000 solution: Ampules and vials containing 1 mg/mL. 1:10,000 solution: Prefilled syringes containing 1 mg in 10 mL (0.1 mg/mL). Auto-injector (EpiPen): 0.5 mg/mL (1:2,000).
Route	IM, SC
Dosage and administration	Adult: Mild allergic reactions and asthma: 0.3–0.5 mg (0.3–0.5 mL of 1:1,000) SC. Anaphylaxis: 0.1 mg (1 mL of 1:10,000) IV/IO over 5 minutes. Pediatric: Mild allergic reactions and asthma: 0.01 mg/kg (0.01 mL/kg) of 1:1,000 solution SC (maximum of 0.3 mL).
Duration of action	Onset: Immediate. Peak effect: Minutes. Duration: Several minutes.
Special considerations	Pregnancy safety: The drug may pose a risk to the human fetus. May cause syncope in asthmatic children. May increase myocardial oxygen demand.
Glucagon	
Class	Hyperglycemic agent, pancreatic hormone, insulin antagonist
Mechanism of action	Increases blood glucose level by stimulating glycogenesis; unknown mechanism of stabilizing cardiac rhythm in beta blocker overdose; minimal positive inotropic and chronotropic response; decreases GI motility and secretions
Indications	Altered level of consciousness when hypoglycemia is present or suspected; may be used as inotropic agent in beta blocker overdose
Contraindications	Hyperglycemia, hypersensitivity
Adverse reactions	Nausea, vomiting, tachycardia, hypertension
Drug interactions	Incompatible in solution with most other substances; no significant drug interactions with other emergency medications
How supplied	1-mg ampules (requires reconstitution with diluent provided)
Route	IM
Dosage and administration	Adult: Hypoglycemia: 0.5–1 mg IM; may repeat in 7–10 minutes. Pediatric: Hypoglycemia: 0.5–1 mg IM (for children < 20 kg).
Duration of action	Onset: 1 minute. Peak effect: 30 minutes. Duration: Variable (generally 9–17 minutes).

(continues)

Table A-1
Drugs, Fluids, and Routes Used at the AEMT Level* (*continued*)

Drugs	
Glucagon	
Special considerations	Pregnancy safety: The drug may pose a risk to the human fetus. Ineffective if glycogen stores depleted; should always be used in conjunction with 50% dextrose whenever possible. If patient does not respond to a second dose of glucagon, 50% dextrose must be administered.
Naloxone (Narcan)	
Class	Narcotic antagonist
Mechanism of action	Competitive inhibition at narcotic receptor sites, reverses respiratory depression secondary to narcotic administration, completely inhibits the effect of morphine and other opioid drugs
Indications	Opiate overdose, coma; complete or partial reversal of CNS and respiratory depression induced by opioids; decreased level of consciousness; coma of unknown origin; narcotic agonist competes for receptor sites with the following: Morphine, heroin, hydromorphone (Dilaudid), methadone, meperidine (Demerol), paregoric, fentanyl (Sublimaze), oxycodone (Percodan), codeine, propoxyphene (Darvon).
Contraindications	Use with caution in narcotic-dependent patients; use with caution in neonates of narcotic-addicted mothers.
Adverse reactions	Withdrawal symptoms in the addicted patient, tachycardia, hypertension, arrhythmias, nausea, vomiting, diaphoresis
Drug interactions	Incompatible with bisulfite and alkaline solutions
How supplied	0.4 mg/mL, 1 mg/mL
Route	IV, intranasal
Dosage and administration	Adult: 0.4–2.0 mg IV, dose titrated to effect; repeat at 5-minute intervals to a maximum dose of 10 mg (medical control may request higher amounts)
Duration of action	Onset: Within 2 minutes. Peak effect: Variable. Duration: 30–60 minutes.
Special considerations	Pregnancy safety: Animal studies suggest the drug is safe to the fetus. Seizures without causal relationship have been reported. May not reverse hypotension. Use caution when administering to narcotic addicts (potential violent behavior).
Nitroglycerin (Nitrostat, Tridil)	
Class	Vasodilator
Mechanism of action	Smooth muscle relaxant acting on vascular, bronchial, uterine, and intestinal smooth muscle; dilation of arterioles and veins in the periphery; reduces preload and afterload; decreases the workload of the heart and, thereby, myocardial oxygen demand
Indications	Acute angina pectoris, ischemic chest pain, hypertension, CHF, pulmonary edema
Contraindications	Hypotension, hypovolemia; intracranial bleeding or head injury; previous administration of Viagra, Revatio, Levitra, Cialis, or similar agents within past 24–36 hours
Adverse reactions	Headache, hypotension, syncope, reflex tachycardia, flushing, nausea, vomiting, diaphoresis, muscle twitching
Drug interactions	Additive effects with other vasodilators
How supplied	Tablets: 0.15 mg (1/400 grain); 0.3 mg (1/200 grain); 0.4 mg (1/150 grain); 0.6 mg (1/100 grain). Nitroglycerin spray: 0.4 mg–0.8 mg under the tongue.
Route	SL (rapid absorption)
Dosage and administration	Adult: Tablets: 0.3–0.4 mg SL; may repeat in 3–5 minutes to maximum of 3 doses. Nitroglycerin spray: 0.4 mg under the tongue; 1–2 sprays.
Duration of action	Onset: 1–3 minutes. Peak effect: 5–10 minutes. Duration: 20–30 minutes or if IV, 1–10 minutes after discontinuation of infusion.

Table A-1
Drugs, Fluids, and Routes Used at the AEMT Level* (continued)

Drugs	
Nitroglycerin (Nitrostat, Tridil)	
Special considerations	Pregnancy safety: The drug may pose a risk to the human fetus. Hypotension more common in geriatric population. Nitroglycerin decomposes if exposed to light or heat; must be kept in airtight containers. Active ingredient may have a stinging effect when administered.
Nitropaste (Nitro-Bid Ointment)	
Class	Vasodilator
Mechanism of action	Same as nitroglycerin
Indications	Angina pectoris and chest pain associated with acute MI
Contraindications	Same as nitroglycerin
Adverse reactions	Same as nitroglycerin
Drug interactions	Same as nitroglycerin
How supplied	2% solution of nitroglycerin in absorbent paste; 20-, 60-g tubes of paste with measuring applicators; transcutaneous units of varying doses
Route	Transcutaneous
Dosage and administration	Adult: Paste: Apply ½" to ¾" (1–2 cm), 15–30 mg, cover with wrap and secure with tape; maximum, 5" (75 mg) per application. Transcutaneous: Apply unit to intact skin (usually chest wall) in varying doses.
Duration of action	Onset: 30 minutes. Peak effect: Variable. Duration: 18–24 hours.
Special considerations	Pregnancy safety: The drug may pose a risk to the human fetus. Avoid using fingers to spread paste. Store paste in cool place with tube tightly capped. Erratic absorption rates are quite common.
Nitrous Oxide: Oxygen (50:50) (Nitronox)	
Class	Gaseous analgesic and anesthetic
Mechanism of action	Exact mechanism unknown; affects CNS phospholipids
Indications	Moderate to severe pain, anxiety, apprehension
Contraindications	Impaired level of consciousness, head injury, inability to comply with instructions; decompression sickness (nitrogen narcosis, air embolism, air transport); undiagnosed abdominal pain or marked distention, bowel obstruction; hypotension, shock, COPD (with history/suspicion of carbon dioxide retention); cyanosis; chest trauma with pneumothorax
Adverse reactions	Dizziness, apnea, expansion of gas-filled pockets, cyanosis, nausea, vomiting, malignant hyperthermia, drowsiness, euphoria
Drug interactions	None of significance
How supplied	D and E cylinders (blue and green) of 50% nitrous oxide and 50% oxygen compressed gas
Route	Inhalation
Dosage and administration	Adult: (Note: Invert cylinder several times before use.) Instruct the patient to inhale deeply through demand valve and mask or mouthpiece. Pediatric: Same as adult.
Duration of action	Onset: 2–5 minutes. Peak effect: Variable. Duration: 2–5 minutes.
Special considerations	Pregnancy safety: Nitrous oxide increases the incidence of spontaneous abortion. Ventilate patient area during use. Nitrous oxide is a nonflammable and nonexplosive gas. Nitrous oxide is ineffective in 20% of the population.

(continues)

Table A-1
Drugs, Fluids, and Routes Used at the AEMT Level* (*continued*)

Drugs	
Oral Glucose (Insta-Glucose)	
Class	Hyperglycemic
Mechanism of action	Provides quickly absorbed glucose to increase blood glucose levels
Indications	Conscious patients with confirmed or suspected hypoglycemia
Contraindications	Decreased level of consciousness, nausea, vomiting
Adverse reactions	Nausea, vomiting
Drug interactions	None
How supplied	Glucola: 300-mL bottles; glucose pastes and gels in various forms
Route	Oral, buccal
Dosage and administration	Adult: Should be sipped slowly by patient until clinical improvement is noted. Pastes or gels may be fed to the patient or placed between the cheek and gum for absorption. Pediatric: Same as adult.
Duration of action	Onset: Immediate. Peak effect: Variable. Duration: Variable.
Special considerations	As noted in Indications section
Oxygen	
Class	Naturally occurring atmospheric gas
Mechanism of action	Reverses hypoxemia
Indications	Confirmed or suspected hypoxemia, ischemic chest pain, respiratory insufficiency, prophylactically during air transport, confirmed or suspected carbon monoxide poisoning, all other causes of decreased tissue oxygenation, decreased level of consciousness, shock of any type or cause
Contraindications	Hyperventilation
Adverse reactions	Respiratory depression in patients with chronic carbon dioxide retention
Drug interactions	None
How supplied	Oxygen cylinders (usually green and white) of 100% compressed oxygen gas
Route	Inhalation
Dosage and administration	Adult: Cardiac arrest and carbon monoxide poisoning: 100%. Hypoxemia: 10–15 L/min via nonrebreathing mask. COPD: 1–6 L/min via nasal cannula or 28%–35% via Venturi mask. Be prepared to provide ventilatory. Support if higher concentrations of oxygen are needed. Pediatric: Same as for adult with exception of premature infant.
Duration of action	Onset: Immediate. Peak effect: Not applicable. Duration: Less than 2 minutes.
Special considerations	Be familiar with liter flow and each type of delivery device used. Supports combustion.
IV Solutions	
Lactated Ringer's (Hartmann's Solution)	
Class	Isotonic crystalloid solution
Mechanism of action	Lactated Ringer's replaces water and electrolytes
Indications	Hypovolemic shock; keep open IV
Contraindications	Should not be used in patients with congestive heart failure or renal failure
Adverse reactions	Rare in therapeutic dosages
Drug interactions	Few in the emergency setting

Table A-1
Drugs, Fluids, and Routes Used at the AEMT Level* *(continued)*

IV Solutions	
Lactated Ringer's (Hartmann's Solution)	
How supplied	250-, 500-, and 1,000-mL bags, IV infusion
Route	IV
Dosage and administration	Hypovolemic shock; titrate according to patient's physiologic response
Duration of action	Short-term therapy
Special considerations	None
5% Dextrose in Water (D$_5$W)	
Class	Hypotonic dextrose-containing solution
Mechanism of action	Provides nutrients in the form of dextrose as well as free water
Indications	IV access for emergency drugs; for dilution of concentrated drugs for IV infusion
Contraindications	Should not be used as a fluid replacement for hypovolemic states
Adverse reactions	Rare in therapeutic dosages
Drug interactions	Should not be used with phenytoin (Dilantin) or amrinone (Inocor)
How supplied	Bags of 50, 100, 150, 250, 500, and 1,000 mL
Route	IV
Dosage and administration	Usually administered through a minidrip (60 drops/mL) set at a rate of "to keep open"
Duration of action	Short-term therapy
Special considerations	None
0.9% Sodium Chloride (Normal Saline)	
Class	Isotonic crystalloid solution
Mechanism of action	Replaces water and electrolytes
Indications	Heat-related problems (heat exhaustion, heat stroke), freshwater drowning, hypovolemia, diabetic ketoacidosis, keep-open IV
Contraindications	Should not be considered in patients with CHF because circulatory overload can be easily induced
Adverse reactions	Rare in therapeutic dosages
Drug interactions	Few in the emergency setting
How supplied	250-, 500-, and 1,000-mL bags; sterile NS for irrigation should not be confused with that designed for IV administration
Route	IV
Dosage and administration	The specific situation being treated will dictate the rate at which normal saline will be administered. In severe heat stroke, diabetic ketoacidosis, and freshwater drowning, it is likely that you will be called on to administer the fluid rapidly. In other cases, it is advisable to administer the fluid at a moderate rate (for example, 100 mL/h).
Duration of action	Short-term therapy
Special considerations	None

*Local protocols vary and may not include all of these drugs, or may include some of the above routes but not others, and drug concentrations may vary. Always follow local protocols regarding medications to administer, forms, routes, and dosages.

Abbreviations: CHF, congestive heart failure; CNS, central nervous system; COPD, chronic obstructive pulmonary disease: CVA, cerebrovascular accident; GI, gastrointestinal; IM, intramuscular; MAOIs, monoamine oxidase inhibitors; MDI, metered-dose inhaler; MI, myocardial infarction; NS, normal saline; NSAIDs, nonsteroidal anti-inflammatory drugs; PO, orally; SC, subcutaneous; SL, sublingual

APPENDIX B

Mathematical Principles Used in Pharmacology

Mathematical Principles Used in Pharmacology

As an AEMT, you will need an understanding of some basic mathematical principles in order to accurately calculate and convert medication dosages. This section reviews some basic principles and then discusses formulas for medication calculations.

The Metric System

The *metric system* is a decimal system based on multiples of ten. It is used to measure length, volume, and weight, which are represented as follows:

- Meter (m): The basic unit of length
- Liter (L): The basic unit of volume
- Gram (g): The basic unit of weight

> *Metric system* A decimal system based on tens for the measurement of length, weight, and volume.

In the metric system, prefixes demonstrate the fraction of the base being used. Commonly used prefixes, from smallest to largest, include the following:

- micro- = 0.000001
- milli- = 0.001
- centi- = 0.01
- kilo- = 1,000.0

TABLE B-1 illustrates the symbols of weight and volume used in the metric system. It is important to be able to recognize these symbols because drugs will be supplied in a variety of weights and volumes and you will be required to convert these weights to volume to administer the appropriate dose of a medication to your patient.

TABLE B-2 illustrates the metric units of weight and volume and their equivalents. Again, you must be able to understand these metric unit equivalents for proper drug conversion and subsequent administration.

To administer the appropriate dose of a medication to a patient, you must be able to convert larger units of volume

Table B-1
Symbols Used in the Metric System

Unit	Symbol
Weight (smallest to largest)	
Microgram	µg (or mcg)
Milligram	mg
Gram	g (or gm)
Kilogram	kg
Volume (smallest to largest)	
Milliliter	mL
Deciliter	dL
Liter	L

Table B-2
Metric Units and Their Equivalents

Unit	Equivalent
Weight (smallest to largest)	
1 µg	0.001 mg
1 mg	1,000 µg
1 g	1,000 mg
1 kg	1,000 g
Volume (smallest to largest)	
1 mL	1 cc*
10 mL	1 dL
1,000 mL	1 L

*Cubic centimeters (cc) is a unit also used to represent milliliters (mL); therefore, 1 cc is the same as 1 mL (1 cc = 1 mL).

to smaller ones (for example, L to mL) and larger units of weight to smaller ones (for example, g to mg). Conversely, you must also be able to convert smaller units of volume to larger ones (for example, mL to L) and smaller units of weight to larger ones (for example, mg to g).

Drugs are packaged in different units of volume and weight; however, the volume (for example, mL) and weight (for example, μg, mg, g) of the drug to be administered is usually only a fraction of the total amount of its packaged form. For example, a physician may order 50 mg of a drug for a patient, but the drug is packaged in grams. Therefore, you must be able to convert grams to milligrams and then determine how much volume is required to achieve the desired dose.

Volume Conversion

In the prehospital setting, you will usually be dealing with only two measurements of volume: milliliters and liters. Since 1 L equals 1,000 mL, simply divide or multiply by 1,000, or move the decimal point three places to the left or right.

When you are converting mL to L, divide the smaller unit of volume by 1,000, or simply move the decimal point three places to the left, as demonstrated in the following examples:

Example 1:
Converting 100 mL to L (100 mL = X L)
$$100 \text{ mL} \div 1,000 = 0.1 \text{ L } or \overleftarrow{100.} = 0.1 \text{ L}$$

Example 2:
Converting 250 mL to L (250 mL = X L)
$$250 \text{ mL} \div 1,000 = 0.25 \text{ L } or \overleftarrow{250.} = 0.25 \text{ L}$$

Conversely, when you are converting L to mL, multiply L by 1,000, or simply move the decimal point three places to the right, as demonstrated in the following examples:

Example 1:
Converting 1.5 L to mL (1.5 L = X mL)
$$1.5 \text{ L} \times 1,000 = 1,500 \text{ mL } or \overrightarrow{1.500} = 1,500 \text{ mL}$$

Example 2:
Converting 25 L to mL (25 L = X mL)
$$25 \text{ L} \times 1,000 = 25,000 \text{ mL } or \overrightarrow{25.000} = 25,000 \text{ mL}$$

Weight Conversion

An AEMT will likely only need to convert weight when assisting a paramedic with administering a medication to a pediatric patient. Converting weight from g to mg is simply a matter of multiplying or dividing by 1,000 or moving the decimal point three places to the right or left. To convert g to mg or mg to μg, multiply the larger unit of weight by 1,000, or simply move the decimal point three places to the right, as demonstrated in the following examples:

Example 1:
Converting 2 g to mg (2 g = X mg)
$$2 \text{ g} \times 1,000 = 2,000 \text{ mg } or \overrightarrow{2.000} = 2,000 \text{ mg}$$

Example 2:
Converting 5 mg to μg (5 mg = X λg)
$$5 \text{ mg} \times 1,000 = 5,000 \text{ μg } or \overrightarrow{5.000} = 5,000 \text{ μg}$$

Transition Tip

When you are converting units of volume, remember these basic rules:

Volume conversion
Smaller to larger (for example, mL to L): Divide the smaller unit by 1,000 or move the decimal point three places to the left.

Larger to smaller (for example L to mL): Multiply the larger number by 1,000 or move the decimal point three places to the right.

Conversely, to convert a smaller unit to a larger unit when the difference is 1,000 (such as mg to g or μg to mg), divide the mg by 1,000, simply move the decimal point three places to the left, as demonstrated in the following examples. Remember that 1 g equals 1,000 mg and 1 mg equals 1,000 μg.

Example 1:
Converting 200 μg to mg (200 μg = X mg)
$$200 \text{ mg} \div 1,000 = 0.2 \text{ mg } or \overleftarrow{200.} = 0.2 \text{ mg}$$

Example 2:
Converting 250 mg to g (250 mg = X g)
$$250 \text{ mg} \div 1,000 = 0.25 \text{ g } or \overleftarrow{250.} = 0.25 \text{ g}$$

Converting Pounds to Kilograms

It would be a luxury if your patients were able to tell you how much they weighed in kilograms (kg); however, the chances of this happening are slim to none. For patients who do not know their weight in pounds or who are unresponsive and unable to provide you with this information, you must do the following:

1. Estimate the patient's weight in pounds (lb)
2. Convert pounds to kilograms (kg)

Although many of the drugs given in emergency medicine are administered in a standard dose (for example, 1 mg of epinephrine), other paramedic-level drugs are administered based on the patient's weight in kilograms (for example, 1 to 1.5 mg/kg of lidocaine). In addition, most drugs administered to pediatric patients are based on their weight in kilograms.

There are two formulas that can be used to convert pounds to kilograms; use the one that is easiest for you to remember.

> Formula 1: Divide the patient's weight in pounds by 2.2 (1 kg = 2.2 lb).

For example, when converting a 170-lb man's weight to kilograms, the formula would be as follows:

$$170 \text{ lb} \div 2.2 = 77.27 \text{ kg}$$

Because the value following the decimal point in the preceding example is less than 0.5, you may round the patient's weight in kg to 77.0. If the value after the decimal point had been greater than 0.5, you would round the weight in kg to 78.0. Although this may seem negligible, it is important to administer the most appropriate amount of the drug to the patient; it's good practice.

> Formula 2: Divide the patient's weight in pounds by 2 and subtract 10%.

For example, when converting a 120-lb woman's weight to kg, the formula would be as follows:

> *Step 1:* 120 lb ÷ 2 = 60 lb
> *Step 2:* 60 lb × 10% = 6
> *Step 3:* 60 − 6 = 54 kg

Calculating Drip Rates

As an AEMT, you will sometimes administer IV fluid such as normal saline, lactated Ringer's, or D_5W. IV fluid hydrates the patient and may treat shock, but it does not include medication. When you administer IV fluid, you will need to calculate the *drip rate*.

> *Drip rate* Number of drops per minute.

One of the easiest ways to calculate drip rates is to use dimensional analysis. Dimensional analysis uses the same simple conversions as equations, and you will not need to memorize the equation! Dimensional analysis allows you to compare seemingly unrelated items by setting up a relationship (that is, a comparison between two items).

An example of a relationship could be a car and the wheels on a car. Every car rides on four wheels, so there are four wheels for every car.

$$\frac{1 \text{ car}}{4 \text{ wheels}} = \frac{4 \text{ wheels}}{1 \text{ car}}$$

Another way to look at these comparisons is as a ratio, which is by nature a relationship. Dimensional analysis uses ratios as conversion factors.

To calculate a drip rate, you need to know:

- Which administration set to use
- Length of time for the infusion
- Amount to flow

You may need the conversion factor of 1 hour equals 60 minutes.

Example:

- Order is given for 250 mL normal saline over 90 minutes.
- IV administration is a macrodrip (10 gtt/mL). Note: gtt is an abbreviation for drops.

In order to determine how many drops per minute should be given. Set up the equation:

$$\frac{? \text{ gtt}}{\text{min}} = \frac{10 \text{ gtt}}{1 \text{ mL}} \times \frac{250 \text{ mL}}{90 \text{ min}}$$

Cancel out what you can and reduce the fractions:

$$\frac{? \text{ gtt}}{\text{min}} = \frac{10 \text{ gtt}}{1 \text{ mL}} \times \frac{250 \text{ mL}}{90 \text{ min}}$$

Multiply and divide:

$$= \frac{250 \text{ gtt}}{9 \text{ min}} = \frac{27.77 \text{ gtt}}{\text{min}} = 28 \text{ gtt/min}$$

You will need to set the drip rate at 28 gtt/min normal saline using a macrodrip administration set to achieve the desired order.

> **Transition Tip**
>
> The volume in milliliters (mL) is the "doctor's order." The drip set is always drops per mL, and the time is always in minutes. Multiply the doctor's order (in mL) times the drip set (in drops/mL) and divide by the time (in minutes). This yields the number of drops per minute.

Another useful formula to remember is a simple drip rate calculation that gives you the number of drops per minute:

$$\frac{(\text{volume in mL}) \times (\text{drip set})}{(\text{time in minutes})} = \frac{\text{gtt}}{\text{min}}$$

> **Transition Tip**
>
> KVO means "keep vein open"; "TKO" means to keep open. Both are abbreviations for rates equal to about 8 to 15 drops/min that are used to allow just enough fluid through the IV line to keep blood from clotting at the end of the catheter.

Calculating Medication Doses

AEMTs are certified to administer certain medications. When you administer a medication, you will need to calculate the dose. There are multiple formulas for calculating medication doses. It is beyond the scope of this appendix to demonstrate every one of these calculation formulas. Therefore, the discussion in this appendix will be limited to formulas that most students find easy to understand. For other calculation formulas, the AEMT is encouraged to consult with his or her instructor or other books on this subject. The method of drug dose calculation demonstrated in this chapter will be based on the following three factors:

1. Desired dose
2. Concentration of the drug available (dose on hand)
3. Volume to be administered

Desired Dose

The desired dose (that is, the drug order) is the amount of a drug that the physician orders you to administer to a patient. It may be expressed as a standard dose (for example, 25 g of dextrose), or it may be expressed as a specific number of grams or milligrams per kilogram of body weight (for example, 0.1 mg/kg is the pediatric dose for naloxone).

Drug Concentrations

After receiving a drug order (that is, the desired dose), you must determine how much of the drug is available. In other words, you must know its *concentration*—the total weight (µg, mg, or g) of the drug contained in a specific volume (mL or L). An example of a common prepackaged drug concentration is 50% dextrose, 25 g/50 mL.

> *Concentration* The total weight of a drug contained in a specific volume of liquid.

Note that drugs are contained in different volumes of solution. This is your *volume on hand*. *However, to administer a drug, you must know the weight of the drug that is present in each milliliter.* This will tell you the concentration of the drug that you have on hand. The formula for calculating this is as follows:

> Total Weight of the Drug ÷ Total Volume in Milliliters
> = Weight per Milliliter

> *Volume on hand* The amount of fluid you have on hand, such as the amount of fluid in an IV bag or the amount of fluid in a vial of medication.

By using the preceding formula and the examples of common prepackaged drugs, you can calculate how much of the drug is contained in each milliliter (dose on hand). For example, if the drug order is for dextrose, 25 g/50 mL, you would calculate the concentration as follows:

> 25 g (total weight) ÷ 50 mL (total volume) = 0.5 g/mL

Volume to Be Administered

After the concentration of the drug present in each milliliter (dose on hand) is determined, you must calculate how much volume is needed to give the amount of the drug ordered (desired dose). Use the following formula to calculate the volume to be administered:

> Desired Dose (mg) ÷ Dose on Hand (mg/mL)
> = Volume to be Administered (mL)

Notice that the desired dose is in mg and the dose on hand is in mg/mL. There may be instances where the desired dose is in a different unit, such as g or µg. Before using the above formula, the units in the desired dose must match the units in the top of the dose-on-hand fraction. If they do not, you will need to do a quick calculation to convert the desired dose units to match the units in the top half of the dose on hand.

On the basis of the preceding formula, you will be able to determine how much volume to give to achieve the required dose. Here is an example:

Example 1:

You are ordered to administer 12.5 g of dextrose to a hypoglycemic patient. You have a prefilled syringe of 50% dextrose containing 25 g in 50 mL. How many milliliters of dextrose will you give?

Step 1: Determine the concentration/dose on hand (in g/mL).

> 25 g ÷ 50 mL = 0.5 g/mL (dose on hand)

Step 2: Determine how much volume to administer.

> 12.5 g (desired dose) ÷ 0.5 g/mL (dose on hand) = 25 mL

You will need to administer 25 mL, or half of the 50-mL syringe.

Example 2:

You are ordered to administer 70 mg of medication "Y" to a patient. The medication is prepared as follows: 100 mg in 5 mL of saline. How many milliliters must you give to achieve the ordered dose?

Step 1: Determine the concentration/dose on hand (in mg/mL).

> 100 mg ÷ 5 mL = 20 mg/mL (dose on hand)

Step 2: Determine how much volume to administer.

> 70 mg (desired dose) ÷ 20 mg/mL (dose on hand)
> = 3.5 mL

You will need to administer 3.5 mL of the medication.

Weight-Based Drug Doses

As previously discussed, some medication doses are based on the patient's weight in kilograms. Determining the appropriate dose for the patient requires simply converting the patient's weight in pounds to kilograms and then proceeding with the formula that was just discussed. Remember, 1 kg equals 2.2 lb. As an AEMT, drugs that you may administer and whose orders may be weight-based include pediatric dosages for dextrose, epinephrine, and naloxone.

The following are some examples of how to calculate the appropriate drug dose based on the patient's weight:

Example 1:

You are ordered to give 0.1 mg/kg of naloxone (Narcan) to your 40-lb pediatric patient. You have a prefilled syringe of the medication containing 100 mg in 10 mL. How many milligrams will you give to this patient? How much volume will you give to achieve the required dose?

Step 1: Convert the patient's weight in pounds to kilograms.

- **Formula 1:** 40 lb ÷ 2.2 = 18.18 kg (round to 18 kg)
- **Formula 2:** 40 lb ÷ 2 = 20 - 10% = 18 kg

Step 2: Determine the desired dose.

$$0.1 \text{ mg/kg} \times 18 \text{ kg} = 1.8 \text{ mg (desired dose)}$$

Step 3: Determine the concentration/dose on hand (in mg/mL).

$$100 \text{ mg} ÷ 10 \text{ mL} = 10 \text{ mg/mL (dose on hand)}$$

Step 4: Determine how much volume to administer.

$$1.8 \text{ mg (desired dose)} ÷ 10 \text{ mg/mL (dose on hand)}$$
$$= 0.18 \text{ mL (round to 0.2 mL)}$$

Example 2:

A 4-year-old boy in asystole requires 0.01 mg/kg of epinephrine. You have a prefilled syringe of epinephrine containing 1 mg in 10 mL. The child's mother tells you that he weighs 35 lb. How many milligrams will you give to this patient (that is, what is the desired dose)? How much volume will you give to achieve the required dose?

Step 1: Convert the patient's weight in pounds to kilograms.

- **Formula 1:** 35 lb ÷ 2.2 = 15.9 kg (round to 16 kg)
- **Formula 2:** 35 lb ÷ 2 = 17.5 - 10% = 15.75 kg (round to 16 kg)

Step 2: Determine the desired dose.

$$0.01 \text{ mg} \times 16 \text{ kg} = 0.16 \text{ mg/kg (desired dose)}$$

Step 3: Determine the concentration/dose on hand (in mg/mL).

$$1 \text{ mg} ÷ 10 \text{ mL} = 0.1 \text{ mg/mL (dose on hand)}$$

Step 4: Determine how much volume to administer.

$$0.16 \text{ mg (desired dose)} ÷ 0.1 \text{ mg/mL (dose on hand)}$$
$$= 1.6 \text{ mL (round to 2 mL)}$$

Transition Tip

It is important to administer the most appropriate dose of a drug to a child. Many parents or caregivers know how much their children weigh in pounds, which you can easily convert to kilograms (1 kg = 2.2 lb). If a parent or caregiver is available, simply ask the child's weight; do not attempt to estimate the child's weight if it is not necessary.

Pediatric Doses

There are numerous methods for determining the appropriate dose of medication for a pediatric patient. Many rescuers use length-based resuscitation tapes; others may carry a field guide with tables or charts for reference. Most drugs used in pediatric emergency medicine are based on the child's weight in kilograms. The calculations for pediatric drug dosing and medication infusions are the same as they are for adults, but the doses and volumes will be obviously smaller.

Glossary

Abbreviations Letters or symbols that take the place of words and are used to shorten notes or documentation.

Abdominal aortic aneurysm (AAA) A condition in which the walls of the aorta in the abdomen weaken and blood leaks into the layers of the vessel, causing it to bulge.

Abruptio placenta A premature separation of the placenta from the wall of the uterus.

Absence seizures The seizures that may be characterized by a brief lapse of attention in which the patient may stare and does not respond; formerly known as a petit mal seizure.

Acidosis A pathologic condition resulting from the accumulation of acids in the body.

Acquired immunodeficiency syndrome (AIDS) The end-stage disease process caused by the human immunodeficiency virus (HIV). A person with this is extremely vulnerable to numerous infections.

Acute chest syndrome A vasoocclusive crisis that can be confused with pneumonia; common signs and symptoms include chest pain, fever, and cough.

Acute coronary syndrome (ACS) A group of symptoms caused by myocardial ischemia that includes angina and myocardial infarction.

Acute myocardial infarction (AMI) Heart attack; death of heart muscle following obstruction of blood flow to it. Acute in this context means "new" or "happening right now."

Acute renal failure (ARF) A sudden decrease in filtration through the glomeruli of the kidneys.

Addiction A state of overwhelming obsession or physical need to continue the use of a drug or agent.

Adolescents Persons who are 12 to 18 years of age.

Adrenergic Pertaining to nerves that release the neurotransmitter norepinephrine or noradrenaline; also pertains to the receptors acted on by norepinephrine.

Advance directive Written documentation that specifies medical treatment for a competent patient should the patient become unable to make decisions; also called a living will.

Advanced EMT (AEMT) An individual who has training in specific aspects of advanced life support, such as intravenous therapy, and the administration of certain emergency medications.

Adventitious breath sounds Abnormal breath sounds such as wheezes, rhonchi, rales, stridor, and pleural friction rubs.

Aerobic metabolism Metabolism that can proceed only in the presence of oxygen.

Afterload The pressure in the aorta against which the left ventricle must pump blood.

Agitated delirium A condition of disorientation, confusion, and possible hallucinations coupled with purposeless restless physical activity.

Agonal gasps Occasional, slow gasps that are ineffective attempts at breathing, occurring after the heart has stopped; sometimes seen in dying patients.

Agonists Substances that mimic the actions of a specific neurotransmitter or hormone by binding to the specific receptor of the naturally occurring substance.

Airborne transmission The spread of an organism in aerosol form.

Alcoholic ketoacidosis The metabolic acidotic state that manifests from the poor nutritional habits associated with chronic alcohol abuse. The liver and the body experience inadequate fuel reserves of glycogen and thus have to switch to fatty acid metabolism.

Alkalosis A pathologic condition resulting from the accumulation of bases in the body.

Allergen A substance that causes an allergic reaction; also referred to as an antigen.

Allergic reaction The body's exaggerated immune response to an internal or surface antigen.

Alpha radiation Type of energy that is emitted from a strong radiologic source; it is the least harmful penetrating type of radiation and cannot travel fast or through most objects.

Alveolar ventilation The volume of air that reaches the alveoli. It is determined by subtracting the amount of dead space air from the tidal volume.

Ampules Small glass containers that are sealed and the contents sterilized.

Anaerobic metabolism Metabolism that takes place in the absence of oxygen; its principal product is lactic acid.

Analgesics A classification for medications that relieve pain, or induce analgesia.

Anaphylactic shock Severe shock caused by an allergic reaction.

Anaphylaxis An extreme, possibly life-threatening systemic allergic reaction that may include shock and respiratory failure. Also known as a hypersensitivity reaction.

Aneurysm A swelling or enlargement of a part of an artery, resulting from weakening of the arterial wall.

Angina pectoris Transient (short-lived) chest discomfort caused by partial or temporary blockage of blood flow to the heart muscle.

Angiotensin-converting enzyme (ACE) inhibitors Medications that suppress the conversion of angiotensin I to angiotensin II.

Antagonists Molecules that block the ability of a given chemical to bind to its receptor, preventing a biologic response; in the pharmacologic sense, drugs that counteract the action of something else.

Anthrax A deadly bacterium (*Bacillus anthracis*) that lays dormant in a spore (protective shell); the germ is released from the spore when exposed to the optimal temperature and moisture. The route of entry into the body may be inhalation, cutaneous, or gastrointestinal (from consuming food that contains spores).

Antiarrhythmic medications The medications used to treat and prevent cardiac rhythm disorders.

Anticholinergic Of or pertaining to blockage of acetylcholine receptors, resulting in inhibition of transmission of parasympathetic nerve impulses.

Anticoagulant drugs The medications used to prevent intravascular thrombosis by preventing blood coagulation in the vascular system.

Anticonvulsant medications The medications used to treat seizures; believed to work by inhibiting the influx of sodium into cells.

Antihypertensives Medications used to control blood pressure.

Antiplatelet agents The medications that interfere with the collection of platelets.

Anuria A complete stop in urine production.

Anxious-avoidant attachment A bond between an infant and his or her parent or caregiver in which the infant is repeatedly rejected and develops an isolated lifestyle that does not depend on the support and care of others.

Aorta The main artery that receives blood from the left ventricle and delivers it to all the other arteries that carry blood to the tissues of the body.

Aortic aneurysm A weakness in the wall of the aorta that makes it susceptible to rupture.

Aortic arch One of three described portions of the aorta; the section of the aorta between the ascending and descending portions that gives rise to the right brachiocephalic (innominate), left common carotid, and left subclavian arteries.

Aortic valve The one-way semilunar valve that regulars blood flow from the left ventricle to the aorta.

Aphasia The inability to understand or produce speech.

Aplastic crisis A condition in which the body stops producing red blood cells; typically caused by infection.

Apnea Absence of breathing; periods of not breathing.

Applied ethics The manner in which principles of ethics are incorporated into professional conduct.

Arrhythmia An irregular or abnormal heart rhythm; also, absence of heart rhythm.

Arterial air embolism Air bubbles in the arterial blood vessels.

Arterial rupture The rupture of an artery. Involvement of a cerebral artery may contribute to interruption of cerebral blood flow.

Arteries The blood vessels that carry blood away from the heart.

Arterioles The smallest branches of arteries leading to the vast network of capillaries.

Arteriosclerosis A disease that is characterized by hardening, thickening, and calcification of the arterial walls.

Ascending aorta The first of three portions of the aorta; originates from the left ventricle and gives rise to two branches, the right and left main coronary arteries.

Aseptic technique A method of cleansing used to prevent contamination of a site when performing an invasive procedure, such as inserting an IV line.

Asthma A disease of the lungs in which muscle spasm in the small air passageways and the production of large amounts of mucus result in airway obstruction.

Asystole Complete absence of heart electrical activity.

Ataxic respirations Irregular, ineffective respirations that may or may not have an identifiable pattern.

Atelectasis Collapse of the alveoli; prevents the use of that portion of the lung for ventilation and oxygenation.

Atherosclerosis A disorder in which cholesterol and calcium build up inside the walls of blood vessels, forming plaque, which eventually leads to partial or complete blockage of blood flow; a plaque can become a site where blood clots can form, detach, and travel elsewhere in the circulatory system (embolize).

Atrioventricular (AV) node The site located in the right atrium adjacent to the septum that is responsible for transiently slowing electrical conduction.

Atrioventricular valves The two valves through which blood flows from the atria to the ventricles.

Atrium One of two (right and left) upper chambers of the heart.

Aura Sensations experienced before an attack occurs; common in seizures and migraine headaches.

Autism A pervasive developmental disorder characterized by impairment of social interaction.

Automaticity The ability of cardiac cells to generate an impulse to contract even when there is no external nervous stimulus.

Autonomic nervous system (ANS) The part of the nervous system that regulates functions that are not controlled consciously, such as digestion and sweating.

Axon A projection from a neuron that makes connections with adjacent cells.

Bacteria Microorganisms that reproduce by binary fission. These single-cell creatures reproduce rapidly. Some can form spores (encysted variants) when environmental conditions are harsh.

Bacterial vaginosis An overgrowth of bacteria in the vagina, characterized by itching, burning, or pain, and possibly a "fishy" foul-smelling discharge.

Barbiturates Potent sedative-hypnotics historically used as sleep aids, antianxiety drugs, and as part of the regimen for seizure control.

Baroreceptors Receptors in the blood vessels, kidneys, brain, and heart that respond to changes in pressure in the heart or main arteries to help maintain blood pressure and homeostasis.

Basilar skull fracture A fracture that typically occurs following diffuse impact to the head (such as in a fall or motor vehicle crash); it generally results from extension of a linear fracture to the base of the skull and can be difficult to diagnose with a radiograph (X-ray).

Behavioral crisis The point at which a person's reactions to events interfere with activities of daily living; the crisis becomes a psychiatric emergency when it causes a major life interruption, such as attempted suicide.

Benzodiazepines Sedative-hypnotic drugs that provide muscle relaxation and mild sedation; includes drugs such as diazepam (Valium) and midazolam (Versed).

Beta blocker A common class of cardiac drugs that blocks beta effects, causing a decrease in the workload of the heart by reducing the speed of contraction and reducing blood pressure.

Beta radiation Type of energy that is emitted from a strong radiologic source; it is slightly more penetrating than alpha radiation and requires a layer of clothing to stop it.

Bilateral A body part or condition that appears on both sides of the midline.

Biotransformation A chemical alteration that a substance undergoes in the body.

Bloodborne pathogens Pathogenic microorganisms that are present in human blood and can cause disease in humans. These pathogens include, but are not limited to, hepatitis B virus and human immunodeficiency virus.

Blowout fracture A fracture of the orbit or of the bones that support the floor of the orbit.

Bolus A term used to describe "in one mass"; in medication administration, a single dose given by the IV route; may be a small or large quantity of a drug.

Bonding The formation of a close, personal relationship.

Botulinum A very potent neurotoxin produced by bacteria. When introduced into the body, it affects the nervous system's ability to function and causes botulism.

Bradypnea A slow respiratory rate.

Bronchial breath sounds Normal breath sounds made by air moving through the bronchi.

Bronchiolitis Inflammation of the bronchioles that usually occurs in children younger than 2 years and is often caused by the respiratory syncytial virus.

Buboes Enlarged lymph nodes (up to the size of a tennis ball) that are characteristic of people infected with the bubonic plague.

Bubonic plague An infection transmitted by infected fleas that is characterized by acute malaise, fever, and the formation of tender, enlarged, inflamed lymph nodes that appear as lesions, called buboes.

Buccal Relating to the cheek or mouth.

Capillaries The tiny blood vessels between the arterioles and venules that permit transfer of oxygen, carbon dioxide, nutrients, and waste between body tissues and the blood.

Carbon dioxide retention A condition characterized by a chronically high level of carbon dioxide in blood as the result of a respiratory disease.

Cardiac glycosides A classification of medications that naturally occur in plant substances and that block certain ionic pumps in the membranes of heart cells, which indirectly increases calcium concentrations; an example is digoxin.

Cardiac output (CO) The amount of blood pumped through the circulatory system in 1 minute.

Cardiac tamponade (pericardial tamponade) Compression of the heart as a result of buildup of blood or other fluid in the pericardial sac, leading to decreased cardiac output.

Cardiogenic shock Shock caused by inadequate function of the heart, or pump failure.

Caustics Chemicals that are acids or alkalis; cause direct chemical injury to the tissues they contact.

Centers for Disease Control and Prevention (CDC) The primary federal agency that conducts and supports public health activities in the United States. The CDC is part of the US Department of Health and Human Services.

Central nervous system (CNS) depression The slowing of the nervous system function of the brain because of delays in nerve cell transmission. Several factors can influence CNS depression including nerve cell permeability, hypoxia, drugs, and injury.

Central venous catheter An intravenous access device used in many types of home care patients, including those receiving chemotherapy, long-term antibiotic or pain management, high-concentration glucose solutions, and hemodialysis.

Cerebral embolism Obstruction of a cerebral artery caused by a clot that was formed elsewhere in the body and traveled to the brain.

Cerebral palsy A group of disorders characterized by poorly controlled body movement.

Cerebral vasodilation Relaxation of cerebral blood vessels that can lead to pooling of blood and inadequate circulation.

Cerebrovascular accident (CVA) An interruption of blood flow to the brain that results in the loss of brain function; also referred to as a stroke or brain attack.

Certification A process in which a person, an institution, or a program is evaluated and recognized as meeting certain predetermined standards to provide safe and ethical care.

Chemical mediators Chemicals that work to cause the immune or allergic response, for example, histamines.

Chemoreceptors Receptors in the blood vessels, kidneys, brain, and heart that respond to changes in chemical composition of the blood to help maintain homeostasis.

Chlamydia A sexually transmitted disease caused by the bacterium *Chlamydia trachomatis*.

Chlorine (CL) The first chemical agent ever used in warfare. It has a distinct odor of bleach, creates a green haze when released as a gas, and initially produces upper airway irritation and a choking sensation.

Cholinergic Fibers in the parasympathetic nervous system that release a chemical called acetylcholine.

Chronic bronchitis Irritation and inflammation of the major lung passageways from either infectious disease or irritants such as smoke.

Chronic obstructive pulmonary disease (COPD) A progressive and irreversible disease of the airway that causes destructive changes in the alveoli and bronchioles in the lungs, resulting in decreased inspiratory and expiratory capacity.

Chronic renal failure (CRF) Progressive and irreversible inadequate kidney function as a result of permanent loss of nephrons.

Chronotropic Affecting the rate of contraction of the heart.

Chronotropic effects Affecting the heart's rate of contraction.

Circumflex coronary artery The two branches of the left main coronary artery.

Civil tort A wrongful act that gives rise to a civil suit.

Clonic phase Seizure movement marked by repetitive muscle contractions and relaxations in rapid succession.

Closed-ended questions Questions that can be answered in short or single-word responses.

Clotting factors Substances in the blood that are necessary for clotting; also called coagulation factors.

Cobra perilaryngeal airway (CobraPLA) A supraglottic airway device with a shape that allows the device to slide easily along the hard palate and to hold the soft tissue away from the laryngeal inlet.

Colostomy A surgical procedure that establishes an opening between the colon and the surface of the body.

Combining form A form created when a root word is combined with a vowel, usually an *o*, but sometimes an *i*.

Combitube A dual-lumen airway device that is inserted blindly; permits ventilation of the patient whether the tube is placed in the esophagus or the trachea.

Common cold A viral infection usually associated with swollen nasal mucous membranes and the production of fluid from the sinuses.

Commotio cordis A blunt chest injury caused by a sudden, direct blow to the chest that occurs during the critical portion of a person's heartbeat.

Communicable disease Any disease that can be spread from person to person or from animal to person.

Complex partial seizures The seizures that involve subtle changes in the level of consciousness that may include confusion, less alertness, hallucinations, and inability to speak.

Concentration The total weight of a drug contained in a specific volume of liquid.

Congestive heart failure (CHF) A disorder in which the heart loses part of its ability to effectively pump blood, usually as a result of damage to the heart muscle and usually resulting in a backup of fluid into the lungs.

Conjunctivitis Inflammation of the conjunctiva.

Consent Permission to render care.

Contamination The presence of infective organisms or foreign bodies on or in objects such as dressings, water, food, needles, wounds, or a patient's body; the spread of a disease-causing agent through direct contact or exposure to a weapon of mass destruction.

Continuous positive airway pressure (CPAP) A method of ventilation used primarily in the treatment of critically ill patients with respiratory distress; can prevent the need for endotracheal intubation.

Contractility The strength of heart muscle contraction.

Contusion A bruise from an injury that causes bleeding beneath the skin without breaking the skin.

Conventional reasoning A type of reasoning in which a child looks for approval from peers and society.

Coronary arteries Arteries that arise from the aorta shortly after it leaves the left ventricle and supply the heart with oxygen and nutrients.

Coronary artery disease The condition that results when atherosclerosis or arteriosclerosis is present in the arterial walls.

Coup-contrecoup brain injury A brain injury that occurs when force is applied to the head and energy transmission through brain tissue causes injury on the opposite side of original impact.

Cross-contamination The spread of a disease-causing agent as a result of coming into contact with another contaminated person.

Cross-tolerance A tolerance to a particular drug that crosses over to other drugs in the same class.

Croup An infectious disease of the upper respiratory system that may cause partial airway obstruction and is characterized by a barking cough; usually seen in children; also called laryngotracheobronchitis.

Cultural imposition A situation in which one person imposes his or her beliefs, values, and practices on another person because the first person believes his or her ideals are superior.

Cumulative effect Action of increased intensity after administration of several doses of a drug.

Cyanide An agent that affects the body's ability to use oxygen; a colorless gas that has an odor similar to almonds. The effects of cyanide poisoning begin on the cellular level and are seen very rapidly at the organ system level.

Cystic fibrosis (CF) A genetic disorder of the endocrine system that makes it difficult for chloride to move through cells; primarily targets the respiratory and digestive systems.

Danger zone (hot zone) An area where people can be exposed to sharp metal edges, broken glass, toxic substances, lethal rays, or ignition or explosion of hazardous materials.

Decerebrate posturing A body position in which the patient extends the arms outward and rotates the lower arms in a palms-down manner, and points the toes; indicates severe brain dysfunction from pressure on the brainstem.

Decorticate posturing A body position in which the patient flexes the arms and curls them toward the chest, flexes the wrists, and points his or her toes; indicates severe brain dysfunction from pressure on the brainstem.

Decubitis ulcers Sores caused by the pressure of skin against a surface for long periods; they can range from a pink discoloration of the skin to a deep wound that may invade into bone or organs. Also known as bedsores.

Delirium A more or less sudden change in mental status marked by the inability to focus, think logically, and maintain attention.

Dementia The slow onset of progressive disorientation, shortened attention span, and loss of cognitive function.

Dependent edema Swelling in the part of the body closest to the ground or the most dependent portion, caused by collection of fluid in the tissues (typically in the sacral area in a bedridden patient); a possible sign of congestive heart failure.

Depressants Agents used to slow brain activity.

Depressed skull fracture A fracture that results from high-energy direct trauma to the head with a blunt object; patients present with neurologic signs (such as loss of consciousness).

Descending aorta One of the three portions of the aorta, it is the longest portion and extends through the thorax and abdomen into the pelvis.

Designated officer The person in the department who is charged with the responsibility of managing exposures and infection control issues.

Developmental disability Insufficient development of the brain, resulting in some level of dysfunction or impairment.

Diabetic ketoacidosis (DKA) A form of hyperglycemia in uncontrolled diabetes in which certain acids accumulate when insulin is not available.

Diastole The relaxation phase of the heart, when the ventricles are filling with blood.

Diffusion The movement of solutes (molecules) from an area of higher concentration to an area of lower concentration.

Diphtheria An infectious disease in which a membrane lining the pharynx is formed that can severely obstruct passage of air into the larynx.

Direct contact Exposure to or transmission of a communicable disease from one person to another by physical contact.

Dirty bomb Nickname for a bomb that is used as a radiologic dispersal device.

Dislocation Disruption of a joint in which ligaments are damaged and the bone ends become completely displaced.

Dissecting aneurysm A condition in which the inner layers of an artery such as the aorta become separated, allowing blood (at high pressures) to flow between the layers.

Dissemination The means that a terrorist uses to spread a disease—for example, poisoning of the water supply or aerosolizing the agent into the air or ventilation system of a building.

Dissociate To lose a hydrogen atom in the presence of water. Acids are classified as strong or weak, depending on how completely they dissociate in water.

Distributive shock A condition that occurs when there is widespread dilation of the small arterioles, small venules, or both.

Diuretic medications Medications designed to promote elimination of excess salt and water by the kidneys.

Dorsal respiratory group (DRG) A portion of the medulla oblongata where the primary respiratory pacemaker is found.

Down syndrome A genetic chromosomal defect that occurs during fetal development and that results in mental retardation as well as certain physical characteristics, such as a round head with a flat occiput and slanted, wide-set eyes.

Drip rate Number of drops per minute.

Dromotropic Affecting the velocity of conduction in the heart.

Dromotropic effects Affecting the heart's velocity of conduction.

Drug antagonism A decrease in the action of a drug by the administration of another drug.

Drug dependence A psychological and sometimes physical state resulting from continued use of a substance, characterized by a compulsion to take the drug on a continuous or periodic basis to experience its effects or to avoid the discomfort of its absence.

Drug interaction A situation in which the effects of one medication alter the response of another medication.

Drug reconstitution Injecting sterile water (or saline) from one vial into another vial containing a powdered form of a drug.

Drugs Chemical agents used in the diagnosis, treatment, and prevention of disease.

DuoDote Auto-Injector A nerve agent kit containing atropine and 2-PAM chloride (pralidoxime chloride); delivered as a single dose through one needle.

Duration of action The amount of time a medication concentration can be expected to remain above the minimum level needed to provide the intended action.

Dysarthria The inability to pronounce speech clearly, often due to loss of the nerves or brain cells that control the small muscles in the larynx.

Dyspnea Shortness of breath or difficulty breathing.

Dysrhythmia An irregular or abnormal heart rhythm.

Early adults Persons who are 19 to 40 years of age.

Ecchymosis Bruising or discoloration associated with bleeding within or under the skin.

Eclampsia Seizures (convulsions) resulting from severe hypertension in a pregnant woman.

Ectopic pregnancy A pregnancy that develops outside the uterus, typically in a fallopian tube.

Edema The presence of abnormally large amounts of fluid between cells in body tissues; causing swelling of the affected area.

Ejection fraction The portion of the blood ejected from the left ventricle during systole.

Emancipated minor A person who is under the legal age in a given state but, because of other circumstances, is legally considered an adult.

Emergency medical responder (EMR) The first trained individual, such as a police officer, firefighter, lifeguard, or other rescuer, to arrive at the scene of an emergency to provide initial medical assistance.

Emergency medical technician (EMT) An individual who has training in basic life support, including automated external defibrillation, use of a definitive airway adjunct, and assisting patients with certain medications.

Emphysema A disease of the lungs in which there is extreme dilation and eventual destruction of pulmonary alveoli with poor exchange of oxygen and carbon dioxide; it is one form of chronic obstructive pulmonary disease.

Endocrine gland Any of the glands that secrete or release hormones—that is, chemicals that are used inside the body.

Endocrine system The body system that regulates metabolism and maintains homeostasis.

Enteral medications Medications that are given through a portion of the gastrointestinal tract.

Epidural hematoma An accumulation of blood between the skull and the dura mater.

Epiglottitis An acute bacterial infection that results in rapid swelling of the epiglottis and surrounding tissues, and that may cause upper airway obstruction; also called acute supraglottic laryngitis.

Esophageal varices A condition in which the amount of pressure within the blood vessels surrounding the esophagus increases, eventually causing the capillary network of the esophagus to leak, which in turn leads to severe hematemesis.

Esophagitis Inflammation of the lining of the esophagus.

Ethics The philosophy of right and wrong, of moral duties, and of ideal professional behavior.

Ethnocentrism A situation in which a person considers his or her own cultural values to be more important when interacting with people of a different culture.

Eviscerate To displace organs outside the body.

Exposure A situation in which a person has had contact with blood, body fluids, tissues, or airborne particles that increases the risk of disease transmission.

Expressed consent A type of consent in which a patient gives specific and direct authorization for provision of care or transport.

External jugular IVs IV access established in the jugular veins of the neck.

External respiration The exchange of gases between the lungs and the blood cells in the pulmonary capillaries; also called pulmonary respiration.

Extrapyramidal symptoms A wide array of symptoms such as involuntary movements, tremors, rigidity, muscle contractions, restlessness, and changes in breathing and heart rate; usually as a result of taking antipsychotic drugs.

False imprisonment The unauthorized confinement of a person that lasts for an appreciable period of time.

Febrile seizures The seizures that result from sudden high fever, particularly in children.

Fibrin A white insoluble protein formed in the clotting process; forms the fibrous component of a blood clot.

Fibrinolytic agent A medication that dissolves blood clots after they have already formed; promotes the digestion of fibrin.

Fick principle States that the movement and use of oxygen in the body are dependent on adequate concentration of inspired oxygen (FIO_2; fraction of inspired oxygen), appropriate movement of oxygen across the alveolar–capillary membrane into the arterial bloodstream, adequate number of red blood cells to carry the oxygen, proper tissue perfusion, and efficient off-loading of oxygen at the tissue level.

Fontanelles Areas in the head where the infant's skull has not fused together; they usually disappear by approximately 18 months of age.

Foodborne transmission The contamination of food or water with an organism that can cause disease.

Forcible restraint The act of physically preventing a person from taking physical action.

Fracture A break in the continuity of a bone.

Functional disorder A disorder in which there is no known physiologic reason for the abnormal functioning of an organ or organ system.

G agents Early nerve agents that were developed by German scientists in the period between World War I and World War II. There are three G agents: sarin, soman, and tabun.

Gamma-hydroxybutyrate (GHB) A sedative and central nervous system depressant.

Gamma (X-ray) radiation Type of energy that is emitted from a strong radiologic source that is far faster and stronger than alpha and beta rays. Gamma rays easily penetrate through the human body and require either several inches of lead or concrete to prevent penetration.

Gastroenteritis A family of conditions resulting from diarrhea, nausea, and vomiting; some have infectious causes.

Gastrostomy tube A tube that is placed directly through the skin into the stomach to provide nutrition for patients who cannot ingest fluids, food, or medication by mouth. Also referred to as a gastric tube or G-tube.

General impression The overall initial impression that determines the priority for patient care; based on the patient's surroundings, the mechanism of injury, signs and symptoms, and the chief complaint.

Golden Period The time from injury to definitive care, during which treatment of shock or traumatic injuries should occur because survival potential is best when care is delivered in this time span.

Gonorrhea A sexually transmitted disease caused by the bacterium *Neisseria gonorrhoeae*.

Guarding Involuntary muscle contractions (spasms) of the abdominal wall in an effort to protect an inflamed or injured abdomen; may be a sign of peritonitis.

Habituation The situation in which there is a physical tolerance and psychological dependence on a drug or drugs.

Half-life The time required by the body, tissue, or organ to metabolize or inactivate half the amount of a substance taken in—an important consideration in determining the proper dose of drug and frequency of administration.

Hazardous materials (HazMat) Any substance that is toxic, poisonous, radioactive, flammable, or explosive and causes injury or death with exposure.

Heart A muscular organ that pumps blood throughout the body.

Hematology The study and prevention of blood-related disorders.

Hematoma A mass of blood in the soft tissues beneath the skin.

Hematopoietic system The system that includes all blood components and the organs involved in their development and production.

Hematuria The presence of blood in the urine.

Hemiparesis Weakness on one side of the body.

Hemoglobin An iron-containing protein within red blood cells that has the ability to combine with and carry oxygen.

Hemolytic crisis A rapid destruction of red blood cells that occurs faster than the body's ability to create new cells.

Hemophilia A congenital abnormality in which the body's ability to clot is impaired, resulting in uncontrollable bleeding.

Hemopneumothorax The accumulation of blood and air in the pleural space of the chest.

Hemorrhagic stroke One of the two main types of stroke; occurs as a result of bleeding inside the brain.

Hemostasis The body's natural blood-clotting mechanism.

Hemothorax A collection of blood in the pleural cavity.

Hepatitis Inflammation of the liver, usually caused by a virus, that causes fever, loss of appetite, jaundice, fatigue, and altered liver function.

Hering-Breuer reflex A protective mechanism that terminates inhalation, thus preventing overexpansion of the lungs.

Herpes simplex Virus caused by human herpes viruses 1 and 2, characterized by small blisters whose location depends on the type of virus. Type 2 results in blisters on the genital area, while type 1 results in blisters in nongenital areas.

Hilus When used in the context of the kidneys, a cleft where the ureters, renal blood vessels, lymphatic vessels, and nerves enter and leave the kidney.

History taking A step within the patient assessment process that provides detail about the patient's chief complaint and an account of the patient's signs and symptoms.

Hollow organs Structures through which materials pass, such as the stomach, small intestines, large intestines, ureters, and bladder.

Homeostasis A tendency to constancy or stability in the body's internal environment.

Host The organism or person attacked by the infecting agent.

Human immunodeficiency virus (HIV) The virus that causes acquired immunodeficiency syndrome (AIDS), which infects the cells in the body's immune system rendering them unable to fight certain types of infection.

Hydrocarbons Compounds made up principally of hydrogen and carbon atom mostly obtained from the distillation of petroleum.

Hypercarbia Increased carbon dioxide level in the bloodstream.

Hyperglycemic crisis Acute and potentially life-threatening complication of diabetes resulting from a combination of problems.

Hyperosmolar hyperglycemic nonketotic coma (HHNC) A metabolic derangement characterized by hyperglycemia, hyperosmolality, dehydration, and an absence of significant ketosis; occurs principally in patients with type 2 diabetes; also called hyperosmolar nonketotic coma (HONK) or HONK/HHNC.

Hyperosmolar hyperglycemic state (HHS) A metabolic derangement that occurs principally in patients with type 2 diabetes; it is characterized by hyperglycemia, hyperosmolarity, and an absence of significant ketosis. HHS was previously called hyperosmolar hyperglycemia nonketotic coma (HHNC). The term was changed because coma occurs in fewer than 20% of patients with HHS.

Hyperosmolar nonketotic coma (HONK) Condition characterized by severe hyperglycemia, hyperosmolality, and dehydration but no ketoacidosis; also called hyperosmolar hyperglycemic nonketotic coma (HHNC) or HONK/HHNC.

Hypersensitivity Abnormal sensitivity; a condition in which there is an exaggerated response by the body to the stimulus of a foreign agent.

Hyperventilation Rapid or deep breathing.

Hypoglycemia A condition characterized by a low blood glucose level.

Hypoglycemic crisis Severe hypoglycemia resulting in changes in mental status.

Hypoperfusion A condition that develops when the circulatory system is not able to deliver sufficient blood and oxygen to body organs, resulting in organ failure and eventual death if untreated.

Hypothermia A condition in which the internal body temperature falls below 95°F (35°C), usually as a result of prolonged exposure to cool or freezing temperatures.

Hypovolemic shock Shock caused by fluid or blood loss.

Hypoxemia A deficiency of oxygen in arterial blood.

Hypoxia A dangerous condition in which the body's cells do not have enough oxygen.

Hypoxic drive A backup system to control respirations when the oxygen level falls. A condition in which chronically low levels of oxygen in the blood stimulate the respiratory drive; it is seen in patients with chronic lung diseases.

Iatrogenic response An adverse condition induced in a patient by the treatment given.

Idiosyncrasy An abnormal sensitivity or reaction to a drug or other substance peculiar to a specific individual.

Idiosyncratic reaction A peculiar or individual response to a drug or medication through unusual susceptibility.

Ileostomy A surgical procedure that creates an opening between the small intestine and the surface of the body.

Immune system The system that protects the body from foreign substances.

Immunity The body's ability to protect itself from acquiring a disease.

Immunosuppressant medications The medications intended to inhibit the body's ability to attack the "foreign" organ or, in the case of autoimmune diseases, the medications that inhibit the body's attack on itself.

Impedance threshold device (ITD) A valve device that is placed between an endotracheal tube and a bag-mask device to limit the amount of air entering the lungs during the recoil phase between chest compressions.

Implied consent A type of consent in which a patient who is unable to give consent is given treatment under the legal assumption that he or she would want treatment.

Incontinence Loss of bowel and bladder control; can be the result of a generalized seizure and other conditions.

Incubation The period of time from when a person is exposed to a disease to when symptoms begin.

Indirect contact Exposure or transmission of disease from one person to another by contact with a contaminated object.

Infants Persons who are from 1 month to 1 year of age.

Infarcted cells The cells that die as a result of loss of blood flow.

Infection The invasion of a host or host tissues by organisms such as bacteria, viruses, or parasites, with or without signs or symptoms of disease.

Infection control Procedures to reduce transmission of infection among patients and health care personnel.

Infectious disease A disease caused by infection or one that is capable of being transmitted with or without direct contact.

Inferior vena cava One of the two largest veins in the body; carries blood from the lower extremities and the pelvic and the abdominal organs to the heart.

Influenza type A A virus that has crossed the animal/human barrier and has infected humans, recently reaching a pandemic level with the H1N1 strain.

Inhalation The active, muscular part of breathing that draws air into the airway and lungs.

Inotropic Affecting the contractility of the heart muscle.

Inotropic effects Affecting the contractility of the heart muscle.

Interference A direct biochemical interaction between two drugs.

Internal cardiac pacemaker A device implanted under the patient's skin to regulate the heart rate in patients with underlying conductive heart conditions.

Internal respiration The exchange of gases between the blood cells and the tissues.

Intracerebral hematoma Bleeding within the brain tissue (parenchyma) itself; also referred to as an intraparenchymal hematoma.

Intracranial pressure (ICP) The pressure within the cranial vault.

Intramuscular (IM) Injection into a muscle; a medication delivery route.

Intranasal A delivery route in which a medication is pushed through a specialized atomizer device called a mucosal atomizer device into a nostril.

Intraosseous (IO) lines A method of delivering fluids or medications into the medullary canal of the bone; used when IV access cannot be quickly obtained.

Intrapulmonary shunting Bypassing of oxygen-poor blood past nonfunctional alveoli to the left side of the heart.

Intravenous (IV) Into a vein; a medication delivery route.

Ionizing radiation Energy that is emitted in the form of rays or particles.

Ischemia A lack of oxygen that deprives tissues of necessary nutrients, resulting from partial or complete blockage of blood flow; potentially reversible because permanent injury has not yet occurred.

Ischemic cells The cells that receive enough blood after an event, such as a cerebrovascular accident, to stay alive but not enough to function properly.

Ischemic stroke One of the two main types of stroke; occurs when blood flow to a particular part of the brain is cut off by a blockage (for example, a clot) inside a blood vessel.

Kehr sign Left shoulder pain caused by blood in the peritoneal cavity.

Ketoacidosis An acidotic state created by the production of ketones via fat metabolism.

Ketones The by-products of fat metabolism when fatty acids are used, rather than glucose, by body cells. An excess can lead to ketoacidosis.

Kidnapping The seizing, confining, abducting, or carrying away of a person by force.

Kidney stones Solid crystalline masses formed in the kidney, resulting from an excess of insoluble salts or uric acid crystallizing in the urine; may become trapped anywhere along the urinary tract.

Kidneys Two retroperitoneal organs that excrete the end products of metabolism as urine and regulate the body's salt and water content.

Kinetic energy The energy of a moving object.

King LT airway A single-lumen airway that is blindly inserted into the esophagus; when properly placed in the esophagus, one cuff seals the esophagus and the other seals the oropharynx.

Kyphosis A forward curling of the back caused by an abnormal increase in the curvature of the spine.

Labored breathing Breathing that requires visibly increased effort; characterized by grunting, stridor, and use of accessory muscles.

Lactic acidosis The metabolic acidotic state resulting from the accumulation of lactic acid during anaerobic cellular metabolism.

Laryngeal mask airway (LMA) An airway device that is inserted into the mouth blindly and comes to rest at the glottic opening. A flexible cuff is inflated, creating an almost airtight seal.

Laryngospasm A severe constriction of the larynx and vocal cords.

Late adults Persons who are 61 years of age or older.

Left anterior descending (LAD) artery One of the two branches of the left main coronary artery that is the largest and shortest of the myocardial blood vessels; this vessel and the circumflex coronary arteries supply blood to the left ventricle and other areas.

Left ventricular assist device A piece of medical equipment that takes over the function of either one or both heart ventricles.

Lewisite (L) A blistering agent that has a rapid onset of symptoms and produces immediate intense pain and discomfort on contact.

Licensure The process by which a competent authority, usually the state, grants permission to practice a job, trade, or profession.

Life expectancy The typical number of years a person can be expected to live.

Linear skull fracture A type of fracture that accounts for 80% of skull fractures; also referred to as a nondisplaced skull fracture. These fractures commonly occur in the temporal-parietal region of the skull and are not associated with deformities to the skull.

Lithium The cornerstone drug for the treatment of bipolar disorder.

Load-distributing band (LDB) A circumferential chest compression device that consists of a constricting band and backboard; it is either electrically or pneumatically driven to compress the heart by putting inward pressure on the thorax.

Macrophages Cells that provide the body's first line of defense in the inflammatory process.

Mallory-Weiss syndrome A condition in which the junction between the esophagus and the stomach tears as a result of prolonged forceful vomiting or retching, causing severe bleeding and, potentially, death.

Mean arterial pressure (MAP) The average pressure against the arterial wall during a cardiac cycle; generally considered to be the same as blood pressure.

Mechanical piston device A device that depresses the sternum via a compressed gas-powered plunger mounted on a backboard.

Mechanism of action The way in which a medication produces the intended response.

Meconium staining The occurrence of a dark green material in the amniotic fluid that can cause lung disease in the newborn.

Mediastinum The space between the lungs that contains the heart, great vessels, trachea, mainstem bronchi, vagus nerve, and part of the esophagus.

Medication A chemical substance that is used to treat or prevent disease or relieve pain.

Meningitis Inflammation of the meninges that cover the spinal cord and the brain.

Meningococcal meningitis An inflammation of the meningeal coverings of the brain and spinal cord; can be highly contagious.

Metabolic acidosis A pathologic condition characterized by a blood pH of less than 7.35; caused by accumulation of acids in the body from a metabolic cause.

Metabolic alkalosis A pathologic condition characterized by a blood pH of greater than 7.45, and resulting from the accumulation of bases in the body from a metabolic cause.

Metabolism (cellular respiration) The biochemical processes that result in production of energy from nutrients within the cells.

Metered-dose inhaler (MDI) A miniature spray canister used to direct medications through the mouth and into the lungs.

Methicillin-resistant Staphylococcus aureus (MRSA) A bacterium that causes infections in different parts of the body and is often resistant to commonly used antibiotics. It can be found on the skin, in surgical wounds, and in the bloodstream, lungs, and urinary tract.

Metric system A decimal system based on tens for the measurement of length, weight, and volume.

Middle adults Persons who are 41 to 60 years of age.

Minute ventilation The volume of air moved through the lungs in 1 minute minus the dead space air; it is calculated by multiplying the tidal volume (minus the dead space air) and the respiratory rate. Also referred to as minute volume.

Monoamine oxidase inhibitors (MAOIs) Psychiatric medication used primarily to treat atypical depression by increasing norepinephrine and serotonin levels in the central nervous system.

Morality A code of conduct that can be defined by society, religion, or a person, affecting character, conduct, and conscience.

Moro reflex A reflex in which, when an infant is caught off guard, the infant opens his or her arms wide, spreads the fingers, and seems to grab at things.

Mucosal atomizer device A device that attaches to the end of a syringe used to spray (atomize) certain medications via the intranasal route.

Multilumen airways Airway devices with a single long tube that can be used for esophageal obturation or endotracheal tube ventilation, depending on where it comes to rest following blind positioning.

Multiple-organ dysfunction syndrome (MODS) A progressive condition usually characterized by combined failure of several organs, such as the lungs, liver, and kidney, along with some clotting mechanisms, which occurs after severe illness or injury.

Multisystem trauma Trauma that affects more than one body system.

Muscarinic cholinergic antagonists Medications that block acetylcholine exclusively at the muscarinic receptors; an example is atropine.

Myocardial contractility The ability of the heart muscle to contract.

Myocardial contusion A bruise of the heart muscle.

National EMS Scope of Practice Model A document created by the National Highway Traffic Safety Administration (NHTSA) that outlines the skills performed by various EMS providers.

National Incident Management System (NIMS) A Department of Homeland Security system designed to enable federal, state, and local governments and private-sector and nongovernmental organizations to effectively and efficiently prepare for, prevent, respond to, and recover from domestic incidents, regardless of cause, size, or complexity, including acts of catastrophic terrorism.

Nebulizer A device for producing a fine spray or mist that is used to deliver inhaled medications.

Neonates Persons who are between birth and 1 month of age.

Nephrons The basic filtering units in the kidneys. The structural and functional units of the kidney that form urine; composed of the glomerulus, the glomerular (Bowman) capsule, the proximal convoluted tubule, loop of Henle, and the distal convoluted tubule.

Nerve agents A class of chemicals called organophosphates; they function by blocking an essential enzyme in the nervous system, which causes the body's organs to become overstimulated and burn out.

Neurogenic shock Circulatory failure caused by paralysis of the nerves that control the size of the blood vessels, leading to widespread dilation; seen in patients with spinal cord injuries.

Neuropathy A group of conditions in which the nerves leaving the spinal cord are damaged, resulting in distortion of signals to or from the brain.

Neurotoxins Biologic agents that are the most deadly substances known to humans; they include botulinum toxin and ricin.

Neurotransmitters The chemicals produced by the body that stimulate electrical reactions in adjacent neurons.

Neutron radiation Type of energy that is emitted from a strong radiologic source; the fastest-moving and most powerful form of radiation. Neutrons easily penetrate through lead and require several feet of concrete to stop them.

Nonbarbiturate hypnotics Medications designed to sedate without the side effects of a barbiturate.

Nonopioid analgesics Medications designed to relieve pain without the side effects of opioids.

Nonsteroidal anti-inflammatory drugs (NSAIDs) Medications with analgesic, anti-inflammatory, and fever-reducing properties.

Obesity A condition in which a person has an excessive amount of body fat.

Obstructive shock Shock that occurs when there is a block to blood flow in the heart or great vessels, causing an insufficient blood supply to the body's tissues.

Occupational Safety and Health Administration (OSHA) The federal regulatory compliance agency that develops, publishes, and enforces guidelines concerning safety in the workplace.

Oliguria A decrease in urine output to the extent that total urine output drops to less than 750 mL/day.

Onset of action The time needed for the concentration of the medication at the target tissue to reach the minimum effective level.

Open-ended questions Questions for which the patient must provide detail to give an answer.

Open pneumothorax An open or penetrating chest wall wound through which air passes during inspiration and expiration, creating a sucking sound; also referred to as a sucking chest wound.

Opioid agonist-antagonists Medications designed to relieve pain without the side effects of opioids.

Opioid agonists Chemicals similar to or derived from the opium plant.

Opioid antagonists A classification of medications that reverse the effects of opioid drugs.

Organic brain syndrome A temporary or permanent dysfunction of the brain, caused by a disturbance in the physical or physiologic functioning of brain tissue.

Organophosphates A class of chemicals found in many insecticides used in agriculture and in the home.

Orthopnea Severe dyspnea experienced when lying down and relieved by sitting up.

Orthostatic vital signs Assessing vital signs in three different patient positions (for example, from a lying position, to a sitting position, then to a standing position) to determine the degree of hypovolemia; also called a tilt test.

Osteoporosis A generalized bone disease in which a reduction in the amount of bone mass leads to compression fractures after minimal trauma; this disease can occur in both men and women, although it is more prevalent in postmenopausal women.

Overdose An excessive quantity of a drug that, when taken or administered, can have toxic or lethal consequences.

Oxygenation The process of delivering oxygen to the blood by diffusion from the alveoli following inhalation into the lungs.

Oxygen saturation (SpO$_2$) The measure of the percentage of hemoglobin binding sites attached to oxygen in arterial blood.

Palmar grasp A reflex that occurs when something is placed in the infant's palm; the infant grasps the object.

Pancreatitis Inflammation of the pancreas.

Paradoxical motion The motion of the chest wall section that is detached in a flail chest; the motion is exactly the opposite of normal motion during breathing (that is, in during inhalation, out during exhalation).

Paramedic An individual who has extensive training in advanced life support, including endotracheal intubation, emergency pharmacology, cardiac monitoring, and other advanced assessment and treatment skills.

Parasympathetic nervous system A subdivision of the autonomic nervous system, involved in control of involuntary, vegetative functions, mediated largely by the vagus nerve through the chemical acetylcholine.

Parasympatholytics Drugs that block the actions of the parasympathetic nervous system; also known as anticholinergics.

Parasympathomimetics Drugs that produce the same effects as those of the parasympathetic nervous system; also known as cholinergics.

Parenteral medications Drug administration through any route other than through the gastrointestinal tract; includes IV, IO, subcutaneous, intramuscular, sublingual, buccal, transcutaneous, intranasal, and inhalation routes.

Partial seizures The seizures affecting a limited portion of the brain.

Pathogen A microorganism that is capable of causing disease in a susceptible host.

Pedal edema Swelling of the feet and ankles caused by collection of fluid in the tissues; a possible sign of congestive heart failure.

Pediatric assessment triangle (PAT) A structured assessment tool that allows the health care provider to rapidly form a general impression of an infant or child without touching him or her; it consists of assessing appearance, work of breathing, and circulation to the skin.

Pelvic inflammatory disease (PID) An infection of the fallopian tubes and the surrounding tissues of the pelvis.

Perfusion The circulation of oxygenated blood to target tissues and organs, and within an organ or tissue, in adequate amounts to meet the cells' current needs.

Peristalsis The wavelike contraction of smooth muscle by which the ureters or other tubular organs propel their contents.

Peritoneal cavity The abdominal cavity.

Peritonitis Inflammation of the peritoneum.

Personal protective equipment (PPE) Clothing or specialized equipment that provides protection to the wearer.

Pertussis (whooping cough) An airborne bacterial infection that causes fever and a "whoop" sound on inspiration after a coughing attack; affects mostly children younger than 6 years; highly contagious through droplet infection.

pH The measure of acidity or alkalinity of a solution.

Pharmacodynamics The study of drugs and their actions on living organisms.

Pharmacokinetics The study of the metabolism and action of drugs with a particular emphasis on the time required for absorption, duration of action, distribution in the body, and method of excretion.

Pharmacology The study of the properties (characteristics) and effects of drugs and medications on the body.

Pharyngeotracheal lumen airway (PtL) A dual-lumen airway device that is inserted blindly into the mouth. The patient can be ventilated whether the tube is placed in the esophagus or into the trachea.

Phosgene A pulmonary agent that is a product of combustion, and that might be generated in a fire at a textile factory or house, or from metalwork or burning Freon. This very potent agent has a delayed onset of symptoms, usually in the range of hours.

Phosgene oxime (CX) A blistering agent that has a rapid onset of symptoms and produces immediate intense pain and discomfort on contact.

Phrenic nerve The nerve that innervates the diaphragm; important for adequate breathing.

Placenta previa A condition in which the placenta develops over and covers the cervix.

Plasma A sticky, yellow fluid that carries the blood cells and nutrients and transports cellular waste material to the organs of excretion.

Platelets Small cells in the blood that are responsible for clot formation; also called thrombocytes.

Pneumonia An inflammation/infection of the lung from a bacterial, viral, or fungal cause.

Pneumonic plague A lung infection, also known as plague pneumonia, that results from inhalation of plague bacteria.

Pneumothorax A partial or complete accumulation of air in the pleural space.

Poison A substance whose chemical action could damage structures or impair function when introduced into the body.

Polypharmacy The use of many drugs by the same patient.

Positive end-expiratory pressure (PEEP) Mechanical maintenance of pressure in the airway at the end of expiration to increase the volume of gas remaining in the lungs.

Postconventional reasoning A type of reasoning in which a child bases decisions on his or her conscience.

Postictal state The period following a seizure that lasts between 5 and 30 minutes, characterized by labored respirations and some degree of altered mental status.

Potential energy The product of mass, gravity, and height, which is converted into kinetic energy and results in injury, such as from a fall.

Potentiation Enhancement of the effect of one drug by another drug.

Precedence The practice of basing current action on lessons, rules, or guidelines derived from previous similar experiences.

Preconventional reasoning A type of reasoning in which a child acts almost purely to avoid punishment and to get what he or she wants.

Preeclampsia A condition of late pregnancy that involves headache, visual changes, and swelling of the hands and feet; also called pregnancy-induced hypertension.

Prefix A word element that appears at the beginning of a word.

Preload The amount of blood returned to the heart to be pumped out; directly affects myocardial contractility.

Preschoolers Persons who are 3 to 6 years of age.

Primary assessment A step within the patient assessment process in which the health care provider identifies and initiates treatment of immediate or potential life threats.

Primary (direct) injury An injury to the brain and its associated structures that is a direct result of impact to the head.

Primary prevention Efforts to prevent an injury or illness from ever occurring.

Pronation The act of extending the arms outward and turning the palms downward.

Protected health information Any information about health status, provision of health care, or payment for health care that can be linked to an individual. This is interpreted rather broadly and includes any part of a patient's medical record or payment history.

Proxemics The study of space between people and its effects on communication.

Psychiatric disorder An illness with psychological or behavioral symptoms and/or impairment in functioning caused by a social, psychological, genetic, physical, chemical, or biologic disturbance.

Psychiatric emergency An emergency in which abnormal behavior threatens an individual's health and safety or the health and safety of another person—for example, when a person becomes suicidal, homicidal, or psychotic.

Psychogenic shock Shock caused by a sudden, temporary reduction in blood supply to the brain that causes fainting (syncope).

Psychosis A mental disorder characterized by the loss of contact with reality.

Public health A branch of health care focused on examining the health needs of entire populations with the goal of preventing health problems.

Pulmonary blast injury Pulmonary trauma resulting from short-range exposure to the detonation of explosives.

Pulmonary circulation The circulatory system in the body that carries blood from the right side of the heart to the lungs and back to the left side of the heart.

Pulmonary edema A buildup of fluid in the lungs, usually a result of congestive heart failure.

Pulmonary ventilation The process of moving air into and out of the lungs through inhalation and exhalation.

Pulmonic valve The semilunar valve that regulates blood flow between the lungs to the left atrium of the heart.

Pulse oximetry An assessment tool that measures oxygen saturation of hemoglobin in the capillary beds.

Pulse pressure The difference between the systolic and diastolic pressures.

Pyelonephritis Inflammation of the kidney and renal pelvis.

Radiologic dispersal device (RDD) Any container that is designed to disperse radioactive material.

Reassessment A step within the patient assessment process that is performed at regular intervals during the assessment process. Its purpose is to identify and treat changes in a patient's condition. An unstable patient should be reassessed every 5 minutes, whereas a stable patient should be reassessed every 15 minutes.

Rebound tenderness Pain that the patient feels when pressure is released as opposed to when pressure is applied; characteristic of appendicitis.

Red blood cells (RBCs) Cells that contain hemoglobin and carry oxygen to the body's tissues; also called erythrocytes.

Refractory A disease or condition that does not respond to treatment.

Renal dialysis A technique for filtering the blood of its toxic wastes, removing excess fluids, and restoring the normal balance of electrolytes.

Renal fascia Dense, fibrous connective tissue that anchors the kidney to the retroperitoneal flank.

Residual volume The air that remains in the lungs after maximal expiration.

Respiration The exchange of gases that occurs at both the pulmonary level and the cellular level. At the pulmonary level, oxygen in the alveoli is exchanged for carbon dioxide in the bloodstream, and the opposite occurs at the cellular level, when oxygen in the bloodstream is exchanged for carbon dioxide in the cells.

Respiratory acidosis A pathologic condition characterized by a blood pH of less than 7.35, caused by accumulation of acids in the body from a respiratory cause.

Respiratory alkalosis A pathologic condition characterized by a blood pH of greater than 7.45 and resulting from the accumulation of bases in the body from a respiratory cause.

Respiratory syncytial virus (RSV) A virus that causes an infection of the lungs and breathing passages; can lead to other serious illnesses that affect the lungs or heart such as bronchiolitis and pneumonia; highly contagious and spread through droplets.

Retractions Movements in which the skin pulls in around the ribs during inspiration.

Revised Trauma Score (RTS) A scoring system used for patients with head trauma.

Ricin A neurotoxin derived from mash that is left from the castor bean; it causes pulmonary edema and respiratory and circulatory failure, leading to death.

Root word The main part or stem of a word.

Rooting reflex A reflex that occurs when something touches an infant's cheek; the infant instinctively turns his or her head toward the touch.

Route of exposure Manner by which a toxic substance enters the body.

Safe zone An area of protection providing safety from the danger zone (hot zone).

Salicylates Aspirin-like drugs.

Saline locks A type of IV access device that allows an active IV site to be maintained without having to run fluids through the vein; also called a buff cap or intermittent site.

Sarin (GB) A nerve agent that is one of the G agents; a highly volatile, colorless and odorless liquid that turns from liquid to gas within seconds to minutes at room temperature.

SARS (severe acute respiratory syndrome) Potentially life-threatening viral infection that usually starts with flulike symptoms.

Scene size-up A step within the patient assessment process that involves a quick assessment of the scene and its surroundings to provide information about scene safety and the mechanism of injury or nature of illness before you enter and begin patient care.

School-age children Persons who are 6 to 12 years of age.

Scope of practice A document that outlines the tasks the AEMT is legally authorized to perform.

Secondary assessment A step within the patient assessment process in which a systematic physical examination of the patient is performed. This examination may be a systematic full-body scan or a systematic assessment that focuses on a certain area or region of the body, often determined through the chief complaint.

Secondary device A type of explosive used by terrorists that is set to explode after the initial bomb goes off.

Secondary (indirect) injury The "aftereffects" of the primary injury. It includes abnormal processes such as cerebral edema, increased intracranial pressure, cerebral ischemia and hypoxia, and infection; onset of these symptoms is often delayed following the primary brain injury.

Secondary prevention Efforts to limit the effects of an injury or illness that cannot be completely prevented.

Secure attachment A bond between an infant and his or her parent or caregiver, in which the infant understands that his or her parents or caregivers will be responsive to his or her needs and take care of him or her when help is needed.

Seizures Episodes often characterized by generalized, unco-ordinated muscular activity associated with loss of consciousness; a convulsion.

Selective serotonin reuptake inhibitors (SSRIs) A class of antidepressants that inhibit the reuptake of serotonin.

Sensitization Developing a sensitivity to a substance that initially caused no allergic reaction.

Sensorineural deafness A permanent lack of hearing caused by a lesion or damage of the inner ear.

Septic shock Shock caused by severe infection, usually a bacterial infection.

Serum sickness A condition in which antigen antibody complexes formed in the bloodstream deposit in sites around the body, most notably in the kidney, with resultant inflammatory reactions.

Severe acute respiratory syndrome (SARS) A potentially life-threatening viral infection that usually starts with flulike symptoms.

Shock A condition in which the circulatory system fails to provide sufficient circulation to enable every body part to perform its function; also called hypoperfusion.

Shunt A tube that drains fluid from the brain to another part of the body outside of the brain, such as the abdomen; it lowers pressure in the brain.

Sickle cell disease A hereditary disease that causes normal, round red blood cells to become oblong, or sickle shaped.

Side effects Any effects of a medication other than the desired ones.

Simple partial seizures The seizures involving the movement of one part of the body or altered sensations in one part of the body; the movement may stay in one body part or spread from one part to another in a wave.

Simple pneumothorax Any pneumothorax that is free from significant physiologic changes and does not cause drastic changes in the vital signs of the patient.

Sinoatrial (SA) node The normal site of the origin of electrical impulses; located high in the right atrium, it is the heart's natural pacemaker.

Smallpox A highly contagious viral disease; it is most contagious when blisters begin to form.

Small-volume nebulizer A respiratory device that holds liquid medicine that is turned into a fine mist. The patient inhales the medication into the airways and lungs as a treatment for conditions like asthma.

Solid organs Solid masses of tissue in which much of the chemical work of the body takes place (eg, the liver, spleen, pancreas, and kidneys).

Soman (GD) A nerve agent that is one of the G agents; it has a fruity odor and is both a contact and inhalation hazard—it can enter the body through either skin absorption or the respiratory tract.

Sphincters Circular muscles that encircle and, by contracting, constrict a duct, tube, or opening. Examples are found within the rectum, bladder, and blood vessels.

Spina bifida A developmental defect in which a portion of the spinal cord or meninges protrudes outside of the vertebrae and possibly even outside of the body, usually at the lower third of the spine in the lumbar area.

Splenic sequestration crisis An acute, painful enlargement of the spleen caused by sickle cell disease.

Sprain A joint injury involving damage to supporting ligaments, and sometimes partial or temporary dislocation of bone ends.

Standard of care How a reasonably prudent person with similar training and experience would act under similar circumstances, with similar equipment, and in the same or similar environment.

Standard precautions Protective measures that have traditionally been developed by the Centers for Disease Control and Prevention for use in dealing with objects, blood, body fluids, and other potential exposure risks of communicable disease.

Starling's law A principle that states that if a muscle is stretched slightly before stimulation to contract, the muscle will contract harder; describes how increased venous return to the heart stretches the ventricles and allows for increased cardiac contractility.

Status asthmaticus A prolonged exacerbation of asthma that does not respond to conventional therapy.

Status epilepticus A condition in which seizures recur every few minutes without a lucid interval or last more than 4 or 5 minutes.

Stimulants An agent that increases the level of body activity.

Strain Stretching or tearing of a muscle; also called a muscle pull.

Stroke A loss of brain function in certain brain cells that do not get enough oxygen during a cerebrovascular accident; usually caused by obstruction of the blood vessels in the brain that feed oxygen to the brain cells.

Stroke volume The volume of blood pumped forward with each ventricular contraction.

Subarachnoid hemorrhage Bleeding into the subarachnoid space, where the cerebrospinal fluid circulates.

Subcutaneous Into the tissue between the skin and muscle; a medication delivery route.

Subcutaneous emphysema A characteristic crackling sensation felt on palpation of the skin, caused by the presence of air in soft tissues.

Subdural hematoma An accumulation of blood beneath the dura mater but outside the brain.

Sublingual Under the tongue; a medication delivery route.

Subluxation A partial or incomplete dislocation of a joint.

Substance abuse The misuse of any substance to produce some desired effect.

Sucking reflex A reflex in which the infant starts sucking when his or her lips are stroked.

Suffix A word element that appears at the end of a word.

Sulfur mustard (H) A vesicant; a brownish-yellowish oily substance that is generally considered very persistent. This agent has the distinct smell of garlic or mustard, is quickly absorbed into the skin and mucous membranes, and begins an irreversible process of damaging the cells.

Summation effect Increased effect that may occur when two drugs that have the same or similar action are given together.

Superior vena cava One of the two largest veins in the body; carries blood from the upper extremities, head, neck, and chest into the heart.

Sympathetic blocking agents Antihypertensive medications that decrease cardiac output and renin secretions.

Sympathetic nervous system Subdivision of the autonomic nervous system that governs the body's fight-or-flight reactions by inducing smooth muscle contraction or relaxation of the blood vessels and bronchioles.

Sympatholytics Drugs that block the actions of the sympathetic nervous system.

Sympathomimetics Drugs that produce the same effects as the hormones of the sympathetic nervous system.

Synapses The gaps between nerve cells across which nervous stimuli are transmitted.

Syncope Fainting, often caused by an interruption of blood flow to the brain.

Synergism Combined effect of two drugs that is greater than the sum of their individual effects.

Systemic circulation The portion of the circulatory system outside of the heart and lungs.

Systemic vascular resistance (SVR) The resistance that blood must overcome to be able to move within the blood vessels; related to the amount of dilation or constriction in the blood vessel.

Systole The contraction, or period of contraction, of the heart, especially that of the ventricles.

Tabun (GA) A nerve agent that is one of the G agents; it has a fruity smell and is unique because the components used to manufacture the agent are easy to acquire and the agent is easy to manufacture.

Tension pneumothorax An accumulation of air or gas in the pleural cavity that progressively increases pressure in the chest, causing collapse of one lung and compressing the heart and great vessels, and leading eventually to circulatory collapse with potentially fatal results.

Teratogenic Poses a risk to the normal development or health of the unborn fetus.

Terminal drop hypothesis The theory that a person's mental function declines in the last 5 years of life.

Termination of action The amount of time after the concentration of a medication falls below the minimum effective level until it is eliminated from the body.

Terrorism As defined by the Federal Code of Regulations, the unlawful use of force and violence against persons or property to intimidate or coerce a government, the civilian population, or any segment thereof, in furtherance of political or social objectives.

Therapeutic communication Verbal and nonverbal communication techniques that encourage patients to express their feelings and to achieve a positive relationship with the patient.

Therapeutic index The difference between the minimum effective concentration and the toxic level of a drug.

Therapeutic threshold The minimal concentration of a drug necessary to cause the desired response.

Thrombin An enzyme that causes the conversion of fibrinogen to fibrin, which binds to the platelet plug, forming the final mature clot.

Thromboembolism A blood clot that has formed within a blood vessel and is floating within the bloodstream.

Thrombophilia A tendency toward the development of blood clots as a result of an abnormality of the coagulation system.

Thrombosis A blood clot, either in the arterial or venous system.

Thrombus In terms of neurologic emergencies, the local clotting of blood in the cerebral arteries that may result in the interruption of cerebral blood flow and subsequent stroke.

Toddlers Persons who are 1 to 3 years of age.

Tolerance Physiologic adaptation to the effects of a drug such that increasingly larger doses of the drug are required to achieve the same effect.

Tonic-clonic seizures The seizures characterized by severe twitching of all of the body's muscles that may last several minutes or more; formerly known as a grand mal seizure.

Tonic phase In a seizure, the steady, rigid muscle contractions with no relaxation.

Toxicology The study of toxic or poisonous substances.

Tracheostomy tube A plastic tube placed within the tracheostomy site (stoma).

Transient ischemic attack (TIA) A disorder of the brain in which brain cells temporarily stop working because of insufficient oxygen, causing strokelike symptoms that resolve completely within 24 hours of onset.

Transmission The way in which an infectious agent is spread: contact, airborne, by vehicles (for example, food or needles), or by vectors.

Traumatic asphyxia A pattern of injuries seen after a severe force is applied to the chest, forcing blood from the great vessels back into the head and neck.

Traumatic brain injury (TBI) A traumatic insult to the brain capable of producing physical, intellectual, emotional, social, and vocational changes.

Tricyclic antidepressants (TCAs) A group of drugs used to treat severe depression and manage pain; minimal dosing errors can cause toxic results.

Trismus The involuntary contraction of the mouth resulting in clenched teeth; occurs during seizures and head injuries.

Trust and mistrust A stage of development from birth to approximately 18 months of age, during which infants develop trust in their parents or caregivers if their world is planned, organized, and routine.

Tuberculosis A chronic bacterial disease caused by *Myobacterium tuberculosis* that usually affects the lungs but also can affect other organs such as the brain or kidneys.

Tympanic membrane The eardrum; a thin, semitransparent membrane in the middle ear that transmits sound vibrations to the internal ear by means of auditory ossicles.

Ulcers Abrasions of the inner lining of the stomach or small intestine.

Uremic frost A powdery buildup of uric acid, especially on the face.

Ureters Small, hollow tubes that carry urine from the kidneys to the bladder.

Urethra The canal that conveys urine from the bladder to outside the body.

Urinary bladder A hollow, muscular sac in the midline of the lower pelvis that stores urine until it is released from the body.

Urinary tract infections (UTIs) Infections, usually of the lower urinary tract (urethra and bladder), which occur when normal flora bacteria or other bacteria enter the urethra and grow.

Urine Liquid waste products filtered out of the body by the urinary system.

V agent (VX) A clear, oily agent that has no odor and looks like baby oil; more than 100 times more lethal than sarin and is extremely persistent.

Vasodilator medications Medications that work on the smooth muscles of the arterioles and/or the veins.

Vasodilatory shock A type of shock related to relaxation of the blood vessels, allowing blood to pool and impairing circulation.

Vasoocclusive crisis Ischemia and pain caused by sickle-shaped red blood cells that obstruct blood flow to a portion of the body.

Vector-borne transmission Spread of a disease-causing organism by an animal or insect to human hosts.

Veins The blood vessels that transport unoxygenated blood back to the heart.

Ventilation The movement of air into and out of the lungs, spontaneously by the patient or with assistance.

Ventral respiratory group (VRG) A portion of the medulla oblongata that is responsible for modulating breathing during speech.

Ventricle One of two lower chambers of the heart.

Venules Very small, thin-walled vessels.

Vesicants Blister agents. Their primary route of entry into the body is through the skin.

Vesicular breath sounds Normal breath sounds made by air moving in and out of the alveoli; heard over a normal lung.

Vials Small glass bottles for medications; may contain single or multiple doses.

Viral hemorrhagic fevers (VHF) A group of diseases that include the Ebola, Rift Valley, and yellow fever viruses, among others. They cause the blood in the body to seep out from the tissues and blood vessels.

Virulence The strength or ability of a pathogen to produce disease.

Viruses Germs that require a living host to multiply and survive.

Visceral discomfort Crampy, aching pain deep within the body, the source of which is usually difficult to pinpoint; common with urologic problems.

Vital capacity The amount of air that can be forcibly expelled from the lungs after breathing in as deeply as possible.

Volume on hand The amount of fluid you have on hand, such as the amount of fluid in an IV bag or the amount of fluid in a vial of medication.

V̇/Q̇ mismatch A measurement that examines how much gas is being moved effectively and how much blood is gaining access to the alveoli.

Weapon of mass destruction (WMD) Any agent designed to bring about mass death, casualties, and/or massive damage to property and infrastructure (bridges, tunnels, airports, and seaports); also known as a weapon of mass casualty.

White blood cells (WBCs) Blood cells that have a role in the body's immune defense mechanisms against infection; also called leukocytes.

Whooping cough An airborne disease caused by bacteria that mostly affects children younger than 6 years and presents with fever and a "whoop" sound that occurs when the patient tries to inhale after a coughing attack; also called pertussis.

Work of breathing An indicator of oxygenation and ventilation; it reflects the patient's attempt to compensate for hypoxia.

Xanthines A classification of medications that affect the respiratory smooth muscle and that relax bronchiole smooth muscles, stimulate cardiac muscle, and stimulate the central nervous system.

Index